Applied Logistic Regression

Applied Logistic Regression

Third Edition

DAVID W. HOSMER, JR.

Professor of Biostatistics (Emeritus)
Division of Biostatistics and Epidemiology
Department of Public Health
School of Public Health and Health Sciences
University of Massachusetts
Amherst, Massachusetts

STANLEY LEMESHOW

Dean, College of Public Health
Professor of Biostatistics
College of Public Health
The Ohio State University
Columbus, Ohio

RODNEY X. STURDIVANT

Colonel, U.S. Army
Academy and Associate Professor
Department of Mathematical Sciences
United States Military Academy
West Point, New York

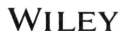

Published by John Wiley & Sons, Inc., Hoboken, New Jersey.
Published simultaneously in Canada.

For general information on our other products and services or for technical support, please contact our Customer Care Department within the United States at (800) 762-2974, outside the United States at (317) 572-3993 or fax (317) 572-4002.

Wiley also publishes its books in a variety of electronic formats. Some content that appears in print may not be available in electronic formats. For more information about Wiley products, visit our web site at www.wiley.com.

Library of Congress Cataloging-in-Publication Data Is Available

Hosmer, David W.
    Applied Logistic Regression / David W. Hosmer, Jr., Stanley Lemeshow, Rodney X. Sturdivant. - 3rd ed.
    Includes bibliographic references and index.
    ISBN 978-0-470-58247-3 (cloth)

Printed in the United States of America

10 9 8 7 6 5 4

To our wives, Trina, Elaine, and Mandy,
and our sons, daughters,
and grandchildren

Contents

Preface to the Third Edition

This third edition of *Applied Logistic Regression* comes 12 years after the 2000 publication of the second edition. During this interval there has been considerable effort researching statistical aspects of the logistic regression model—particularly when the outcomes are correlated. At the same time, capabilities of computer software packages to fit models grew impressively to the point where they now provide access to nearly every aspect of model development a researcher might need. As is well-recognized in the statistical community, the inherent danger of this easy-to-use software is that investigators have at their disposal powerful computational tools, about which they may have only limited understanding. It is our hope that this third edition will help bridge the gap between the outstanding theoretical developments and the need to apply these methods to diverse fields of inquiry.

As was the case in the first two editions, the primary objective of the third edition is to provide an introduction to the underlying theory of the logistic regression model, with a major focus on the application, using real data sets, of the available methods to explore the relationship between a categorical outcome variable and a set of covariates. The materials in this book have evolved over the past 12 years as a result of our teaching and consulting experiences. We have used this book to teach parts of graduate level survey courses, quarter- or semester-long courses, as well as focused short courses to working professionals. We assume that students have a solid foundation in linear regression methodology and contingency table analysis. The positive feedback we have received from students or professionals taking courses using this book or using it for self-learning or reference, provides us with some assurance that the approach we used in the first two editions worked reasonably well; therefore, we have followed that approach in this new edition.

The approach we take is to develop the logistic regression model from a regression analysis point of view. This is accomplished by approaching logistic regression in a manner analogous to what would be considered good statistical practice for linear regression. This differs from the approach used by other authors who have begun their discussion from a contingency table point of view. While the contingency table approach may facilitate the interpretation of the results, we believe that it obscures the regression aspects of the analysis. Thus, discussion of the interpretation of the model is deferred until the regression approach to the analysis is firmly established.

To a large extent, there are no major differences between the many software packages that include logistic regression modeling. When a particular approach is available in a limited number of packages, it will be noted in this text. In general, analyses in this book have been performed using STATA [Stata Corp. (2011)]. This easy-to-use package combines excellent graphics and analysis routines; is fast; is compatible across Macintosh, Windows and UNIX platforms; and interacts well with Microsoft Word. Other major statistical packages employed at various points during the preparation of this text include SAS [SAS Institute Inc. (2009)], OpenBUGS [Lunn et al. (2009)] and R [R Development Core Team (2010)]. For all intents and purposes the results produced were the same regardless of which package we used. Reported numeric results have been rounded from figures obtained from computer output and thus may differ slightly from those that would be obtained in a replication of our analyses or from calculations based on the reported results. When features or capabilities of the programs differed in an important way, we noted them by the names given rather than by their bibliographic citation.

We feel that this new edition benefits greatly from the addition of a number of key topics. These include the following:

1. An expanded presentation of numerous new techniques for model-building, including methods for determining the scale of continuous covariates and assessing model performance.

2. An expanded presentation of regression modeling of complex sample survey data.

3. An expanded development of the use of logistic regression modeling in matched studies, as well as with multinomial and ordinal scaled responses.

4. A new chapter dealing with models and methods for correlated categorical response data.

5. A new chapter developing a number of important applications either missing or expanded from the previous editions. These include propensity score methods, exact methods for logistic regression, sample size issues, Bayesian logistic regression, and other link functions for binary outcome regression models. This chapter concludes with sections dealing with the epidemiologic concepts of mediation and additive interaction.

As was the case for the second edition, all of the data sets used in the text are available at a web site at John Wiley & Sons, Inc.

http://wiley.mpstechnologies.com/wiley/BOBContent/searchLPBobContent.do

In addition, the data may also be found, by permission of John Wiley & Sons Inc., in the archive of statistical data sets maintained at the University of Massachusetts at http://www.umass.edu/statdata/statdata in the logistic regression section.

We would like to express our sincere thanks and appreciation to our colleagues, students, and staff at all of the institutions we have been fortunate to have been affiliated with since the first edition was conceived more than 25 years ago. This includes not only our primary university affiliations but also the locations where we spent extended sabbatical leaves and special research assignments. For this edition we would like to offer special thanks to Sharon Schwartz and Melanie Wall from Columbia University who took the lead in writing the two final sections of the book dealing with mediation and additive interaction. We benefited greatly from their expertise in applying these methods in epidemiologic settings. We greatly appreciate the efforts of Danielle Sullivan, a PhD candidate in biostatistics at Ohio State, for assisting in the preparation of the index for this book. Colleagues in the Division of Biostatistics and the Division of Epidemiology at Ohio State were helpful in their review of selected sections of the book. These include Bo Lu for his insights on propensity score methods and David Murray, Sigrún Alba Jóhannesdóttir, and Morten Schmidt for their thoughts concerning the sections on mediation analysis and additive interaction. Data sets form the basis for the way we present our materials and these are often hard to come by. We are very grateful to Karla Zadnik, Donald O. Mutti, Loraine T. Sinnott, and Lisa A. Jones-Jordan from The Ohio State University College of Optometry as well as to the Collaborative Longitudinal Evaluation of Ethnicity and Refractive Error (CLEERE) Study Group for making the myopia data available to us. We would also like to acknowledge Cynthia A. Fontanella from the College of Social Work at Ohio State for making both the Adolescent Placement and the Polypharmacy data sets available to us. A special thank you to Gary Phillips from the Center for Biostatistics at OSU for helping us identify these valuable data sets (that he was the first one to analyze) as well as for his assistance with some programming issues with Stata. We thank Gordon Fitzgerald of the Center for Outcomes Research (COR) at the University of Massachusetts / Worcester for his help in obtaining the small subset of data used in this text from the Global Longitudinal Study of Osteoporosis in Women (GLOW) Study's main data set. In addition, we thank him for his many helpful comments on the use of propensity scores in logistic regression modeling. We thank Turner Osler for providing us with the small subset of data obtained from a large data set he abstracted from the National Burn Repository 2007 Report, that we used for the burn injury analyses. In many instances the data sets we used were modified from the original data sets in ways to allow us to illustrate important modeling techniques. As such, we issue a general disclaimer here, and do so again throughout the text, that results presented in this text do not apply to the original data.

Before we began this revision, numerous individuals reviewed our proposal anonymously and made many helpful suggestions. They confirmed that what we planned to include in this book would be of use to them in their research and teaching. We thank these individuals and, for the most part, addressed their comments. Many of these reviewers suggested that we include computer code to run logistic regression in a variety of packages, especially R. We decided not to do this for two reasons: we are not statistical computing specialists and did not want to have to spend time responding to email queries on our code. Also, capabilities of computer packages change rapidly and we realized that whatever we decided to include here would likely be out of date before the book was even published. We refer readers interested in code specific to various packages to a web site maintained by Academic Technology Services (ATS) at UCLA where they use a variety of statistical packages to replicate the analyses for the examples in the second edition of this text as well as numerous other statistical texts. The link to this web site is http://www.ats.ucla.edu/stat/.

Finally, we would like to thank Steve Quigley, Susanne Steitz-Filler, Sari Friedman and the production staff at John Wiley & Sons Inc. for their help in bringing this project to completion.

DAVID W. HOSMER, JR.
STANLEY LEMESHOW
RODNEY X. STURDIVANT*

Stowe, Vermont
Columbus, Ohio
West Point, New York
January 2013

---

*The views expressed in this book are those of the author and do not reflect the official policy or position of the Department of the Army, Department of Defense, or the U.S. Government.

CHAPTER 1

Introduction to the Logistic Regression Model

1.1 INTRODUCTION

Regression methods have become an integral component of any data analysis concerned with describing the relationship between a response variable and one or more explanatory variables. Quite often the outcome variable is discrete, taking on two or more possible values. The logistic regression model is the most frequently used regression model for the analysis of these data.

Before beginning a thorough study of the logistic regression model it is important to understand that the goal of an analysis using this model is the same as that of any other regression model used in statistics, that is, to find the best fitting and most parsimonious, clinically interpretable model to describe the relationship between an outcome (dependent or response) variable and a set of independent (predictor or explanatory) variables. The independent variables are often called *covariates*. The most common example of modeling, and one assumed to be familiar to the readers of this text, is the usual linear regression model where the outcome variable is assumed to be continuous.

What distinguishes a logistic regression model from the linear regression model is that the outcome variable in logistic regression is *binary* or *dichotomous*. This difference between logistic and linear regression is reflected both in the form of the model and its assumptions. Once this difference is accounted for, the methods employed in an analysis using logistic regression follow, more or less, the same general principles used in linear regression. Thus, the techniques used in linear regression analysis motivate our approach to logistic regression. We illustrate both the similarities and differences between logistic regression and linear regression with an example.

Applied Logistic Regression, Third Edition.
David W. Hosmer, Jr., Stanley Lemeshow, and Rodney X. Sturdivant.
© 2013 John Wiley & Sons, Inc. Published 2013 by John Wiley & Sons, Inc.

Example 1: Table 1.1 lists the age in years (AGE), and presence or absence of evidence of significant coronary heart disease (CHD) for 100 subjects in a hypothetical study of risk factors for heart disease. The table also contains an identifier variable (ID) and an age group variable (AGEGRP). The outcome variable is CHD, which is coded with a value of "0" to indicate that CHD is absent, or "1" to indicate that it is present in the individual. In general, any two values could be used, but we have found it most convenient to use zero and one. We refer to this data set as the CHDAGE data.

   It is of interest to explore the relationship between AGE and the presence or absence of CHD in this group. Had our outcome variable been continuous rather than binary, we probably would begin by forming a scatterplot of the outcome versus the independent variable. We would use this scatterplot to provide an impression of the nature and strength of any relationship between the outcome and the independent variable. A scatterplot of the data in Table 1.1 is given in Figure 1.1.

   In this scatterplot, all points fall on one of two parallel lines representing the absence of CHD $(y = 0)$ or the presence of CHD $(y = 1)$. There is some tendency for the individuals with no evidence of CHD to be younger than those with evidence of CHD. While this plot does depict the dichotomous nature of the outcome variable quite clearly, it does not provide a clear picture of the nature of the relationship between CHD and AGE.

   The main problem with Figure 1.1 is that the variability in CHD at all ages is large. This makes it difficult to see any functional relationship between AGE and CHD. One common method of removing some variation, while still maintaining the structure of the relationship between the outcome and the independent variable, is to create intervals for the independent variable and compute the mean of the outcome variable within each group. We use this strategy by grouping age into the categories (AGEGRP) defined in Table 1.1. Table 1.2 contains, for each age group, the frequency of occurrence of each outcome, as well as the percent with CHD present.

   By examining this table, a clearer picture of the relationship begins to emerge. It shows that as age increases, the proportion (mean) of individuals with evidence of CHD increases. Figure 1.2 presents a plot of the percent of individuals with CHD versus the midpoint of each age interval. This plot provides considerable insight into the relationship between CHD and AGE in this study, but the functional form for this relationship needs to be described. The plot in this figure is similar to what one might obtain if this same process of grouping and averaging were performed in a linear regression. We note two important differences.

   The first difference concerns the nature of the relationship between the outcome and independent variables. In any regression problem the key quantity is the mean value of the outcome variable, given the value of the independent variable. This quantity is called the *conditional mean* and is expressed as "$E(Y|x)$" where Y denotes the outcome variable and x denotes a specific value of the independent variable. The quantity $E(Y|x)$ is read "the expected value of Y, given the value x". In linear regression we assume that this mean may be expressed as an equation

Table 1.1   Age, Age Group, and Coronary Heart Disease
(CHD) Status of 100 Subjects

ID	AGE	AGEGRP	CHD
1	20	1	0
2	23	1	0
3	24	1	0
4	25	1	0
5	25	1	1
6	26	1	0
7	26	1	0
8	28	1	0
9	28	1	0
10	29	1	0
11	30	2	0
12	30	2	0
13	30	2	0
14	30	2	0
15	30	2	0
16	30	2	1
17	32	2	0
18	32	2	0
19	33	2	0
20	33	2	0
21	34	2	0
22	34	2	0
23	34	2	1
24	34	2	0
25	34	2	0
26	35	3	0
27	35	3	0
28	36	3	0
29	36	3	1
30	36	3	0
31	37	3	0
32	37	3	1
33	37	3	0
34	38	3	0
35	38	3	0
36	39	3	0
37	39	3	1
38	40	4	0
39	40	4	1
40	41	4	0
41	41	4	0
42	42	4	0
43	42	4	0
44	42	4	0

(*continued*)

Table 1.1 (*Continued*)

ID	AGE	AGEGRP	CHD
45	42	4	1
46	43	4	0
47	43	4	0
48	43	4	1
49	44	4	0
50	44	4	0
51	44	4	1
52	44	4	1
53	45	5	0
54	45	5	1
55	46	5	0
56	46	5	1
57	47	5	0
58	47	5	0
59	47	5	1
60	48	5	0
61	48	5	1
62	48	5	1
63	49	5	0
64	49	5	0
65	49	5	1
66	50	6	0
67	50	6	1
68	51	6	0
69	52	6	0
70	52	6	1
71	53	6	1
72	53	6	1
73	54	6	1
74	55	7	0
75	55	7	1
76	55	7	1
77	56	7	1
78	56	7	1
79	56	7	1
80	57	7	0
81	57	7	0
82	57	7	1
83	57	7	1
84	57	7	1
85	57	7	1
86	58	7	0
87	58	7	1
88	58	7	1
89	59	7	1
90	59	7	1

Table 1.1 (*Continued*)

ID	AGE	AGEGRP	CHD
91	60	8	0
92	60	8	1
93	61	8	1
94	62	8	1
95	62	8	1
96	63	8	1
97	64	8	0
98	64	8	1
99	65	8	1
100	69	8	1

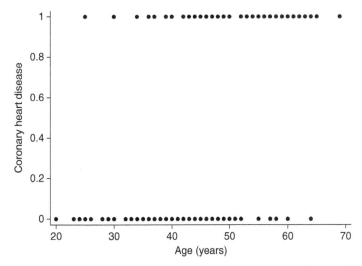

Figure 1.1 Scatterplot of presence or absence of coronary heart disease (CHD) by AGE for 100 subjects.

linear in x (or some transformation of x or Y), such as

$$E(Y|x) = \beta_0 + \beta_1 x.$$

This expression implies that it is possible for $E(Y|x)$ to take on any value as x ranges between $-\infty$ and $+\infty$.

The column labeled "Mean" in Table 1.2 provides an estimate of $E(Y|x)$. We assume, for purposes of exposition, that the estimated values plotted in Figure 1.2 are close enough to the true values of $E(Y|x)$ to provide a reasonable assessment of the functional relationship between CHD and AGE. With a dichotomous outcome variable, the conditional mean must be greater than or equal to zero and less than

Table 1.2 Frequency Table of Age Group by CHD

| Age Group | n | Coronary Heart Disease | | Mean |
		Absent	Present	
20–29	10	9	1	0.100
30–34	15	13	2	0.133
35–39	12	9	3	0.250
40–44	15	10	5	0.333
45–49	13	7	6	0.462
50–54	8	3	5	0.625
55–59	17	4	13	0.765
60–69	10	2	8	0.800
Total	100	57	43	0.430

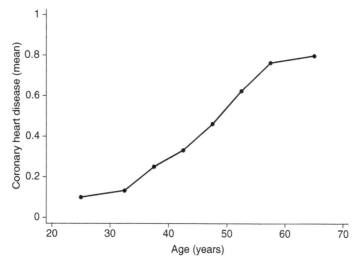

Figure 1.2 Plot of the percentage of subjects with CHD in each AGE group.

or equal to one (i.e., $0 \leq E(Y|x) \leq 1$). This can be seen in Figure 1.2. In addition, the plot shows that this mean approaches zero and one "gradually". The change in the $E(Y|x)$ per unit change in x becomes progressively smaller as the conditional mean gets closer to zero or one. The curve is said to be *S-shaped* and resembles a plot of the cumulative distribution of a continuous random variable. Thus, it should not seem surprising that some well-known cumulative distributions have been used to provide a model for $E(Y|x)$ in the case when Y is dichotomous. The model we use is based on the logistic distribution.

Many distribution functions have been proposed for use in the analysis of a dichotomous outcome variable. Cox and Snell (1989) discuss some of these. There are two primary reasons for choosing the logistic distribution. First, from a mathematical point of view, it is an extremely flexible and easily used function. Second, its model parameters provide the basis for clinically meaningful estimates of effect. A detailed discussion of the interpretation of the model parameters is given in Chapter 3.

In order to simplify notation, we use the quantity $\pi(x) = E(Y|x)$ to represent the conditional mean of Y given x when the logistic distribution is used. The specific form of the logistic regression model we use is:

$$\pi(x) = \frac{e^{\beta_0 + \beta_1 x}}{1 + e^{\beta_0 + \beta_1 x}}. \tag{1.1}$$

A transformation of $\pi(x)$ that is central to our study of logistic regression is the *logit transformation*. This transformation is defined, in terms of $\pi(x)$, as:

$$g(x) = \ln\left[\frac{\pi(x)}{1 - \pi(x)}\right]$$
$$= \beta_0 + \beta_1 x.$$

The importance of this transformation is that $g(x)$ has many of the desirable properties of a linear regression model. The logit, $g(x)$, is linear in its parameters, may be continuous, and may range from $-\infty$ to $+\infty$, depending on the range of x.

The second important difference between the linear and logistic regression models concerns the conditional distribution of the outcome variable. In the linear regression model we assume that an observation of the outcome variable may be expressed as $y = E(Y|x) + \varepsilon$. The quantity ε is called the *error* and expresses an observation's deviation from the conditional mean. The most common assumption is that ε follows a normal distribution with mean zero and some variance that is constant across levels of the independent variable. It follows that the conditional distribution of the outcome variable given x is normal with mean $E(Y|x)$, and a variance that is constant. This is not the case with a dichotomous outcome variable. In this situation, we may express the value of the outcome variable given x as $y = \pi(x) + \varepsilon$. Here the quantity ε may assume one of two possible values. If $y = 1$ then $\varepsilon = 1 - \pi(x)$ with probability $\pi(x)$, and if $y = 0$ then $\varepsilon = -\pi(x)$ with probability $1 - \pi(x)$. Thus, ε has a distribution with mean zero and variance equal to $\pi(x)[1 - \pi(x)]$. That is, the conditional distribution of the outcome variable follows a binomial distribution with probability given by the conditional mean, $\pi(x)$.

In summary, we have shown that in a regression analysis when the outcome variable is dichotomous:

1. The model for the conditional mean of the regression equation must be bounded between zero and one. The logistic regression model, $\pi(x)$, given in equation (1.1), satisfies this constraint.
2. The binomial, not the normal, distribution describes the distribution of the errors and is the statistical distribution on which the analysis is based.

3. The principles that guide an analysis using linear regression also guide us in logistic regression.

1.2 FITTING THE LOGISTIC REGRESSION MODEL

Suppose we have a sample of n independent observations of the pair (x_i, y_i), $i = 1, 2, \ldots, n$, where y_i denotes the value of a dichotomous outcome variable and x_i is the value of the independent variable for the ith subject. Furthermore, assume that the outcome variable has been coded as 0 or 1, representing the absence or the presence of the characteristic, respectively. This coding for a dichotomous outcome is used throughout the text. Fitting the logistic regression model in equation (1.1) to a set of data requires that we estimate the values of β_0 and β_1, the unknown parameters.

In linear regression, the method used most often for estimating unknown parameters is *least squares*. In that method we choose those values of β_0 and β_1 that minimize the sum-of-squared deviations of the observed values of Y from the predicted values based on the model. Under the usual assumptions for linear regression the method of least squares yields estimators with a number of desirable statistical properties. Unfortunately, when the method of least squares is applied to a model with a dichotomous outcome, the estimators no longer have these same properties.

The general method of estimation that leads to the least squares function under the linear regression model (when the error terms are normally distributed) is called *maximum likelihood*. This method provides the foundation for our approach to estimation with the logistic regression model throughout this text. In a general sense, the method of maximum likelihood yields values for the unknown parameters that maximize the probability of obtaining the observed set of data. In order to apply this method we must first construct a function, called the *likelihood function*. This function expresses the probability of the observed data as a function of the unknown parameters. The *maximum likelihood estimators* of the parameters are the values that maximize this function. Thus, the resulting estimators are those that agree most closely with the observed data. We now describe how to find these values for the logistic regression model.

If Y is coded as 0 or 1 then the expression for $\pi(x)$ given in equation (1.1) provides (for an arbitrary value of $\boldsymbol{\beta} = (\beta_0, \beta_1)$, the vector of parameters) the conditional probability that Y is equal to 1 given x. This is denoted as $\pi(x)$. It follows that the quantity $1 - \pi(x)$ gives the conditional probability that Y is equal to zero given x, $\Pr(Y = 0|x)$. Thus, for those pairs (x_i, y_i), where $y_i = 1$, the contribution to the likelihood function is $\pi(x_i)$, and for those pairs where $y_i = 0$, the contribution to the likelihood function is $1 - \pi(x_i)$, where the quantity $\pi(x_i)$ denotes the value of $\pi(x)$ computed at x_i. A convenient way to express the contribution to the likelihood function for the pair (x_i, y_i) is through the expression

$$\pi(x_i)^{y_i}[1 - \pi(x_i)]^{1-y_i}. \tag{1.2}$$

As the observations are assumed to be independent, the likelihood function is obtained as the product of the terms given in equation (1.2) as follows:

$$l(\beta) = \prod_{i=1}^{n} \pi(x_i)^{y_i} [1 - \pi(x_i)]^{1-y_i}. \tag{1.3}$$

The principle of maximum likelihood states that we use as our estimate of β the value that maximizes the expression in equation (1.3). However, it is easier mathematically to work with the log of equation (1.3). This expression, the *log-likelihood*, is defined as

$$L(\beta) = \ln[l(\beta)] = \sum_{i=1}^{n} \{y_i \ln[\pi(x_i)] + (1 - y_i) \ln[1 - \pi(x_i)]\}. \tag{1.4}$$

To find the value of β that maximizes $L(\beta)$ we differentiate $L(\beta)$ with respect to β_0 and β_1 and set the resulting expressions equal to zero. These equations, known as the *likelihood equations*, are

$$\sum [y_i - \pi(x_i)] = 0 \tag{1.5}$$

and

$$\sum x_i [y_i - \pi(x_i)] = 0. \tag{1.6}$$

In equations (1.5) and (1.6) it is understood that the summation is over i varying from 1 to n. (The practice of suppressing the index and range of summation, when these are clear, is followed throughout this text.)

In linear regression, the likelihood equations, obtained by differentiating the sum-of-squared deviations function with respect to β are linear in the unknown parameters and thus are easily solved. For logistic regression the expressions in equations (1.5) and (1.6) are nonlinear in β_0 and β_1, and thus require special methods for their solution. These methods are iterative in nature and have been programmed into logistic regression software. For the moment, we need not be concerned about these iterative methods and view them as a computational detail that is taken care of for us. The interested reader may consult the text by McCullagh and Nelder (1989) for a general discussion of the methods used by most programs. In particular, they show that the solution to equations (1.5) and (1.6) may be obtained using an iterative weighted least squares procedure.

The value of β given by the solution to equations (1.5) and (1.6) is called the *maximum likelihood estimate* and is denoted as $\hat{\beta}$. In general, the use of the symbol "$\hat{\ }$" denotes the maximum likelihood estimate of the respective quantity. For example, $\hat{\pi}(x_i)$ is the maximum likelihood estimate of $\pi(x_i)$. This quantity provides an estimate of the conditional probability that Y is equal to 1, given that x is equal to x_i. As such, it represents the fitted or predicted value for the logistic regression model. An interesting consequence of equation (1.5) is that

$$\sum_{i=1}^{n} y_i = \sum_{i=1}^{n} \hat{\pi}(x_i).$$

Table 1.3   Results of Fitting the Logistic Regression Model to the CHDAGE Data, $n = 100$

Variable	Coeff.	Std. Err.	z	p
Age	0.111	0.0241	4.61	<0.001
Constant	−5.309	1.1337	−4.68	<0.001

Log-likelihood = −53.676546.

That is, the sum of the observed values of y is equal to the sum of the predicted (expected) values. We use this property in later chapters when we discuss assessing the fit of the model.

As an example, consider the data given in Table 1.1. Use of a logistic regression software package, with continuous variable AGE as the independent variable, produces the output in Table 1.3.

The maximum likelihood estimates of β_0 and β_1 are $\hat{\beta}_0 = -5.309$ and $\hat{\beta}_1 = 0.111$. The fitted values are given by the equation

$$\hat{\pi}(x) = \frac{e^{-5.309+0.111\times \text{AGE}}}{1 + e^{-5.309+0.111\times \text{AGE}}} \tag{1.7}$$

and the estimated logit, $\hat{g}(x)$, is given by the equation

$$\hat{g}(x) = -5.309 + 0.111 \times \text{AGE}. \tag{1.8}$$

The log-likelihood given in Table 1.3 is the value of equation (1.4) computed using $\hat{\beta}_0$ and $\hat{\beta}_1$.

Three additional columns are present in Table 1.3. One contains estimates of the standard errors of the estimated coefficients, the next column displays the ratios of the estimated coefficients to their estimated standard errors, and the last column displays a p-value. These quantities are discussed in the next section.

Following the fitting of the model we begin to evaluate its adequacy.

1.3   TESTING FOR THE SIGNIFICANCE OF THE COEFFICIENTS

In practice, the modeling of a set of data, as we show in Chapters 4, 7, and 8, is a much more complex process than one of simply fitting and testing. The methods we present in this section, while simplistic, do provide essential building blocks for the more complex process.

After estimating the coefficients, our first look at the fitted model commonly concerns an assessment of the significance of the variables in the model. This usually involves formulation and testing of a statistical hypothesis to determine whether the independent variables in the model are "significantly" related to the outcome variable. The method for performing this test is quite general, and differs from one type of model to the next only in the specific details. We begin by discussing the general approach for a single independent variable. The multivariable case is considered in Chapter 2.

One approach to testing for the significance of the coefficient of a variable in any model relates to the following question. *Does the model that includes the variable in question tell us more about the outcome (or response) variable than a model that does not include that variable?* This question is answered by comparing the observed values of the response variable to those predicted by each of two models; the first with, and the second without, the variable in question. The mathematical function used to compare the observed and predicted values depends on the particular problem. If the predicted values with the variable in the model are better, or more accurate in some sense, than when the variable is not in the model, then we feel that the variable in question is "significant". It is important to note that we are not considering the question of whether the predicted values are an accurate representation of the observed values in an absolute sense (this is called *goodness of fit*). Instead, our question is posed in a relative sense. The assessment of goodness of fit is a more complex question that is discussed in detail in Chapter 5.

The general method for assessing significance of variables is easily illustrated in the linear regression model, and its use there motivates the approach used for logistic regression. A comparison of the two approaches highlights the differences between modeling continuous and dichotomous response variables.

In linear regression, one assesses the significance of the slope coefficient by forming what is referred to as an *analysis of variance table*. This table partitions the total sum-of-squared deviations of observations about their mean into two parts: (1) the sum-of-squared deviations of observations about the regression line SSE (or *residual sum-of-squares*) and (2) the sum-of-squares of predicted values, based on the regression model, about the mean of the dependent variable SSR (or *due regression sum-of-squares*). This is just a convenient way of displaying the comparison of observed to predicted values under two models. In linear regression, the comparison of observed and predicted values is based on the square of the distance between the two. If y_i denotes the observed value and $\hat{y}_i$ denotes the predicted value for the ith individual under the model, then the statistic used to evaluate this comparison is

$$\text{SSE} = \sum_{i=1}^{n} (y_i - \hat{y}_i)^2.$$

Under the model not containing the independent variable in question the only parameter is β_0, and $\hat{\beta}_0 = \overline{y}$, the mean of the response variable. In this case, $\hat{y}_i = \overline{y}$ and SSE is equal to the total sum-of-squares. When we include the independent variable in the model, any decrease in SSE is due to the fact that the slope coefficient for the independent variable is not zero. The change in the value of SSE is due to the regression source of variability, denoted SSR. That is,

$$\text{SSR} = \left[\sum_{i=1}^{n} (y_i - \overline{y}_i)^2 \right] - \left[\sum_{i=1}^{n} (y_i - \hat{y}_i)^2 \right].$$

In linear regression, interest focuses on the size of SSR. A large value suggests that the independent variable is important, whereas a small value suggests that the independent variable is not helpful in predicting the response.

The guiding principle with logistic regression is the same: compare observed values of the response variable to predicted values obtained from models, with and without the variable in question. In logistic regression, comparison of observed to predicted values is based on the log-likelihood function defined in equation (1.4). To better understand this comparison, it is helpful conceptually to think of an observed value of the response variable as also being a predicted value resulting from a saturated model. A saturated model is one that contains as many parameters as there are data points. (A simple example of a saturated model is fitting a linear regression model when there are only two data points, $n = 2$.)

The comparison of observed to predicted values using the likelihood function is based on the following expression:

$$D = -2\ln\left[\frac{(\text{likelihood of the fitted model})}{(\text{likelihood of the saturated model})}\right]. \tag{1.9}$$

The quantity inside the large brackets in the expression above is called the *likelihood ratio*. Using minus twice its log is necessary to obtain a quantity whose distribution is known and can therefore be used for hypothesis testing purposes. Such a test is called the *likelihood ratio test*. Using equation (1.4), equation (1.9) becomes

$$D = -2\sum_{i=1}^{n}\left[y_i\ln\left(\frac{\hat{\pi}_i}{y_i}\right) + (1-y_i)\ln\left(\frac{1-\hat{\pi}_i}{1-y_i}\right)\right], \tag{1.10}$$

where $\hat{\pi}_i = \hat{\pi}(x_i)$.

The statistic, D, in equation (1.10) is called the *deviance*, and for logistic regression, it plays the same role that the residual sum-of-squares plays in linear regression. In fact, the deviance as shown in equation (1.10), when computed for linear regression, is identically equal to the SSE.

Furthermore, in a setting as shown in Table 1.1, where the values of the outcome variable are either 0 or 1, the likelihood of the saturated model is identically equal to 1.0. Specifically, it follows from the definition of a saturated model that $\hat{\pi}_i = y_i$ and the likelihood is

$$l(\text{saturated model}) = \prod_{i=1}^{n} y_i^{y_i} \times (1-y_i)^{(1-y_i)} = 1.0.$$

Thus it follows from equation (1.9) that the deviance is

$$D = -2\ln(\text{likelihood of the fitted model}). \tag{1.11}$$

Some software packages report the value of the deviance in equation (1.11) rather than the log-likelihood for the fitted model. In the context of testing for the significance of a fitted model, we want to emphasize that we think of the deviance in the same way that we think of the residual sum-of-squares in linear regression.

In particular, to assess the significance of an independent variable we compare the value of D with and without the independent variable in the equation. The change in D due to the inclusion of the independent variable in the model is:

$$G = D(\text{model without the variable}) - D(\text{model with the variable}).$$

This statistic, G, plays the same role in logistic regression that the numerator of the partial F-test does in linear regression. Because the likelihood of the saturated model is always common to both values of D being differenced, G can be expressed as

$$G = -2 \ln \left[\frac{(\text{likelihood without the variable})}{(\text{likelihood with the variable})} \right]. \tag{1.12}$$

For the specific case of a single independent variable, it is easy to show that when the variable is not in the model, the maximum likelihood estimate of β_0 is $\ln(n_1/n_0)$ where $n_1 = \sum y_i$ and $n_0 = \sum(1 - y_i)$ and the predicted probability for all subjects is constant, and equal to n_1/n. In this setting, the value of G is:

$$G = -2 \ln \left[\frac{\left(\frac{n_1}{n}\right)^{n_1} \left(\frac{n_0}{n}\right)^{n_0}}{\prod\limits_{i=1}^{n} \hat{\pi}_i^{y_i} (1 - \hat{\pi}_i)^{(1-y_i)}} \right], \tag{1.13}$$

or

$$G = 2 \left\{ \sum_{i=1}^{n} \left[y_i \ln \left(\hat{\pi}_i \right) + (1 - y_i) \ln(1 - \hat{\pi}_i) \right] \right.$$
$$\left. - \left[n_1 \ln \left(n_1 \right) + n_0 \ln(n_0) - n \ln(n) \right] \right\}. \tag{1.14}$$

Under the hypothesis that β_1 is equal to zero, the statistic G follows a chi-square distribution with 1 degree of freedom. Additional mathematical assumptions are needed; however, for the above case they are rather nonrestrictive, and involve having a sufficiently large sample size, n, and enough subjects with both $y = 0$ and $y = 1$. We discuss in later chapters that, as far as sample size is concerned, the key determinant is $\min(n_0, n_1)$.

As an example, we consider the model fit to the data in Table 1.1, whose estimated coefficients and log-likelihood are given in Table 1.3. For these data the sample size is sufficiently large as $n_1 = 43$ and $n_0 = 57$. Evaluating G as shown in equation (1.14) yields

$$G = 2\{-53.677 - [43 \ln(43) + 57 \ln(57) - 100 \ln(100)]\}$$
$$= 2[-53.677 - (-68.331)] = 29.31.$$

The first term in this expression is the *log-likelihood* from the model containing age (see Table 1.3), and the remainder of the expression simply substitutes n_1 and n_0 into the second part of equation (1.14). We use the symbol $\chi^2(v)$ to denote a chi-square random variable with v degrees of freedom. Using this notation, the *p*-value associated with this test is $P[\chi^2(1) > 29.31] < 0.001$; thus, we have convincing evidence that AGE is a significant variable in predicting CHD. This is merely a statement of the statistical evidence for this variable. Other important factors to consider before concluding that the variable is clinically important would include the appropriateness of the fitted model, as well as inclusion of other potentially important variables.

As all logistic regression software report either the value of the log-likelihood or the value of D, it is easy to check for the significance of the addition of new terms to the model or to verify a reported value of G. In the simple case of a single independent variable, we first fit a model containing only the constant term. Next, we fit a model containing the independent variable along with the constant. This gives rise to another log-likelihood. The likelihood ratio test is obtained by multiplying the difference between these two values by -2.

In the current example, the log-likelihood for the model containing only a constant term is -68.331. Fitting a model containing the independent variable (AGE) along with the constant term results in the log-likelihood shown in Table 1.3 of -53.677. Multiplying the difference in these log-likelihoods by -2 gives

$$-2 \times [-68.331 - (-53.677)] = -2 \times (-14.655) = 29.31.$$

This result, along with the associated *p*-value for the chi-square distribution, is commonly reported in logistic regression software packages.

There are two other statistically equivalent tests: the Wald test and the Score test. The assumptions needed for each of these is the same as those of the likelihood ratio test in equation (1.14). A more complete discussion of these three tests and their assumptions may be found in Rao (1973).

The Wald test is equal to the ratio of the maximum likelihood estimate of the slope parameter, $\hat{\beta}_1$, to an estimate of its standard error. Under the null hypothesis and the sample size assumptions, this ratio follows a standard normal distribution. While we have not yet formally discussed how the estimates of the standard errors of the estimated parameters are obtained, they are routinely printed out by computer software. For example, the Wald test for the coefficient for AGE in Table 1.3 is provided in the column headed z and is

$$W = \frac{\hat{\beta}_1}{\widehat{SE}(\hat{\beta}_1)} = \frac{0.111}{0.024} = 4.61.$$

The two-tailed *p*-value, provided in the last column of Table 1.3, is $P(|z| > 4.61) < 0.001$, where z denotes a random variable following the standard normal distribution. Some software packages display the statistic $W^2 = z^2$, which is distributed as chi-square with 1 degree of freedom. Hauck and Donner (1977) examined the performance of the Wald test and found that it behaved in an aberrant manner, often failing to reject the null hypothesis when the coefficient was significant using the likelihood ratio test. Thus, they recommended (and we agree) that the likelihood ratio test is preferred. We note that while the assertions of Hauk and Donner are true, we have never seen huge differences in the values of G and W^2. In practice, the more troubling situation is when the values are close, and one test has $p < 0.05$ and the other has $p > 0.05$. When this occurs, we use the p-value from the likelihood ratio test.

A test for the significance of a variable that does not require computing the estimate of the coefficient is the score test. Proponents of the score test cite this reduced computational effort as its major advantage. Use of the test is limited by the fact that it is not available in many software packages. The score test is based on the distribution theory of the derivatives of the log-likelihood. In general, this is a multivariate test requiring matrix calculations that are discussed in Chapter 2.

In the univariate case, this test is based on the conditional distribution of the derivative in equation (1.6), given the derivative in equation (1.5). In this case, we can write down an expression for the Score test. The test uses the value of equation (1.6) computed using $\beta_0 = \ln(n_1/n_0)$ and $\beta_1 = 0$. As noted earlier, under these parameter values, $\hat{\pi} = n_1/n = \bar{y}$ and the left-hand side of equation (1.6) becomes $\sum x_i(y_i - \bar{y})$. It may be shown that the estimated variance is $\bar{y}(1 - \bar{y})\sum(x_i - \bar{x})^2$. The test statistic for the score test (ST) is

$$ST = \frac{\displaystyle\sum_{i=1}^{n} x_i(y_i - \bar{y})}{\sqrt{\bar{y}(1 - \bar{y})\displaystyle\sum_{i=1}^{n}(x_i - \bar{x})^2}}.$$

As an example of the score test, consider the model fit to the data in Table 1.1. The value of the test statistic for this example is

$$ST = \frac{296.66}{\sqrt{3333.742}} = 5.14$$

and the two tailed p-value is $P(|z| > 5.14) < 0.001$. We note that, for this example, the values of the three test statistics are nearly the same (*note*: $\sqrt{G} = 5.41$).

In summary, the method for testing the significance of the coefficient of a variable in logistic regression is similar to the approach used in linear regression; however, it is based on the likelihood function for a dichotomous outcome variable under the logistic regression model.

1.4 CONFIDENCE INTERVAL ESTIMATION

An important adjunct to testing for significance of the model, discussed in Section 1.3, is calculation and interpretation of confidence intervals for parameters of interest. As is the case in linear regression we can obtain these for the slope, intercept and the "line" (i.e., the logit). In some settings it may be of interest to provide interval estimates for the fitted values (i.e., the predicted probabilities).

The basis for construction of the interval estimators is the same statistical theory we used to formulate the tests for significance of the model. In particular, the confidence interval estimators for the slope and intercept are, most often, based on their respective Wald tests and are sometimes referred to as *Wald-based confidence intervals*. The endpoints of a $100(1-\alpha)\%$ confidence interval for the slope coefficient are

$$\hat{\beta}_1 \pm z_{1-\alpha/2}\widehat{SE}(\hat{\beta}_1) \tag{1.15}$$

and for the intercept they are

$$\hat{\beta}_0 \pm z_{1-\alpha/2}\widehat{SE}(\hat{\beta}_0) \tag{1.16}$$

where $z_{1-\alpha/2}$ is the upper $100(1-\alpha/2)\%$ point from the standard normal distribution and $\widehat{SE}(\cdot)$ denotes a model-based estimator of the standard error of the respective parameter estimator. We defer discussion of the actual formula used for calculating the estimators of the standard errors to Chapter 2. For the moment, we use the fact that estimated values are provided in the output following the fit of a model and, in addition, many packages also provide the endpoints of the interval estimates.

As an example, consider the model fit to the data in Table 1.1 regressing AGE on the presence or absence of CHD. The results are presented in Table 1.3. The endpoints of a 95 percent confidence interval for the slope coefficient from equation (1.15) are $0.111 \pm 1.96 \times 0.0241$, yielding the interval $(0.064, 0.158)$. We defer a detailed discussion of the interpretation of these results to Chapter 3. Briefly, the results suggest that the change in the log-odds of CHD per one year increase in age is 0.111 and the change could be as little as 0.064 or as much as 0.158 with 95 percent confidence.

As is the case with any regression model, the constant term provides an estimate of the response at $x = 0$ unless the independent variable has been centered at some clinically meaningful value. In our example, the constant provides an estimate of the log-odds ratio of CHD at zero years of age. As a result, the constant term, by itself, has no useful clinical interpretation. In any event, from equation (1.16), the endpoints of a 95 percent confidence interval for the constant are $-5.309 \pm 1.96 \times 1.1337$, yielding the interval $(-7.531, -3.087)$.

The logit is the linear part of the logistic regression model and, as such, is most similar to the fitted line in a linear regression model. The estimator of the logit is

$$\hat{g}(x) = \hat{\beta}_0 + \hat{\beta}_1 x. \tag{1.17}$$

The estimator of the variance of the estimator of the logit requires obtaining the variance of a sum. In this case it is

$$\widehat{Var}[\hat{g}(x)] = \widehat{Var}(\hat{\beta}_0) + x^2\widehat{Var}(\hat{\beta}_1) + 2x\widehat{Cov}(\hat{\beta}_0, \hat{\beta}_1). \tag{1.18}$$

In general, the variance of a sum is equal to the sum of the variance of each term and twice the covariance of each possible pair of terms formed from the

Table 1.4 Estimated Covariance Matrix of the Estimated Coefficients in Table 1.3

	Age	Constant
Age	0.000579	
Constant	−0.026677	1.28517

components of the sum. The endpoints of a $100(1 - \alpha)\%$ *Wald-based confidence interval* for the logit are

$$\hat{g}(x) \pm z_{1-\alpha/2}\widehat{SE}[\hat{g}(x)], \qquad (1.19)$$

where $\widehat{SE}[\hat{g}(x)]$ is the positive square root of the variance estimator in equation (1.18).

The estimated logit for the fitted model in Table 1.3 is shown in equation (1.8). In order to evaluate equation (1.18) for a specific age we need the estimated covariance matrix. This matrix can be obtained from the output from all logistic regression software packages. How it is displayed varies from package to package, but the triangular form shown in Table 1.4 is a common one.

The estimated logit from equation (1.8) for a subject of age 50 is

$$\hat{g}(50) = -5.31 + 0.111 \times 50 = 0.240,$$

the estimated variance, using equation (1.18) and the results in Table 1.4, is

$$\widehat{Var}[\hat{g}(50)] = 1.28517 + (50)^2 \times 0.000579 + 2 \times 50 \times (-0.026677) = 0.0650$$

and the estimated standard error is $\widehat{SE}[\hat{g}(50)] = 0.2549$. Thus the end points of a 95 percent confidence interval for the logit at age 50 are

$$0.240 \pm 1.96 \times 0.2550 = (-0.260, 0.740).$$

We discuss the interpretation and use of the estimated logit in providing estimates of odds ratios in Chapter 3.

The estimator of the logit and its confidence interval provide the basis for the estimator of the fitted value, in this case the logistic probability, and its associated confidence interval. In particular, using equation (1.7) at age 50 the estimated logistic probability is

$$\hat{\pi}(50) = \frac{e^{\hat{g}(50)}}{1 + e^{\hat{g}(50)}} = \frac{e^{-5.31+0.111\times50}}{1+e^{-5.31+0.111\times50}} = 0.560 \qquad (1.20)$$

and the endpoints of a 95 percent confidence interval are obtained from the respective endpoints of the confidence interval for the logit. The endpoints of the $100(1 - \alpha)\%$ *Wald-based confidence interval* for the fitted value are

$$\frac{e^{\hat{g}(x)\pm z_{1-\alpha/2}\widehat{SE}[\hat{g}(x)]}}{1 + e^{\hat{g}(x)\pm z_{1-\alpha/2}\widehat{SE}[\hat{g}(x)]}}. \qquad (1.21)$$

Using the example at age 50 to demonstrate the calculations, the lower limit is

$$\frac{e^{-0.260}}{1 + e^{-0.260}} = 0.435,$$

and the upper limit is

$$\frac{e^{0.740}}{1 + e^{0.740}} = 0.677.$$

We have found that a major mistake often made by data analysts new to logistic regression modeling is to try and apply estimates on the probability scale to individual subjects. The fitted value computed in equation (1.20) is analogous to a particular point on the line obtained from a linear regression. In linear regression each point on the fitted line provides an estimate of the mean of the dependent variable in a population of subjects with covariate value "x". Thus the value of 0.56 in equation (1.20) is an estimate of the mean (i.e., proportion) of 50-year-old subjects in the population sampled that have evidence of CHD. An individual 50-year-old subject either does or does not have evidence of CHD. The confidence interval suggests that this mean could be between 0.435 and 0.677 with 95 percent confidence. We discuss the use and interpretation of fitted values in greater detail in Chapter 3.

One application of fitted logistic regression models that has received a lot of attention in the subject matter literature is using model-based fitted values similar to the one in equation (1.20) to predict the value of a binary dependent value in individual subjects. This process is called *classification* and has a long history in statistics where it is referred to as *discriminant analysis*. We discuss the classification problem in detail in Chapter 4. We also discuss discriminant analysis within the context of a method for obtaining estimators of the coefficients in the next section.

The *coverage*[*][†] of the Wald-based confidence interval estimators in equations (1.15) and (1.16) depends on the assumption that the distribution of the maximum likelihood estimators is normal. Potential sensitivity to this assumption is the main reason that the likelihood ratio test is recommended over the Wald test for assessing the significance of individual coefficients, as well as for the overall model. In settings where the number of events ($y = 1$) and/or the sample size is small the normality assumption is suspect and a log-likelihood function-based confidence interval can have better coverage. Until recently routines to compute these intervals were not available in most software packages. Cox and Snell (1989, p. 179–183) discuss the theory behind likelihood intervals, and Venzon and Moolgavkar (1988) describe an efficient way to calculate the end points.

---

[*]The remainder of this section is more advanced material that can be skipped on first reading of the text.

[†]The term coverage of an interval estimator refers to the percent of time confidence intervals computed in a similar manner contain the true parameter value. Research has shown that when the normality assumption does not hold, Wald-based confidence intervals can be too narrow and thus contain the true parameter with a smaller percentage than the stated confidence coefficient.

Royston (2007) describes a STATA [StataCorp (2011)] routine that implements the Venzon and Moolgavkar method that we use for the examples in this text. The SAS package's logistic regression procedure [SAS Institute Inc. (2009)] has the option to obtain likelihood confidence intervals.

The *likelihood-based confidence interval* estimator for a coefficient can be concisely described as the interval of values, β^*, for which the likelihood ratio test would fail to reject the hypothesis, $H_0 : \beta = \beta^*$, at the stated $1 - \alpha$ percent significance level. The two end points, β_{lower} and β_{upper}, of this interval for a coefficient are defined as follows:

$$2[l(\hat{\beta}) - l_p(\beta_{upper})] = 2[l(\hat{\beta}) - l_p(\beta_{lower})] = \chi^2_{1-\alpha}(1), \qquad (1.22)$$

where $l(\hat{\beta})$ is the value of the log-likelihood of the fitted model and $l_p(\beta)$ is the value of the *profile log-likelihood*. A value of the profile log-likelihood is computed by first specifying/fixing a value for the coefficient of interest, for example the slope coefficient for age, and then finding the value of the intercept coefficient, using the Venzon and Moolgavkar method, that maximizes the log-likelihood. This process is repeated over a grid of values of the specified coefficient, for example, values of β^*, until the solutions to equation (1.22) are found. The results can be presented graphically or in standard interval form. We illustrate both in the example below.

As an example, we show in Figure 1.3 a plot of the profile log-likelihood for the coefficient for AGE using the CHDAGE data in Table 1.1. The end points of the 95 percent likelihood interval are $\beta_{lower} = 0.067$ and $\beta_{upper} = 0.162$ and are shown in the figure where the two vertical lines intersect the "x" axis. The horizontal line in the figure is drawn at the value

$$-55.5964 = -53.6756 - \left(\frac{3.8416}{2}\right),$$

where -53.6756 is the value of the log-likelihood of the fitted model from Table 1.3 and 3.8416 is the 95th percentile of the chi-square distribution with 1 degree of freedom.

The quantity "Asymmetry" in Figure 1.3 is a measure of asymmetry of the profile log-likelihood that is the difference between the lengths of the upper part of the interval, $\beta_{upper} - \hat{\beta}$, to the lower part, $\hat{\beta} - \beta_{lower}$, as a percent of the total length, $\beta_{upper} - \beta_{lower}$. In the example the value is

$$A = 100 \times \frac{(0.162 - 0.111) - (0.111 - 0.067)}{(0.162 - 0.067)} \cong 7.5\%.$$

As the upper and lower endpoints of the Wald-based confidence interval in equation (1.15) are equidistant from the maximum likelihood estimator, it has asymmetry $A = 0$.

In this example, the Wald-based confidence interval for the coefficient for age is $(0.064, 0.158)$. The likelihood interval is $(0.067, 0.162)$, which is only 1.1% wider than the Wald-based interval. So there is not a great deal of pure numeric difference in the two intervals and the asymmetry is small. In settings where there

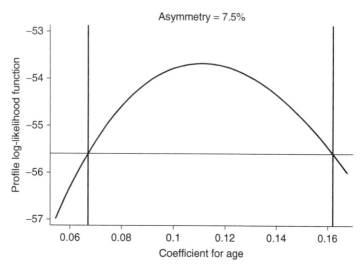

Figure 1.3   Plot of the profile log-likelihood for the coefficient for AGE in the CHDAGE data.

is greater asymmetry in the likelihood-based interval there can be more substantial differences between the two intervals. We return to this point in Chapter 3 where we discuss the interpretation of estimated coefficients. In addition, we include an exercise at the end of this chapter where there is a pronounced difference between the Wald and likelihood confidence interval estimators.

Methods to extend the likelihood intervals to functions of more than one coefficient such as the estimated logit function and probability are not available in current software packages.

1.5   OTHER ESTIMATION METHODS

The method of maximum likelihood described in Section 1.2 is the estimation method used in the logistic regression routines of the major software packages. However, two other methods have been and may still be used for estimating the coefficients. These methods are: (1) noniterative weighted least squares, and (2) discriminant function analysis.

A linear models approach to the analysis of categorical data proposed by Grizzle et al. (1969) [Grizzle, Starmer, and Koch (GSK) method] uses estimators based on noniterative weighted least squares. They demonstrate that the logistic regression model is an example of a general class of models that can be handled by their methods. We should add that the maximum likelihood estimators are usually calculated using an iterative reweighted least squares algorithm, and are also technically "least squares" estimators. The GSK method requires one iteration and is used in SAS's GENMOD procedure to fit a logistic regression model containing only categorical covariates.

A major limitation of the GSK method is that we must have an estimate of $\pi(x)$ that is not zero or 1 for most values of x. An example where we could use both maximum likelihood and GSK's noniterative weighted least squares is the data in Table 1.2. In cases such as this, the two methods are *asymptotically equivalent*, meaning that as n gets large, the distributional properties of the two estimators become identical. The GSK method could not be used with the data in Table 1.1.

The discriminant function approach to estimation of the coefficients is of historical importance as it was popularized by Cornfield (1962) in some of the earliest work on logistic regression. These estimators take their name from the fact that the posterior probability in the usual discriminant function model is the logistic regression function given in equation (1.1). More precisely, if the independent variable, X, follows a normal distribution within each of two groups (subpopulations) defined by the two values of Y and has different means and the same variance, then the conditional distribution of Y given $X = x$ is the logistic regression model. That is, if

$$X|Y \sim N(\mu_j, \sigma^2), j = 0, 1$$

then $P(Y = 1|x) = \pi(x)$. The symbol "$\sim$" is read "is distributed" and the "$N(\mu, \sigma^2)$" denotes the normal distribution with mean equal to μ and variance equal to σ^2. Under these assumptions it is easy to show [Lachenbruch (1975)] that the logistic coefficients are

$$\beta_0 = \ln\left(\frac{\theta_1}{\theta_0}\right) - 0.5(\mu_1^2 - \mu_0^2)/\sigma^2 \tag{1.23}$$

and

$$\beta_1 = (\mu_1 - \mu_0)/\sigma^2, \tag{1.24}$$

where $\theta_j = P(Y = j), j = 0, 1$. The discriminant function estimators of β_0 and β_1 are obtained by substituting estimators for $\mu_j, \theta_j, j = 0, 1$ and σ^2 into the above equations. The estimators usually used are $\hat{\mu}_j = \overline{x}_j$, the mean of x in the subgroup defined by $y = j, j = 0, 1, \theta_1 = n_1/n$ the mean of y with $\hat{\theta}_0 = 1 - \hat{\theta}_1$ and

$$\hat{\sigma}^2 = [(n_0 - 1)s_0^2 + (n_1 - 1)s_1^2]/(n_0 + n_1 - 2),$$

where s_j^2 is the unbiased estimator of σ^2 computed within the subgroup of the data defined by $y = j, j = 0, 1$. The above expressions are for a single variable x and multivariable expressions are presented in Chapter 2.

It is natural to ask why, if the discriminant function estimators are so easy to compute, they are not used in place of the maximum likelihood estimators? Halpern et al. (1971) and Hosmer et al. (1983) compared the two methods when the model contains a mixture of continuous and discrete variables, with the general conclusion that the discriminant function estimators are sensitive to the assumption of normality. In particular, the estimators of the coefficients for non-normally distributed variables are biased away from zero when the coefficient is, in fact, different from zero. The practical implication of this is that for dichotomous independent variables (that occur in many situations), the discriminant function estimators overestimate the magnitude of the coefficient. Lyles et al. (2009) describe a clever linear regression-based approach to compute the discriminant function estimator of the coefficient for a single continuous variable that, when their assumptions of normality hold, has better statistical properties than the maximum likelihood estimator. We discuss their multivariable extension and some of its practical limitations in Chapter 2.

At this point it may be helpful to delineate more carefully the various uses of the term *maximum likelihood*, as it applies to the estimation of the logistic regression coefficients. Under the assumptions of the discriminant function model stated above, the estimators obtained from equations (1.23) and (1.24) are maximum likelihood estimators. The estimators obtained from equations (1.5) and (1.6) are based on the conditional distribution of Y given X and, as such, are technically "conditional maximum likelihood estimators". It is common practice to drop the word "conditional" when describing the estimators given in equations (1.5) and (1.6). In this text, we use the word *conditional* to describe estimators in logistic regression with matched data as discussed in Chapter 7.

In summary there are alternative methods of estimation for some data configurations that are computationally quicker; however, we use the maximum likelihood method described in Section 1.2 throughout the rest of this text.

1.6 DATA SETS USED IN EXAMPLES AND EXERCISES

A number of different data sets are used in the examples as well as the exercises for the purpose of demonstrating various aspects of logistic regression modeling. Six of the data sets used throughout the text are described below. Other data sets are introduced as needed in later chapters. Some of the data sets were used in the previous editions of this text, for example the ICU and Low Birth Weight data, while others are new to this edition. All data sets used in this text may be obtained from links to web sites at John Wiley & Sons Inc. and the University of Massachusetts given in the Preface.

1.6.1 The ICU Study

The ICU study data set consists of a sample of 200 subjects who were part of a much larger study on survival of patients following admission to an adult intensive care unit (ICU). The major goal of this study was to develop a logistic regression model to predict the probability of survival to hospital discharge of these patients. A number of publications have appeared that have focused on various facets of this problem. The reader wishing to learn more about the clinical aspects of this study should start with Lemeshow et al. (1988). For a more up-to-date discussion of modeling the outcome of ICU patients the reader is referred to Lemeshow and Le Gall (1994) and to Lemeshow et al. (1993). The actual observed variable values have been modified to protect subject confidentiality. A code sheet for the variables to be considered in this text is given in Table 1.5. We refer to this data set as the ICU data.

Table 1.5 Code Sheet for the Variables in the ICU Data

Variable	Description	Codes/Values	Name
1	Identification code	ID number	ID
2	Vital status at hospital discharge	0 = Lived	STA
		1 = Died	
3	Age	Years	AGE
4	Gender	0 = Male	GENDER
		1 = Female	
5	Race	1 = White	RACE
		2 = Black	
		3 = Other	
6	Service at ICU admission	0 = Medical	SER
		1 = Surgical	
7	Cancer part of present problem	0 = No	CAN
		1 = Yes	
8	History of chronic renal failure	0 = No	CRN
		1 = Yes	
9	Infection probable at ICU admission	0 = No	INF
		1 = Yes	
10	CPR prior to ICU admission	0 = No	CPR
		1 = Yes	
11	Systolic blood pressure at ICU admission	mm Hg	SYS
12	Heart rate at ICU admission	Beats/min	HRA
13	Previous admission to an ICU within 6 months	0 = No	PRE
		1 = Yes	
14	Type of admission	0 = Elective	TYPE
		1 = Emergency	
15	Long bone, multiple, neck, single area, or hip fracture	0 = No	FRA
		1 = Yes	
16	PO_2 from initial blood gases	0 = >60	PO2
		1 = ≤60	
17	PH from initial blood gases	0 = ≥7.25	PH
		1 = <7.25	
18	PCO_2 from initial blood gases	0 = ≤45	PCO
		1 = >45	
19	Bicarbonate from initial blood gases	0 = ≥18	BIC
		1 = <18	
20	Creatinine from initial blood gases	0 = ≤2.0	CRE
		1 = >2.0	
21	Level of consciousness at ICU admission	0 = No coma or deep stupor	LOC
		1 = Deep stupor	
		2 = Coma	

Table 1.6   Code Sheet for the Variables in the Low Birth Weight Data

Variable	Description	Codes/Values	Name
1	Identification code	1–189	ID
2	Low birth weight	0 = ≥2500 g	LOW
		1 = <2500 g	
3	Age of mother	Years	AGE
4	Weight of mother at last menstrual period	Pounds	LWT
5	Race	1 = White	RACE
		2 = Black	
		3 = Other	
6	Smoking status during pregnancy	0 = No	SMOKE
		1 = Yes	
7	History of premature labor	0 = None	PTL
		1 = One	
		2 = Two, etc.	
8	History of hypertension	0 = No	HT
		1 = Yes	
9	Presence of uterine irritability	0 = No	UI
		1 = Yes	
10	Number of physician visits during the first trimester	0 = None	FTV
		1 = One	
		2 = Two, etc.	
11	Recorded birth weight	Grams	BWT

1.6.2   The Low Birth Weight Study

Low birth weight, defined as birth weight less than 2500 grams, is an outcome that has been of concern to physicians for years. This is because of the fact that infant mortality rates and birth defect rates are higher for low birth weight babies. A woman's behavior during pregnancy (including diet, smoking habits, and receiving prenatal care) can greatly alter the chances of carrying the baby to term, and, consequently, of delivering a baby of normal birth weight.

Data were collected as part of a larger study at Baystate Medical Center in Springfield, Massachusetts. This data set contains information on 189 births to women seen in the obstetrics clinic. Fifty-nine of these births were low birth weight. The variables identified in the code sheet given in Table 1.6 have been shown to be associated with low birth weight in the obstetrical literature. The goal of the current study was to determine whether these variables were risk factors in the clinic population being served by Baystate Medical Center. Actual observed variable values have been modified to protect subject confidentiality. We refer to this data set as the LOWBWT data.

1.6.3   The Global Longitudinal Study of Osteoporosis in Women

The Global Longitudinal Study of Osteoporosis in Women (GLOW) is an international study of osteoporosis in women over 55 years of age being coordinated at the

Table 1.7 Code Sheet for Variables in the GLOW Study

Variable	Description	Codes/Values	Name
1	Identification code	1−n	SUB_ID
2	Study site	1–6	SITE_ID
3	Physician ID code	128 unique codes	PHY_ID
4	History of prior fracture	1 = Yes 0 = No	PRIORFRAC
5	Age at enrollment	Years	AGE
6	Weight at enrollment	Kilograms	WEIGHT
7	Height at enrollment	Centimeters	HEIGHT
8	Body mass index	kg/m^2	BMI
9	Menopause before age 45	1 = Yes 0 = No	PREMENO
10	Mother had hip fracture	1 = Yes 0 = No	MOMFRAC
11	Arms are needed to stand from a chair	1 = Yes 0 = No	ARMASSIST
12	Former or current smoker	1 = Yes 0 = No	SMOKE
13	Self-reported risk of fracture	1 = Less than others of the same age 2 = Same as others of the same age 3 = Greater than others of the same age	RATERISK
14	Fracture risk score	Composite risk score[a]	FRACSCORE
15	Any fracture in first year	1 = Yes 0 = No	FRACTURE

[a]FRACSCORE = $0 \times (AGE \leq 60) + 1 \times (60 < AGE \leq 65) + 2 \times (65 < AGE \leq 70) + 3 \times (70 < AGE \leq 75) + 4 \times (75 < AGE \leq 80) + 5 \times (80 < AGE \leq 85) + 6 \times (AGE > 85) + (PRIORFRAC = 1) + (MOMFRAC = 1) + (WEIGHT < 56.8) + 2 \times (ARMASSIST = 1) + (SMOKE = 1)$.

Center for Outcomes Research (COR) at the University of Massachusetts/Worcester by its Director, Dr. Frederick Anderson, Jr. The study has enrolled over 60,000 women aged 55 and older in ten countries. The major goals of the study are to use the data to provide insights into the management of fracture risk, patient experience with prevention and treatment of fractures and distribution of risk factors among older women on an international scale over the follow up period. Complete details on the study as well as a list of GLOW publications may be found at the Center for Outcomes Research web site, www.outcomes-umassmed.org/glow.

Data used here come from six sites in the United States and include a few selected potential risk factors for fracture from the baseline questionnaire. The outcome variable is any fracture in the first year of follow up. The incident first-year fracture rate among the 21,000 subjects enrolled in these six sites is about 4 percent. In order to have a data set of a manageable size, $n = 500$, for this text we have over sampled the fractures and under sampled the non-fractures. As a result associations and conclusions from modeling these data do not apply to the study cohort as a whole. Data have been modified to protect subject confidentiality. We thank Dr. Gordon Fitzgerald of COR for his help in obtaining these data sets. A code sheet for the variables is shown in Table 1.7. This data set is named the GLOW500 data.

1.6.4 The Adolescent Placement Study

Fontanella et al. (2008) present results from a study of determinants of aftercare placement for psychiatrically hospitalized adolescents and have made the data, suitably modified to protect confidentiality, available to us. It is not our intent to repeat

Table 1.8 Code Sheet for Variables in the Adolescent Placement Study

Variable	Description	Codes/Values	Name
1	Identification code	1–508	ID
2	Placement	0 = Outpatient	PLACE
		1 = Day treatment	
		2 = Intermediate residential	
		3 = Residential	
3	Placement combined	0 = Outpatient or day treatment	PLACE3
		1 = Intermediate residential	
		2 = Residential	
3	Age at admission	Years	AGE
4	Race	0 = White	RACE
		1 = Nonwhite	
5	Gender	0 = Female	GENDER
		1 = Male	
6	Neuropsychiatric disturbance	0 = None	NEURO
		1 = Mild	
		2 = Moderate	
		3 = Severe	
7	Emotional disturbance	0 = Not severe	EMOT
		1 = Severe	
8	Danger to others	0 = Unlikely	DANGER
		1 = Possible	
		2 = Probable	
		3 = Likely	
9	Elopement risk	0 = No risk	ELOPE
		1 = At risk	
10	Length of hospitalization	Days	LOS
11	Behavioral symptoms score[a]	0–9	BEHAV
12	State custody	0 = No	CUSTD
		1 = Yes	
13	History of violence	0 = No	VIOL
		1 = Yes	

[a]Behavioral symptom score is based on the sum of three symptom subscales (oppositional behavior, impulsivity, and conduct disorder) from the CSPI.

the detailed analyses reported in their paper, but rather to use the data to motivate and describe methods for modeling a multinomial or ordinal scaled outcome using logistic regression models. As such, we selected a subset of variables, which are described in Table 1.8. This data set is referred to as the *APS data*.

1.6.5 The Burn Injury Study

The April 2008 release (Version 4.0) of the National Burn Repository research dataset (National Burn Repository 2007 Report, Dataset Version 4.0 accessed on 12/05/2008 at: http://www.ameriburn.org/2007NBRAnnualReport.pdf) includes information on a total of 306,304 burn related hospitalizations that occurred between 1973 and 2007. Available information included patient demographics, total burn surface area, presence of inhalation injury, and blinded trauma center identifiers. The outcome of interest is survival to hospital discharge. Osler et al. (2010) selected a subset of approximately 40,000 subjects treated between 2000 and 2007 at 40 different burn facilities to develop a new predictive logistic regression model (see the paper for the details on how this subset was selected). To obtain a much smaller data set for use in this text we over sampled subjects who died in hospital and under sampled subjects who lived to obtain a data set with $n = 1000$ and achieve a sample with 15 percent in hospital mortality. As such, all analyses and inferences contained in this text do not apply to the sample of 40,000, the original data from the registry or the population of burn injury patients as a whole. These data are used here to illustrate methods when prediction is the final goal as well as to demonstrate various model building techniques. The variables are described in Table 1.9 and the data are referred to as the *BURN1000 data*.

Table 1.9 Code Sheet for Variables in the Burn Study

Variable	Description	Codes/Values	Name
1	Identification code	1–1000	ID
2	Burn facility	1–40	FACILITY
3	Hospital discharge status	0 = Alive 1 = Dead	DEATH
4	Age at admission	Years	AGE
5	Gender	0 = Female 1 = Male	GENDER
6	Race	0 = Non-White 1 = White	RACE
7	Total burn surface area	0–100%	TBSA
8	Burn involved inhalation injury	0 = No 1 = Yes	INH_INJ
9	Flame involved in burn injury	0 = No 1 = Yes	FLAME

Table 1.10   Code Sheet for Variables in the Myopia Study

Variable	Variable Description	Values/Labels	Variable Name
1	Subject identifier	Integer (range 1–1503)	ID
2	Year subject entered the study	Year	STUDYYEAR
3	Myopia within the first 5 yr of follow up[a]	0 = No 1 = Yes	MYOPIC
4	Age at first visit	Years	AGE
5	Gender	0 = Male 1 = Female	GENDER
6	Spherical equivalent refraction[b]	Diopter	SPHEQ
7	Axial length[c]	mm	AL
8	Anterior chamber depth[d]	mm	ACD
9	Lens thickness[e]	mm	LT
10	Vitreous chamber depth[f]	mm	VCD
11	How many hours per week outside of school the child spent engaging in sports/outdoor activities	Hours per week	SPORTHR
12	How many hours per week outside of school the child spent reading for pleasure	Hours per week	READHR
13	How many hours per week outside of school the child spent playing video/computer games or working on the computer	Hours per week	COMPHR
14	How many hours per week outside of school the child spent reading or studying for school assignments	Hours per week	STUDYHR
15	How many hours per week outside of school the child spent watching television	Hours per week	TVHR
16	Composite of near-work activities	Hours per week	DIOPTERHR
17	Was the subject's mother myopic?[g]	0 = No 1 = Yes	MOMMY
18	Was the subject's father myopic?	0 = No 1 = Yes	DADMY

[a]MYOPIC is defined as SPHEQ <= −0.75D.

[b]A measure of the eye's effective focusing power. Eyes that are "normal" (don't require glasses or contact lenses) have spherical equivalents between −0.25 diopters (D) and +1.00 D. The more negative the spherical equivalent, the more myopic the subject.

[c]The length of eye from front to back.

[d]The length from front to back of the aqueous-containing space of the eye between the cornea and the iris.

[e]The length from front to back of the crystalline lens.

[f]The length from front to back of the aqueous-containing space of the eye in front of the retina.

[g]DIOPTERHR = 3 × (READHR + STUDYHR) + 2 × COMPHR + TVHR.

Table 1.11   Variables in the Modified NHANES Data Set

Variable	Description	Code/values	Name
1	Identification code	1–6482	ID
2	Gender	0 = Male, 1 = Female	GENDER
3	Age at screening	Years	AGE
4	Marital status	1 = Married 2 = Widowed 3 = Divorced 4 = Separated 5 = Never married 6 = Living together	MARSTAT
5	Statistical weight	4084.478–153810.3	SAMPLEWT
6	Pseudo-PSU	1, 2	PSU
7	Pseudo-stratum	1–15	STRATA
8	Total cholesterol	mg/dl	TCHOL
9	HDL-cholesterol	mg/dl	HDL
10	Systolic blood pressure	mm Hg	SYSBP
11	Diastolic blood pressure	mm Hg	DBP
12	Weight	kg	WT
13	Standing height	cm	HT
14	Body mass index	kg/m^2	BMI
15	Vigorous work activity	0 = Yes, 1 = No	VIGWRK
16	Moderate work activity	0 = Yes, 1 = No	MODWRK
17	Walk or bicycle	0 = Yes, 1 = No	WLKBIK
18	Vigorous recreational activities	0 = Yes, 1 = No	VIGRECEXR
19	Moderate recreational activities	0 = Yes, 1 = No	MODRECEXR
20	Minutes of sedentary activity per week	Minutes	SEDMIN
21	BMI > 35	0 = No, 1 = Yes	OBESE

1.6.6   The Myopia Study

Myopia, more commonly referred to as *nearsightedness*, is an eye condition where an individual has difficulty seeing things at a distance. This condition is primarily because the eyeball is too long. In an eye that sees normally, the image of what is being viewed is transmitted to the back portion of the eye, or retina, and hits the retina to form a clear picture. In the myopic eye, the image focuses in front of the retina, so the resultant image on the retina itself is blurry. The blurry image creates problems with a variety of distance viewing tasks (e.g., reading the blackboard,

Table 1.12   Code Sheet for the Variables in the Polypharmacy Data Set

Variable	Description	Codes/Values	Name
1	Subject ID	ID number 1–500	ID
2	Outcome; taking drugs from more than three different classes	0 = Not taking drugs from more than three classes 1 = Taking drugs from more than three classes	POLYPHARMACY
3	Number of outpatient mental health visits (MHV)	0 = None 1 = One to five 2 = Six to fourteen 3 = Greater than 14	MHV4
4	Number of inpatient mental health visits (MHV)	0 = None 1 = One 2 = More than one	INPTMHV3
5	Year	2002–2008	YEAR
6	Group	1 = Covered families and children (CFC) 2 = Aged, blind or disabled (ABD) 3 = Foster care (FOS)	GROUP
7	Location	0 = Urban 1 = Rural	URBAN
8	Comorbidity	0 = No 1 = Yes	COMORBID
9	Any primary diagnosis (bipolar, depression, etc.)	0 = No 1 = Yes	ANYPRIM
10	Number of primary diagnosis	0 = None 1 = One 2 = More than one	NUMPRIMRC
11	Gender	0 = Female 1 = Male	GENDER
12	Race	0 = White 1 = Black 2 = Other	RACE
13	Ethnic category	0 = NonHispanic 1 = Hispanic	ETHNIC
14	Age	Years and months (two decimal places)	AGE

doing homework, driving, playing sports) and requires wearing glasses or contact lenses to correct the problem. Myopia onset is typically between the ages of 8 and 12 years with cessation of the underlying eye growth that causes it by age 15–16 years.

The risk factors for the development of myopia have been debated for a long time and include genetic factors (e.g., family history of myopia) and the amount and type of visual activity that a child performs (e.g., studying, reading, TV watching, computer or video game playing, and sports/outdoor activity). There is strong evidence that having myopic parents increases the chance that a child will become myopic, and weaker evidence that certain types of visual activities (called *near work*, e.g., reading) increase the chance that a child will become myopic.

These data are a subset of data from the Orinda Longitudinal Study of Myopia (OLSM), a cohort study of ocular component development and risk factors for the onset of myopia in children, which evolved into the Collaborative Longitudinal Evaluation of Ethnicity and Refractive Error (CLEERE) Study, and both OLSM and CLEERE were funded by the National Institutes of Health/National Eye Institute. OLSM was based at the University of California, Berkeley [see Zadnik et al. (1993, 1994)]. Data collection began in the 1989–1990 school year and continued annually through the 2000–2001 school year. All data about the parts that make up the eye (the ocular components) were collected during an examination during the school day. Data on family history and visual activities were collected yearly in a survey completed by a parent or guardian.

The dataset used in this text is from 618 of the subjects who had at least five years of followup and were not myopic when they entered the study. All data are from their initial exam and includes 17 variables. In addition to the ocular data there is information on age at entry, year of entry, family history of myopia and hours of various visual activities. The ocular data come from a subject's right eye. A subject was coded as myopic if they became myopic at any time during the first five years of followup. We refer to this data set, in Table 1.10, as the MYOPIA data.

1.6.7 The NHANES Study

The National Health and Nutrition Examination Survey (NHANES), a major effort of the National Center for Health Statistics, was conceived in the early 1960s to provide nationally representative and reliable data on the health and nutritional status of adults and children in the United States. NHANES has since evolved into a ongoing survey program that provides the best available national estimates of the prevalence of, and risk factors for, targeted diseases in the United States population. The survey collects interview and physical exam data on a nationally representative, multistage probability sample of about 5,000 persons each year, who are chosen to be representative of the civilian, non-institutionalized, population in the US.

For purposes of illustrating fitting logistic regression models to sample survey data in Section 6.4 we chose selected variables, shown in Table 1.11, from the 2009–2010 cycle of the National Health and Nutrition Examination Study [NHANES III Reference Manuals and Reports (2012)] and made some modifications to the data. We refer to this data set as the NHANES data.

1.6.8 The Polypharmacy Study

In Chapter 9, we illustrate model building with correlated data using data on polypharmacy described in Table 1.12. The outcome of interest is whether the patient is taking drugs from three or more different classes (POLYPHARMACY), and researchers were interested in identifying factors associated with this outcome. We selected a sample of 500 subjects from among only those subjects with observations in each of the seven years data were collected. Based on the suggestions of the principal investigator, we initially treated the covariates for number of inpatient and outpatient mental health visits (MHVs) with categories described in Table 1.12. In addition we added a random number of months to the age, which was recorded only in terms of the year in the original data set. As our data set is a sample, the results in this section do not apply to the original study. We refer to this data set as the POLYPHARM data.

EXERCISES

1. In the ICU data described in Section 1.6.1 the primary outcome variable is vital status at hospital discharge, STA. Clinicians associated with the study felt that a key determinant of survival was the patient's age at admission, AGE.

    (a) Write down the equation for the logistic regression model of STA on AGE. Write down the equation for the logit transformation of this logistic regression model. What characteristic of the outcome variable, STA, leads us to consider the logistic regression model as opposed to the usual linear regression model to describe the relationship between STA and AGE?

    (b) Form a scatterplot of STA versus AGE.

    (c) Using the intervals (15, 24), (25, 34), (35, 44), (45, 54), (55, 64), (65, 74), (75, 84), (85, 94) for age, compute the STA mean over subjects within each age interval. Plot these values of mean STA versus the midpoint of the age interval using the same set of axes as was used in 1(b). Note: this plot may done "by hand" on a printed copy of the plot from 1(b).

    (d) Write down an expression for the likelihood and log-likelihood for the logistic regression model in Exercise 1(a) using the ungrouped, $n = 200$, data. Obtain expressions for the two likelihood equations.

    (e) Using a logistic regression package of your choice obtain the maximum likelihood estimates of the parameters of the logistic regression model in Exercise 1(a). These estimates should be based on the ungrouped, $n = 200$, data. Using these estimates, write down the equation for the fitted values, that is, the estimated logistic probabilities. Plot the equation for the fitted values on the axes used in the scatterplots in 1(b) and 1(c).

    (f) Using the results of the output from the logistic regression package used for 1(e), assess the significance of the slope coefficient for AGE using the likelihood ratio test, the Wald test, and if possible, the score test. What assumptions are needed for the p-values computed for each of these tests to be valid? Are the results of these tests consistent with one another? What is the value of the deviance for the fitted model?

    (g) Using the results from 1(e) compute 95 percent confidence intervals for the slope coefficient for AGE. Write a sentence interpreting this confidence.

    (h) Obtain from the package used to fit the model in 1(e) the estimated covari-
ance matrix. Compute the logit and estimated logistic probability for a
60-year-old subject. Evaluate the endpoints of the 95 percent confidence
intervals for the logit and estimated logistic probability. Write a sentence
interpreting the estimated probability and its confidence interval.

2. In the Myopia Study described in Section 1.6.2, one variable that is clearly
important is the initial value of spherical equivalent refraction·(SPHREQ).
Repeat steps (a)–(g) of Exercise 1, but for 2(c) use eight intervals containing
approximately equal numbers of subjects (i.e., cut points at 12.5%, 25%, ...,
etc.).

3. Using the data from the ICU study create a dichotomous variable NONWHITE
(NONWHITE $= 1$ if RACE $= 2$ or 3 and NONWHITE $= 0$ if RACE $= 1$).
Fit the logistic regression of STA on NONWHITE and show that the 95 percent profile likelihood confidence interval for the coefficient for nonwhite has
asymmetry of -13% and that this interval is 26% wider than the Wald-based
interval. This example points out that even when the sample size and number
of events are large $n = 200$, and $n_1 = 40$ there can be substantial asymmetry
and differences between the two interval estimators. Explain why this is the
case in this example.

CHAPTER 2

The Multiple Logistic Regression Model

2.1 INTRODUCTION

In Chapter 1 we introduced the logistic regression model in the context of a model containing a single variable. As in the case of linear regression, the strength of the logistic regression model is its ability to handle many variables, some of which may be on different measurement scales. In this chapter, we generalize the model to one with more than one independent variable (i.e., the multivariable or multiple logistic regression model). Central to the consideration of the multiple logistic models is estimating the coefficients and testing for their significance. We use the same approach discussed in Chapter 1 for the univariable setting. An additional modeling consideration, which is introduced in this chapter, is using design variables for modeling discrete, nominal scale, independent variables. In all cases, we assume that there is a predetermined collection of variables to be examined. We consider statistical methods for selecting variables in Chapter 4.

2.2 THE MULTIPLE LOGISTIC REGRESSION MODEL

Consider a collection of p independent variables denoted by the vector $\mathbf{x}' = (x_1, x_2, \ldots, x_p)$. For the moment we assume that each of these variables is at least interval scaled. Let the conditional probability that the outcome is present be denoted by $\Pr(Y = 1|\mathbf{x}) = \pi(\mathbf{x})$. The logit of the multiple logistic regression model is given by the equation

$$g(\mathbf{x}) = \ln\left(\frac{\pi(\mathbf{x})}{1 - \pi(\mathbf{x})}\right) = \beta_0 + \beta_1 x_1 + \beta_2 x_2 + \cdots + \beta_p x_p \qquad (2.1)$$

Applied Logistic Regression, Third Edition.
David W. Hosmer, Jr., Stanley Lemeshow, and Rodney X. Sturdivant.
© 2013 John Wiley & Sons, Inc. Published 2013 by John Wiley & Sons, Inc.

where, for the multiple logistic regression model,

$$\pi(\mathbf{x}) = \frac{e^{g(\mathbf{x})}}{1 + e^{g(\mathbf{x})}}. \tag{2.2}$$

If some of the independent variables are discrete, nominal scale variables such as race, sex, treatment group, and so forth, it is inappropriate to include them in the model as if they were interval scale variables. The numbers used to represent the various levels of these nominal scale variables are merely identifiers, and have no numeric significance. In this situation, the method of choice is to use a collection of *design variables* (or *dummy variables*). Suppose, for example, that one of the independent variables is race, which has been coded as "white," "black," and "other." In this case, two design variables are necessary. One possible coding strategy is that when the respondent is "white," the two design variables, D_1 and D_2, would both be set equal to zero; when the respondent is "black," D_1 would be set equal to 1 while D_2 would still equal 0; when the race of the respondent is "other," we would use $D_1 = 0$ and $D_2 = 1$. Table 2.1 illustrates this coding of the design variables.

Every logistic regression software package we use has the capability to generate design variables, and some provide a choice of several different methods. We discuss different strategies for creation and interpretation of the coefficients for the design variables in detail in Chapter 3.

In general, if a nominal scaled variable has k possible values, then $k - 1$ design variables are needed. The reason for using one less than the number of values is that, unless stated otherwise, our models have a constant term. To illustrate the notation used for design variables in this text, suppose that the jth independent variable x_j has k_j levels. The $k_j - 1$ design variables will be denoted as D_{jl} and the coefficients for these design variables will be denoted as $\beta_{jl}, l = 1, 2, \ldots, k_j - 1$. Thus, the logit for a model with p variables, with the jth variable being discrete is

$$g(\mathbf{x}) = \beta_0 + \beta_1 x_1 + \cdots + \sum_{l=1}^{k_j-1} \beta_{jl} D_{jl} + \beta_p x_p.$$

With a few exceptions, we suppress the summation and double subscripting needed to indicate when design variables are being used when discussing the multiple logistic regression model.

Table 2.1   An Example of the Coding of the Design Variables for Race, Coded at Three Levels

RACE	D_1	D_2
White	0	0
Black	1	0
Other	0	1

2.3 FITTING THE MULTIPLE LOGISTIC REGRESSION MODEL

Assume that we have a sample of n independent observations $(\mathbf{x}_i, y_i), i = 1, 2, \ldots, n$. As in the univariable case, fitting the model requires that we obtain estimates of the vector $\boldsymbol{\beta}' = (\beta_0, \beta_1, \ldots, \beta_p)$. The method of estimation used in the multivariable case is the same as in the univariable situation – maximum likelihood. The likelihood function is nearly identical to that given in equation (1.3) with the only change being that $\pi(\mathbf{x})$ is now defined as in equation (2.1). There will be $p + 1$ likelihood equations that are obtained by differentiating the log-likelihood function with respect to the $p + 1$ coefficients. The likelihood equations that result may be expressed as follows:

$$\sum_{i=1}^{n}[y_i - \pi(\mathbf{x}_i)] = 0$$

and

$$\sum_{i=1}^{n}x_{ij}[y_i - \pi(\mathbf{x}_i)] = 0$$

for $j = 1, 2, \ldots, p$.

As in the univariable model, the solution of the likelihood equations requires software that is available in virtually every statistical software package. Let $\hat{\boldsymbol{\beta}}$ denote the solution to these equations. Thus, the fitted values for the multiple logistic regression model are $\hat{\pi}(\mathbf{x}_i)$, the value of the expression in equation (2.2) computed using $\hat{\boldsymbol{\beta}}$ and $\mathbf{x}_i$.

In the previous chapter only a brief mention was made of the method for estimating the standard errors of the estimated coefficients. Now that the logistic regression model has been generalized, both in concept and notation to the multivariable case, we consider estimation of standard errors in more detail.

The method of estimating the variances and covariances of the estimated coefficients follows from well-developed theory of maximum likelihood estimation [see, e.g., Rao, (1973)]. This theory states that the estimators are obtained from the matrix of second partial derivatives of the log-likelihood function. These partial derivatives have the following general form

$$\frac{\partial^2 L(\beta)}{\partial \beta_j^2} = -\sum_{i=1}^{n}x_{ij}^2\pi_i(1 - \pi_i) \qquad (2.3)$$

and

$$\frac{\partial^2 L(\beta)}{\partial \beta_j \partial \beta_l} = -\sum_{i=1}^{n}x_{ij}x_{il}\pi_i(1 - \pi_i) \qquad (2.4)$$

for $j, l = 0, 1, 2, \ldots, p$ where π_i denotes $\pi(\mathbf{x}_i)$. Let the $(p + 1) \times (p + 1)$ matrix containing the negative of the terms given in equations (2.3) and (2.4) be denoted as $\mathbf{I}(\boldsymbol{\beta})$. This matrix is called the *observed information matrix*. The variances and covariances of the estimated coefficients are obtained from the inverse of this matrix, which we denote as $\text{Var}(\boldsymbol{\beta}) = \mathbf{I}^{-1}(\boldsymbol{\beta})$. Except in very special cases it is not possible to write down an explicit expression for the elements in this matrix. Hence, we will use the notation $\text{Var}(\beta_j)$ to denote the jth diagonal element of this matrix, which is the variance of $\hat{\beta}_j$, and $\text{Cov}(\beta_j, \beta_l)$ to denote an arbitrary off-diagonal element, which is the covariance of $\hat{\beta}_j$ and $\hat{\beta}_l$. The estimators of the variances and covariances, which will be denoted by $\widehat{\text{Var}}(\hat{\boldsymbol{\beta}})$, are obtained by evaluating $\text{Var}(\boldsymbol{\beta})$ at $\hat{\boldsymbol{\beta}}$. We use $\widehat{\text{Var}}(\hat{\beta}_j)$ and $\widehat{\text{Cov}}(\hat{\beta}_j, \hat{\beta}_l)$, $j, l = 0, 1, 2, \ldots, p$ to denote the values in this matrix. For the most part, we only use the estimated standard errors of the estimated coefficients, which we denote as

$$\widehat{\text{SE}}(\hat{\beta}_j) = [\widehat{\text{Var}}(\hat{\beta}_j)]^{1/2} \tag{2.5}$$

for $j = 0, 1, 2, \ldots, p$. We use this notation in developing methods for coefficient testing and confidence interval estimation.

A formulation of the information matrix that is useful when discussing model fitting and assessment of fit is $\hat{\mathbf{I}}(\hat{\boldsymbol{\beta}}) = \mathbf{X}'\hat{\mathbf{V}}\mathbf{X}$ where $\mathbf{X}$ is an n by $p + 1$ matrix containing the data for each subject and $\mathbf{V}$ is an n by n diagonal matrix with general element $\hat{\pi}_i(1 - \hat{\pi}_i)$. That is, the matrix $\mathbf{X}$ is

$$\mathbf{X} = \begin{bmatrix} 1 & x_{11} & x_{12} & \cdots & x_{1p} \\ 1 & x_{21} & x_{22} & \cdots & x_{2p} \\ \vdots & \vdots & \vdots & \ddots & \vdots \\ 1 & x_{n1} & x_{n2} & \cdots & x_{np} \end{bmatrix}$$

and the matrix $\mathbf{V}$ is

$$\hat{\mathbf{V}} = \begin{bmatrix} \hat{\pi}_1(1 - \hat{\pi}_1) & 0 & \cdots & 0 \\ 0 & \hat{\pi}_2(1 - \hat{\pi}_2) & \cdots & 0 \\ \vdots & 0 & \ddots & \vdots \\ 0 & \cdots & 0 & \hat{\pi}_n(1 - \hat{\pi}_n) \end{bmatrix},$$

where $\hat{\pi}_i = \hat{\pi}(\mathbf{x}_i)$ is value of equation (2.2) using $\hat{\boldsymbol{\beta}}$ and the covariates of subject i, $\mathbf{x}_i$.

Before proceeding further, we present an example that illustrates the formulation of a multiple logistic regression model and the estimation of its coefficients using a subset of the variables from the data for the Global Longitudinal Study of Osteoporosis in Women (GLOW) study described in Section 1.6.3. The code sheet for the full data set is given in Table 1.7. As discussed in Section 1.6.3, one goal of this study is to evaluate risk factors for fracture during follow up.

The GLOW data set used in this text has information on 500 women, $n_1 = 125$ of whom had a fracture during the first year of follow up and $n_0 = 375$ who did not have a fracture. As an example, we consider five variables thought to be of importance that are age at enrollment (AGE), weight at enrollment (WEIGHT), history of a previous fracture (PRIORFRAC), whether or not the woman experienced

Table 2.2   Fitted Multiple Logistic Regression Model of Fracture in the First Year of Follow Up (FRACTURE) on Age, Weight, Prior Fracture (PRIORFRAC), Early Menopause (PREMENO), and Self-Reported Risk of Fracture (RATERISK) from the GLOW Study, $n = 500$

Variable	Coeff.	Std. Err.	z	p	95% CI
AGE	0.050	0.0134	3.74	<0.001	0.024, 0.076
WEIGHT	0.004	0.0069	0.59	0.556	−0.009, 0.018
PRIORFRAC	0.679	0.2424	2.80	0.005	0.204, 1.155
PREMENO	0.187	0.2767	0.68	0.499	−0.355, 0.729
RATERISK2	0.534	0.2759	1.94	0.053	−0.006, 1.075
RATERISK3	0.874	0.2892	3.02	0.003	0.307, 1.441
Constant	−5.606	1.2207	−4.59	<0.001	−7.998, −3.213

Log-Likelihood = −259.03768

menopause before or after age 45 (PREMENO) and self-reported risk of fracture relative to women of the same age (RATERISK) coded at three levels: less, same or more risk. In this example, the variable RATERISK is modeled using the two design variables in Table 2.1. The results of fitting the multiple logistic regression model to these data are shown in Table 2.2.

In Table 2.2 the estimated coefficients for the two design variables for RATERISK are indicated by RATERISK2 and RATERISK3. The estimated logit is given in the following equation:

$$\hat{g}(\mathbf{x}) = -5.606 + 0.050 \times \text{AGE} + 0.004 \times \text{WEIGHT}$$

$$+ 0.679 \times \text{PRIORFRAC} + 0.187 \times \text{PREMENO}$$

$$+ 0.534 \times \text{RATERISK}\,2 + 0.874 \times \text{RATERISK}\,3$$

and the associated estimated logistic probabilities are found by using equation (2.2).

2.4   TESTING FOR THE SIGNIFICANCE OF THE MODEL

Once we have fit a particular multiple (multivariable) logistic regression model, we begin the process of model assessment. As in the univariable case presented in Chapter 1, the first step in this process is usually to assess the significance of the variables in the model. The likelihood ratio test for overall significance of the p coefficients for the independent variables in the model is performed in exactly the same manner as in the univariable case. The test is based on the statistic G given in equation (1.12). The only difference is that the fitted values, $\hat{\pi}$, under the model are based on the fitted model containing $p + 1$ parameters, $\hat{\boldsymbol{\beta}}$. Under the null hypothesis that the p "slope" coefficients for the covariates in the model are equal to zero, the distribution of G is chi-square with p degrees of freedom.

Consider the fitted model whose estimated coefficients are given in Table 2.2. For that model, the value of the log-likelihood, shown at the bottom of the table, is $L = -259.0377$. The log-likelihood for the constant only model may be obtained by evaluating the numerator of equation (1.13) or by fitting the constant only model. Either method yields the log-likelihood $L = -281.1676$. Thus the value of the likelihood ratio test is, from equation (1.12),

$$G = -2[-281.1676 - (-259.0377)] = 44.2598$$

and the p-value for the test is $P[\chi^2(6) > 44.2598] \leq 0.0001$, which is significant at well beyond the $\alpha = 0.05$ level. We reject the null hypothesis in this case and conclude that at least one or more of the p coefficients are different from zero, an interpretation analogous to the F-test used in multiple linear regression.

Before concluding that any or all of the coefficients are nonzero, we may look at the univariable Wald test statistics,

$$W_j = \frac{\hat{\beta}_j}{\widehat{SE}(\hat{\beta}_j)}.$$

These are shown in the fourth column, labeled z, in Table 2.2. Under the hypothesis that an individual coefficient is zero, these statistics will follow the standard normal distribution. The p-values computed under this hypothesis are shown in the fifth column of Table 2.2. If we use a level of significance of 0.05, then we would conclude that the variables AGE, history of prior fracture (PRIORFRAC) and self-reported rate of risk (RATERISK) are statistically significant, while WEIGHT and early menopause (PREMENO) are not significant.

As our goal is to obtain the best fitting model while minimizing the number of parameters, the next logical step is to fit a reduced model containing only those variables thought to be significant and compare that reduced model to the full model containing all of the variables. The results of fitting the reduced model are given in Table 2.3.

The difference between the two models is the exclusion of the variables WEIGHT and early menopause (PREMENO) from the full model. The likelihood

Table 2.3   Fitted Multiple Logistic Regression Model of Fracture in the First Year of Follow Up (FRACTURE) on AGE, Prior Fracture (PRIORFRAC), and Self-Reported Risk of Fracture (RATERISK) from the GLOW Study, $n = 500$

Variable	Coeff.	Std. Err.	z	p	95% CI
AGE	0.046	0.0124	3.69	<0.001	0.022, 0.070
PRIORFRAC	0.700	0.2412	2.90	0.004	0.228, 1.173
RATERISK2	0.549	0.2750	1.99	0.046	0.010, 1.088
RATERISK3	0.866	0.2862	3.02	0.002	0.305, 1.427
Constant	-4.991	0.9027	-5.53	<0.001	-6.760, -3.221

Log-Likelihood $= -259.4494$

ratio test comparing these two models is obtained using the definition of G given in equation (1.12). It has a distribution that is chi-square with 2 degrees of freedom under the hypothesis that the coefficients for both excluded variables are equal to zero. The value of the test statistic comparing the model in Table 2.3 to the one in Table 2.2 is

$$G = -2[-259.4494 - (-259.0377)] = 0.8324$$

which, with 2 degrees of freedom, has a p-value of $P[\chi^2(2) > 0.8324] = 0.663$. As the p-value is large, exceeding 0.05, we conclude that the full model is no better than the reduced model. That is, there is little statistical justification for including WEIGHT and PREMENO in the model. However, we must not base our models entirely on tests of statistical significance. As we discuss in Chapters 4 and 5, there are numerous other considerations that influence our decision to include or exclude variables from a model.

Whenever a categorical independent variable is included (or excluded) from a model, all of its design variables should be included (or excluded); to do otherwise implies that we have recoded the variable. For example, if we only include design variable D_1 as defined in Table 2.1, then the self-reported risk of fracture is entered into the model as a dichotomous variable coded as 0 (for less risk than others of the same age) and 1 (for the same or more risk than others of the same age). If k is the number of levels of a categorical variable, then the contribution to the degrees of freedom for the likelihood ratio test for the exclusion of this variable is $k - 1$. For example, if we exclude self-reported risk from the model and it is coded at three levels using the design variables shown in Table 2.1, then there are 2 degrees of freedom for the test, one for each design variable.

Because of the multiple degrees of freedom we must be careful in our use of the Wald (W) statistics to assess the significance of the coefficients. For example, if the W statistics for both coefficients exceed 2, then we could reasonably conclude that the design variables are significant. Alternatively, if one coefficient has a W statistic of 3.0 and the other a value of 0.1, then we cannot be sure about the contribution of the variable to the model. As both design variables for RATERISK are significant we can be fairly certain that the 2 degree of freedom test is also significant. We leave the details as an exercise, but for now it suffices to report that the $p < 0.001$ for the likelihood ratio test for the removal of RATERISK from the model in Table 2.3.

In the previous chapter we described, for the univariable model, two other tests equivalent to the likelihood ratio test for assessing the significance of the model: the Wald test and the Score test. At this point, we briefly discuss the multivariable versions of these tests, as their use appears occasionally in the literature. These tests are available in some software packages. For example, SAS computes both the likelihood ratio and score tests for a fitted model and STATA has the capability to easily perform the Wald test. For the most part we use likelihood ratio tests in this text because, as noted earlier, the quantities needed to carry it out may be obtained from all computer packages.

The multivariable analog of the Wald test is obtained from the following vector-matrix calculation:

$$W = \hat{\boldsymbol{\beta}}'[\widehat{\mathrm{Var}}(\hat{\boldsymbol{\beta}})]^{-1}\hat{\boldsymbol{\beta}}$$
$$= \hat{\boldsymbol{\beta}}'(\mathbf{X}'\hat{\mathbf{V}}\mathbf{X})\hat{\boldsymbol{\beta}},$$

which is distributed as chi-square with $p+1$ degrees of freedom under the hypothesis that each of the $p+1$ coefficients is equal to zero. The multivariable Wald test, equivalent to the likelihood ratio test for the significance of the fitted model, is based on just the p slope coefficients and is obtained by eliminating $\hat{\beta}_0$ from $\hat{\boldsymbol{\beta}}$ and the relevant row (first or last) and column (first or last) from $(\mathbf{X}'\hat{\mathbf{V}}\mathbf{X})$. As the evaluation of this test requires an extra step to perform vector-matrix operations and to obtain $\hat{\boldsymbol{\beta}}$, there is no gain over the likelihood ratio test for determining the significance of the model. Extensions of the Wald test that can be used to examine functions of the coefficients are quite useful and are illustrated in subsequent chapters. The value of the multivariable Wald test for the fitted model in Table 2.3 is $W = 39.88$, which, with 4 degrees of freedom, corresponds to $p < 0.001$. Hence, both the likelihood ratio test and the Wald test reject the hypothesis that the model is not significant. In this particular example the value of the multivariable Wald test is smaller than the likelihood ratio test, but this is not always the case.

The multivariable analog of the Score test for the significance of the model is based on the distribution of the p derivatives of $L(\boldsymbol{\beta})$ with respect to $\boldsymbol{\beta}$. The computation of this test is of the same order of complication as the Wald test. To define it in detail would require introduction of additional notation that would find little use in the remainder of this text. Thus, we refer the interested reader to Cox and Hinkley (1974) or Dobson (2002). We do note that the score test is computed by some statistical packages (e.g., the logistic procedure in SAS).

2.5 CONFIDENCE INTERVAL ESTIMATION

We discussed confidence interval estimators for the coefficients, the logit and the logistic probabilities for the univariable logistic regression model in Section 1.4. The methods used for confidence interval estimators for a multivariable model are essentially the same.

The endpoints for a $100(1-\alpha)\%$ Wald-based confidence interval for the coefficients are obtained from equation (1.15) for slope coefficients and from equation (1.16) for the constant term. For example, using the fitted model presented in Table 2.3, the 95 percent confidence interval for the coefficient of AGE is

$$0.046 \pm 1.96 \times 0.0124 = (0.022, 0.070),$$

which are exactly the values in the last column of Table 2.3, labeled "95% Conf. Int.". The interpretation of this interval is that we are 95 percent confident that the increase in the log-odds per one-year increase in age is between 0.022 and 0.070. As we noted in Section 1.4 many software packages (e.g., STATA) automatically provide confidence intervals for all model coefficients in the output. Confidence intervals for the other coefficients shown in Table 2.3 are calculated in a similar manner. We also calculated the profile likelihood confidence interval estimator discussed at the end of Section 1.4 for each of the variables in Table 2.3, and they differed from their respective Wald-based confidence intervals at most by 0.3 percent and as a result, are not shown.

The confidence interval estimator for the logit is a bit more complicated for the multiple variable model than the result presented in equation (1.19). The basic idea is the same; only there are now more terms involved in the summation. It follows that a general expression for the estimator of the logit for a model containing p covariates is

$$\hat{g}(\mathbf{x}) = \hat{\beta}_0 + \hat{\beta}_1 x_1 + \hat{\beta}_2 x_2 + \cdots + \hat{\beta}_p x_p. \tag{2.6}$$

An alternative way to express the estimator of the logit in equation (2.6) is through the use of vector notation as $\hat{g}(\mathbf{x}) = \mathbf{x}'\hat{\boldsymbol{\beta}}$, where the vector $\hat{\boldsymbol{\beta}}' = (\hat{\beta}_0, \hat{\beta}_1, \hat{\beta}_2, \ldots, \hat{\beta}_p)$ denotes the estimator of the $p+1$ coefficients and the vector $\mathbf{x}' = (x_0, x_1, x_2, \ldots, x_p)$ represents a set of values of the p-covariates in the model and the constant, $x_0 = 1$.

It follows from equation (1.18) that an expression for the estimator of the variance of the estimator of the logit in equation (2.6) is

$$\widehat{\text{Var}}[\hat{g}(\mathbf{x})] = \sum_{j=0}^{p} x_j^2 \widehat{\text{Var}}(\hat{\beta}_j) + \sum_{j=0}^{p} \sum_{k=j+1}^{p} 2x_j x_k \widehat{\text{Cov}}(\hat{\beta}_j, \hat{\beta}_k). \tag{2.7}$$

We can express this result much more concisely by using the matrix expression for the estimator of the variance of the estimator of the coefficients. From the expression for the observed information matrix, we have that

$$\widehat{\text{Var}}(\hat{\boldsymbol{\beta}}) = (\mathbf{X}'\hat{\mathbf{V}}\mathbf{X})^{-1}. \tag{2.8}$$

It follows from equation (2.8) that an equivalent expression for the estimator in equation (2.7) is

$$\widehat{\text{Var}}[\hat{g}(\mathbf{x})] = \mathbf{x}'\widehat{\text{Var}}(\hat{\boldsymbol{\beta}})\mathbf{x}$$

$$= \mathbf{x}'(\mathbf{X}'\hat{\mathbf{V}}\mathbf{X})^{-1}\mathbf{x}. \tag{2.9}$$

Fortunately, all good logistic regression software packages provide the option for the user to create a new variable containing the estimated values of equation (2.9) or the standard error for all observed values of the covariates of subjects in the data set. This feature eliminates the computational burden associated with the matrix calculations in equation (2.9) and allows the user to routinely calculate fitted values and confidence interval estimates. However, it is useful to illustrate the details of the calculations.

Using the model in Table 2.3, the estimated logit for a 65-year-old woman with a prior fracture (PRIORFRAC $= 1$) who thinks that her risk is the same as other women of her age is

$$\hat{g}(\text{AGE} = 65, \text{PRIORFRAC} = 1, \text{RATERISK} = 2)$$
$$= -4.991 + 0.046 \times 65 + 0.700 \times 1 + 0.549 \times 1 + 0.866 \times 0$$
$$= -0.752$$

and the estimated logistic probability is

$$\hat{\pi}(\text{AGE} = 65, \text{PRIORFRAC} = 1, \text{RATERISK} = 2) = \frac{e^{-0.752}}{1 + e^{-0.752}} = 0.320.$$

The interpretation of this fitted value is that the estimated proportion of 65-year-old women with a prior fracture, who rate their risk of fracture as the same as women of their age having a facture in the next year is 0.320.

In order to use equation (2.7) to estimate the variance of this estimated logit we need the estimated covariance matrix, which is shown in Table 2.4. The expression for the estimated variance of the logit is

$$\widehat{\text{Var}}[\hat{g}(\text{AGE} = 65, \text{PRIORFRAC} = 1, \text{RATERISK} = 2)]$$
$$= \widehat{\text{Var}}(\hat{\beta}_0) + (65)^2 \times \widehat{\text{Var}}(\hat{\beta}_1) + (1)^2 \times \widehat{\text{Var}}(\hat{\beta}_2) + (1)^2 \times \widehat{\text{Var}}(\hat{\beta}_3) + 2 \times 65$$
$$\times \widehat{\text{Cov}}(\hat{\beta}_0, \hat{\beta}_1) + 2 \times 1 \times \widehat{\text{Cov}}(\hat{\beta}_0, \hat{\beta}_2) + 2 \times 1 \times \widehat{\text{Cov}}(\hat{\beta}_0, \hat{\beta}_3) + 2 \times 65 \times 1$$
$$\times \widehat{\text{Cov}}(\hat{\beta}_1, \hat{\beta}_2) + 2 \times 65 \times 1 \times \widehat{\text{Cov}}(\hat{\beta}_1, \hat{\beta}_3) + 2 \times 1 \times 1 \times \widehat{\text{Cov}}(\hat{\beta}_2, \hat{\beta}_3),$$

which when evaluated using the values in Table 2.4 is

$$\widehat{\text{Var}}[\hat{g}(\text{AGE} = 65, \text{PRIORFRAC} = 1, \text{RATERISK} = 2)]$$
$$= 0.81487 + (65)^2 \times 0.00015 + 1 \times 0.05816 + 1 \times 0.07563$$
$$+ 2 \times 65(-0.01089) + 2 \times 1 \times 0.04450 + 2 \times 1 \times (-0.06039) + 2 \times 65$$
$$\times 1 \times (-0.00083) + 2 \times 65 \times 1 \times 0.00022 + 2 \times 1 \times 1 \times (-0.00313)$$
$$= 0.04937.$$

Table 2.4 Estimated Covariance Matrix of the Estimated Coefficients in Table 2.3

	AGE	PRIORFRAC	RATERISK2	RATERISK3	Constant
AGE	0.00015				
PRIROFRAC	−0.00083	0.05816			
RATERISK2	0.00022	−0.00313	0.07563		
RATERISK3	0.00054	−0.01184	0.04624	0.08191	
Constant	−0.01089	0.04450	−0.06039	−0.08055	0.81487

The standard error is

$$\widehat{SE}[\hat{g}(\text{AGE} = 65, \text{PRIORFRAC} = 1, \text{RATERISK} = 2)] = \sqrt{0.04937} = 0.22220$$

and the 95 percent confidence interval for the estimated logit is

$$-0.752 \pm 1.96 \times 0.22220 = (-1.18751, -0.31648).$$

The associated confidence interval for the fitted value is $(0.234, 0.422)$. We defer discussion and interpretation of the estimated logit, fitted values and their respective confidence intervals until Chapter 3.

2.6 OTHER ESTIMATION METHODS

In Section 1.5, we discussed the discriminant function estimators of the coefficients of the logistic regression model and note here that it may also be employed in the multivariable case. This approach to estimation of the logistic regression coefficients is based on the assumption that the distribution of the independent variables, given the value of the outcome variable, is multivariate normal. Two points should be kept in mind: (i) the assumption of multivariate normality is rarely, if ever, satisfied in practice because of the frequent occurrence of categorical independent variables, and (ii) the discriminant function estimators of the coefficients for non-normally distributed independent variables, especially dichotomous variables, will be biased away from zero when the true coefficient is nonzero. For these reasons, in general, we do not recommend the use of this method. However, these estimators are of historical importance as a number of the classic papers in the applied literature [such as Truett et al. (1967)] used them. These estimators are easily computed and in the absence of a logistic regression program, could be used as a first approximation to parameter estimates. Thus, it seems worthwhile to include the relevant formulae for their computation. An exception to the general recommendation is when the focus is on the effect of a single continuous variable and all other variables in the model are there for adjustment, a concept we discuss in the next chapter. In this special setting Lyles et al. (2009) show how one may compute the discriminant function estimator of this single coefficient through an easily performed linear regression.

Specifically, the assumptions for the discriminant function approach are that the conditional distribution of $\mathbf{X}$ (the vector of p covariate random variables) given the outcome variable, $Y = y$, is multivariate normal with a mean vector that depends on y, but a covariance matrix that does not. Using notation defined in Section 1.5 we have that $(\mathbf{X}|y = j) \sim N(\mu_j, \Sigma)$ where μ_j contains the means of the p independent variables for the subpopulation defined by $y = j$ and Σ is the $p \times p$ covariance matrix of these variables. Under these assumptions, $\Pr(Y = 1|\mathbf{x}) = \pi(\mathbf{x})$, where the coefficients are given by:

$$\beta_0 = \ln\left(\frac{\theta_1}{\theta_0}\right) - 0.5(\mu_1 - \mu_0)'\Sigma^{-1}(\mu_1 + \mu_0) \qquad (2.10)$$

and

$$\boldsymbol{\beta} = (\mu_1 - \mu_0)' \Sigma^{-1}, \qquad (2.11)$$

where $\theta_1 = \Pr(Y = 1)$ and $\theta_0 = 1 - \theta_1$ denote the proportion of the population with y equal to 1 or 0, respectively. Equations (2.10) and (2.11) are the multivariable analogs of equations (1.23) and (1.24).

The discriminant function estimators of β_0 and $\boldsymbol{\beta}$ are found by substituting estimators for μ_j, $j = 0, 1, \Sigma$, and θ_1 into equations (2.10) and (2.11). The estimators most often used are the maximum likelihood estimators under the multivariate normal model. That is, we let

$$\hat{\mu}_j = \bar{\mathbf{x}}_j,$$

the mean of $\mathbf{x}$ in the subgroup of the sample with $y = j$, $j = 0, 1$.

The estimator of the covariance matrix, Σ, is the multivariable extension of the pooled sample variance given in Section 1.5. This may be represented as

$$\mathbf{S} = \frac{(n_0 - 1)\mathbf{S}_0 + (n_1 - 1)\mathbf{S}_1}{(n_0 + n_1 - 2)},$$

where $\mathbf{S}_j$, $j = 0, 1$ is the $p \times p$ matrix of the usual unbiased estimators of the variances and covariances computed within the subgroup defined by $y = j$, $j = 0, 1$.

Because of the bias in the discriminant function estimators when normality does not hold, they should be used only when logistic regression software is not available, and then only in preliminary analyses. Any final analyses should be based on the maximum likelihood estimators of the coefficients.

EXERCISES

1. In Section 2.4 we stated, but did not provide details for, the likelihood ratio test for the addition of weight and early menopause to the model containing AGE, prior fracture (PRIORFRAC) and self-reported risk (RATERISK).

    (a) Using the GLOW500 data and a logistic regression package verify the values of the coefficients for the models shown in Table 2.2 and Table 2.3.

    (b) Perform the likelihood ratio test comparing these two models [i.e., the test for the contribution of WEIGHT and early menopause (PREMENO) to a model containing AGE, prior fracture (PRIORFRAC) and self-reported risk (RATERISK)].

2. Use the ICU data described in Section 1.6.1 and consider the multiple logistic regression model of vital status, STA, on age (AGE), cancer part of the present problem (CAN), CPR prior to ICU admission (CPR), infection probable at ICU admission (INF), and race (RACE).

    (a) The variable race is coded at three levels. Prepare a table showing the coding of the two design variables necessary for including this variable in a logistic regression model.

(b) Write down the equation for the logistic regression model of STA on AGE, CAN, CPR, INF, and RACE. Write down the equation for the logit transformation of this logistic regression model. How many parameters does this model contain?

(c) Write down an expression for the likelihood and log-likelihood for the logistic regression model in Exercise 2(b). How many likelihood equations are there? Write down an expression for a typical likelihood equation for this problem.

(d) Using a logistic regression package, obtain the maximum likelihood estimates of the parameters of the logistic regression model in Exercise 2(b). Using these estimates write down the equation for the fitted values (i.e., the estimated logistic probabilities).

(e) Using the results of the output from the logistic regression package used in Exercise 2(d), assess the significance of the slope coefficients for the variables in the model using the likelihood ratio test. What assumptions are needed for the p-values computed for this test to be valid? What is the value of the deviance for the fitted model?

(f) Use the Wald statistics to obtain an approximation to the significance of the individual slope coefficients for the variables in the model. Fit a reduced model that eliminates those variables with nonsignificant Wald statistics. Assess the joint (conditional) significance of the variables excluded from the model. Present the results of fitting the reduced model in a table.

(g) Using the results from Exercise 2(f), compute 95 percent confidence intervals for all coefficients in the model. Write a sentence interpreting the confidence intervals for the nonconstant covariates.

(h) Obtain the estimated covariance matrix for the final model fit in Exercise 2(f). Choose a set of values for the covariates in that model and estimate the logit and logistic probability for a subject with these characteristics. Compute 95 percent confidence intervals for the logit and estimated logistic probability. Write a sentence or two interpreting the estimated probability and its confidence interval.

3. Use the Myopia Study data described in Section 1.6.6 and use MYOPIC as the outcome and as possible variables for a model: AGE, GENDER, family history of myopia (MOMMY and DADMY), number of hours playing sports (SPORTHR) and number of hours watching television (TVHR).

(a) Repeat parts 2(b)–2(h) of Exercise 2.

(b) Verify that there is little difference between the Wald-based and profile likelihood intervals for the variables in the model in part 3(a).

CHAPTER 3

Interpretation of the Fitted Logistic Regression Model

3.1 INTRODUCTION

In Chapters 1 and 2 we discussed the methods for fitting and testing for the significance of the logistic regression model. After fitting a model the emphasis shifts from the computation and assessment of significance of the estimated coefficients to the interpretation of their values. Strictly speaking, an assessment of the adequacy of the fitted model should precede any attempt at interpreting it. In the case of logistic regression, the methods for assessment of fit are rather technical in nature and thus are deferred until Chapter 5, at which time the reader should have a good working knowledge of the logistic regression model. Thus, we begin this chapter assuming that a logistic regression model has been fit, that the variables in the model are significant in either a clinical or statistical sense, and that the model fits according to some statistical measure of fit.

The interpretation of any fitted model requires that we be able to draw practical inferences from the estimated coefficients in the model. The question being addressed is: *What do the estimated coefficients in the model tell us about the research questions that motivated the study?* For most statistical models this involves the estimated coefficients for the independent variables in the model. In most instances, the intercept coefficient is of little interest. The estimated coefficients for the independent variables represent the slope (i.e., rate of change) of a function of the dependent variable per unit of change in the independent variable. Thus, interpretation involves two issues: determining the functional relationship between the dependent variable and the independent variable, and appropriately defining the unit of change for the independent variable.

The first step is to determine what function of the dependent variable yields a linear function of the independent variables. This is called the *link function* [see

Applied Logistic Regression, Third Edition.
David W. Hosmer, Jr., Stanley Lemeshow, and Rodney X. Sturdivant.
© 2013 John Wiley & Sons, Inc. Published 2013 by John Wiley & Sons, Inc.

McCullagh and Nelder (1989), or Dobson (2002)]. In the case of a linear regression model, the link function is the identity function as the dependent variable, by definition, is linear in the parameters. (For those unfamiliar with the term *identity function*, it is the function $y = y$.) In the logistic regression model the link function is the logit transformation $g(x) = \ln\{\pi(x)/[1 - \pi(x)]\} = \beta_0 + \beta_1 x$.

For a linear regression model recall that the slope coefficient, β_1, is equal to the difference between the value of the dependent variable at $x + 1$ and the value of the dependent variable at x, for any value of x. For example, the linear regression model at x is $y(x) = \beta_0 + \beta_1 x$. It follows that the slope coefficient is $\beta_1 = y(x + 1) - y(x)$. In this case, the interpretation of the slope coefficient is that it is the change in the outcome variable corresponding to a one-unit change in the independent variable. For example, in a regression of weight on height of male adolescents if the slope is 5 then we would conclude that an increase of 1 inch in height is associated with an increase of 5 pounds in weight.

In the logistic regression model, the slope coefficient is the change in the logit corresponding to a change of one unit in the independent variable [i.e., $\beta_1 = g(x + 1) - g(x)$]. Proper interpretation of the coefficient in a logistic regression model depends on being able to place meaning on the difference between two values of the logit function. This difference is discussed in detail on a case-by-case basis as it relates directly to the definition and meaning of a one-unit change in the independent variable. In the following sections of this chapter we consider the interpretation of the coefficients for a univariable logistic regression model for each of the possible measurement scales of the independent variable. We discuss interpretation of the coefficients from multivariable models and the probabilities from a fitted logistic model. We also compare the results of a logistic regression analysis to a stratified contingency table analysis that is common in epidemiological research. We conclude the chapter with a discussion of the construction, use and interpretation of the propensity score.

3.2 DICHOTOMOUS INDEPENDENT VARIABLE

We begin by discussing the interpretation of logistic regression coefficients in the situation where the independent variable is nominal scaled and dichotomous (i.e., measured at two levels). This case provides the conceptual foundation for all the other situations.

We assume that the independent variable, x, is coded as either 0 or 1. The difference in the logit for a subject with $x = 1$ and $x = 0$ is

$$g(1) - g(0) = (\beta_0 + \beta_1 \times 1) - (\beta_0 + \beta_1 \times 0) = (\beta_0 + \beta_1) - (\beta_0) = \beta_1.$$

The algebra shown in this equation is rather straightforward. The rationale for presenting it in this level of detail is to emphasize that four steps are required to obtain the correct expression of the coefficient(s) and hence, the correct interpretation of the coefficient(s). In some settings, like the current one, these steps are quite straightforward, but in the examples in Section 3.3 they are not so obvious.

The first three of the four steps are: (1) define the two values of the covariate to be compared (e.g., $x = 1$ and $x = 0$); (2) substitute these two values into the equation for the logit [e.g., $g(1)$ and $g(0)$], and (3) calculate the difference in the two equations [e.g., $g(1) - g(0)$]. As shown, for a dichotomous covariate coded 0 and 1 the result at the end of step 3 is equal to β_1. Thus, the slope coefficient, or logit difference, is the difference between the log of the odds when $x = 1$ and the log of the odds when $x = 0$. The practical problem is that change on the scale of the log-odds is hard to explain and it may not be especially meaningful to a subject-matter audience. In order to provide a more meaningful interpretation we need to introduce the *odds ratio* as a measure of association.

The possible values of the logistic probabilities from a model containing a single dichotomous covariate coded 0 and 1 are displayed in the 2×2 table, shown in Table 3.1. The *odds* of the outcome being present among individuals with $x = 1$ is $\pi(1)/[1 - \pi(1)]$. Similarly, the odds of the outcome being present among individuals with $x = 0$ is $\pi(0)/[1 - \pi(0)]$. The *odds ratio*, denoted OR, is the ratio of the odds for $x = 1$ to the odds for $x = 0$, and is given by the equation

$$\text{OR} = \frac{\dfrac{\pi(1)}{[1 - \pi(1)]}}{\dfrac{\pi(0)}{[1 - \pi(0)]}}. \tag{3.1}$$

Substituting the expressions for the logistic regression model probabilities in Table 3.1 into equation (3.1) we obtain

$$\text{OR} = \frac{\left(\dfrac{e^{\beta_0 + \beta_1}}{1 + e^{\beta_0 + \beta_1}}\right)}{\left(\dfrac{1}{1 + e^{\beta_0 + \beta_1}}\right)} \Big/ \frac{\left(\dfrac{e^{\beta_0}}{1 + e^{\beta_0}}\right)}{\left(\dfrac{1}{1 + e^{\beta_0}}\right)}$$

$$= \frac{e^{\beta_0 + \beta_1}}{e^{\beta_0}}$$

$$= e^{(\beta_0 + \beta_1) - \beta_0}$$

$$= e^{\beta_1}.$$

Hence, for a logistic regression model with a dichotomous independent variable coded 0 and 1, the relationship between the odds ratio and the regression coefficient is

$$\text{OR} = e^{\beta_1}. \tag{3.2}$$

This illustrates the fourth step in interpreting the effect of a covariate, namely exponentiate the logit difference computed in step 3 to obtain an odds ratio.

Table 3.1 Values of the Logistic Regression Model when the Independent Variable Is Dichotomous

	Independent Variable (x)	
Outcome Variable (y)	$x = 1$	$x = 0$
$y = 1$	$\pi(1) = \dfrac{e^{\beta_0+\beta_1}}{1+e^{\beta_0+\beta_1}}$	$\pi(0) = \dfrac{e^{\beta_0}}{1+e^{\beta_0}}$
$y = 0$	$1 - \pi(1) = \dfrac{1}{1+e^{\beta_0+\beta_1}}$	$1 - \pi(0) = \dfrac{1}{1+e^{\beta_0}}$
Total	1.0	1.0

The odds ratio is widely used as a measure of association as it approximates how much more likely or unlikely (in terms of odds) it is for the outcome to be present among those subjects with $x = 1$ as compared to those subjects with $x = 0$. For example, if the outcome, Y, denotes the presence or absence of lung cancer and if X denotes whether the subject is a smoker, then an OR $= 2$ is interpreted to mean that the odds of lung cancer among smokers is two times greater than the odds of lung cancer among the nonsmokers in this study population. As another example, suppose that the outcome, Y, is the presence or absence of heart disease and X denotes whether or not the person engages in regular strenuous physical exercise. If the odds ratio is OR $= 0.5$, then the odds of heart disease among those subjects who exercise is one-half the odds of heart disease for those subjects who do not exercise in the study population. This simple relationship between the coefficient and the odds ratio is the fundamental reason logistic regression has proven to be such a powerful analytic research tool.

In certain settings, the odds ratio can approximate another measure of association called the relative risk, which is the ratio of the two outcome probabilities, RR $= \pi(1)/\pi(0)$. It follows from equation (3.1) that the odds ratio approximates the relative risk if $[1 - \pi(0)]/[1 - \pi(1)] \approx 1$. This holds when $\pi(x)$ is small for both $x = 0$ and $x = 1$, often referred to in medical/epidemiological research as the *rare disease assumption*.

Readers who have not had experience with the odds ratio as a measure of association would be advised to spend some time reading about this measure in one of the following texts: Breslow and Day (1980), Rothman et al. (2008), Aschengrau and Seage (2008), Lilienfeld and Stolley (1994), and Oleckno (2008).

An example from the GLOW study described in Section 1.6.3 and used in Chapter 2 may help clarify how the odds ratio is estimated from the results of a fitted logistic regression model and from a 2×2 contingency table. To review, the outcome variable is having a fracture (FRACTURE) in the first year of follow-up. Here we use having had a fracture between the age of 45 and enrollment in the study (PRIORFRAC) as the dichotomous independent variable. The result of cross-classifying fracture during follow-up by prior fracture is presented in Table 3.2.

The frequencies in Table 3.2 tell us that there were 52 subjects with values $(x = 1, y = 1)$, 73 with $(x = 0, y = 1)$, 74 with $(x = 1, y = 0)$, and 301 with

Table 3.2 Cross-Classification of Prior Fracture and Fracture During Follow-Up in the GLOW Study, $n = 500$

Fracture During	Prior Fracture (x)		Total
Follow-Up (y)	Yes (1)	No (0)	Total
Present (1)	52	73	125
Absent (0)	74	301	375
Total	126	374	500

Table 3.3 Results of Fitting the Logistic Regression Model of Fracture (FRACTURE) on Prior Fracture (PRIORFRAC) Using the Data in Table 3.2

Variable	Coeff.	Std. Err.	z	p	95% CI
PRIORFRAC	1.064	0.2231	4.77	<0.001	0.627, 1.501
Constant	−1.417	0.1305	−10.86	<0.001	−1.672, −1.161

Log-likelihood = −270.03397.

$(x = 0, y = 0)$. The results of fitting a logistic regression model containing the dichotomous covariate PRIORFRAC are shown in Table 3.3.

The estimate of the odds ratio using equation (3.2) and the estimated coefficient for PRIORFRAC in Table 3.3 is $\widehat{OR} = e^{1.064} = 2.9$. Readers who have had some previous experience with the odds ratio undoubtedly wonder why we used a logistic regression package to estimate the odds ratio, when we easily could have computed it directly as the cross-product ratio from the frequencies in Table 3.2, namely,

$$\widehat{OR} = \frac{52 \times 301}{74 \times 73} = 2.897.$$

The tremendous advantage of using logistic regression will surface when additional independent variables are included in the logistic regression model.

Thus, we see that the slope coefficient from the fitted logistic regression model is $\hat{\beta}_1 = \ln[(52 \times 301)/(74 \times 73)] = 1.0638$. This emphasizes the fact that logistic regression is, even in the simplest possible case, a regression analysis. The fact that the data may be presented in terms of a contingency table just aids in the interpretation of the estimated coefficients as the log of the odds ratio.

Along with the point estimate of a parameter, it is always a good idea to use a confidence interval estimate to provide additional information about the parameter value. In the case of the odds ratio from a 2×2 table (corresponding to a fitted logistic regression model with a single dichotomous covariate) there is an extensive literature focused on the problem of confidence interval estimation for the odds ratio when the sample size is small. The reader who wishes to learn more about the available exact and approximate methods should see the papers by Fleiss (1979), and Gart and Thomas (1972). Breslow and Day (1980), Kleinbaum et al. (1982), and Rothman et al. (2008) discuss inference with small samples. We discuss the small sample setting in Section 10.3.

As we noted earlier, the odds ratio is usually the parameter of interest derived from a fitted logistic regression due to its ease of interpretation. However, its estimator, $\widehat{OR}$, tends to have a distribution that is highly skewed to the right. This is due to the fact that its range is between 0 and ∞, with the null value equaling 1. In theory, for extremely large sample sizes, the distribution of $\widehat{OR}$ would be normal. Unfortunately, this sample size requirement typically exceeds that of most studies. Hence, inferences are usually based on the sampling distribution of $\ln(\widehat{OR}) = \hat{\beta}_1$, which tends to follow a normal distribution for much smaller sample sizes. We obtain a $100 \times (1 - \alpha)\%$ confidence interval estimator for the odds ratio by first calculating the endpoints of a confidence interval estimator for the log-odds ratio (i.e., β_1) and then exponentiating the endpoints of this interval. In general, the endpoints are given by the expression

$$\exp[\hat{\beta}_1 \pm z_{1-\alpha/2} \times \widehat{SE}(\hat{\beta}_1)].$$

As an example, consider the estimation of the odds ratio for the dichotomized variable PRIORFRAC. Using the results in Table 3.3 the point estimate is $\widehat{OR} = 2.9$ and the 95% confidence interval is

$$\exp(1.064 \pm 1.96 \times 0.2231) = (1.87, 4.49).$$

This interval is typical of many confidence intervals for odds ratios when the point estimate exceeds 1, in that it is skewed to the right from the point estimate. This confidence interval suggests that the odds of a fracture during follow-up among women with a prior fracture could be as little as 1.9 times or much as 4.5 times the odds for women without a prior fracture, at the 95% level of confidence.

We discussed the profile likelihood confidence interval estimator for a logistic regression coefficient in Section 1.4. The resulting profile likelihood confidence interval for the odds ratio in this example is nearly identical to the Wald based interval given earlier and thus is not presented. There is an exercise at the end of the chapter where this is not the case.

Because of the importance of the odds ratio as a measure of association, many software packages automatically provide point and confidence interval estimates based on the exponentiation of each coefficient in a fitted logistic regression model. The user must be aware that these automatically reported quantities provide estimates of odds ratios of interest in only a few special cases (e.g., a dichotomous variable coded 0 and 1 that is not involved in any interactions with other variables), a point we return to in the next section. One major goal of this chapter is to show, using the four steps noted earlier, that one may obtain point and confidence interval estimates of odds ratios, regardless of the complexity of the fitted model.

Before concluding the dichotomous variable case, it is important to consider the effect that coding has on computing the estimator of odds ratios. In the previous discussion we noted that the estimator is $\widehat{OR} = \exp(\hat{\beta}_1)$ and that this is correct as long as one codes the independent variable as 0 or 1 (or any two values that differ by one). Any other coding requires that one calculate the value of the logit difference for the specific coding used and then exponentiate this difference, essentially following the four steps, not just blindly exponentiating the estimator of the coefficient.

We illustrate the setting of alternate coding in detail, as it helps emphasize the four steps in the general method for computing estimators of odds ratios from a fitted logistic regression model. Suppose that our dichotomous covariate is coded using values a and b and that, at Step 1, we would like to estimate the odds ratio for the covariate at level a versus b. Next, at Step 2, we substitute the two values of the covariate into the equation for the logit to obtain $\hat{g}(a) = \hat{\beta}_0 + \hat{\beta}_1 a$ and $\hat{g}(b) = \hat{\beta}_0 + \hat{\beta}_1 b$. For Step 3, we compute the difference in the two equations and algebraically simplify to obtain the expression for the log-odds as

$$
\begin{aligned}
\ln[\widehat{OR}(a, b)] &= \hat{g}(x = a) - \hat{g}(x = b) \\
&= (\hat{\beta}_0 + \hat{\beta}_1 \times a) - (\hat{\beta}_0 + \hat{\beta}_1 \times b) \\
&= \hat{\beta}_1 \times (a - b).
\end{aligned}
\tag{3.3}
$$

At Step 4 we exponentiate the equation obtained in Step 3, shown in this case in equation (3.3), to obtain our estimator of the odds ratio, namely

$$
\widehat{OR}(a, b) = \exp[\hat{\beta}_1 \times (a - b)].
\tag{3.4}
$$

In equations (3.3) and (3.4) the notation $\widehat{OR}(a, b)$ denotes the specific odds ratio

$$
\widehat{OR}(a, b) = \frac{\dfrac{\hat{\pi}(x = a)}{[1 - \hat{\pi}(x = a)]}}{\dfrac{\hat{\pi}(x = b)}{[1 - \hat{\pi}(x = b)]}}.
\tag{3.5}
$$

In the usual case when $a = 1$ and $b = 0$ we suppress a and b and simply use $\widehat{OR}$.

Some software packages offer a choice of methods for coding design variables. The "0–1 coding" is the one most often used and is referred to as *reference cell* coding. The reference cell method typically assigns the value of 0 to the lower code for x and 1 to the higher code. For example, if gender was coded as 1 = male and 2 = female, then the resulting design variable under this method, D, would be coded 0 = male and 1 = female. Exponentiation of the estimated coefficient for D would estimate the odds ratio of female relative to male. This same result would have been obtained had sex been coded originally as 0 = male and 1 = female, and then treating the variable gender as if it were interval scaled.

Another coding method is frequently referred to as *deviation from means* coding. This method assigns the value of −1 to the lower code, and a value of 1 to the higher code. The coding for the variable gender discussed earlier is shown in Table 3.4. Suppose we wish to estimate the odds ratio of female versus male when deviation from means coding is used. We do this by using the results of the general

Table 3.4 Illustration of the Coding of the Design Variable Using the Deviation from Means Method

Gender (Code)	Design Variable (D)
Male (1)	−1
Female (2)	1

four-step method that results in equations (3.3) and (3.4),

$$\ln[\widehat{OR}(\text{female,male})] = \hat{g}(\text{female}) - \hat{g}(\text{male})$$

$$= \hat{g}(D = 1) - \hat{g}(D = -1)$$

$$= [\hat{\beta}_0 + \hat{\beta}_1 \times (D = 1)] - [\hat{\beta}_0 + \hat{\beta}_1 \times (D = -1)]$$

$$= 2\hat{\beta}_1,$$

and the estimated odds ratio is $\widehat{OR}(\text{female,male}) = \exp(2\hat{\beta}_1)$. Thus, if we had exponentiated the coefficient from the computer output we would have obtained the wrong estimate of the odds ratio. This points out quite clearly that we must pay close attention to the method used to code the design variables.

The method of coding also influences the calculation of the endpoints of the confidence interval. For the example using deviation from means coding, the estimated standard error needed for confidence interval estimation is $\widehat{SE}(2\hat{\beta}_1) = 2\widehat{SE}(\hat{\beta}_1)$. Thus the endpoints of the confidence interval are

$$\exp[2\hat{\beta}_1 \pm z_{1-\alpha/2} 2\widehat{SE}(\hat{\beta}_1)].$$

In general, the endpoints of the confidence interval for the odds ratio given in equation (3.5) are

$$\exp[\hat{\beta}_1(a - b) \pm z_{1-\alpha/2}|a - b| \times \widehat{SE}(\hat{\beta}_1)],$$

where $|a - b|$ is the absolute value of $(a - b)$. (This is necessary because a might be less than b.) As we have control of how we code our dichotomous variables, we recommend that, when interest focuses on the odds ratio, they be coded as 0 or 1 for analysis purposes.

In summary, for a dichotomous variable the parameter of interest in most, if not all, applied settings is the odds ratio. An estimate of this parameter may be obtained from a fitted logistic regression model by exponentiating the estimated coefficient. In a setting where the coding is not 0 or 1, the estimate may be found by simply following the four steps described in this section. The relationship between the logistic regression coefficient and the odds ratio provides the foundation for our interpretation of all logistic regression results.

3.3 POLYCHOTOMOUS INDEPENDENT VARIABLE

Suppose that instead of two categories the independent variable has $k > 2$ distinct values. For example, we may have variables that denote the county of residence within a state, the clinic used for primary health care within a city, or race. Each of these variables has a fixed number of discrete values and the scale of measurement is nominal. We saw in Chapter 2 that it is inappropriate to model a nominal scale variable as if it were an interval scale variable. Therefore, we must form a set of design variables to represent the categories of the variable. In this section we present methods for creating design variables for polychotomous independent variables. The choice of a particular method depends to some extent on the goals of the analysis and the stage of model development.

We begin by extending the method shown in Section 3.2 for a dichotomous variable. In the GLOW study the covariate self-reported risk is coded at three levels (less, same, and more). The cross tabulation of it with fracture during follow-up (FRACTURE) is shown in Table 3.5. In addition we show the estimated odds ratio, its 95% confidence interval and log-odds ratio for same and more versus less risk. The extension to a situation where the variable has more than three levels is not conceptually different so all the examples in this section use $k = 3$.

At the bottom of Table 3.5, the odds ratio is given for the groups "same risk" and "more risk," as compared to the reference group, "less risk." For example, for the "same risk" group the estimated odds ratio is $\widehat{OR}(\text{Same, Less}) = (48 \times 139)/(28 \times 138) = 1.73$. The log of each odds ratio is given in the last row of Table 3.5. The example in this table is typical of what is found in the literature presenting univariable results for a nominal scaled variable. Note that the reference group is indicated by a value of 1 for the odds ratio. These same estimates and confidence intervals for the odds ratio are also easily obtained from a logistic regression program with an appropriate choice of design variables. The method for specifying the design variables involves setting all of them equal to 0 for the reference group, and then setting a single design variable equal to 1 for each of the other groups. This is illustrated in Table 3.6. As noted in Section 3.2 this method is usually referred to as *reference cell* coding and is the default method in many statistical software packages. However, not all packages use the lowest code as the referent group. In particular, the SPSS [SPSS for Windows, Release 20.0 (2012)] package's default coding is to use the highest code as the referent value.

Table 3.5 Cross-Classification of Fracture During Follow-Up (FRACTURE) by Self-Reported Rate of Risk (RATERISK) from the GLOW Study, $n = 500$

FRACTURE	RATERISK			Total
	Less	Same	More	
Yes	28	48	49	125
No	139	138	98	375
Total	167	186	147	500
Odds Ratio	1	1.73	2.48	
95% CI		(1.02, 2.91)	(1.46, 4.22)	
$\ln(\widehat{OR})$	0.0	0.55	0.91	

Table 3.6   Specification of the Design Variables for RATERISK Using Reference Cell Coding with Less as the Reference Group

RATERISK (Code)	RATERISK2	RATERISK3
Less (1)	0	0
Same (2)	1	0
More (3)	0	1

Table 3.7   Results of Fitting the Logistic Regression Model to the Data in Table 3.5 Using the Design Variables in Table 3.6

Variable	Coeff.	Std. Err.	z	p	95% CI
RATERISK2	0.546	0.2664	2.05	0.040	0.024, 1.068
RATERISK3	0.909	0.2711	3.35	0.001	0.378, 1.441
Constant	−1.602	0.2071	−7.74	<0.001	−2.008, −1.196

Log-likelihood = −275.28917

Use of any logistic regression program with design variables coded as shown in Table 3.6 yields the estimated logistic regression coefficients given in Table 3.7.

When we compare the estimated coefficients in Table 3.7 to the log-odds ratios in Table 3.5 we find that

$$\ln[\widehat{OR}(\text{Same, Less})] = \hat{\beta}_1 = 0.546,$$

and

$$\ln[\widehat{OR}(\text{More, Less})] = \hat{\beta}_2 = 0.909.$$

Did this happen by chance? We can check this by using the first three of the four-step procedure, described in Section 3.2, as follows:

Step 1: We want to compare levels Same to Less;
Step 2: The logit for Same is

$$\hat{g}(\text{Same}) = \hat{\beta}_0 + \hat{\beta}_1 \times (\text{RATERISK2} = 1) + \hat{\beta}_2 \times (\text{RATERISK3} = 0),$$

and the logit for Less is

$$\hat{g}(\text{Less}) = \hat{\beta}_0 + \hat{\beta}_1 \times (\text{RATERISK2} = 0) + \hat{\beta}_2 \times (\text{RATERISK3} = 0);$$

Step 3: The logit difference is

$$\ln[\widehat{OR}(\text{Same, Less})] = \hat{g}(\text{Same}) - \hat{g}(\text{Less})$$
$$= [\hat{\beta}_0 + \hat{\beta}_1 \times 1 + \hat{\beta}_2 \times 0] - [\hat{\beta}_0 + \hat{\beta}_1 \times 0 + \hat{\beta}_2 \times 0]$$
$$= \hat{\beta}_1.$$

Similar calculations demonstrate that the estimated coefficient for RATERISK3 from the logistic regression in Table 3.7 is equal to the log-odds ratio computed from the data in Table 3.5.

A comment about the estimated standard errors may be helpful at this point. In the univariable case the estimates of the standard errors found in the logistic regression output are identical to the estimates obtained using the cell frequencies from the contingency table. For example, the estimated standard error of the estimated coefficient for the design variable RATERISK2 is

$$\widehat{SE}(\hat{\beta}_1) = \left[\frac{1}{48} + \frac{1}{139} + \frac{1}{28} + \frac{1}{138} \right]^{0.5} = 0.2664.$$

Confidence limits for the odds ratios are obtained using the same approach used in Section 3.2 for a dichotomous variable. We begin by computing the confidence limits for the log-odds ratio (the logistic regression coefficient) and then exponentiate these limits to obtain limits for the odds ratio. In general, the limits for a $100(1 - \alpha)\%$ confidence interval for the jth coefficient, β_j, are of the form

$$\hat{\beta}_j \pm z_{1-\alpha/2} \times \widehat{SE}(\hat{\beta}_j).$$

These are shown in the right most column of Table 3.7. The corresponding limits for the odds ratio, obtained by exponentiating these limits, are as follows:

$$\exp[\hat{\beta}_j \pm z_{1-\alpha/2} \times \widehat{SE}(\hat{\beta}_j)]. \tag{3.6}$$

The confidence limits given in Table 3.5 in the row beneath the estimated odds ratios are obtained using equation (3.6) with the estimated coefficients and standard errors in Table 3.7 for $j = 1, 2$ with $\alpha = 0.05$.

Reference cell coding is the most commonly employed coding method appearing in the literature. The primary reason for the widespread use of this method is the interest in estimating the odds of an "exposed" group relative to that of a "control" or "unexposed" group.

As discussed in Section 3.2 a second method of coding design variables is called *deviation from means* coding. This coding expresses an effect as the deviation of the "group mean" from the "overall mean." In the case of logistic regression, the "group mean" is the logit for the group and the "overall mean" is the average logit over all groups. This method of coding is obtained by setting the value of all the design variables equal to -1 for one of the categories, and then using the 0, 1 coding for the remainder of the categories. Use of the deviation from means coding for RATERISK shown in Table 3.8 yields the estimated logistic regression coefficients in Table 3.9.

In order to interpret the estimated coefficients in Table 3.9 we need to refer to Table 3.5 and calculate the logit for each of the three categories of RATERISK. These are:

$$\hat{g}_1 = \ln \left(\frac{\frac{28}{167}}{\frac{139}{167}} \right) = \ln \left(\frac{28}{139} \right) = -1.602,$$

Table 3.8 Specification of the Design Variables for RATERISK Using Deviation from Means Coding

	Design Variables	
Rate Risk (Code)	RATERISK2D	RATERISK3D
Less (1)	−1	−1
Same (2)	1	0
More (3)	0	1

Table 3.9 Results of Fitting the Logistic Regression Model to the Data in Table 3.5 Using the Design Variables in Table 3.8

Variable	Coeff.	Std. Err.	z	p	95% CI
RATERISK2D	0.061	0.1437	0.43	0.671	−0.221, 0.343
RATERISK3D	0.424	0.1466	2.89	0.004	0.137, 0.711
Constant	−1.117	0.1062	−10.51	<0.001	−1.325, −0.909

Log-likelihood = −275.28917

$$\hat{g}_2 = \ln\left(\frac{\frac{48}{186}}{\frac{138}{186}}\right) = \ln\left(\frac{48}{138}\right) = -1.056,$$

$$\hat{g}_3 = \ln\left(\frac{\frac{49}{147}}{\frac{98}{147}}\right) = \ln\left(\frac{49}{98}\right) = -1.056,$$

and the average of these three logits

$$\overline{g} = \sum_{i=1}^{3} \frac{\hat{g}_i}{3} = -1.117.$$

The estimated coefficient for design variable RATERISK2D in Table 3.9 is $\hat{g}_2 - \overline{g} = (-1.056) - (-1.117) = 0.061$ and for RATERISK3D it is $\hat{g}_3 - \overline{g} = (-0.693) - (-1.117) = 0.424$. The general expression for the estimated coefficient for the jth design variable using deviation from means coding is $\hat{g}_j - \overline{g}$.

The interpretation of the estimated coefficients from deviation from means coding is not as easy or clear as when reference cell coding is used. Exponentiation of the estimated coefficients yields the ratio of the odds for the particular group to the geometric mean of the odds. Specifically, for RATERISK2D in Table 3.9 we have

$$\exp(0.061) = \exp(\hat{g}_2 - \overline{g})$$

$$= \frac{\exp(\hat{g}_2)}{\exp\left(\sum \hat{g}_j/3\right)}$$

$$= \frac{(48/138)}{[(28/139) \times (49/138) \times (49/98)]^{0.333}}$$

$$= 1.06.$$

This number, 1.06, is not a true odds ratio because the quantities in the numerator and denominator do not represent the odds for two distinct categories. The exponentiation of the estimated coefficient expresses the odds relative to the geometric mean odds. The interpretation of this value depends on whether the geometric mean odds is at all meaningful in the context of the study.

The estimated coefficients obtained using deviation from means coding can be used to estimate the odds ratio for one category relative to a reference category. The equation for the estimate is more complicated than the one obtained using the reference cell coding. However, it provides an excellent example of how application of the four-step method can always yield the odds ratio of interest.

Step 1: Suppose we want to estimate the odds ratio of RATERISK = 2 (Same) versus RATERISK = 1 (Less).

Step 2: Using the coding for design variables given in Table 3.8 the logit at RATERISK = 2 is

$$\hat{g}(\text{RATERISK} = 2) = \hat{\beta}_0 + \hat{\beta}_1 \times (\text{RATERISK2}D = 1)$$
$$+ \hat{\beta}_2 \times (\text{RATERISK3}D = 0),$$

and the logit at RATERISK = 1 is

$$\hat{g}(\text{RATERISK}=1) = \hat{\beta}_0 + \hat{\beta}_1 \times (\text{RATERISK2}D = -1)$$
$$+ \hat{\beta}_2 \times (\text{RATERISK3}D = -1).$$

Step 3: The difference between the two logit functions is

$$\hat{g}(\text{RATERISK} = 2) - \hat{g}(\text{RATERISK} = 1) =$$
$$[\hat{\beta}_0 + \hat{\beta}_1 \times (\text{RATERISK2}D = 1) + \hat{\beta}_2 \times (\text{RATERISK3}D = 0)]$$
$$- [\hat{\beta}_0 + \hat{\beta}_1 \times (\text{RATERISK2}D = -1) + \hat{\beta}_2 \times (\text{RATERISK3}D = -1)]$$
$$= 2\hat{\beta}_1 + \hat{\beta}_2. \tag{3.7}$$

Step 4: The estimator of the odds ratio is obtained as the exponentiation of the logit difference calculated in Step 3 and is

$$\widehat{\text{OR}}(\text{Same, Less}) = e^{2\hat{\beta}_1+\hat{\beta}_2}.$$

To obtain a confidence interval we must estimate the variance of the logit difference in equation (3.7). In this example, the estimator is

$$\widehat{\text{Var}}[\hat{g}(\text{RATERISK} = 2) - \hat{g}(\text{RATERISK} = 1)]$$

$$= 4 \times \widehat{\text{Var}}(\hat{\beta}_1) + \widehat{\text{Var}}(\hat{\beta}_2) + 4 \times \widehat{\text{Cov}}(\hat{\beta}_1, \hat{\beta}_2). \tag{3.8}$$

Values for each of the estimators in equation (3.8) may be obtained from the output from logistic regression software. Confidence intervals for the odds ratio are obtained by exponentiating the endpoints of the confidence limits for the logit difference in equation (3.7). Evaluation of equation (3.7) for the current example gives

$$\hat{g}(\text{RATERISK} = 2) - \hat{g}(\text{RATERISK} = 1) = 2 \times 0.061 + 0.424$$

$$= 0.546.$$

The estimate of the variance is obtained by evaluating equation (3.8), which, for the current example, yields

$$\widehat{\text{Var}}[\hat{g}(\text{RATERISK} = 2) - \hat{g}(\text{RATERISK} = 1)]$$

$$= 4 \times 0.02065 + 0.02149 - 4 \times 0.00828 = 0.07097,$$

and the estimated standard error is

$$\widehat{\text{SE}}[\hat{g}(\text{RATERISK} = 2) - \hat{g}(\text{RATERISK} = 1)] = 0.2664.$$

We note that the values of the estimated logit difference (i.e., the log-odds ratio), 0.546, and the estimated standard error, 0.2664, are identical to the values of the estimated coefficient and standard error for RATERISK2D in Table 3.7. This is expected, as the design variables used to obtain the estimated coefficients in Table 3.7 were formulated specifically to yield the log-odds ratio of Same versus Less.

It should be apparent that, if the objective is to obtain odds ratios, use of deviation from means coding for design variables is computationally much more complex than reference cell coding. However, if the objective is to flag (through the Wald tests) which of the subgroups differ from the average, the deviation from means strategy can be extremely effective.

In summary, we have shown that discrete nominal scale variables are included properly into the analysis only when they have been recoded into design variables. The particular choice of design variables depends on the application, though the reference cell coding is the easiest to interpret, has a direct relationship to the odds ratio, and thus is the one used in the remainder of this text.

3.4 CONTINUOUS INDEPENDENT VARIABLE

When a logistic regression model contains a continuous independent variable, interpretation of the estimated coefficient depends on how it is entered into the model and the particular units of the variable. For purposes of developing the method to interpret the coefficient for a continuous variable, we assume that the logit is linear in the variable. We note that this linearity assumption is key and methods for examining this assumption are presented in Chapter 4.

Under the assumption that the logit is linear in the continuous covariate, x, the equation for the logit is $g(x) = \beta_0 + \beta_1 x$. Application of the four steps to obtain the estimator of the odds ratio yields the following: (1) suppose that we are interested in the odds ratio for a one-unit increment in the covariate, i.e., $x + 1$ versus x; (2) it follows from the equation for the logit at x that the logit at $x + 1$ is $g(x + 1) = \beta_0 + \beta_1(x + 1)$; (3) hence the estimator of the logit difference is

$$\hat{g}(x + 1) - \hat{g}(x) = \hat{\beta}_1;$$

and (4) the estimator of odds ratio is $\widehat{OR} = \exp(\hat{\beta}_1)$. This estimator has exactly the same form as the estimator in equation (3.2) for a dichotomous covariate. The problem is that a value of "1" is not likely to be clinically interesting for a continuous covariate. For example, a 1-year increase in age or a 1-pound increase in body weight for adults is probably too small to be considered an important change. A change of 10 years or 10 pounds might be more interesting. On the other hand, if the range of a covariate is only from 0 to 1, then a change of 1 is too large and a change of 0.01 or 0.05 is more realistic. Hence, to provide a useful interpretation for continuous covariates we need to develop a method for point and interval estimation of the odds ratio for an arbitrary change of "c" units in the covariate.

Following the first three steps, we find that the estimator of the log-odds ratio for a change of c units in x is $\hat{g}(x + c) - \hat{g}(x) = c\hat{\beta}_1$ and (5) the estimator odds ratio is $\widehat{OR}(x + c, x) = \exp(c\hat{\beta}_1)$, more concisely denoted as $\widehat{OR}(c)$. The estimator of the standard error of $c\hat{\beta}_1$ is $\widehat{SE}(c\hat{\beta}_1) = |c|\widehat{SE}(\hat{\beta}_1)$, where "$|c|$" denotes the absolute value of c. We need to use the absolute value as c could be negative. Hence, the endpoints of the $100(1 - \alpha)\%$ confidence interval estimate are

$$\exp[c\hat{\beta}_1 \pm z_{1-\alpha/2}|c|\widehat{SE}(\hat{\beta}_1)].$$

As both the point estimate and endpoints of the confidence interval depend on the choice of c, the particular value of c should be clearly specified in all tables and calculations. The rather arbitrary nature of the choice of c may be troublesome to some. For example, why use a change of 10 years when 5 or 15 or even 20 years may be equally good? We, of course, could use any reasonable value; but the goal must be kept in mind: to provide the reader of your analysis with a clear indication of how the odds of the outcome change with the variable in question. For most continuous covariates changes in multiples of 2, 5, or 10 may be most meaningful and easily understood.

As an example, we show the results in Table 1.3 of a logistic regression of AGE on CHD status using the data in Table 1.1. The estimated logit is $\hat{g}(AGE) = -5.310 + 0.111 \times AGE$. The estimated odds ratio for an increase of 10 years in age is $\widehat{OR}(10) = \exp(10 \times 0.111) = 3.03$. Thus, for every increase of 10 years in age, the odds of CHD being present is estimated to increase 3.03 times. The validity of this statement is questionable, because the increase in the odds of CHD for a 40-year-old compared to a 30-year-old may be quite different from the odds for a 60-year-old compared to a 50-year-old. This is the unavoidable dilemma when a continuous covariate is modeled linearly in the logit and motivates the importance of examining the linearity assumption for continuous covariates. As already noted, we consider this in detail in Chapter 4. The endpoints of a 95% confidence interval for this odds ratio are

$$\exp(10 \times 0.111 \pm 1.96 \times 10 \times 0.024) = (1.90, 4.86).$$

In summary, the interpretation of the estimated odds ratio for a continuous variable is similar to that of nominal scale variables. The main difference is that a meaningful change must be defined for the continuous variable.

3.5 MULTIVARIABLE MODELS

In the previous sections in this chapter we discussed the interpretation of an esti-mated logistic regression coefficient in the case when there is a single variable in the fitted model. Fitting a series of univariable models, although useful for a pre-liminary analysis, rarely provides an adequate or complete analysis of the data in a study because the independent variables are usually associated with one another and may have different distributions within levels of the outcome variable. Thus, one generally uses a multivariable analysis for a more comprehensive modeling of the data. One goal of such an analysis is to *statistically adjust* the estimated effect of each variable in the model for differences in the distributions of and associa-tions among the other independent variables in the model. Applying this concept to a multivariable logistic regression model, we may surmise that each estimated coefficient provides an estimate of the log-odds adjusting for the other variables in the model.

Another important aspect of multivariable modeling is to assess to what extent, if at all, the estimate of the log-odds of one independent variable changes, depending on the value of another independent variable. When the odds ratio for one variable is not constant over the levels of another variable, the two variables are said to have a *statistical interaction*. In some applied disciplines statistical interaction is referred to as *effect modification*. This terminology is used to describe the fact that the log-odds of one variable is modified or changed by values of the other variable. In this section we consider, in considerable detail, the concepts of statistical adjustment and interaction and illustrate estimation of odds ratios under each case with examples.

A full understanding of estimating the log-odds or coefficients from a multi-variable logistic regression model requires that we have a clear understanding of what is actually meant by the term *adjusting, statistically, for other variables in the model*. In some fields variables that are used to adjust the effects of others are called *confounders* and adjustment for them is called *controlling for confounding*. We begin by examining statistical adjustment in the context of the usual linear regression model, and then extend the concept to the logistic regression model.

To begin, we consider a multivariable model that contains two independent variables: one dichotomous and one continuous, but primary interest is focused on estimating the effect of the dichotomous variable on the outcome variable. This situation is frequently encountered in epidemiological and medical research when an exposure to a risk factor is recorded as being either present or absent, and we wish to adjust for a continuous variable such as age. The analogous situation in linear regression is called *analysis of covariance*.

Suppose we wish to compare the mean weight of two groups of boys. It is known that weight is associated with many characteristics, one of which is age. Assume that on all characteristics, except age, the two groups have nearly identical distributions. If the age distribution is also the same for the two groups, then a univariable analysis of group comparing the mean weight of the two groups would suffice. This analysis would provide us with a correct estimate of the difference in the mean weight of the two groups. However, if one group was, on average, much younger than the other group, then a comparison of the two groups would be meaningless, because a portion of any difference observed would be due to the differences in mean age. It would not be possible to determine the effect of group without first eliminating the discrepancy in the distribution of age in the two groups.

This situation is described graphically in Figure 3.1. In the figure it is assumed that the true relationship between age and mean weight is linear, with the same significant nonzero slope in each group. Both of these assumptions would usually be tested in an analysis of covariance before making any inferences about group differences. We defer a discussion of methods to examine these assumptions until Chapter 4, as they are an integral part of modeling with logistic regression. Here, we proceed as if these assumptions have been checked and are supported by the data.

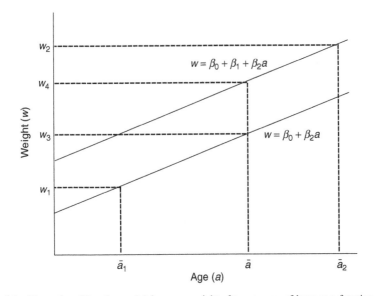

Figure 3.1 Figure describing the model for mean weight of two groups of boys as a function of age.

The statistical model that describes the situation in Figure 3.1 states that the value of mean weight, w, may be expressed as $w = \beta_0 + \beta_1 x + \beta_2 a$, where $x = 0$ for group 1 and $x = 1$ for group 2 and "a" denotes age. In this model the parameter β_1 represents the true difference in weight between the two groups, as it is the vertical distance between the two lines at any age. The coefficient β_2 is the change in weight per year of age. Suppose, as shown in Figure 3.1, that the mean age of group 1 is $\bar{a}_1$ and the mean age of group 2 is $\bar{a}_2$. Comparison of the mean weight of group 1 to the mean weight of group 2 amounts to a comparison of w_1 to w_2. In terms of the model this difference is

$$(w_2 - w_1) = (\beta_0 + \beta_1 + \beta_2 \bar{a}_1) - (\beta_0 + \beta_2 \bar{a}_0)$$
$$= \beta_1 + \beta_2 (\bar{a}_1 - \bar{a}_0).$$

This comparison involves not only the true difference between the groups, β_1, but a component, $\beta_2 (\bar{a}_2 - \bar{a}_1)$, which reflects the difference between the mean ages of the groups and the association of age and weight.

The process of statistically adjusting for age involves comparing the two groups at some common value of age. The value usually used is the overall mean of the two groups, which, for the example, is denoted by $\bar{a}$ in Figure 3.1. Hence, comparing group 2 to group 1 at the mean age is, in terms of the model, a comparison of w_4 to w_3. This difference is

$$(w_4 - w_3) = (\beta_0 + \beta_1 + \beta_2 \bar{a}) - (\beta_0 + \beta_2 \bar{a})$$
$$= \beta_1 + \beta_2 (\bar{a} - \bar{a})$$
$$= \beta_1,$$

which is the true difference between the mean weight of two groups. In theory any common value of age could be used, as it would yield the same difference, β_1. The choice of the overall mean makes sense for two reasons: it is clinically reasonable and lies within the range where we believe the association between age and weight is linear and constant within each group.

Consider the same situation shown in Figure 3.1, but instead of weight being the outcome variable, assume it is a dichotomous variable and that the vertical axis now denotes the logit or log-odds of the outcome (i.e., in the figure w denotes the log-odds). That is, the logit of the outcome is given by the equation $g(x, a) = \beta_0 + \beta_1 x + \beta_2 a$. Under this logit model the univariable comparison of the log-odds of the two groups is approximately $(w_2 - w_1) = \beta_1 + \beta_2 (\bar{a}_2 - \bar{a}_1)$. This would incorrectly estimate the effect of group on the log-odds due to the difference in the distribution of age. To account or adjust for this difference, we include age in the model and calculate the logit difference at a common value of age, such as the combined mean, $\bar{a}$. This logit difference is, using the figure,

$$(w_4 - w_3) = g(x = 1, a = \bar{a}) - g(x = 0, a = \bar{a})$$
$$= (\beta_0 + \beta_1 + \beta_2 \bar{a}) - (\beta_0 + \beta_2 \bar{a})$$
$$= \beta_1.$$

The natural question to ask is: What conditions are required for the unadjusted difference $(w_2 - w_1)$ to be the same as the adjusted difference $(w_4 - w_3)$? Stated in terms of the model, the question is, under what conditions is $\beta_1 + \beta_2(\bar{a}_2 - \bar{a}_1) = \beta_1$? This is true if age is not associated with the outcome, $\beta_2 = 0$, or if the mean age of the two groups is the same, $(\bar{a}_2 - \bar{a}_1) = 0$. Conversely, the unadjusted and adjusted logit differences are not the same if $\beta_2(\bar{a}_2 - \bar{a}_1) \neq 0$, which only happens when both β_2 and $(\bar{a}_2 - \bar{a}_1)$ are nonzero.

As the amount of statistical adjustment or control for confounding is a function of two quantities β_2 and $(\bar{a}_2 - \bar{a}_1)$ we cannot determine whether x is a confounder simply by using a significance test of β_2. Also, in an applied setting it is impractical to calculate $(\bar{a}_2 - \bar{a}_1)$ or its equivalent for every possible pair of variables. Instead, we use some approximations. First, we fit a model containing only d (i.e., the model excludes the adjustment covariate, a. Denote the estimate of the coefficient of d from this model as $\hat{\theta}_1$. Next, we fit a model containing d along with the adjustment covariate, a. Denote the estimates of the coefficients from this model as $\hat{\beta}_1$ and $\hat{\beta}_2$ respectively. Under the model the estimate $\hat{\theta}_1$ should be approximately equal to $\hat{\beta}_1 + \hat{\beta}_2(\bar{a}_2 - \bar{a}_1)$. Hence the difference between the unadjusted and adjusted estimates of the effect of d, $(\hat{\theta}_1 - \hat{\beta}_1)$, should approximate the theoretical amount of adjustment, $\beta_2(\bar{a}_2 - \bar{a}_1)$. As the amount of adjustment is more of a relative than an absolute quantity, we scale it by dividing by $\hat{\beta}_1$ to obtain a measure we call *delta-beta-hat-percent*, defined as

$$\Delta\hat{\beta}\% = 100\frac{(\hat{\theta}_1 - \hat{\beta}_1)}{\hat{\beta}_1}. \tag{3.9}$$

Thus, the amount of adjustment is expressed as a percentage of the adjusted log-odds ratio. Some colleagues we have worked with scale differently, preferring to divide by $\hat{\theta}_1$. The disadvantage of this scaling is that both numerator and denominator now contain the amount of adjustment. The rule of thumb that we use in practice to conclude that a covariate is needed in the model to adjust the effect of another covariate is $\Delta\hat{\beta}\% > 20$. Some of our colleagues prefer to use 10% whereas others use 25%. What is important is that one calculate $\Delta\hat{\beta}\%$ and make some sort of assessment as to whether it is large enough to make a practical difference in the estimate of the log-odds ratio. Examples of the calculation and interpretation of $\Delta\hat{\beta}\%$ may be found at the end of this section and in Chapter 4.

Statistical adjustment when the variables are all dichotomous, polychotomous, continuous, or a mixture of these is identical to that just described for the case of one dichotomous and one continuous variable. The advantage of the setting we described is that it lends itself nicely to the graphical description shown in Figure 3.1.

One point must be kept clearly in mind when interpreting statistically adjusted log-odds ratios and odds ratios. The effectiveness of the adjustment is entirely dependent on the assumptions of linearity in each covariate and constant slopes. Departures from either or both of these assumptions may render the adjustment useless. One commonly occurring departure is the setting where there is a statistical interaction.

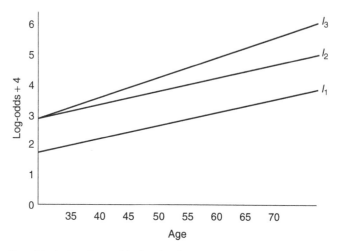

Figure 3.2 Plot of the logit under models showing the presence and absence of statistical interaction.

The simplest and most commonly used model for including a statistical interaction is one in which the logit is also linear in the second group, but with a different slope. Alternative models can be formulated that allow for a nonlinear relationship within each group. Regardless, a statistical interaction is incorporated by the inclusion of product terms of the general form "$d \times x$."

In order to more easily explain statistical interaction we plot three different logit functions in Figure 3.2, where 4 has been added to make the plotting more convenient. Suppose the plotted functions come from a setting where the outcome variable is the presence or absence of CHD, the risk factor is GENDER, and the covariate is AGE. Suppose that the line labeled l_1 corresponds to the logit for females as a function of age and l_2 represents the logit for males. These two lines are parallel to each other, indicating that the relationship between AGE and CHD is the same for males and females. In this situation there is no interaction and the log-odds ratio for GENDER (male versus female), controlling for AGE, is given by the difference between line l_2 and l_1, $l_2 - l_1$. This difference is equal to the vertical distance between the two lines, which, because the lines are parallel, is the same for all ages.

Suppose instead that the logit for males is the line l_3. This line is steeper than the line l_1, for females, indicating that the relationship between AGE and CHD for males is different from that of females. When this occurs we say that there is an interaction between AGE and GENDER. The estimate of the log-odds ratios for GENDER (males versus females) controlling for age is still given by the vertical distance between the lines, $l_3 - l_1$, but this difference now *depends* on the age at which the comparison is made. Thus, we cannot estimate the odds ratio for GENDER without first specifying the AGE at which the comparison is being made. In other words, age *modifies the effect* of gender, so in this terminology age is called an *effect modifier*.

Suppose we continue to consider models with the pair of independent variables d (dichotomous) and x (continuous). The role of x with respect to the effect of d in the model can be one of three possibilities.

1. There is no statistical adjustment or interaction. The covariate, x, is not a confounder or an effect modifier.
2. There is statistical adjustment but no statistical interaction. The covariate, x, is a confounder but not an effect modifier.
3. There is statistical interaction. The covariate, x, is an effect modifier.

We present an example of each of the three possibilities using data from the studies described in Section 1.6. In each example we fit three models: (i) a model that contains only d; (ii) a model that contains d and x; and (iii) a model that contains d, x and their statistical interaction, $d \times x$. We use the results of the three fitted models to decide which model is the best one to use in practice.

We begin with an example where there is neither statistical adjustment nor statistical interaction. The data we use come from the GLOW study described in Section 1.6.3. The outcome variable is having a fracture during the first year of follow up (FRACTURE). For the dichotomous variable, we use variable history of prior fracture (PRIORFRAC) and for the continuous covariate, we use height in centimeters (HEIGHT). The results from the three fitted models are presented in Table 3.10. In discussing the results from the examples we use significance levels from the Wald statistics. In all cases the same conclusions would be reached had we used likelihood ratio tests.

The Wald Statistic for the coefficient of PRIORFRAC in Model 1 is significant with $p < 0.001$. When we add HEIGHT to the model the Wald statistics are significant at the 1% level for both covariates. Note that there is little change in the

Table 3.10 Estimated Logistic Regression Coefficients, Standard Errors, Wald Statistics, p-Values and 95% CIs from Three Models Showing No Statistical Adjustment and No Statistical Interaction from the GLOW Study, $n = 500$

Model	Variable	Coeff.	Std. Err.	z	p	95% CI	
1	PRIORFRAC	1.064	0.2231	4.77	<0.001	0.627,	1.501
	Constant	−1.417	0.1305	−10.86	<0.001	−1.672,	−1.161
2	PRIORFRAC	1.012	0.2254	4.49	<0.001	0.570,	1.454
	HEIGHT	−0.045	0.0174	−2.61	0.009	−0.079,	−0.011
	Constant	5.785	2.7980	2.07	0.039	0.301,	11.269
3	PRIORFRAC	−3.055	5.7904	−0.53	0.598	−14.404,	8.294
	HEIGHT	−0.054	0.0219	−2.49	0.013	−0.097,	−0.012
	PRIORFRAC × HEIGHT	0.025	0.0361	0.70	0.482	−0.045,	0.096
	Constant	7.361	3.5102	2.10	0.036	0.481,	14.241

estimate of the coefficient for PRIORFRAC as

$$\Delta\hat{\beta}\% = 100 \times \frac{(1.064 - 1.012)}{1.012}$$
$$= 5.1,$$

indicating that inclusion of HEIGHT does not statistically adjust the coefficient of PRIORFRAC. Thus we conclude that, in these data, height it is not a confounder of prior fracture. The fact that the coefficient for HEIGHT is significant, $\hat{\beta}_2 \neq 0$, implies that the mean HEIGHT for the two PRIORFRAC groups must be similar. In fact they are with values of 161.7 and 161.2 cm. Under the dichotomous–continuous covariate model we showed that the univariable model coefficient should be approximately $\hat{\beta}_1 + \hat{\beta}_2(\bar{x}_1 - \bar{x}_0)$. Evaluating this expression we obtain a value of

$$1.08 = 1.012 - 0.045(160.2 - 161.7),$$

which is quite close to the value of the estimate from the univariable model of 1.064.

The statistical interaction of prior fracture (PRIORFRAC) and height (HEIGHT) is added to Model 2 to obtain Model 3. The Wald statistic for the added product term has $p = 0.492$, and thus is not significant. In these data height is not an effect modifier of prior fracture. Hence, the choice is between Model 1 and Model 2. Even though the estimate of the effect of prior fracture is basically the same for the two models, we would choose Model 2 as height (HEIGHT) is not only statistically significant in Model 2, but is an important clinical covariate as well. One would estimate the odds ratio for prior fracture using the results from Model 2 and follow the methods discussed in Section 3.2 for a dichotomous covariate coded 0 or 1.

In the next example we illustrate a setting where there is statistical adjustment but no statistical interaction. The data come from the Myopia study described in Section 1.6.6. The outcome variable is becoming myopic in the first 5 years of follow-up (MYOPIC). We use gender (GENDER) as the dichotomous variable and spherical equivalent refraction at enrollment (SPHEQ) as the continuous covariate. The results of the three fitted models are presented in Table 3.11.

The Wald test for the coefficient of GENDER in Model 1 is not significant with $p = 0.127$, which presents an interesting dilemma that occurs reasonably often in practice. We know that gender can be an important covariate, but it is not significant in the univariable model. Thus, under some model building methods it might not be considered for a multivariable model. We address this situation explicitly in Chapter 4 where we discuss *purposeful selection* of covariates. For this example, suppose we proceed on to Model 2 where we add SPHEQ. The Wald test for SPHEQ is significant with $p < 0.001$. We note that the value of the estimated coefficient for GENDER has increased from 0.366 to 0.558. In addition, it is now significant with a Wald statistic significance level of $p = 0.050$. The percentage

Table 3.11 Estimated Logistic Regression Coefficients, Standard Errors, Wald Statistics, _p_-Values and 95% CIs from Three Models Showing Statistical Adjustment and No Statistical Interaction from the Myopia Study, _n_ = 618

Model	Variable	Coeff.	Std. Err.	z	p	95% CI
1	GENDER	0.366	0.2404	1.52	0.127	−0.105, 0.838
	Constant	−2.083	0.1792	−11.62	<0.001	−2.434, −1.732
2	GENDER	0.558	0.2851	1.96	0.050	−0.001, 1.117
	SPHEQ	−3.845	0.4171	−9.22	<0.001	−4.662, −3.027
	Constant	−0.226	0.2527	−0.89	0.371	−0.721, 0.269
3	GENDER	0.492	0.4157	1.18	0.237	−0.323, 1.306
	SPHEQ	−3.948	0.6353	−6.21	<0.001	−5.193, −2.703
	GENDER × SPHEQ	0.185	0.8422	0.22	0.826	−1.466, 1.836
	Constant	−0.191	0.2999	−0.64	0.524	−0.779, 0.397

difference in the two estimated coefficients is

$$\Delta \hat{\beta}\% = 100 \frac{(0.366 - 0.588)}{0.588}$$
$$= -37.6.$$

Why did this happen? The mean value of SPHEQ for males is 0.781 and the mean for females is 0.821, which, although not identical, are similar in value. However, the estimated coefficient for SPHEQ is quite large and negative. Putting the two parts together under the dichotomous–continuous covariate model, the univariable estimated coefficient for GENDER is approximately

$$0.430 = 0.588 - 3.845(0.822 - 0.781),$$

which is larger than the actual univariable estimated value of 0.366. Thus we conclude that the univariable coefficient underestimates the effect of GENDER due to the fact that females tended to have larger values of spherical equivalent refraction and it is strongly negatively related to myopia.

When we add the statistical interaction of gender and spherical equivalent refraction, GENDER × SPHEQ, to the model, its estimated coefficient by Wald test is not significant with $p = 0.185$, as shown in the last row of Table 3.11. We use the estimated coefficient from Model 2 and the methods from Section 3.2 to estimate the odds ratio of gender. In this case we use Model 2 as it adjusts for SPHEQ.

In the third example we illustrate a setting where there is statistical interaction. The data we use come from the GLOW study, used earlier in the first example. Again, we use as the dichotomous variable history of prior fracture (PRIORFRAC). In this example the continuous covariate is age (AGE). The results of the three fitted models are presented in Table 3.12.

In this example we are going to see that age could be described as being both a confounder and an effect modifier. To describe age in this way is somewhat

Table 3.12   Estimated Logistic Regression Coefficients, Standard Errors, Wald Statistics, p-Values and 95% CIs from Three Models Showing Statistical Adjustment and Statistical Interaction from the GLOW Study, $n = 500$

Model	Variable	Coeff.	Std. Err.	z	p	95% CI
1	PRIORFRAC	1.064	0.2231	4.77	<0.001	0.627, 1.501
	Constant	−1.417	0.1305	−10.86	<0.001	−1.672, −1.161
2	PRIORFRAC	0.839	0.2342	3.58	<0.001	0.380, 1.298
	AGE	0.041	0.0122	3.38	0.001	0.017, 0.065
	Constant	−4.214	0.8478	−4.97	<0.001	−5.876, −2.553
3	PRIORFRAC	4.961	1.8102	2.74	0.006	1.413, 8.509
	AGE	0.063	0.0155	4.04	<0.001	0.032, 0.093
	PRIORFRAC × AGE	−0.057	0.0250	−2.29	0.022	−0.106, −0.008
	Constant	−5.689	1.0841	−5.25	<0.001	−7.814, −3.565

misleading and some would argue it is incorrect. So we qualify this by noting that if the analysis stopped, incorrectly, at Model 2 there is evidence of statistical adjustment. However, in Model 3 we show that there is a significant statistical interaction, whereupon Model 2 is no longer relevant. In many, if not all, practical analyses of data a vital step in modeling is deciding which model is best: the adjustment model, Model 2, or the interaction model, Model 3. We discuss this in detail in Chapter 4.

The Wald test for prior fracture (PRIORFRAC) in Model 1 is highly significant with $p < 0.001$. When we add age (AGE), Model 2, the coefficient for PRIORFRAC continues to be highly significant with $p = 0.006$. The percentage change in the coefficient for PRIORFRAC from Model 1 to Model 2 is

$$\Delta\hat{\beta}\% = 100\frac{(1.064 - 0.839)}{0.839}$$
$$= 26.8.$$

Thus the coefficient from the univariable model overestimates the effect by 26.8%. Hence, at this point, we could conclude that adding age (AGE) to the model provides an important statistical adjustment to the effect of prior fracture (PRIORFRAC). Looking at the two factors required for adjustment, the mean age of those without a prior fracture is 67.0 whereas the mean for those with a prior fracture is 73.1 and the coefficient for AGE is statistically significant. Under the dichotomous–continuous covariate model, the univariable estimated coefficient for PRIORFRAC is approximately

$$1.089 = 0.839 + 0.041(73.1 - 67.0),$$

which is quite close to the univariable value from Model 1 of 1.064.

When the interaction term, PRIORFRAC×AGE, is added to Model 2 to obtain Model 3 we see that the Wald statistic for its coefficient is statistically significant with $p = 0.022$. Thus, there is considerable evidence of a statistical interaction between these two covariates. We are commonly asked if it is appropriate to drop the main effects and include only the interaction term in the model. In our opinion this is not appropriate, as the model must contain both main effects when the interaction is significant in order to correctly estimate odds ratios of interest.

Another commonly asked question is whether the change in the main effect coefficient for the dichotomous covariate from Model 2 to Model 3 is evidence of confounding or statistical adjustment? The answer is "no," because once an interaction is included in a model one is no longer able to estimate an adjusted odds ratio that applies to all values of the adjusting covariate. Odds ratios, as we show shortly, are estimated at specific values of the interacting covariate. In the interaction model the main effect coefficient provides an estimate of the log-odds at the value of 0 for the other covariate.

When a model contains an interaction term the only sure way to obtain the correct expression of model coefficients to estimate an odds ratio is to carefully follow the four-step method. As the estimates depend on the values of the adjusting covariate one has the option to present them graphically or in a table. We illustrate both. Although the four-step process is more complicated when an interaction term is present than it is for an adjustment model (i.e., Model 2), the results may be more interesting for subject-matter scientists.

To start, suppose we would like to estimate the odds ratio for prior fracture at some arbitrary choice of age, say "a." The four steps are as follows:

Step 1: The two sets of values of the covariates are (PRIORFRAC $= 1$, AGE $= a$) compared to (PRIORFRAC $= 0$, AGE $= a$).

Step 2: Substituting these values into the general expression for the estimated logit under Model 3 we obtain:

$$\hat{g}(\text{PRIORFRAC} = 1, \text{AGE} = a) = \hat{\beta}_0 + \hat{\beta}_1 \times 1 + \hat{\beta}_2 \times a + \hat{\beta}_3 \times 1 \times a,$$

and

$$\hat{g}(\text{PRIORFRAC} = 0, \text{AGE} = a) = \hat{\beta}_0 + \hat{\beta}_1 \times 0 + \hat{\beta}_2 \times a + \hat{\beta}_3 \times 0 \times a$$
$$= \hat{\beta}_0 + \hat{\beta}_2 \times a.$$

Step 3: Taking the difference in the two functions in Step 2 and algebraically simplifying we obtain:

$$[\hat{g}(\text{PRIORFRAC} = 1, \text{AGE} = a) - \hat{g}(\text{PRIORFRAC} = 0, \text{AGE} = a)]$$
$$= [(\hat{\beta}_0 + \hat{\beta}_1 \times 1 + \hat{\beta}_2 \times a + \hat{\beta}_3 \times 1 \times a) - (\hat{\beta}_0 + \hat{\beta}_2 \times a)]$$
$$= \hat{\beta}_1 + \hat{\beta}_3 \times a. \tag{3.10}$$

This is the correct function of the coefficients to exponentiate in Step 4 to estimate the odds ratio for prior fracture, specifically at AGE $= a$. Note that this expression involves the coefficients for both the main effect and interaction terms.

Step 4: Exponentiating the result of Steps 3 we obtain

$$\widehat{\text{OR}}[(\text{PRIORFRAC} = 1, \text{AGE} = a), (\text{PRIORFRAC} = 0, \text{AGE} = a)]$$

$$= \exp[\hat{\beta}_1 + \hat{\beta}_3 \times a]. \tag{3.11}$$

Following a point made earlier, we see from equation (3.11) that $\exp(\hat{\beta}_1)$ is the AGE $= 0$ estimate of the odds ratio for PRIORFRAC (a quantity that is obviously not clinically relevant in a study of women 55 and older).

As noted earlier, we have the choice at this point to either tabulate or graph the results. As this is our first example of a model with an interaction we delve into it in more detail than one might typically do in practice. The easiest way to see the nature of the interaction is to plot the two logit functions in Step 2 as a function of age, which we present in Figure 3.3.

The upper line in Figure 3.3 is a plot of the log-odds for subjects with a prior fracture, which from Model 3 in Table 3.12 and equation (3.10) is

$$\hat{g}(\text{PRIORFRAC} = 1, \text{AGE} = a)$$

$$= -5.689 + 4.961 \times 1 + 0.063 \times a - 0.057 \times a \times 1 = -0.728 + 0.006 \times a.$$

The lower line is the logit for subjects without a prior fracture and is

$$\hat{g}(\text{PRIORFRAC} = 0, \text{AGE} = a)$$

$$= -5.689 + 4.961 \times 0 + 0.063 \times a - 0.057 \times a \times 0 = -5.689 + 0.063 \times a.$$

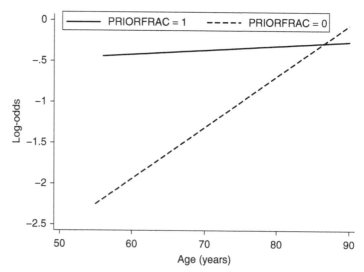

Figure 3.3 Plot of the estimated logit as a function of age for subjects with PRIORFRAC $= 1$ and PRIORFRAC $= 0$.

The log-odds ratio is given in equation (3.10) and is the vertical distance between the two lines in Figure 3.3 at a specific age, a, and is equal to

$$\ln\{\widehat{OR}[(PRIORFRAC = 1, AGE = a), (PRIORFRAC = 0, AGE = a)]\}$$
$$= 4.961 - 0.057 \times a.$$

This function is plotted in Figure 3.4.

We have included the 95% confidence bands in Figure 3.4. These are calculated, using equation (3.10), at each observed value of age as

$$(\hat{\beta}_1 + \hat{\beta}_3 \times a) \pm 1.96 \times \widehat{SE}(\hat{\beta}_1 + \hat{\beta}_3 \times a), \tag{3.12}$$

where

$$\widehat{SE}(\hat{\beta}_1 + \hat{\beta}_3 \times a) = [\widehat{Var}(\hat{\beta}_1) + a^2\widehat{Var}(\hat{\beta}_3) + 2a\widehat{Cov}(\hat{\beta}_1, \hat{\beta}_3)]^{0.5}. \tag{3.13}$$

The actual plotted values in Figure 3.4 are obtained by substituting the estimates of the coefficients from Model 3 in Table 3.12 and the values of the estimated covariance matrix of the estimated coefficients (not shown) into equations (3.12) and (3.13). One should note that the form of the plot in Figure 3.4 is similar to the plot of a linear regression model with its confidence bands being narrower in the middle at about the mean age, 68.6, and wider at the extremes. We added a line at log-odds ratio of 0 to the figure to aid interpretation. We see that the lower confidence limit crosses the 0-line at 78 years. This means that the log-odds ratio is not significantly different from 0 for ages greater than or equal to 78.

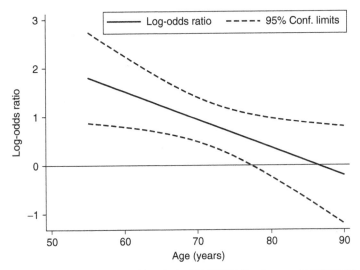

Figure 3.4 Plot of the estimated log-odds ratio for PRIORFRAC = 1 versus PRIORFRAC = 0 as a function of age, with 95% confidence bands.

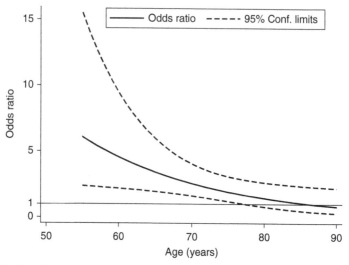

Figure 3.5 Plot of the estimated odds ratio for PRIORFRAC = 1 versus PRIORFRAC = 0 as a function of age, with 95% confidence bands.

Figure 3.5 presents the plot of the estimated odds ratio and its confidence limits. This is accomplished by exponentiating the values on the three lines in Figure 3.4. A horizontal line at 1.0 is added to aid interpretation. We see that the estimated odds ratio decreases from a value of about 6 at 55 years and becomes insignificant at 78 years, where the lower confidence limit line drops below 1.0. The problem with the plot is that the upper confidence limits are so large at ages below about 60 that the rest of the lines become compressed and are difficult to read with any accuracy. This is often the case in an interaction model with a continuous covariate and for this reason, in practice, we prefer a plot of the log-odds ratio.

The advantage of a plot is that it describes, in a general way, how the estimated log-odds ratios or odds ratios change as a function of the plotted covariate. It is, however, not as useful as a table for obtaining specific values. We show in Table 3.13 estimates of the odds ratio and confidence intervals at ages 55, 60, 65, 70, and 80 years of age. These values are obtained by first evaluating equations (3.12) and (3.13) at each of the ages and then exponentiating the values.

The values in Table 3.13 provide more detail on how the odds ratio for prior fracture decreases as a function of age from 6.1 at age 55 to the point where it becomes not statistically significant at age 80 (actually 78). Note that had we incorrectly used Model 2 we would have stated that the "age-adjusted" odds ratio is $2.3 = \exp(0.839)$, implying that this estimate was valid for all ages. In fact, we can see from the results in Table 3.13, this is only true for age approximately equal to 72.

In summary, the examples in this section demonstrate that evidence for a covariate being necessary in a model to adjust for the effect of another variable cannot be determined by a statistical test. It is a judgmental decision based on the change

Table 3.13 Estimated Odds Ratios for Prior Fracture
as a Function of Age from Model 3 in Table 3.12

Age	Odds Ratio	95% CI
55	6.1	2.38, 15.53
60	4.6	2.20, 9.49
65	3.4	1.96, 5.99
70	2.6	1.63, 4.06
75	1.9	1.20, 3.11
80	1.4	0.79, 2.65

in the estimate of a coefficient. When there is a statistically significant interaction statistical adjustment is no longer an issue as one must estimate the odds ratio at specific values of the covariate. These are most easily calculated by carefully following the four-step method.

3.6 PRESENTATION AND INTERPRETATION OF THE FITTED VALUES

In previous sections of this chapter we discussed using the logistic regression model coefficients to estimate odds ratios and construct confidence intervals in a number of settings typically encountered in practice. In our experience this accounts for the vast majority of the use of logistic regression modeling in applied settings. However, there are situations where the fitted values (i.e., the estimated probabilities) from the model are equally, if not more, important. For example, Groeger et al. (1998) used logistic regression modeling methods to estimate a patient's probability of hospital mortality after admission to an intensive care unit. We discussed in Sections 1.4 and 2.5 the methods for computing a fitted value and its confidence interval estimate. In this section, we expand this work to include graphical presentations of fitted values. In addition we discuss prediction of the outcome for a subject not in the estimation sample.

Settings where predicted probabilities are of interest tend be those where there is a reasonably wide range in the values. Conversely, if the range is too narrow graphs of fitted values tend to look like straight lines and thus are not much different, though on a different scale, than plots of fitted logits shown in Section 3.5 and add little to the analysis. Among the data sets described in Section 1.6 the Burn Study (Section 1.6.5) has the widest range of fitted values and we use it for the example in this section.

Suppose we fit a model containing the total burn surface area (TBSA) and burn involved an inhalation injury (INH_INJ). Furthermore, suppose we are interested in describing, graphically, the effect of these two covariates on the estimated probabilities. We encourage the reader to review the details in Section 1.6.5 on how these data were sampled from a much larger data set. The results of the fit are shown in Table 3.14.

Table 3.14   Fitted Multiple Logistic Regression Model of Death from a Burn Injury (DEATH) on TBSA and Inhalation Injury Involved (INH_INJ) from the Burn Study, $n = 1000$

Variable	Coeff.	Std. Err.	z	p	95% CI
TBSA	0.073	0.0072	10.11	<0.001	0.059, 0.087
INH_INJ	1.290	0.2926	4.41	<0.001	0.716, 1.863
Constant	−3.380	0.1776	−19.03	<0.001	−3.728, −3.031

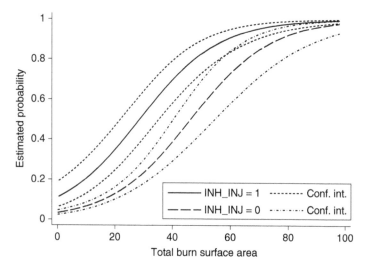

Figure 3.6   Plot of the fitted values from the model in Table 3.14 and their 95% confidence bands.

Both burn area and inhalation injury are highly significant and, after controlling for TBSA, the estimated odds ratio for inhalation injury is 3.63 (95% confidence interval: 2.05, 6.45). Clearly, involvement of an inhalation injury greatly increases the odds of dying, but how could we express the effect of this variable on the probability of dying? In this example, the model is not complicated and contains the continuous covariate TBSA, thus a plot of the fitted values versus burn area for those with and without inhalation injury involvement provides a simple graphical summary of the effect of the two covariates. This is shown in Figure 3.6 along with the 95% confidence bands.

The plotted curves in Figure 3.6 show that the estimated probability of death from a burn injury ranges from about 0.03 (3%) for a small burn with no inhalation injury involvement to almost 1.0 (100%) for subjects with a burn area of more than 95%. The plotted confidence bands for two fitted value curves show that inhalation injury involvement greatly increases the estimated probability of death, particularly when the burn area is between 20% and 60%. For burn area greater than 70% the estimated probability curves converge and approach 1.0. In this range the estimated probabilities are so large that inhalation injury cannot add much. Note that we have described the difference in the two curves as an additive difference rather than a relative difference. Under the fitted model the relative difference (i.e., the estimated odds ratio) for inhalation injury involvement is 18.7 at all estimated probabilities. We discuss summary measures that use fitted values to describe model performance in Chapter 5.

Using the methods described at the end of Section 2.5 and the results in Table 3.14 the required calculations to obtain the values plotted in Figure 3.6 are as follows. First, we calculate the two fitted logit functions:

$$\hat{g}_1(a) = \hat{g}(\text{TBSA} = a, \text{INH\_INJ} = 1)$$
$$= -3.380 + 0.073 \times a + 1.290 \times 1$$
$$= -2.090 + 0.073 \times a,$$

$$\hat{g}_0(a) = \hat{g}(\text{TBSA} = a, \text{INH\_INJ} = 0)$$
$$= -3.380 + 0.073 \times a + 1.290 \times 0$$
$$= -3.380 + 0.073 \times a.$$

Next, we compute the estimator of the variance of each estimated logit:

$$\widehat{\text{Var}}[\hat{g}_1(a)] = 0.03154 + (a^2) \times 0.00005199 + (1^2) \times 0.08561 - 2 \times a$$
$$\times 0.0008339 - 2 \times 1 \times 0.007801 \times 1 - 2 \times a \times 1 \times 0.0006466$$
$$= 0.1093 - a \times 0.01727 + (a)^2 \times 0.00005199,$$

and

$$\widehat{\text{Var}}[\hat{g}_0(a)] = 0.03154 + (a^2) \times 0.00005199 + (0^2) \times 0.08561 - 2 \times a \times 0.0008339$$
$$- 2 \times 0 \times 007801 \times 0 - 2 \times a \times 0 \times 0.0006466$$
$$= 0.03154 - a \times 0.00001667 + (a)^2 \times 0.00005199,$$

where the values of the various estimated variances and covariances are obtained from the estimated covariance matrix of the estimated parameters in the fitted model (not shown but available from all software packages). Hence the two sets of fitted values as a function of burn area are

$$\hat{\pi}_j(a) = \frac{e^{\hat{g}_j(a)}}{1 + e^{\hat{g}_j(a)}}, \qquad j = 0, 1, \tag{3.14}$$

and their lower (l) and upper (u) confidence bands are obtained from

$$\hat{\pi}_j^l(a), \hat{\pi}_j^u(a) = \frac{e^{\hat{g}_j(a) \pm 1.96\widehat{\text{SE}}(\hat{g}_j(a))}}{1 + e^{\hat{g}_j(a) \pm 1.96\widehat{\text{SE}}(\hat{g}_j(a))}}, \qquad j = 0, 1, \tag{3.15}$$

where $\widehat{\text{SE}}(g) = \sqrt{\widehat{\text{Var}}(g)}$.

We now focus our attention on the fitted value and confidence interval for the single set of values (TBSA = 30, INH_INJ = 1). As these two values are among those in the data set we can obtain them from those used in the plot in Figure 3.6. In fact, the estimated probability is 0.52 with 95% confidence interval $(0.41, 0.64)$. The interpretation is that among patients admitted with a burn area of 40% and inhalation injury involvement the model estimates that 52% would die and it could be between 41% and 64% with 95% confidence.

If the covariate values that we would like estimates for are within the range of those in the observed data set but not specifically present (e.g., TBSA = 64, INH_INJ = 1) then we use the expressions for $\hat{g}_1(a)$ and $\widehat{\text{Var}}[\hat{g}_1(a)]$ with these values and use the results to evaluate equations (3.14) and (3.15).

The fitted model in Table 3.14 is much simpler than one typically uses to model data in a practical multivariable data set. To extend the bivariable example in Table 3.14 we show in Table 3.15 the fit of a model that adds age (AGE), gender (GENDER), race (RACE) and flame involved in the burn injury (FLAME) to the model. Suppose that all variables are kept in the model for either clinical or statistical reasons. We would like to plot the estimated probability of death as a function of burn area (same as Figure 3.6) and inhalation injury but now controlling for the other four covariates in the model.

In order to control for the additional covariates we could choose "typical" values for each (e.g., median age and 0 for the three dichotomous covariates). However, these values may not provide a logit that is, in some sense, at the median or middle of the log-odds of death for these covariates. What we propose is to calculate a modified logit that subtracts the contribution of burn area and inhalation injury from the logit and uses its median value as a way to control for the additional model covariates. Specially, the logit for the fitted model in Table 3.15 is

$$\hat{g}(\mathbf{x}) = -7.695 + 0.089 \times \text{TBSA} + 1.365 \times \text{INH\_INJ} + 0.083 \times \text{AGE}$$
$$- 0.201 \times \text{GENDER} + 0.583 \times \text{FLAME} - 0.701 \times \text{RACE}.$$

Table 3.15 Fitted Multiple Logistic Regression Model of Death from a Burn Injury (DEATH) on Total Body Surface Area (TBSA), Inhalation Injury (INH_INJ), Age (AGE), Gender (GENDER), Race (RACE), and Flame Involved (FLAME) from the Burn Study, $n = 1000$

Variable	Coeff.	Std. Err.	z	p	95% CI	
TBSA	0.089	0.0091	9.83	<0.001	0.072,	0.107
INH_INJ	1.365	0.3618	3.77	<0.001	0.656,	2.074
AGE	0.083	0.0086	9.61	<0.001	0.066,	0.100
GENDER	−0.201	0.3078	−0.65	0.513	−0.805,	0.402
FLAME	0.583	0.3545	1.64	0.100	−0.112,	1.277
RACE	−0.701	0.3098	−2.26	0.024	−1.309,	−0.094
Constant	−7.695	0.6912	−11.13	<0.001	−9.050,	−6.341

Our proposed modified logit is

$$\widehat{gm}(\mathbf{x}) = \hat{g}(\mathbf{x}) - (+0.089 \times \text{TBSA} + 1.365 \times \text{INH\_INJ}),$$

and the median value of $\widehat{gm}(\mathbf{x})$ over the 1000 subjects is $\widehat{gm}_{50} = -5.349$. Here we use $\mathbf{x}$ to generically denote the covariates. Next we calculate the adjusted logit for the two inhalation injury groups as a function of burn area as

$$\hat{g}_1(a) = \widehat{gm}_{50} + 0.089 \times \text{TBSA} + 1.365 \times 1$$

$$= -5.349 + 0.089 \times \text{TBSA} + 1.365$$

$$= -3.984 + 0.089 \times \text{TBSA},$$

and

$$\hat{g}_0(a) = \widehat{gm}_{50} + 0.089 \times \text{TBSA} + 1.365 \times 0$$

$$= -5.349 + 0.089 \times \text{TBSA} + 0$$

$$= -5.349 + 0.089 \times \text{TBSA}.$$

The estimated probabilities are computed using equation (3.14) and are plotted in Figure 3.7.

The plot in Figure 3.7 shows, quite clearly, how having an inhalation injury increases the probability of death over the range of burn area. A specific value is easily obtained by substituting in values for TBSA and INH_INJ into the equation for the logit. For example, for the pair (TBSA = 40, INH_INJ = 0) the value of the logit is

$$\hat{g}_0(a) = -5.349 + 0.089 \times 40$$

$$= -1.789,$$

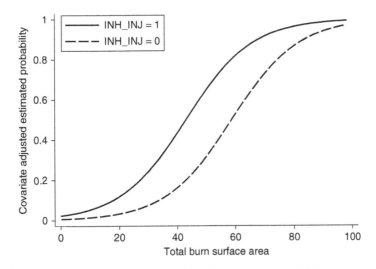

Figure 3.7 Plot of the covariate adjusted fitted values from the model in Table 3.15.

and the covariate adjusted probability is

$$\hat{\pi}_0(40) = \frac{e^{-1.789}}{1 + e^{-1.789}}$$

$$= 0.143.$$

Using the modified logit $\widehat{gm}(\mathbf{x})$ avoids having to choose specific values for the covariates. Using its median value adjusts at a middle level of log-odds for these covariates. However, as we have not used specific covariate values, an extension of the expression for $\widehat{Var}[\hat{g}_j(a)]$ can no longer be evaluated and thus confidence bands based on it are not possible to compute. Confidence bands can be obtained with some additional programming and using a resampling method called bootstrapping. As this topic is beyond the technical level of this text, we do not consider it further here.

As is the case with any regression model we must take care not to extend model-based inferences beyond the observed range of the data. It is also important to keep in mind that any estimate is only as good as the model upon which it is based. In this section we did not attend to many of the important model building details that are discussed in Chapter 4. We have implicitly assumed that these steps have been performed.

3.7 A COMPARISON OF LOGISTIC REGRESSION AND STRATIFIED ANALYSIS FOR 2 × 2 TABLES

Many users of logistic regression, especially those coming from a background in epidemiology, have performed stratified analyses of 2 × 2 tables to assess interaction and to control confounding. The essential objective of such analyses is to produce an adjusted odds ratio. This is accomplished by first determining whether the odds ratios are constant, or homogeneous, over a number of strata. If the odds ratios are constant, then a stratified odds ratio estimator such as the Mantel–Haenszel estimator or the weighted logit-based estimator is computed. This same analysis may also be performed using the logistic regression modeling techniques discussed in Sections 3.5 and 3.6. In this section we compare these two approaches. An example from the Burn Study illustrates the similarities and differences in the two approaches.

Consider an analysis of the risk factor whether a flame was involved in the burn injury (FLAME) on the outcome variable vital status at hospital discharge (DEATH). The crude (or unadjusted) odds ratio computed from the 2 × 2 table shown in Table 3.16, cross-classifying the outcome variable DEATH with FLAME, is $\widehat{OR} = 7.35$.

As we have seen earlier in this chapter, total body surface area burned (TBSA) is an important determinant of patient survival. Examination of the distribution of TBSA shows that the 25th, 50th, and 75th percentiles of body surface area are 2.5%, 6%, and 16%, respectively. Using these quartiles, Table 3.17 presents the cross tabulation of DEATH by FLAME within each of the four quartiles of TBSA.

Table 3.16 Cross-Classification of Vital Status at Hospital Discharge (DEATH) by Whether a Flame Was Involved in the Burn Injury (FLAME)

		FLAME		
		0	1	Total
DEATH	0	451	399	850
	1	20	130	150
Total		471	529	1000

Table 3.17 Cross-Classification of DEATH by FLAME Stratified by TBSA Quartile Groups

			FLAME		
TBSA			0	1	Total
TBSA < 2.5%	DEATH	0	168	73	241
		1	3	2	5
		Total	171	75	246
2.5% ≤ TBSA < 6%	DEATH	0	124	101	225
		1	2	6	8
		Total	126	107	233
6% ≤ TBSA < 16%	DEATH	0	117	134	251
		1	5	14	19
		Total	122	148	270
TBSA ≥ 16%	DEATH	0	42	91	133
		1	10	108	118
		Total	52	199	251

We can use these tables as the basis for computing either the Mantel–Haenszel estimate or the logit-based estimate of the odds ratio.

The Mantel–Haenszel estimator is a weighted average of the stratum specific odds ratios, $\widehat{OR}_i = (a_i \times d_i)/(b_i \times c_i)$, where a_i, b_i, c_i, and d_i are the observed cell frequencies in the 2×2 table for stratum i. For example, in stratum 1, $a_1 = 168$, $b_1 = 73$, $c_1 = 3$, and $d_1 = 2$, and the total number of subjects is $N_1 = 246$. The Mantel–Haenszel estimator of the odds ratio is defined in this case as follows:

$$\widehat{OR}_{MH} = \frac{\sum \dfrac{a_i \times d_i}{N_i}}{\sum \dfrac{b_i \times c_i}{N_i}}. \tag{3.16}$$

Evaluating equation (3.16) using the data in Table 3.17 yields the Mantel–Haenszel estimate

$$\widehat{OR}_{MH} = \frac{28.697}{7.864} = 3.65.$$

Table 3.18 Tabulation of the Estimated Odds Ratios, ln(Estimated Odds Ratios), Estimated Variance of the ln(Estimated Odds Ratios), and the Inverse of the Estimated Variance, w, for FLAME Within Each Quartile of TBSA

	Quartile of TBSA			
	1	2	3	4
$\widehat{OR}$	1.534	3.683	2.445	4.985
$\ln(\widehat{OR})$	0.428	1.304	0.894	1.606
$\widehat{Var}[\ln(\widehat{OR})]$	0.853	0.685	0.287	0.144
w	1.172	1.461	3.479	6.942

The logit-based summary estimator of the odds ratio is a weighted average of the stratum specific log-odds ratios where each weight is the inverse of the variance of the stratum specific log-odds ratio,

$$\widehat{OR}_L = \exp\left[\frac{\sum w_i \ln\left(\widehat{OR}_i\right)}{\sum w_i}\right]. \tag{3.17}$$

Table 3.18 presents the estimated odds ratio, log-odds ratio, estimate of the variance of the log-odds ratio and the weight, w.

The logit-based estimator based on the data in Table 3.18 is

$$\widehat{OR}_L = \exp\left(\frac{16.667}{13.054}\right) = 3.585,$$

which is slightly smaller than the Mantel–Haenszel estimate. In general, the Mantel–Haenszel estimator and the logit-based estimator are similar when the data are not too sparse within the strata. One considerable advantage of the Mantel–Haenszel estimator is that it may be computed when some of the cell entries are 0.

It is important to note that these estimators provide a correct estimate of the effect of the risk factor only when the odds ratio is constant across the strata. Thus, a crucial step in the stratified analysis is to assess the validity of this assumption. Statistical tests of this assumption are based on a comparison of the stratum specific estimates to an overall estimate computed under the assumption that the odds ratio is, in fact, constant. The simplest and most easily computed test of the homogeneity of the odds ratios across strata is based on a weighted sum of the squared deviations of the stratum specific log-odds ratios from their weighted mean. This test statistic, in terms of the current notation, is

$$X_H^2 = \sum\{w_i[\ln(\widehat{OR}_i) - \ln(\widehat{OR}_L)]^2\}. \tag{3.18}$$

Under the hypothesis that the odds ratios are constant, X_H^2 has a chi-square distribution with degrees of freedom equal to the number of strata minus 1. Thus, we would reject the homogeneity assumption when X_H^2 is large.

Using the data in Table 3.18 we have $X_H^2 = 2.11$ which, with 3 degrees of freedom, yields a p-value of 0.5492. Thus, the logit-based test of homogeneity indicates that the four groups, based on the quartiles of the distribution of TBSA, are within sampling variation of each other. It should be noted that the p-value calculated from the chi-square distribution is accurate only when the sample sizes are not too small within each stratum. This condition holds in this example.

Another test that also may be calculated by hand, but not as easily, is discussed in Breslow and Day (1980) and is corrected by Tarone (1985). This test compares the value of a_i to an estimated expected value, $\hat{e}_i$, calculated under the assumption that the odds ratio is constant in all strata. As noted by Breslow (1996) the correct formula for the test statistic is

$$X_{BD}^2 = \sum \frac{(a_i - \hat{e}_i)^2}{\hat{v}_i} - \frac{\left[\sum (a_i) - \sum (\hat{e}_i)\right]^2}{\sum (\hat{v}_i)}. \tag{3.19}$$

We note that some packages, for example, STATA, calculate the first part of equation (3.19) as the Breslow–Day test and the entire expression in equation (3.19) as the Tarone test. The quantity $\hat{e}_i$ is one of the two solutions to the following quadratic equation:

$$\widehat{OR} = \frac{(\hat{e}_i)(n_{1i} - m_{0i} + \hat{e}_i)}{(n_{0i} - \hat{e}_i)(m_{0i} - \hat{e}_i)}, \tag{3.20}$$

where $n_{0i} = a_i + b_i$, $m_{0i} = a_i + c_i$, and $n_{1i} = c_i + d_i$. The two solutions for $\hat{e}_i$ in equation (3.20) are found by evaluating the following expressions

$$\frac{-s_i + \sqrt{s_i^2 - 4 \times r \times t_i}}{2 \times r} \quad \text{and} \quad \frac{-s_i - \sqrt{s_i^2 - 4 \times r \times t_i}}{2 \times r}, \tag{3.21}$$

where $r = 1 - \widehat{OR}$, $s_i = (n_{1i} - m_{0i}) + (\widehat{OR})(m_{0i} + n_{0i})$, and $t_i = -(\widehat{OR})(n_{0i} m_{0i})$, but only one of them yields an estimated frequency that is positive and less than both n_{0i} and m_{0i}.

The quantity $\widehat{OR}$ in equation (3.20) is an estimate of the common odds ratio and either $\widehat{OR}_L$ or $\widehat{OR}_{MH}$ may be used, but the default used in most packages is the Mantel–Haenszel estimator. The quantity $\hat{v}_i$ is an estimate of the variance of a_i computed under the assumption of a common odds ratio and is

$$\hat{v}_i = \left(\frac{1}{\hat{e}_i} + \frac{1}{n_{0i} - \hat{e}_i} + \frac{1}{m_{0i} - \hat{e}_i} + \frac{1}{n_{1i} - m_{0i} + \hat{e}_i}\right)^{-1}. \tag{3.22}$$

If we use the value of the Mantel–Haenszel estimate, $\widehat{OR}_{MH} = 3.65$ to compute the Breslow–Day test in equation (3.19) then $X_{BD}^2 = 2.18$ ($p = 0.5366$), which is similar to the value of the logit-based test.

The same analysis may be performed much more easily by fitting three logistic regression models. In model 1 we include only the variable FLAME. We then

Table 3.19   Estimated Logistic Regression Coefficients for the Variable FLAME, Log-Likelihood, the Likelihood Ratio Test Statistic (G), and Resulting p-Value for Estimation of the Stratified Odds Ratio and Assessment of Homogeneity of Odds Ratios across Strata Defined by Quartiles of TBSA

Model	FLAME	Log-Likelihood	G	df	p
1	1.994	−258.34			
2	1.296	−288.64	178.17	3	<0.001
3		−287.57	2.14	3	0.545

add the three design variables representing the four quartiles of TBSA to obtain model 2. For model 3 we add the three TBSA × FLAME interaction terms. The results of fitting these models are shown in Table 3.19. As we are primarily interested in the estimates of the coefficient for FLAME, the estimates of the coefficients for TBSA and the FLAME × TBSA interactions are not shown in Table 3.19.

Using the estimated coefficients in Table 3.19 we have the following estimated odds ratios. The crude odds ratio is $\widehat{OR}$ = exp(1.994) = 7.35. Adjusting for TBSA, the stratified estimate is $\widehat{OR}$ = exp(1.2958) = 3.65. This value is the maximum likelihood estimate of the estimated odds ratio, and it is similar in value to both the Mantel–Haenszel estimate, $\widehat{OR}_{MH}$ = 3.65, and the logit-based estimate, $\widehat{OR}_L$ = 3.59. The change in the estimate of the odds ratio from the crude to the adjusted is 7.35 to 3.65, indicating considerable confounding due to TBSA.

Assessment of the homogeneity of the odds ratios across the strata is based on the likelihood ratio test of model 2 versus model 3. The value of this statistic from Table 3.19 is $G = 2.14$. This statistic is compared to a chi-square distribution with 3 degrees of freedom, as three interaction terms were added to model 2 to obtain model 3. This test statistic is comparable to the ones from the logit-based test, X_H^2 (=2.11), and the Breslow–Day test, X_{BD}^2 (=2.18), each with 3 degrees of freedom.

The previously described analysis based on likelihood ratio tests may be used when the data have either been grouped into contingency tables in advance of the analysis, such as those shown in Table 3.17, or have remained in casewise form. When the data have been grouped, as we did in the example from the burn data, it is possible to point out other similarities between classical analysis of stratified 2 × 2 tables and an analysis using logistic regression. Day and Byar (1979) have shown that the 1 degree of freedom Mantel–Haenszel test of the hypothesis that the stratum specific odds ratios are 1 is identical to the Score test for the exposure variable when added to a logistic regression model already containing the stratification variable. This test statistic may be easily obtained from a logistic regression package with the capability to perform Score tests such as SAS.

Thus, use of the logistic regression model provides a fast and effective way to obtain a stratified odds ratio estimator and to assess easily the assumption of homogeneity of odds ratios across strata.

EXERCISES

1. Consider the ICU data described in Section 1.6.1 and use as the outcome variable vital status (STA) and infection probable at ICU admission (INF) as a covariate.

   (a) Demonstrate that the value of the log-odds ratio obtained from the cross-classification of STA by INF is identical to the estimated slope coefficient from the logistic regression of STA on INF. Verify that the estimated standard error of the estimated slope coefficient for INF obtained from the logistic regression package is identical to the square root of the sum of the inverse of the cell frequencies from the cross-classification of STA by INF. Use either set of computations, contingency table, or logistic regression, to obtain the 95% confidence interval for the odds ratio.

   (b) For purposes of illustration, use a data transformation statement to recode, for this problem only, the variable INF as follows: $4 = $ No and $2 = $ Yes. Perform the logistic regression of STA on INF (recoded). Use the four-step method to calculate the estimate of the odds ratio of INF $=$ Yes versus INF $=$ No. Use the results from the fitted logistic regression model to obtain the 95% confidence interval for the odds ratio. Note that they are the same limits as obtained in Exercise 1(a).

2. Consider data from the Low Birth Weight Study described in Section 1.6.2 and use as the outcome variable low birth weight (LOW) and race of the mother (RACE) as the covariate.

   (a) Prepare a table showing the coding of the two design variables for RACE using the value RACE $= 1$, white, as the reference group. Show that the estimated log-odds ratios obtained from the cross-classification of LOW by RACE, using RACE $= 1$ as the reference group, are identical to estimated slope coefficients for the two design variables from the logistic regression of LOW on RACE. Verify that the estimated standard errors of the estimated slope coefficients for the two design variables for RACE are identical to the square root of the sum of the inverse of the cell frequencies from the cross-classification of LOW by RACE used to calculate the odds ratio. Use either set of computations to compute the 95% confidence interval for the odds ratios. Note that in this example the results are significant at the 10 but not 5% level of significance. Explain circumstances under which you would choose to keep RACE in a statistical model and ones when you might not keep it.

   (b) Create design variables for RACE using the deviation from means coding typically employed in ANOVA. Perform the logistic regression of LOW on RACE. Use the four-step method to compute the estimate of the odds ratio RACE $= 2$ versus RACE $= 1$ and RACE $= 3$ versus RACE $= 1$. Are these estimates the same as those computed in 2(a)? Use the results of the logistic regression to obtain the 95% confidence interval for the odds ratios and verify that they are the same limits as obtained in 2(a). In this example you need the estimated covariance matrix for the estimated coefficients to obtain the estimated variances of the two log-odds ratios.

3. In the ICU data vital status at discharge (STA) is the outcome variable and consider history of chronic renal failure (CRN) as the factor of interest. Using logistic regression, demonstrate and then explain why age (AGE) is needed to adjust the effect of CRN. Using logistic regression modeling, demonstrate that there is no statistical interaction between age (AGE) and history of chronic renal failure (CRN).

4. Repeat problem 3 using cancer part of the present problem (CAN) as the factor of interest and type of admission (TYP) as a potential adjustment and interaction variable.

5. In the Burn Injury Data described in Section 1.6.5 vital status at hospital discharge (DEATH) is the outcome variable.
    (a) Show that age (AGE) is not a confounder of the effect of inhalation injury (INH_INJ) but is an effect modifier.
    (b) Using the interactions model from part 5(a) and the four-step method prepare a table with estimates of the odds ratio and 95% confidence interval for inhalation injury for ages 20, 40, 60, and 80.
    (c) Using the interaction model from part 5(a) prepare a graph of the estimate of the odds ratio for inhalation injury as a function of age.
    (d) Add 95% confidence bands to the graph in part 5(c).

6. The outcome variable in the Myopia Study described in Section 1.6.6 is becoming myopic during the first five years of follow up (MYOPIC). Consider a logistic regression model containing spherical equivalent refraction (SHPQ), gender (GENDER), sports hours (SPORTHR), reading hours (RESDHR), computer hours (COMPHR), study hours (STUDYHR) and television hours (TVHR). Graph the fitted logistic probability of becoming myopic for males and females as a function of spherical equivalent refraction (SHPQ) adjusted for all other variables in the model.

7. In the Low Birth Weight Study described in Section 1.6.2, determine the crude odds ratio of smoking (SMOKE) on the outcome low birthweight (LOW). Stratify on RACE and note the odds ratios within the three strata. Do the odds ratios appear to be homogeneous across strata? Compute the Mantel–Haenszel and logit-based estimates of the odds ratio. How do these compare to the crude estimate? Determine whether homogeneity of the odds ratios across strata holds through the use of the chi-square test of homogeneity and the Breslow–Day test. Finally, use a logistic regression analysis to compute the adjusted odds ratio and to determine whether the odds ratios were homogeneous across strata. How do these results compare to the ones you obtained using the more classical categorical data approach?

CHAPTER 4

Model-Building Strategies and Methods for Logistic Regression

4.1 INTRODUCTION

In previous chapters we focused on estimating, testing, and interpreting the coefficients and fitted values from a logistic regression model. The examples discussed were characterized by having few independent variables, and there was perceived to be only one possible model. While there may be situations where this is the case, it is more typical that there are many independent variables that could potentially be included in the model. Hence, we need to develop a strategy and associated methods for handling these more complex situations.

The goal of any method is to select those variables that result in a "best" model within the scientific context of the problem. In order to achieve this goal we must have: (i) a basic plan for selecting the variables for the model and (ii) a set of methods for assessing the adequacy of the model both in terms of its individual variables and its overall performance. In this chapter and the next we discuss methods that address both of these areas.

The methods to be discussed in this chapter are not to be used as a substitute, but rather as an addition to clear and careful thought. Successful modeling of a complex data set is part science, part statistical methods, and part experience and common sense. It is our goal to provide the reader with a paradigm that, when applied thoughtfully, yields the best possible model within the constraints of the available data.

4.2 PURPOSEFUL SELECTION OF COVARIATES

The criteria for including a variable in a model may vary from one problem to the next and from one scientific discipline to another. The traditional approach to

Applied Logistic Regression, Third Edition.
David W. Hosmer, Jr., Stanley Lemeshow, and Rodney X. Sturdivant.
© 2013 John Wiley & Sons, Inc. Published 2013 by John Wiley & Sons, Inc.

statistical model building involves seeking the most parsimonious model that still accurately reflects the true outcome experience of the data. The rationale for minimizing the number of variables in the model is that the resultant model is more likely to be numerically stable, and is more easily adopted for use. The more variables included in a model, the greater the estimated standard errors become, and the more dependent the model becomes on the observed data. Epidemiologic methodologists suggest including all clinically and intuitively relevant variables in the model, regardless of their "statistical significance." The rationale for this approach is to provide as complete control of confounding as possible within the given data set. This is based on the fact that it is possible for individual variables not to exhibit strong confounding, but when taken collectively, considerable confounding can be present in the data, see Rothman et al. (2008), Maldonado and Greenland (1993), Greenland (1989), and Miettinen (1976). The major problem with this approach is that the model may be "overfit," producing numerically unstable estimates. Overfitting is typically characterized by unrealistically large estimated coefficients and/or estimated standard errors. This may be especially troublesome in problems where the number of variables in the model is large relative to the number of subjects and/or when the overall proportion responding ($y = 1$) is close to either 0 or 1. In an excellent tutorial paper, Harrell et al. (1996) discuss overfitting along with other model building issues.

The following seven steps describe a method of selecting variables that we call purposeful selection. The rationale behind the method is that it follows the steps that many applied investigators employ when examining a set of data and then building a multivariable regression model.

Step 1: Purposeful selection begins with a careful univariable analysis of each independent variable. For categorical variables we suggest doing this via a standard contingency table analysis of the outcome ($y = 0, 1$) versus the k levels of the independent variable. The usual likelihood ratio chi-square test with $k - 1$ degrees of freedom is exactly equal to the value of the likelihood ratio test for the significance of the coefficients for the $k - 1$ design variables in a univariable logistic regression model that contains that single independent variable. Since the Pearson chi-square test is asymptotically equivalent to the likelihood ratio chi-square test, it may also be used. In addition to the overall test, it is a good idea, for those variables exhibiting at least a moderate level of association, to estimate the individual odds ratios (along with confidence limits) using one of the levels as the reference group.

Particular attention should be paid to any contingency table with a zero (frequency) cell, since in that situation, most standard logistic regression software packages will fail to converge and produce a point estimate for one of the odds ratios of either zero or infinity. An intermediate strategy for dealing with this problem is to collapse categories of the independent variable in some sensible fashion to eliminate the zero cell. If the covariate with the zero cell turns out to be statistically significant, we can revisit the problem at a later stage using one of the special programs discussed in Section 10.3. Fortunately, the zero cell problem does not occur too frequently.

For continuous variables, the best univariable analysis involves fitting a univariable logistic regression model to obtain the estimated coefficient, the estimated standard error, the likelihood ratio test for the significance of the coefficient, and the univariable Wald statistic. An alternative analysis, which is nearly equivalent at the univariable level and that may be preferred in an applied setting, is based on the two-sample t-test. Descriptive statistics available from this analysis generally include group means, standard deviations, the t statistic, and its p-value. The similarity of this approach to the logistic regression analysis follows from the fact that the univariable linear discriminant function estimate of the logistic regression coefficient is

$$\frac{(\overline{x}_1 - \overline{x}_0)}{s_p^2} = \frac{t}{s_p}\sqrt{\frac{1}{n_1} + \frac{1}{n_0}}$$

and that the linear discriminant function and the maximum likelihood estimate of the logistic regression coefficient are usually quite close when the independent variable is approximately normally distributed within each of the outcome groups, $y = 0, 1$, [see Halpern et al. (1971)]. Thus, the univariable analysis based on the t-test can be used to determine whether the variable should be included in the model since the p-value should be of the same order of magnitude as that of the Wald statistic, Score test, or likelihood ratio test from logistic regression.

Through the use of these univariable analyses we identify, as candidates for a first multivariable model, any variable whose univariable test has a p-value less than 0.25 along with all variables of known clinical importance.

Our recommendation for using a significance level as high as 0.20 or 0.25 as a screening criterion for initial variable selection is based on the work by Bendel and Afifi (1977) on linear regression and on the work by Mickey and Greenland (1989) on logistic regression. These authors show that use of a more traditional level (such as 0.05) often fails to identify variables known to be important. Use of the higher level has the disadvantage of including variables that are of questionable importance at this initial stage of model development. For this reason, it is important to review all variables added to a model critically before a decision is reached regarding the final model.

Step 2: Fit the multivariable model containing all covariates identified for inclusion at Step 1. Following the fit of this model, we assess the importance of each covariate using the p-value of its Wald statistic. Variables that do not contribute, at traditional levels of statistical significance, should be eliminated and a new model fit. The new, smaller, model should be compared to the old, larger, model using the partial likelihood ratio test. This is especially important if more than one term has been removed from the model, which is always the case when a categorical variable with more than two levels has been included using two or more design variables that appear to be not significant. Also, one must pay attention to make sure that the samples used to fit the larger and smaller models are the same. This becomes an issue when there are missing data. We discuss strategies for handling missing data in Section 10.4.

Step 3: Following the fit of the smaller, reduced model we compare the values of the estimated coefficients in the smaller model to their respective values from the larger model. In particular, we should be concerned about any variable whose coefficient has changed markedly in magnitude [e.g., having a value of $\Delta\hat{\beta} > 20\%$, see equation (3.9)]. This indicates that one or more of the excluded variables are important in the sense of providing a needed adjustment of the effect of the variables that remained in the model. Such variable(s) should be added back into the model. This process of deleting, refitting, and verifying continues, cycling through Step 2 and Step 3, until it appears that all of the important variables are included in the model and those excluded are clinically and/or statistically unimportant. In this process we recommend that one should proceed slowly by deleting only a few covariates at a time.

Step 4: Add each variable not selected in Step 1 to the model obtained at the conclusion of cycling through Step 2 and Step 3, one at a time, and check its significance either by the Wald statistic *p*-value or the partial likelihood ratio test, if it is a categorical variable with more than two levels. This step is vital for identifying variables that, by themselves, are not significantly related to the outcome but make an important contribution in the presence of other variables. We refer to the model at the end of Step 4 as the *preliminary main effects model*.

Step 5: Once we have obtained a model that we feel contains the essential variables, we examine more closely the variables in the model. The question of the appropriate categories for categorical variables should have been addressed during the univariable analysis in Step 1. For each continuous variable in this model we must check the assumption that the logit increases/decreases linearly as a function of the covariate. There are a number of techniques and methods to do this and we discuss them in Section 4.2.1. We refer to the model at the end of Step 5 as the *main effects model*.

Step 6: Once we have the main effects model, we check for interactions among the variables in the model. In any model, as discussed and illustrated with examples in Section 3.5, an interaction between two variables implies that the effect of each variable is not constant over levels of the other variable. As noted in Section 3.5, the final decision as to whether an interaction term should be included in a model should be based on statistical as well as practical considerations. Any interaction term in the model must make sense from a clinical perspective.

We address the clinical plausibility issue by creating a list of possible pairs of variables in the model that have some realistic possibility of interacting with each other. The interaction variables are created as the arithmetic product of the pairs of main effect variables. This can result in more than one interaction term. For example, the interaction of two categorical variables, each with three levels (i.e., two dummy variables), generates four interaction variables. We add the interactions, one at a time, to the main effects model from Step 5. (This may involve adding more than one term at a time to the model.) We then assess the statistical significance of the interaction using a likelihood ratio test. Unlike main effects where we consider adjustment as well as significance, we only consider the statistical significance of interactions and as such, they must contribute to the model at traditional levels, such as 5% or even 1%. Inclusion of an interaction term in the model that is not significant typically just increases the estimated standard errors without much change in the point estimates of effect.

Following the univariable analysis of the interaction terms we add each interaction that was significant to the model at the end of Step 5. We then follow Step 2 to simplify the model, considering only the removal of the interaction terms, not any main effects. At this point we view the main effect terms as being "locked" and they cannot be removed from the model. One implication of "locking the main effects" is that we do not consider statistical adjustment, $\Delta\hat{\beta}\%$, when winnowing insignificant interactions.

We refer to the model at the conclusion of Step 6 as the *preliminary final model*.

Step 7: Before any model becomes the final model we must assess its adequacy and check its fit. We discuss these methods in Chapter 5. Note that regardless of what method is used to obtain a multivariable statistical model, purposeful selection or any of the other methods discussed in this chapter, one must perform Step 7 before using the fitted model for inferential purposes.

Bursac et al. (2008) studied the properties of purposeful selection compared to stepwise selection via simulations. The results showed that purposeful selection retained significant covariates and also included covariates that were confounders of other model covariates in a manner superior to stepwise selection.

As noted above, the issue of variable selection is made more complicated by different analytic philosophies as well as by different statistical methods. One school of thought argues for the inclusion of all scientifically relevant variables into the multivariable model regardless of the results of univariable analyses. In general, the appropriateness of the decision to begin the multivariable model with all possible variables depends on the overall sample size and the number in each outcome group relative to the total number of candidate variables. When the data are adequate to support such an analysis it may be useful to begin the multivariable modeling from this point. However, when the data are inadequate, this approach can produce a numerically unstable multivariable model, discussed in greater detail in Section 4.5. In this case the Wald statistics should not be used to select variables because of the unstable nature of the results. Instead, we should select a subset of variables based on results of the univariable analyses and refine the definition of "scientifically relevant."

Another approach to variable selection is to use a stepwise method in which variables are selected either for inclusion or exclusion from the model in a sequential fashion based solely on statistical criteria. There are two main versions of the stepwise procedure: (i) forward selection with a test for backward elimination and (ii) backward elimination followed by a test for forward selection. The algorithms used to define these procedures in logistic regression are discussed in Section 4.3. The stepwise approach is useful and intuitively appealing in that it builds models in a sequential fashion and it allows for the examination of a collection of models that might not otherwise have been examined.

"Best subsets selection" is a selection method that has not been used extensively in logistic regression. With this procedure a number of models containing one, two, three variables, and so on, are examined to determine which are considered the "best" according to some specified criteria. Best subsets linear regression software has been available for a number of years. A parallel theory has been worked out for nonnormal errors models [Lawless and Singhal (1978, 1987a, 1987b)]. We show in Section 4.4 how logistic regression may be performed using any best subsets linear regression program.

Stepwise, best subsets, and other mechanical selection procedures have been criticized because they can yield a biologically implausible model [Greenland (1989)] and can select irrelevant, or noise, variables [Flack and Chang (1987); Griffiths and Pope (1987)]. They may also fail to select variables that narrowly fail to achieve the pre-designated threshold for inclusion into a model. The problem is not the fact that the computer can select such models, but rather that the judgment of the analyst is taken out of the process and, as a result, has no opportunity to scrutinize the resulting model carefully before the final, best model is reported. The wide availability and ease with which stepwise methods can be used has undoubtedly reduced some analysts to the role of assisting the computer in model selection rather than the more appropriate alternative. It is only when the analyst understands the strengths, and especially the limitations of the methods that these methods can serve as useful tools in the model-building process. The analyst, not the computer, is ultimately responsible for the review and evaluation of the model.

4.2.1 Methods to Examine the Scale of a Continuous Covariate in the Logit

An important step in refining the main effects model is to determine whether the model is linear in the logit for each continuous variable. In this section we discuss four methods to address this assumption: (i) smoothed scatter plots, (ii) design variables, (iii) fractional polynomials and (iv) spline functions.

As a first step, it is useful to begin checking linearity in the logit with a smoothed scatterplot. This plot is helpful, not only as a graphical assessment of linearity but also as a tool for identifying extreme (large or small) observations that could unduly influence the assessment of linearity when using fractional polynomials or spline functions. One simple and easily computed form of a smoothed scatterplot was illustrated in Figure 1.2 using the data in Table 1.2. Other more complicated methods that have greater precision are preferred at this stage.

Kay and Little (1986) illustrate the use of a method proposed by Copas (1983). This method requires computing a smoothed value for the response variable for each subject that is a weighted average of the values of the outcome variable over all subjects. The weight for each subject is a continuous decreasing function of the distance of the value of the covariate for the subject under consideration from the value of the covariate for all other cases. For example, for covariate x for the ith subject we compute the smoothed value as

$$\overline{y}_{si} = \frac{\displaystyle\sum_{j=i_l}^{i_u} w(x_i, x_j) y_j}{\displaystyle\sum_{j=i_l}^{i_u} w(x_i, x_j)},$$

where $w(x_i, x_j)$ represents a particular weight function. For example, if we use STATA's scatterplot lowess smooth command, with the mean option and bandwidth k, then

$$w(x_i, x_j) = \left[1 - \left(\frac{|x_i - x_j|^3}{\Delta} \right) \right]^3,$$

where Δ is defined so that the maximum value for the weight is ≤ 1 and the two indices defining the summation, i_l and i_u, include the k percent of the n subjects with x values closest to x_i. Other weight functions are possible as well as additional smoothing using locally weighted least squares regression, which is actually the default in STATA.

In general, when using STATA, we use the default bandwidth of $k = 0.8$ and obtain the plot of the triplet $(x_i, y_i, \overline{y}_{si})$, that is, the observed and smoothed values of y on the same set of axes. The shape of the smoothed plot should provide some idea about the parametric relationship between the outcome and the covariate. Some packages, such as STATA's lowess command, provide the option of plotting the smoothed values, $(x_i, \overline{l}_{si})$ where $\overline{l}_{si} = \ln[\overline{y}_{si}/(1 - \overline{y}_{si})]$, that is, plotting on the logit scale, thus making it a little easier to make decisions about linearity in the logit. The advantage of the smoothed scatter plot is that, if it looks linear then the logit is likely linear in the covariate. One disadvantage of the smoothed scatter plot is that if it does not look linear, most of us lack the experience to guess, with any reliability, what function would satisfactorily reflect the displayed nonlinearity. The parametric approaches discussed below are useful here since they specify a best nonlinear transformation. Another disadvantage is that a smoothed scatterplot does not easily extend to multivariable models.

The second suggested method is one that is easily performed in all statistical packages and may be used with a multivariable model. The steps are as follows: (i) using the descriptive statistics capabilities of your statistical package, obtain the quartiles of the distribution of the continuous variable; (ii) create a categorical variable with four levels using three cutpoints based on the quartiles. We note that many other grouping strategies can be used but the one based on quartiles seems to work well in practice; (iii) fit the multivariable model replacing the continuous variable with the four-level categorical variable. To do this, one includes three design variables that use the lowest quartile as the reference group; (iv) following the fit of the model, plot the three estimated coefficients versus the midpoints of the upper three quartiles. In addition, plot a coefficient equal to zero at the midpoint of the first quartile. To aid in the interpretation connect the four plotted points with straight lines. Visually inspect the plot. If it does not look linear then choose the most logical parametric shape(s) for the scale of the variable.

The next step is to refit the model using the possible parametric forms suggested by the plot and choose one that is significantly different from the linear model and makes clinical sense. It is possible that two or more different parameterizations of the covariate may yield similar results in the sense that they are significantly different from the linear model. However, it is our experience that one of the possible models will be more appealing clinically, thus yielding more easily interpreted parameter estimates.

The advantage of the first two methods is that they are graphical and easily performed. The disadvantage, as noted, is that it is sometimes difficult to postulate a parametric form from either a somewhat noisy plot (method 1) or from only four points (method 2).

The third method is an analytic approach based on the use of fractional polynomials as developed by Royston and Altman (1994). Since that key paper, Royston and colleagues have researched this method extensively and have written numerous papers providing guidance to applied investigators. For example, see Royston et al. (1999) and Sauerbrei and Royston (1999). The recent text on the method by Royston and Sauerbrei (2008) provides a detailed and highly readable account of the method along with its extensions and contains numerous numerical examples. Readers looking for more details are urged to consult this reference.

The essential idea is that we wish to determine what value of x^p yields the best model for the covariate. In theory, we could incorporate the power, p, as an additional parameter in the estimation procedure. However, this greatly increases the numerical complexity of the estimation problem. Royston and Altman (1994) propose replacing full maximum likelihood estimation of the power by a search through a small but reasonable set of possible values. The method is described in the second edition of this text, Hosmer and Lemeshow (2000) and Hosmer et al. (2008) provide a brief, but updated introduction to fractional polynomials when fitting a proportional hazards regression model. This material provides the basis for the discussion.

The method of fractional polynomials may be used with a multivariable logistic regression model, but for the sake of simplicity, we describe the procedure using a model with a single continuous covariate. The equation for a logit, that is linear in the covariate, is

$$g(x, \boldsymbol{\beta}) = \beta_0 + \beta_1 x,$$

where $\boldsymbol{\beta}$, in general, denotes the vector of model coefficients. One way to generalize this function is to specify it as

$$g(x, \boldsymbol{\beta}) = \beta_0 + \sum_{j=1}^{J} \beta_j \times F_j(x),$$

where the functions $F_j(x)$ are a particular type of power function. The value of the first function is $F_1(x) = x^{p_1}$. In theory, the power, p_1, could be any number, but in most applied settings it makes sense to try to use something simple. Royston and Altman (1994) propose restricting the power to be among those in the set $\wp = \{-2, -1, -0.5, 0, 0.5, 1, 2, 3\}$, where $p_1 = 0$ denotes the log of the variable. The remaining functions are defined as

$$F_j(x) = \begin{cases} x^{p_j}, & p_j \neq p_{j-1} \\ F_{j-1}(x)\ln(x), & p_j = p_{j-1} \end{cases}$$

for $j = 2, \ldots, J$ and restricting powers to those in $\wp$. For example, if we chose $J = 2$ with $p_1 = 0$ and $p_2 = -0.5$, then the logit is

$$g(x, \boldsymbol{\beta}) = \beta_0 + \beta_1 \ln(x) + \beta_2 \frac{1}{\sqrt{x}}.$$

As another example, if we chose $J = 2$ with $p_1 = 2$ and $p_2 = 2$, then the logit is

$$g(x, \boldsymbol{\beta}) = \beta_0 + \beta_1 x^2 + \beta_2 x^2 \ln(x).$$

The model is quadratic in x when $J = 2$ with $p_1 = 1$ and $p_2 = 2$. Again, we could allow the covariate to enter the model with any number of functions, J, but in most applied settings an adequate transformation is found if we use $J = 1$ or 2.

Implementation of the method requires, for $J = 1$, fitting 8 models, that is $p_1 \in \wp$. The best model is the one with the largest log-likelihood (or smallest deviance). The process is repeated with $J = 2$ by fitting the 36 models obtained from the distinct pairs of powers (i.e., $(p_1, p_2) \in \wp \times \wp$) and the best model is again the one with the largest log-likelihood (or smallest deviance).

The relevant question is whether either of the two best models is significantly better than the linear model. Let $L(1)$ denote the log-likelihood for the linear model (i.e., $J = 1$ and $p_1 = 1$) and let $L(p_1)$ denote the log-likelihood for the best $J = 1$ model and $L(p_1, p_2)$ denote the log-likelihood for the best $J = 2$ model. Royston and Altman (1994) and Ambler and Royston (2001) suggest, and verify with simulations, that each term in the fractional polynomial model contributes approximately 2 degrees of freedom to the model, effectively one for the power and one for the coefficient. Thus, the partial likelihood ratio test comparing the linear model to the best $J = 1$ model,

$$G(1, p_1) = -2\{L(1) - L(p_1)\},$$

is approximately distributed as chi-square with one degree of freedom under the null hypothesis that the logit is linear in x. The partial likelihood ratio test comparing the best $J = 1$ model to the best $J = 2$ model,

$$G[p_1, (p_1, p_2)] = -2\{L(p_1) - L(p_1, p_2)\},$$

is approximately distributed as chi-square with 2 degrees of freedom under the hypothesis that the $J = 2$ model is not significantly different from the $J = 1$ model.

Similarly, the partial likelihood ratio test comparing the linear model to the best $J = 2$ model is distributed approximately as chi-square with 3 degrees of freedom. (Note: to keep the notation simple, we use p_1 to denote the best power both when $J = 1$ and as the first of the two powers for $J = 2$. These are not likely to be the same numeric value in practice.)

In an applied setting we can use the partial likelihood ratio test in two ways to determine whether a transformation is significantly better than the linear model: a closed test and a sequential test [see Sauerbrei et al. (2006) and cited references]. We note that Sauerbrei, Meier-Hirmer, Benner, and Royston consider a model that does not contain x as the base model. We use the linear model as the base model since, at the end of step 3, we have eliminated all statistically nonsignificant or clinically unimportant covariates.

The closed test procedure begins by comparing the best two-term fractional polynomial model to the linear model using $G[1, (p_1, p_2)]$. If this test is not significant, at a typical level such as 0.05, then we stop and use the linear model. If the test is significant then the best two-term fractional polynomial model is compared to the best one-term fractional polynomial model using $G[p_1, (p_1, p_2)]$. If this test is significant then we select the two-term model; otherwise select the one-term model.

The sequential test procedure begins by comparing the best two-term fractional polynomial model to the best one-term fractional polynomial model using $G[p_1, (p_1, p_2)]$. If this test is significant we select the two-term model. If it is not significant then we compare the best one-term fractional polynomial model to the linear model using $G[1, (p_1, p_2)]$. If the test is significant then we select the best one-term model; otherwise we use the linear model.

Ambler and Royston (2001) examined the type I error rates of the two testing methods via simulations and concluded that the closed test is better than the sequential test at maintaining the overall error rate. Thus, we use the closed test method in this text.

Whenever a one or two-term model is selected we highly recommend that the resulting functional form be critically examined for subject matter plausibility. The best way to do this is by plotting the fitted model versus the covariate. We explain how to do this and illustrate it with the examples later in this chapter. One should always ask the obvious question: Does the functional form of the fractional polynomial transformation make sense within the context of the study? If it really does not make sense then we suggest using the linear model or possibly another fractional polynomial model. In almost every example we have encountered, where one of the two best fractional polynomial models is better than the linear model there is another fractional polynomial model that is also better whose deviance is trivially larger than the selected best model. This other model may provide a more clinically acceptable transformation. For example, assume that the closed test procedure selects the two-term model with powers (2, 3). This transformation may have a deviance that is not much smaller than that of the two-term quadratic model (1, 2). From a subject matter perspective the quadratic model may make more sense and be more easily explained than the best model. In this case we would not hesitate to use the quadratic model.

The only software package that has fully implemented the method of fractional polynomials within the distributed package is STATA. In addition to the method described above, STATA's fractional polynomial routine offers the user considerable flexibility in expanding the set of powers, $\wp$, searched; however, in most settings the default set of values should be more than adequate. STATA's implementation also includes valuable graphical displays of the transformed model. Sauerbrei et al. (2006) provide links to obtain macros for SAS and R code that can be used to perform all the fractional polynomial analyses done with STATA in this text.

So far the discussion of fractional polynomials has been in the setting of a simple univariable logistic regression model. In practice, most models are multivariable and can contain numerous continuous covariates, each of which must be checked for linearity. The approach we described above, where we checked for linearity one variable at a time, is the one we use in Step 5 of purposeful selection.

Royston and Ambler (1998, 1999) extended the original fractional polynomial software to incorporate an iterative examination for scale with multivariable models. The default method incorporates recommendations discussed in detail in Sauerbrei and Royston (1999). Multivariable modeling using fractional polynomials is available in distributed STATA and can be performed in SAS and R using the macros and code that can be obtained from links in Sauerbrei et al. (2006). We describe model building using multivariable fractional polynomials in Section 4.3.3.

We have found, in our practice, a level of reluctance by applied investigators to use fractional polynomial transformations, regardless of how much clinical sense they might make, because they think the model is too complicated to estimate odds ratios. We showed in Section 3.5 that by carefully following the four-step procedure for estimating odds ratios, one is able to obtain the correct expression involving the model coefficients to estimate any odds ratio, no matter how complicated the model might be.

The fourth method of checking for linearity in the logit is via spline functions. Spline functions have been used in statistical applications to model nonlinear functions for a long time; well before the advent of computers and modern statistical software brought computer intensive methods to the desk top [see, for example, Poirier (1973), who cites pioneering work on these functions by Schoenberg (1946)]. Harrell (2001, pp. 18–24) presents a concise mathematical treatment of the spline function methods we discuss in this section. Royston and Sauerbrei (2008, Chapter 9) compare spline functions to fractional polynomials.

The basic idea behind spline functions is to mathematically mimic the use of the draftsman's spline to fit a series of smooth curves that are joined at specified points, called "knots". In this section we consider linear and restricted cubic spines as these are the ones commonly available in statistical packages (e.g., STATA and SAS).

We begin our discussion by considering linear splines based on three knots. We discuss how to choose the number of knots and where these knots should be placed shortly. The linear spline variables used in the fit can be parameterized with coefficients representing the slope in each interval, or alternatively, by the slope in the first interval and the change in the slope from the previous interval. We use the former parameterization, in which case the definitions of the four spline variables formed from three knots are as follows:

$$x_1 = \min(X, k_1)$$

and

$$x_j = \max[\min(X, k_j), k_{j-1}] - k_{j-1}, j = 2, \ldots, 4$$

where k_1, k_2 and k_3 are the three knots. The four linear spline variables used in the fit are as follows:

$$x_{l1} = \begin{cases} X, & \text{if } X < k_1, \\ k_1, & \text{if } k_1 \leq X, \end{cases}$$

$$x_{l2} = \begin{cases} 0, & \text{if } X < k_1, \\ X - k_1, & \text{if } k_1 \leq X < k_2, \\ k_2 - k_1, & \text{if } k_2 \leq X, \end{cases}$$

$$x_{l3} = \begin{cases} 0, & \text{if } X < k_2, \\ X - k_2, & \text{if } k_2 \leq X < k_3, \\ k_3 - k_2, & \text{if } k_3 \leq X, \end{cases}$$

$$x_{l4} = \begin{cases} 0, & \text{if } X < k_3, \\ X - k_3, & \text{if } k_3 \leq X, \end{cases}$$

where the subscript "l" stands for linear spline.

The equation of the logit is

$$g(\mathbf{x}_l, \boldsymbol{\beta}_l) = \beta_{l0} + \beta_{l1}x_{l1} + \beta_{l2}x_{l2} + \beta_{l3}x_{l3} + \beta_{l4}x_{l4}. \qquad (4.1)$$

Under the model in equation (4.1) the equation of the logit in the four intervals defined by the three knots is as follows:

$$g(\mathbf{x}_l, \boldsymbol{\beta}_l)$$

$$= \begin{cases} \beta_{l0} + \beta_{l1}X & \text{if } X < k_1, \\ \beta_{l0} + \beta_{l1}k_1 + \beta_{l2}(X - k_1) & \\ \quad = [\beta_{l0} + \beta_{l1}k_1 - \beta_{l2}k_2] + \beta_{l2}X & \text{if } k_1 \leq X < k_2, \\ \beta_{l0} + \beta_{l1}k_1 + \beta_{l2}(k_2 - k_1) + \beta_{l3}(X - k_3) & \\ \quad = [\beta_{l0} + \beta_{l1}k_1 + \beta_{l2}(k_2 - k_1) - \beta_{l3}k_3] + \beta_{l3}X & \text{if } k_2 \leq X < k_3, \\ \beta_{l0} + \beta_{l1}k_1 + \beta_{l2}(k_2 - k_1) + \beta_{l3}(k_3 - k_2) + \beta_{l4}(X - k_3) & \\ \quad = [\beta_{l0} + \beta_{l1}k_1 + \beta_{l2}(k_2 - k_1) + \beta_{l3}(k_3 - k_2) - \beta_{l4}k_3] + \beta_{l4}X & \text{if } k_3 \leq X. \end{cases}$$

Thus, the slopes of the lines in the four intervals are given by β_{lj}, $j = 1, 2, 3, 4$ and the four intercepts are functions of β_{lj}, $j = 0, 1, 2, 3, 4$ and the three knots.

While linear spline functions, like those in equation (4.1), are relatively easy and simple to describe they may not be sufficiently flexible to model a complex non-linear relationship between an outcome and a covariate. In these settings restricted cubic splines are a good choice. In this approach the spline functions are linear in the first and last intervals and are cubic functions in between, but join at the knots. Restricting the functions to be linear in the tails serves to eliminate wild fluctuations than can be a result of a few extreme data points. The definitions of the restricted cubic spline variables, used by STATA, formed from three knots are as follows:

$$x_{c1} = X,$$

and

$$
\begin{aligned}
x_{c2} &= \frac{1}{(k_3 - k_1)^2} \times \left\{ (X - k_1)_+^3 - (k_3 - k_2)^{-1} \left[(X - k_2)_+^3 (k_3 - k_1) \right. \right. \\
&\left. \left. - (X - k_3)_+^3 (k_2 - k_1) \right] \right\} \\
&= \frac{1}{(k_3 - k_1)^2} \times \left\{ (X - k_1)_+^3 - \frac{(X - k_2)_+^3 (k_3 - k_1)}{(k_3 - k_2)} + \frac{(X - k_3)_+^3 (k_2 - k_1)}{(k_3 - k_2)} \right\},
\end{aligned}
$$

where the function $(u)_+$ is defined as

$$(u)_+ = \begin{cases} 0, & u \le 0 \\ u, & u > 0 \end{cases}$$

and the logit is

$$g(\mathbf{x}_c, \boldsymbol{\beta}_c) = \beta_{c0} + \beta_{c1} x_{c1} + \beta_{c2} x_{c2}. \qquad (4.2)$$

The restricted cubic spline covariate, x_{c2}, is obviously much more complex and more difficult to understand from its formula than the linear spline covariates. The value of this covariate in each of the four intervals is as follows:

$$
x_{c2} = \begin{cases}
0 & \text{if } X < k_1, \\[2mm]
\frac{(X-k_1)^3}{(k_3-k_1)^2} = \frac{X_*^3}{c^2} & \text{if } k_1 \le X < k_2, \\[2mm]
\frac{1}{(k_3-k_1)^2} \left\{ (X-k_1)^3 - \frac{(X-k_2)^3(k_3-k_1)}{(k_3-k_2)} \right\} & \\
\quad = -\frac{a}{bc^2} \{ X_*^3 - 3cX_*^2 + 3acX_* - a^2 c \} & \text{if } k_2 \le X < k_3, \\[2mm]
\frac{1}{(k_3-k_1)^2} \left\{ (X-k_1)^3 - \frac{(X-k_2)^3(k_3-k_1)}{(k_3-k_2)} + \frac{(X-k_3)^3(k_2-k_1)}{(k_3-k_2)} \right\} & \text{if } k_3 \le X, \\
\quad = \frac{a}{c}[3X_* - (a+c)] &
\end{cases}
$$

where

$$X_* = X - k_1, \ a = k_2 - k_1, \ b = k_3 - k_2, \text{ and } \ c = a + b. \qquad (4.3)$$

Obviously, one could use as many or as few knots as one wished. The more knots one chooses the more flexible the resulting fit, but at a price of more parameters to estimate. In most applications three to five knots are sufficient. One could choose the knots to be equally spaced over the range of the covariate. For example, if the range of the covariate was from 0 to 50 and one wanted four knots then one could choose values 10, 20, 30, and 40. One might choose equally spaced percentiles,

Table 4.1 Distribution Percentiles Defining Placement of Knots for Splines

# of Knots	Percentiles					
3	10	50	90			
4	5	35	65	95		
5	5	27.5	50	73.5	95	
6	5	23	41	59	77	95
7	2.5	18.33	34.17	65.83	81.67	97.5

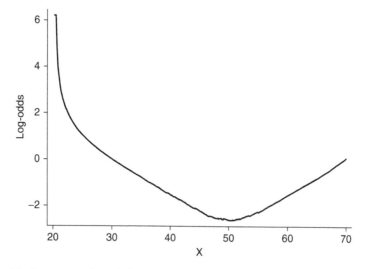

Figure 4.1   Lowess smooth on the log-odds scale of outcome Y versus the covariate X, $n = 500$.

for example, the 25th, 50th and 75th for three knots. Alternatively, Harrell (2001) provides percentiles, for three to seven knots, that have been shown in simulations to provide a good fit to wide range of shapes. These are given in Table 4.1.

Before we use purposeful selection with one of our data sets to build a model we present an example illustrating each of the four methods to examine the scale of a continuous covariate. The data are hypothetical and have been generated with a slightly asymmetric but quadratic-like shape. The data are available as Scale_Example and contain 500 observations of a continuous covariate, X, ranging from 20 to 70 and a binary outcome, Y, coded 0 and 1.

The first method discussed in this section is the graphical presentation of the lowess smooth of the outcome versus the covariate. This was computed in STATA and is shown in Figure 4.1. Recall that the lowess smooth provides a nonparametric description of the relationship between the logit or log-odds and the covariate. Hence, if there is any nonlinearity in the relationship it should be apparent in this plot. In fact, in this example, the departure from linearity is easily seen in Figure 4.1. The relationship is clearly asymmetric in shape. However, describing its shape mathematically from the figure would represent a challenge that is beyond the capabilities of most readers (and even the authors) of this book. Hence, the lowess smooth, while quite useful for displaying nonlinearity in the logit does not lend itself well to modeling decisions about what the correct scale might actually be.

When faced with a complex relationship like the one shown in Figure 4.1 subject matter investigators might decide to categorize the covariate into four groups, effectively using the quartile design variables. We categorized X into four groups using cutpoints of 32, 44, and 56, which are the quartiles rounded to whole numbers. The estimated coefficients and standard errors for this logistic model are presented in Table 4.2. As described earlier, to check linearity in the logit we would plot each of the coefficients versus the midpoint of the interval, using 0.0 as the coefficient for the first quartile. Were we to present this plot it would show the log-odds ratios [each point comparing the log-odds for each quartile to the log-odds for the first quartile (i.e., the reference group)]. However, to compare the lowess smooth to the fitted model in Table 4.2 we need to plot its linear predictor (i.e., the logit, or log-odds). To plot the fitted logit values computed from the model in Table 4.2 we compute the following:

$$\text{logit}(X) = \beta_0 + \beta_1 \times (X\_2) + \beta_2 \times (X\_3) + \beta_3 \times (X\_4)$$

$$= \begin{cases} 0.754 - 2.213\,(0) - 4.451(0) - 1.992(0) & \text{if } X < 32 \\ 0.754 - 2.213\,(1) - 4.451(0) - 1.992(0) & \text{if } 32 \leq X < 44 \\ 0.754 - 2.213\,(0) - 4.451(1) - 1.992(0) & \text{if } 44 \leq X < 56 \\ 0.754 - 2.213\,(0) - 4.451(0) - 1.992(1) & \text{if } 56 \leq X. \end{cases}$$

This provides the values needed for the step function seen in Figure 4.2.

Next, we fit the model using linear splines with knots at 32, 44, and 56. The fit of the model using four linear splines in equation (4.1) is shown in Table 4.3. Due to the way the spline variables were created the coefficients estimate the slope of the logit in each interval. The magnitude of the slopes agrees with the plot in Figure 4.1, in that they become progressively less negative and then positive.

In order to compare the three approaches illustrated so far, we plot each on the same set of axes in Figure 4.2. In addition, we plot the value of the linear spline fit at each of the three knots. In order to better compare the linear spline fit to the fit from the quartile design variables, we plot the mean value of the logit from the linear spline fit within each quartile versus the midpoint of the quartile. In looking

Table 4.2   Results of Fitting the Logistic Regression Model with Quartile Design Variables (X_j), $n = 500$

Variable	Coeff.	Std. Err.	z	p
X_2	−2.213	0.3006	−7.36	<0.001
X_3	−4.451	0.6151	−7.24	<0.001
X_4	−1.992	0.2850	−6.99	<0.001
Constant	0.754	0.1917	3.93	<0.001

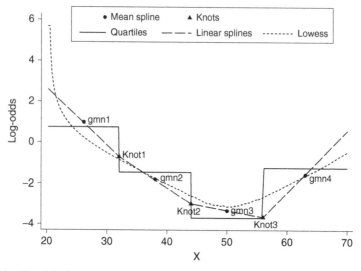

Figure 4.2   Plot of the fitted model using quartiles (——), linear splines (– –), and the lowess smooth (--). Also shown are the three knots (Knot j, △) and the mean of the linear spline fit within each quartile (gmn j, •), $n = 500$.

Table 4.3   Results of Fitting the Logistic Regression Model with Linear Spline Variables at Knots 32, 44, and 56, $n = 500$

Variable	Coeff.	Std. Err.	z	p
x_{l1}	−0.280	0.0552	−5.08	<0.001
x_{l2}	−0.191	0.0542	−3.52	<0.001
x_{l3}	−0.055	0.0673	−0.81	0.418
x_{l4}	0.302	0.0591	5.12	<0.001
Constant	8.263	1.5619	5.29	<0.001

at the plot several things become apparent: The fits from the linear splines and quartile design variables follow the lowess smooth to the extent that their inherent discreteness allows. The fit from the quartile design variables approximates quite closely the mean of the fit from the linear splines. So, in essence, one might say that using quartile design variables is a "poor man's" linear spline fit. Lastly, both fits are just too discrete to help suggest a model that could capture the nonlinearity seen in the lowess smooth.

In order to better explore the complicated nonlinear relationship between the logit of Y and X we display the results of using fractional polynomials in Table 4.4. The values in the column "Dev. Dif." present the difference between the deviance from the model defined by the row and that of the two-term model in the last row. This is the closed test procedure. The fact that the p-values are <0.001 in each row tells us that the two-term fractional polynomial $(2, 2)$ is significantly different (better) than the model fit in each row. In particular, it is better than both the

Table 4.4 Results of the Fractional Polynomial Analysis

X	df	Deviance	Dev. Dif.	p	Powers
Not in model	0	592.953	206.085	<0.001	
Linear	1	521.007	134.14	<0.001	1
$m = 1$	2	452.668	65.8	<0.001	−2
$m = 2$	4	386.868			2 2

linear fit and the one-term fractional polynomial model with power −2. Hence, from a purely statistical view point we would choose the two-term model. Recall the powers (2, 2) means that this model contains X^2 and $X^2 \times \ln(X)$. The fit of this model is shown in Table 4.5.

The results in Table 4.5 indicate that the coefficients for both fractional polynomial variables are significant, but it is difficult to tell what the shape of the resulting logit as a function of the covariate X would be by simply looking at the coefficients. (Note that we divided X by 10 in calculating $Xfp1$ and $Xfp2$ so that the estimated coefficients are not excessively small.) The best and easiest way to make some judgment about shape is to examine the plot of the function. This is shown as the solid line in Figure 4.3.

Next, we fit the model with restricted cubic splines. The results are presented in Table 4.6. The first thing we note about the fit in Table 4.6 is that both estimated coefficients are significant, but are of a completely different magnitude than those for the fractional polynomial model in Table 4.5. Again, the only way to really understand the fit is via a plot. Figure 4.3 now includes the fit from the restricted cubic spline model and the lowess smooth in addition to the fractional polynomial model described earlier.

It is difficult to see from the plots in Figure 4.3 which of the two models fits better in the sense of mimicking the lowess fit. However, the deviance of the fractional polynomial model is 386.868 while that of the restricted cubic spline model is 395.128, a difference of 8.260, which suggests that the fractional polynomial model has the better fit. We also note that the fractional polynomial model appears to model the asymmetry better than the restricted cubic spline model. The knots used correspond to the quartiles and not the 10th, 50th, and 90th percentiles as suggested in Table 4.1. The fit using these knots (24, 44, and 66) had just a slightly

Table 4.5 Results of Fitting the Two-Term Fractional Polynomial (2, 2) Model, $n = 500$

Variable	Coeff.	Std. Err.	z	p
$Xfp1$	−1.883	0.1751	−10.75	<0.001
$Xfp2$	0.892	0.0843	10.58	<0.001
Constant	7.959	0.7874	10.11	<0.001

$Xfp1 = (X/10)^2$ and $Xfp2 = (X/10)^2 \times \ln(X/10)$

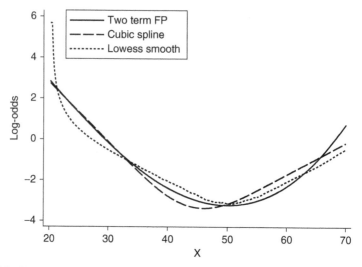

Figure 4.3 Plot of the fitted model using the two-term fractional polynomial (——), restricted cubic splines (– –), and the lowess smooth (--).

Table 4.6   Results of Fitting the Restricted Cubic Spline Model with Knots at 32, 33, and 56, $n = 500$

Variable	Coeff.	Std. Err.	z	p
x_{c1}	−0.292	0.0274	−10.67	<0.001
x_{c2}	0.298	0.0313	9.51	<0.001
Constant	8.639	0.8706	9.92	<0.001

smaller deviance, 391.646. Using four knots placed at the percentiles in Table 4.1 yields a model with effectively the same deviance as the fractional polynomial model, but at a cost of more parameters and much more complex parameterization of X. Hence our conclusion is that, based on statistical considerations, the two-term fractional polynomial model provides the better nonlinear fit from among the models explored. The phrase "statistical considerations" is an important qualifier, as the resulting shape of the logit must make clinical sense before it is used in further modeling. One other point, which we do not illustrate here, is that estimating odds ratios is considerably easier with fractional polynomial models than it is with restricted cubic spline models. Thus, if the goal is to model a nonlinear logit and to then estimate odds ratios for this covariate we highly recommend using fractional polynomials over restricted cubic splines. On the other hand if the goal is simply to model nonlinearity in the logit to control for confounding without odds ratio estimation then restricted cubic splines offer the possibility to model a quite complex relationship without actually having to specify its parametric form.

One special type of "continuous" variable that occurs reasonably often in practice is one that has many values at "zero". Consider a study in which subjects are asked to report their lifetime use of cigarettes. All the nonsmokers report a value of zero. A one-half pack-a-day smoker for 20 years has a value of approximately 73,000 cigarettes. What makes this covariate unusual is the fact that the zero value occurs with a frequency much greater than expected for a fully continuous distribution. In addition, the nonzero values typically exhibit right skewness. Robertson et al. (1994) show that the correct way to model such a covariate is to include two terms, one that is dichotomous recording zero versus nonzero and one for the actual recorded value. Thus, the logit for such a model is

$$g(x, \beta) = \beta_0 + \beta_1 d + \beta_2 x,$$

where $d = 0$ if $x = 0$ and $d = 1$ if $x > 0$. The advantage of this parameterization is that it allows us to model two different odds ratios. The odds ratio comparing a nonsmoker to a smoker with x^* lifetime cigarettes is

$$OR(x = x^*, x = 0) = e^{\beta_1 + \beta_2 x^*}$$

and the odds ratio for an increase of c in lifetime cigarettes is

$$OR(x = x + c, x = x) = e^{\beta_2 c}.$$

Note that during the modeling process we still need to check the scale in the logit for the positive values of the covariate. Since the distribution of x is typically skewed, fractional polynomial analysis often suggests using the one-term transformations $\ln(x)$ or $\sqrt{x}$. As noted above, odds ratios can be estimated by following the four step method discussed in Chapter 3.

4.2.2 Examples of Purposeful Selection

Example 1: The GLOW Study. For our first example of purposeful selection we use the GLOW500 data. This study is described in detail in Section 1.6.3 and the variables are described in Table 1.7. Before beginning, we remind the reader that these data are a sample from the much larger GLOW study. In particular, we over sampled fractures to obtain a modest sized data set where meaningful model building would be possible. This analysis provides a good example of an analysis designed to identify risk factors for a specified binary outcome. In this example, the outcome is fracture during the first year of follow up. Among the 500 women in this data set 125 (25%) had an incident fracture.

> *Step 1:* The first step in purposeful selection is to fit a univariable logistic regression model for each covariate. The results of this analysis are shown in Table 4.7. Note that in this table, each row presents the results for the estimated regression coefficient(s) from a model containing only that covariate.

Table 4.7 Results of Fitting Univariable Logistic Regression Models in the GLOW Data, $n = 500$

	Coeff.	Std. Err.	$\widehat{OR}$	95% CI	G	p
AGE	0.053	0.0116	1.30[a]	1.16, 1.46	21.27	<0.001
WEIGHT	−0.0052	0.0064	0.97[b]	0.91, 1.04	0.67	0.415
HEIGHT	−0.052	0.0171	0.60[c]	0.43, 0.83	9.53	0.002
BMI	0.006	0.0172	1.03[d]	0.87, 1.22	0.11	0.738
PRIORFRAC	1.064	0.2231	2.90	1.87, 4.49	22.27	<0.001
PREMENO	0.051	0.2592	1.05	0.63, 1.75	0.04	0.845
MOMFRAC	0.661	0.2810	1.94	1.12, 3.36	5.27	0.022
ARMASSIST	0.709	0.2098	2.03	1.35, 3.07	11.41	0.001
SMOKE	−0.308	0.4358	0.74	0.31, 1.73	0.53	0.469
RATERISK						
RATERISK_2	0.546	0.2664	1.73	1.02, 2.91	11.76	0.003
RATERISK_3	0.909	0.2711	2.48	1.46, 4.22		

[a]Odds Ratio for a 5-year increase in AGE.
[b]Odds Ratio for a 5 kg increase in WEIGHT.
[c]Odds Ratio for a 10 cm increase in HEIGHT.
[d]Odds Ratio for a 5 kg/m^2 increase in BMI.

Table 4.8 Results of Fitting the Multivariable Model with All Covariates Significant at the 0.25 Level in the Univariable Analysis in the GLOW Data, $n = 500$

	Coeff.	Std. Err.	z	p	95% CI
AGE	0.034	0.0130	2.63	0.008	0.009, 0.060
HEIGHT	−0.044	0.0183	−2.40	0.016	−0.080, −0.008
PRIORFRAC	0.645	0.2461	2.62	0.009	0.163, 1.128
MOMFRAC	0.621	0.3070	2.02	0.043	0.020, 1.223
ARMASSIST	0.446	0.2328	1.91	0.056	−0.011, 0.902
RATERISK_2	0.422	0.2792	1.51	0.131	−0.1253, 0.969
RATERISK_3	0.707	0.2934	2.41	0.016	0.132, 1.282
Constant	2.709	3.2299	0.84	0.402	−3.621, 9.040

Step 2: We now fit our first multivariable model that contains all covariates that are significant in univariable analysis at the 25% level. The results of this fit are shown in Table 4.8. Once this model is fit we examine each covariate to ascertain its continued significance, at traditional levels, in the model. We see that the covariate with the largest *p*-value that is greater than 0.05 is for RATERISK2, the design/dummy variable that compares women with RATERISK = 2 to women with RATERISK = 1. The likelihood ratio test for the exclusion of self-reported risk of fracture (i.e., deleting RATERISK_2 and RATERISK_3 from the model) is $G = 5.96$, which with two degrees of freedom, yields $p = 0.051$, nearly significant at the 0.05 level.

Step 3: Next we check to see if covariate(s) removed from the model in Step 2 confound or are needed to adjust the effects of covariates remaining in the model. In results not shown, we find that the largest percent change is 17% for the coefficient of ARMASSIST. This does not exceed our criterion of 20%. Thus, we see that while self-reported rate of risk is not a confounder it is an important covariate. No other covariates are candidates for exclusion and thus, we continue using the model in Table 4.8.

Step 4: On univariable analysis the covariates for weight (WEIGHT), body mass index (BMI), early menopause (PREMENO) and smoking (SMOKE) were not significant. When each of these covariates is added, one at a time, to the model in Table 4.8 its coefficient did not become significant. The only change of note is that the significance of BMI changed from 0.752 to 0.334. Thus the next step is to check the assumption of linearity in the logit of continuous covariates age and height.

Before moving to step 5 we consider another possible model. Since the coefficient for RATERISK_2 is not significant, one possibility is to combine levels 1 and 2, self-reported risk less than or the same as other women, into a new reference category. The advantage of this is that the new covariate is dichotomous, but we loose information about the specific log-odds of categories 1 and 2. On consultation with subject matter investigators, it was thought that combining these two categories is reasonable. Hence we fit this model and its results are shown in Table 4.9. In this model, the coefficient for the covariate RATERISK_3 now provides the estimate of the log of the odds ratio comparing the odds of fracture for individuals in level 3 to that of the combined group consisting of levels 1 and 2.

Step 5: At this point we have our preliminary main effects model and must now check for the scale of the logit for continuous covariates age and height. We presented four different methods in Section 4.2.1: the lowess smooth, quartile design variables, fractional polynomials and spline functions. In most applied settings we would always use the lowess smooth and fractional polynomials and also do so here. We also illustrate the design variable approach, as it is always an option. We reserve use of spline functions to settings where the best two-term fractional polynomial model does not seem to provide an adequate representation of the what we see in the lowess smooth.

Table 4.9   Results of Fitting the Multivariable Model after Collapsing Rate Risk into Two Categories, $n = 500$

	Coeff.	Std. Err.	z	p	95% CI	
AGE	0.033	0.0129	2.56	0.010	0.008,	0.059
HEIGHT	−0.046	0.0181	−2.55	0.011	−0.082,	−0.011
PRIORFRAC	0.664	0.2452	2.71	0.007	0.184,	1.145
MOMFRAC	0.664	0.3056	2.17	0.030	0.065,	1.263
ARMASSIST	0.473	0.2313	2.04	0.041	0.019,	0.926
RATERISK_3	0.458	0.2381	1.92	0.054	−0.009,	0.925
Constant	3.407	3.1770	1.07	0.284	−2.820,	9.633

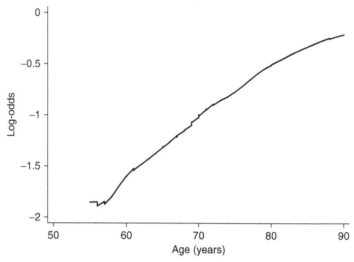

Figure 4.4 Lowess smooth on the log-odds scale of the outcome, fracture during the first year of follow-up, versus AGE, $n = 500$.

Table 4.10   Results of the Quartile Design Variable Analyses of AGE (x) from the Multivariable Model Containing the Variables Shown in the Model in Table 4.9

Quartile	1	2	3	4
Range	$x < 62$	$62 \leq x < 68$	$68 \leq x < 77$	$77 \leq x$
Midpoint	58.5	65	72.5	83.5
Coeff.	0.0	0.610	0.590	0.970
95% CI		−0.059, 1.278	−0.050, 1.229	0.311, 1.629

The lowess smooth for the outcome fracture versus age on the logit or log-odds scale is shown in Figure 4.4. Other than an inconsequential wiggle over age less than about 58, the plotted lowess smooth appears nearly linear, suggesting that there is no reason to suspect that the logit is not linear in age.

Next we examine the scale of age in the logit using quartile design variables. The results of the fit for age when it is replaced with quartile design variables in the multivariable model (Table 4.9) are shown in Table 4.10 and are plotted in Figure 4.5.

The confidence intervals for the coefficients in Table 4.10 for quartiles two and three each contain one, while that for the fourth quartile does not contain one. This suggests that the log-odds for fracture does not seem to increase significantly until after about age 72. Based on these results one might be tempted to replace age, as represented by a continuous variable, with a dichotomous variable that uses the design variable for the fourth quartile. This portrays a slightly different picture than that seen in Figure 4.4, where the lowess smoothed logit increases gradually over the entire range of age. We return to this point after performing the fractional polynomial analysis of age.

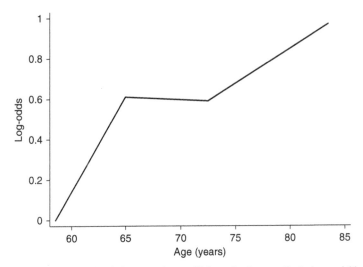

Figure 4.5 Plot of estimated logistic regression coefficients for the quartile design variables versus approximate quartile midpoints of AGE.

Table 4.11 Results of the Fractional Polynomial Analysis of AGE

	df	Deviance	Dev. dif.	p	Powers
Not in Model	0	516.421	7.468	0.113	
Linear	1	509.818	0.865	0.834	1
$m = 1$	2	509.257	0.304	0.859	-2
$m = 2$	4	508.953			3 3

The results of the fractional polynomial analysis are shown in Table 4.11. In general, when we perform a fractional polynomial analysis we proceed under the assumption that we have already decided that it is important to have the covariate in the model. Hence, we tend to ignore the results in the first row that compares the best two-term fractional polynomial model to the model not containing the covariate. The first test we look at is the one in the second row that compares the best two-term fractional polynomial model to the model treating the covariate as linear in the logit, indicated by "1" in the Powers column. In Table 4.11 the value of the likelihood ratio test is given in the "Dev. Dif." column and its p-value is in the "p" column. In this case, the test is not significant as $p = 0.834$, leading to the conclusion that the best fractional polynomial transformation is not better than the linear model. While the closed test procedure stops at this point, we always examine the results in the last two rows to see what transformations have been selected and to make sure we have not missed anything. In this case, all signs point toward treating age as linear in the logit.

The fact that the lowess smooth looks quite linear and that the supporting results from the factional polynomial analysis suggest that nothing new could be learned about the scale of the logit in AGE from a spline variable analysis. Hence, we choose not to use it.

We remarked in discussing the plot of the quartile design variables that one might elect to dichotomize AGE at the fourth quartile. Categorization of a continuous covariate is, unfortunately, a relatively common practice in many applied fields. The temptation of its simplicity seems, in the minds of proponents, to outweigh the considerable loss of information about the covariate in such a strategy. See Royston et al. (2006) for a full discussion of the pitfalls of dichotomizing a continuous covariate. In results we do not show, but leave as an exercise, the deviance from the model using the dichotomous version of AGE is larger than that of the model in Table 4.9. Thus our decision is to treat AGE as continuous and linear in the logit.

Next we examine the continuous variable HEIGHT to determine whether it is linear in the logit. The plots of two lowess smooths on the logit scale are shown in Figure 4.6. The solid line corresponds to the smooth using all 500 subjects, while the dashed line is the smooth when one subject with a height of 199 cm is excluded. We excluded this subject to see what effect she had on the shape of the smooth. Neither smooth appears to be linear for heights less than 180 cm. The question is whether this represents a "significant" departure from linear. We examine this question using both quartile design variables and fractional polynomials (as shown in Figure 4.7).

The plot of the estimated coefficients from the quartile design variables for height shown in Figure 4.7 are based on fitting a model with $n = 500$, as the 199 cm tall woman has little effect on the coefficient in the last column of Table 4.12. The plot

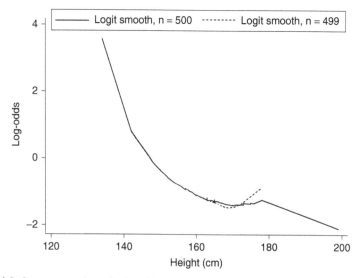

Figure 4.6 Lowess smooth on the log-odds scale of the outcome, fracture during the first year of follow up, versus HEIGHT, $n = 500$ (solid) and $n = 499$ (dashed).

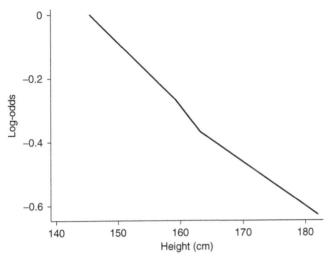

Figure 4.7 Plot of estimated logistic regression coefficients for the quartile design variables versus approximate quartile midpoints of HEIGHT.

Table 4.12   Results of the Quartile Design Variable Analyses of HEIGHT from the Multivariable Model Containing the Variables Shown in the Model in Table 4.9

Quartile	1	2	3	4
Range	$x \leq 157$	$157 < x \leq 161.5$	$161.5 < x \leq 165$	$x > 165$
Midpoint	145.5	159.25	163.25	182
Coeff.	0.0	−0.266	−0.369	−0.628
95% CI		−0.861, 0.329	−0.964, 0.226	−1.255, −0.001

Table 4.13   Results of the Fractional Polynomial Analysis of HEIGHT

	df	Deviance	Dev. Dif.	p	Powers
Not in Model	0	516.558	8.574	0.073	
Linear	1	509.818	1.834	0.608	1
$m = 1$	2	509.137	1.154	0.562	−2
$m = 2$	4	507.984			−2 −2

is strikingly linear, giving a different impression of the parametric form than what is seen in Figure 4.6.

We turn to fractional polynomials to sort out the discrepancies seen in Figure 4.6 and Figure 4.7. These results are shown in Table 4.13 where we see that the two-term fractional polynomial with powers $(-2, -2)$ is far from significantly different from the linear model. We ran the analysis excluding the 199 cm woman and the results are not appreciably different from those in Table 4.13. Hence our conclusion is to treat HEIGHT as linear in the logit. For the time being, we are going to retain

Table 4.14   **Log-Likelihood, Likelihood Ratio Test (G, df = 1), and p-Value for the Addition of the Interactions to the Main Effects Model**

Interaction	Log-Likelihood	G	p
Main Effects Model	−254.9089		
AGE*HEIGHT	−254.8422	0.13	0.715
AGE*PRIORFRAC	−252.3921	5.03	0.025
AGE*MOMFRAC	−254.8395	0.14	0.710
AGE*ARMASSIST	−254.8358	0.15	0.702
AGE*RATERISK3	−254.3857	1.05	0.306
HEIGHT*PRIORFRAC	−254.8024	0.21	0.645
HEIGHT*MOMFRAC	−253.7043	2.41	0.121
HEIGHT*ARMASSIST	−254.1112	1.60	0.207
HEIGHT*RATERISK3	−254.4218	0.97	0.324
PRIORFRAC*MOMFRAC	−253.5093	2.80	0.094
PRIORFRAC*ARMASSIST	−254.7962	0.23	0.635
PRIORFRAC*RATERISK3	−254.8476	0.12	0.726
MOMFRAC*ARMASSIST	−252.5179	4.78	0.029
MOMFRAC*RATERISK3	−254.6423	0.53	0.465
ARMASSIST*RATERISK3	−253.7923	2.23	0.135

the 199 cm woman in the analysis, waiting until we examine her influence using diagnostic statistics in Chapter 5. Hence our final main effects model is the one whose fit is shown in Table 4.9.

> *Step 6:* The next step in the purposeful selection procedure is to explore possible interactions among the main effects. The subject matter investigators felt that each pair of main effects represents a plausible interaction. Hence, we fit models that individually added each of the 15 possible interactions to the main effects model. The results are summarized in Table 4.14. Three interactions are significant at the 10 percent level: Age by prior fracture (PRIORFRAC), prior fracture by mother had a fracture (MOMFRAC) and mother had a fracture by arms needed to rise from a chair (ARMASSIST). We note that prior fracture and mother having had a fracture are involved in two of the three significant interactions.

> The next step is to fit a model containing the main effects and the three significant interactions. The results of this fit are shown in Table 4.15. The three degree of freedom likelihood ratio test of the interactions model in Table 4.15 versus the main effects model in Table 4.9 is $G = 11.03$ with $p = 0.012$. Thus, in aggregate, the interactions contribute to the model. However, one interaction, prior fracture by mother's fracture, is not significant with a Wald statistic $p = 0.191$. Next, we fit the model excluding this interaction and the results are shown in Table 4.16.

The estimated coefficients in the interactions model in Table 4.16 are, with one exception, significant at the five percent level. The exception is the estimated coefficient for the dichotomized self-reported risk of fracture, RATERISK3

Table 4.15 Results of Fitting the Multivariable Model with the Addition of Three Interactions, $n = 500$

	Coeff.	Std. Err.	z	p	95% CI	
AGE	0.058	0.0166	3.49	0.000	0.025,	0.091
HEIGHT	−0.049	0.0184	−2.65	0.008	−0.085,	−0.013
PRIORFRAC	4.598	1.8780	2.45	0.014	0.917,	8.278
MOMFRAC	1.472	0.4229	3.48	0.000	0.644,	2.301
ARMASSIST	0.626	0.2538	2.46	0.014	0.128,	1.123
RATERISK3	0.474	0.2410	1.97	0.049	0.002,	0.947
AGE*PRIORFRAC	−0.053	0.0259	−2.05	0.040	−0.104,	−0.002
PRIORFRAC*MOMFRAC	−0.847	0.6475	−1.31	0.191	−2.116,	0.422
MOMFRAC*ARMASSIST	−1.167	0.6168	−1.89	0.058	−2.376,	0.042
Constant	1.959	3.3272	0.59	0.556	−4.562,	8.481

Table 4.16 Results of Fitting the Multivariable Model with the Significant Interactions, $n = 500$

	Coeff.	Std. Err.	z	p	95% CI	
AGE	0.057	0.0165	3.47	0.001	0.025,	0.090
HEIGHT	−0.047	0.0183	−2.55	0.011	−0.083,	−0.011
PRIORFRAC	4.612	1.8802	2.45	0.014	0.927,	8.297
MOMFRAC	1.247	0.3930	3.17	0.002	0.476,	2.017
ARMASSIST	0.644	0.2519	2.56	0.011	0.150,	1.138
RATERISK3	0.469	0.2408	1.95	0.051	−0.003,	0.941
AGE*PRIORFRAC	−0.055	0.0259	−2.13	0.033	−0.106,	−0.004
MOMFRAC*ARMASSIST	−1.281	0.6230	−2.06	0.040	−2.502,	−0.059
Constant	1.717	3.3218	0.52	0.605	−4.793,	8.228

(1 = more, 0 = same or less) with $p = 0.051$. We elect to retain this in the model since the covariate is clinically important and its significance is nearly five percent. Hence the model in Table 4.16 is our preliminary final model. Its fit, adherence to model assumptions and assessment for influence of individual subjects is examined in Chapter 5. Following this assessment we present the results of the model in terms of odds ratios for estimates of the effect of each covariate on fracture during the first year of follow up.

In summary, our first example of model building using purposeful selection with the GLOW data illustrated: selecting variables, examining the scale in the logit for two continuous covariates and selecting and refining interactions. The resulting model in Table 4.16 is, in a sense, relatively simple in that it contains only two interactions. There was no statistical evidence of nonlinearity in the logit for the two continuous covariates.

Example 2: The Burn Injury Study. The second example is one where the goal is to obtain a model that could be used for estimating the probability of the response, as well as, to some extent, for quantifying the effect of individual risk factors. We use the Burn Injury Study data described in Section 1.6.5 and Table 1.9. The data, BURN1000, contain information on a burn injury for 1000 subjects, 150 of whom died. As noted in Section 1.6.5 these data were sampled from a much larger data set and deaths were over sampled. Since the goal is to develop a model to estimate the probability of death from burn injury we would like a parsimonious model that would be likely to perform well in another data set. As we show later, these data illustrate some of the challenges that one can face when modeling a continuous covariate that is nonlinear in the logit. There are only six covariates and we have a large total sample size (1000) and number of outcomes (150), so rather than perform steps 1 and 2, we begin by fitting the model containing all covariates. The results of this fit are shown in Table 4.17.

In Table 4.17 the Wald test for the coefficient for GENDER is not significant with $p = 0.513$ and that of FLAME has $p = 0.100$. When we delete GENDER and refit the model the significance of the Wald test for FLAME becomes $p = 0.094$ and there is no evidence of confounding by GENDER. After consultation with an experienced burn surgeon, we decided to remove FLAME from the model for the reason that there are many different ways that flame could be involved with a burn injury and using simple yes or no coding is not precise enough to be helpful. In addition, we are striving for a model that is as parsimonious as possible. Thus our preliminary main effects model contains only four covariates: age (AGE), burn surface area (TBSA), race (RACE: 0 = non-white, 1 = white) and inhalation injury involved (INH_INJ, 0 = no, 1 = yes). The results of this fit are shown in Table 4.18.

Table 4.17   Results of Fitting a Multivariable Model to the Burn Injury Data Containing All Available Covariates, $n = 1000$

	Coeff.	Std. Err.	z	p	95% CI
AGE	0.083	0.0086	9.61	<0.001	0.066, 0.100
TBSA	0.089	0.0091	9.83	<0.001	0.072, 0.107
GENDER	−0.201	0.3078	−0.65	0.513	−0.805, 0.402
RACE	−0.701	0.3098	−2.26	0.024	−1.309, −0.094
INH_INJ	1.365	0.3618	3.77	<0.001	0.656, 2.074
FLAME	0.583	0.3545	1.64	0.100	−0.112, 1.277
Constant	−7.695	0.6912	−11.13	<0.001	−9.050, −6.341

Table 4.18   Preliminary Main Effects Model for the Burn Injury Data, $n = 1000$

	Coeff.	Std. Err.	z	p	95% CI
AGE	0.084	0.0085	9.95	<0.001	0.068, 0.101
TBSA	0.090	0.0091	9.95	<0.001	0.073, 0.108
RACE	−0.624	0.2989	−2.09	0.037	−1.209, −0.038
INH_INJ	1.523	0.3512	4.34	<0.001	0.835, 2.211
Constant	−7.595	0.6090	−12.47	<0.001	−8.788, −6.401

Table 4.19   Results of the Quartile Design Variable Analyses of the Scale of AGE

Quartile	1	2	3	4
Range	$x \le 10.8$	$10.8 < x \le 31.9$	$31.9 < x \le 51.2$	$51.2 < x$
Midpoint	5.45	21.35	41.55	70.45
Coeff.	0.0	−0.483	1.139	3.770
95% CI		−1.994, 1.029	−0.066, 2.343	2.629, 4.912

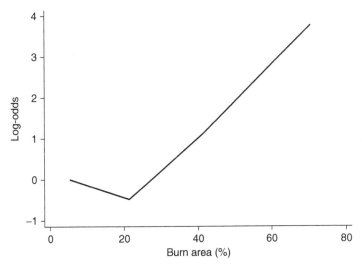

Figure 4.8 Plot of estimated logistic regression coefficients for the quartile design variables versus approximate quartile midpoints of AGE.

The next step is to examine the scale in the logit for age and burn surface area. We begin by considering age in the multivariable model in Table 4.18. The estimated coefficients for the quartile design variables are presented in Table 4.19 and plotted versus the quartile midpoints in Figure 4.8.

Only the estimated coefficient for the fourth versus the first quartile is significant. However, the plot shows that the log-odds of dying decreases and then increases, which makes clinical sense as subjects between 15 and 25, all things being equal, are known to have better outcomes than those who are younger or older. Next, we explore this in detail using the lowess smooth, fractional polynomials and restricted cubic splines.

The results of the fractional polynomial analysis of age are presented in Table 4.20. The p-values show that the two-term fractional polynomial model is better than the linear model at the 10% level but not different from the one-term fractional polynomial model. We know that a one-term fractional polynomial model is monotonic, so cannot be of the shape seen in Figure 4.8. Hence, at this point, we are going to consider both the one-term ($m = 1$) and two-term ($m = 2$)

Table 4.20   Results of the Fractional Polynomial Analysis of AGE

	df	Deviance	Dev. Dif.	p	Powers
Not in Model	0	520.362	187.147	<0.001	
Linear	1	339.785	6.569	0.087	1
$m = 1$	2	336.849	3.634	0.163	2
$m = 2$	4	333.215			3 3

fractional polynomial models as possible parameterizations of the scale of age in the logit.

Before moving on, we offer a few further comments on the models in Table 4.20. First, the model in the $m = 2$ row is the one with the numerically smallest deviance among the 36 two-term models fit. By using the "log" option in STATA we can obtain the value of the deviance for all models fit. Using this feature (output not shown) we find that there are three other two-term models [powers: $(1, 0.5)$, $(1, 1)$, and $(2, 3)$] with a deviance that differs by at most 0.7 from the best model. Note that the powers of these three models are, in a sense, no more easily interpreted than the best model's powers of $(3, 3)$. Thus, there is no compelling reason to use any one of those as an alternative to the $(3, 3)$ model. A natural follow up question is: If the best one-term model uses power 2, then, is the quadratic model $(1, 2)$ an option? In this case, the deviance for the quadratic model is 335.368, which is not significantly different from the deviance for the power 2 model as $G = 1.47$ and $p = 0.225$. Also, the second best one-term model is the linear model.

Hence, by using STATA's log option we have found another model, powers 1 and 2, that may be more easily interpreted than the best fractional polynomial model. If the goal of the analysis is to estimate measures of effect for risk factors for death following a burn injury then it would make good sense to use the quadratic model as it is more easily interpreted than the power 2 model by a subject matter audience. However, our modeling goal is not effect estimation but rather estimation of the probability of death following a burn injury. For the latter goal the smaller model, power 2, may be better than the larger model, powers 1 and 2. Also, we still have additional steps in model building to perform: examining the scale of percent body surface area burned in the logit and assess the need to include interactions. In practice we would likely perform the remaining steps for both parameterizations of age. Then we would assess model adequacy and performance using the methods discussed in Chapter 5 and choose the better of the two models. This is not practical in a text so we are going to proceed with the smaller, power 2 model and leave parallel model development and evaluation, using the quadratic parameterization of age as an exercise for the reader.

Next, we try modeling age using restricted cubic splines. We found (in work we do not show here but leave as an exercise) that the best spline model is one with four knots at the percentiles in Table 4.1. The values of these four knots are: 1.1, 19, 44.37, and 78.87 years of age. The fit of this model is shown in Table 4.21, where AGESPL1, AGESPL2, and AGESPL3 are the three restricted cubic splines

Table 4.21 Fit Modeling AGE with Restricted Cubic Splines Formed from Four Knots at 1.1, 19, 44.37 and 78.87 Years, $n = 1000$

	Coeff.	Std. Err.	z	p	95% CI
AGESPL1	−0.063	0.0608	−1.04	0.297	−0.182, 0.056
AGESPL2	0.507	0.2644	1.92	0.055	−0.011, 1.026
AGESPL3	−0.921	0.5208	−1.77	0.077	−1.941, 0.100
TBSA	0.091	0.0092	9.92	<0.001	0.073, 0.109
RACE	−0.562	0.3065	−1.83	0.067	−1.163, 0.039
INH_INJ	1.516	0.3565	4.25	<0.001	0.817, 2.215
Constant	−5.721	0.7578	−7.55	<0.001	−7.206, −4.236

in AGE created from the four knots using an extension of the three-knot spline variable shown in equation (4.3).

In order to compare the shape of the logit in AGE for the two fractional polynomial models and the cubic spline model compared to the lowess smooth we plot all four logit functions versus age. The three parametric logit functions were scaled so that their average is the same as the average of the lowess smoothed logit. The purpose of this is to obtain a plot where the four curves are more easily compared. As an example, what we calculated to plot for the cubic spline is

$$gspl = -0.063 \times AGESPL1 + 0.507 \times AGESPL2 - 0.921 \times AGESPL3.$$

We calculated the mean of $gspl$ and then added a constant to it so its mean would be equal to the mean of the lowess smooth. Similar calculations were performed using the estimated coefficient of AGE^2 to obtain $gfp1$, the mean adjusted one-term fractional polynomial model in AGE^2 and for $gfp2$, the mean adjusted two-term fractional polynomial model in AGE^3 and $AGE^3 \times \ln(AGE)$. These are shown in Figure 4.9.

We begin by comparing the four functions in the neighborhood of 20 years of age. The upper most of the four curves is the lowess smoothed logit, followed by the one-term fractional polynomial and the two-term fractional polynomial model. The lowest value results from the fit of the restricted cubic spline model. We see that the lowess smooth is nearly linear. The two fractional polynomial models are both increasing functions of age and are similar to each other, supporting $p = 0.163$ from Table 4.20. The plot of the restricted cubic spline fit has a dip, reaching its minimum at about 17 years of age and then it increases and nearly coincides with the two-term fractional polynomial model for age greater than 40. The plot of the restricted cubic spline also has the same form as the plot of the estimated coefficients from the quartile design variables in Figure 4.8.

The plots in Figure 4.9 leave us with some difficult choices. The most reasonable clinical model is the one using restricted cubic splines. However, it comes at the cost of having to use the three complex spline variables that are not easily explained, except in a figure, to clinicians. Thus, the effect of age would have to be estimated using the four-step procedure discussed in Chapter 3. The algebra necessary to

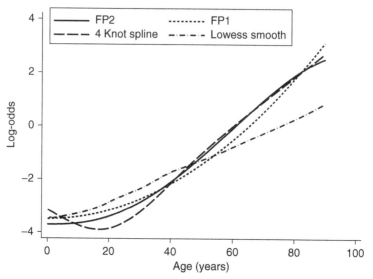

Figure 4.9   Plot of estimated logit from fits based on one (- - -) and two-term (——) fractional polynomials, restricted cubic spline (– – –), and the lowess smooth ($-\dot{c}-\dot{c}-$) of AGE. All fitted logistic
regression models contain TBSA, RACE and INH_INJ.

obtain the difference in the logits is quite complicated and would yield an extremely
complex equation in the spline variables and the three estimated coefficients in
Table 4.21. Hence, although this is a problem that has a solution and the method
for obtaining it is straightforward, the work involved is formidable. We note that
once done it could be programmed. Thus, if our goal was simply to model these
data we would choose to proceed with the restricted cubic splines. However, from
a practical point of view, our goal is to obtain a clinically interpretable model to
estimate the probability of death following a burn injury for potential use with
new data. Hence our decision is to use the simple one-term fractional polynomial
model as it is better than the linear model and as good as the two-term fractional
polynomial model.

Before we leave consideration of the functional form in age we discuss a statistical measure that is commonly used to compare models with different numbers of
parameters, the Akaike Information Criterion (AIC), Akaike (1974). This measure
is defined as

$$\text{AIC} = -2 \times L + 2 \times (p + 1), \tag{4.4}$$

where L is the log-likelihood of the fitted model and p is the number of regression coefficients estimated for nonconstant covariates. Note that in Chapters 1
and 2 we defined the deviance of the fitted model as $D = -2 \times L$, thus AIC $=$
$D + 2 \times (p + 1)$. In general, lower values of AIC are preferred to larger ones. In
the current example, the deviance from the fitted one-term fractional polynomial
model is $D = 336.842$. The model has five coefficients: an intercept and one each
for AGE^2, TBSA, RACE, and INH_INJ. For testing purposes the transformation,

Table 4.22 Results of the Quartile Design Variable Analyses of the Scale of TBSA

Quartile	1	2	3	4
Range	$x \leq 2.5$	$2.5 < x \leq 6$	$6 < x \leq 16$	$x > 16$
Midpoint	1.3	4.25	11.0	57.0
Coeff.	0.0	0.512	1.216	3.851
95% CI		$-0.729, 1.752$	$0.059, 2.372$	$2.758, 4.943$

power 2, is also considered as an estimated parameter. Hence, in this case we need to add $12 = 2 \times (4 + 1 + 1)$ to the deviance not $10 = 2 \times (4 + 1)$, yielding AIC = 348.842. The value of the deviance for the spline model is $D = 331.923$. This model contains seven parameters, thus AIC = 345.923, which is smaller than the AIC for the one-term factional polynomial model. Hence, all things being equal, we would prefer the spline to the one-term fractional polynomial model. However, all things are not really equal so the considerably greater complexity of the spline model leads us to choose the one-term fractional polynomial model, even though it has a larger value of AIC. There is no statistical test to compare values of AIC.

Now that we have decided what transformation to use for age we apply the same methods to check the scale of burn area (TBSA) in the logit. At this point, we are often asked if it is better to use the transformed version of a previously examined covariate or the untransformed form. In our practice, we have not seen a set of data where using different forms gives different results. We discuss a multivariable fractional polynomial selection method in Section 4.5 that uses an iterative process using all transforms from previous iterations. So, in the current example, we follow the guidelines for purposeful selection and use AGE (untransformed) when examining the scale of burn area.

We begin by replacing TBSA in the model with the quartile-based design variables. Results for the estimated coefficients are given in Table 4.22 and plotted versus the quartile midpoint in Figure 4.10. The plot shows some departure from linearity over the first three quartiles, from 0 to 11%. Since the fourth quartile covers such a wide range we cannot see any nonlinearity in the plot beyond 11%.

The next step is to use fractional polynomials, the results of which are shown in Table 4.23. The best two-term fractional polynomial has powers -2 and 0.5. It is significantly better than the linear model with $p = 0.013$ but is not better than the one-term fractional polynomial with power 0.5, the square root ($p = 0.772$). Hence, we select the one-term transformation as best. We note that the shape of the plot in Figure 4.10 in the region less than 11% looks like a square root plot. The shape also is consistent with the burn surgeon's clinical impression of the effect of the size of burn area on mortality. The fit of this model is presented in Table 4.24.

With such straightforward and clinically plausible results from the fractional polynomial analysis we would, likely, not bother with a restricted cubic splines analysis. However, as another opportunity to demonstrate this method, we include this analysis. For TBSA, splines from three knots at the 10th (1%), 50th (6%),

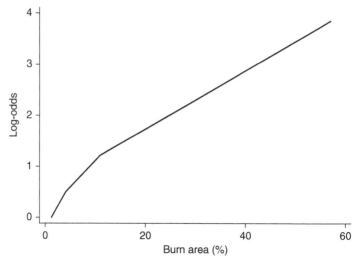

Figure 4.10 Plot of estimated logistic regression coefficients for the quartile design variables versus approximate quartile midpoints of TBSA.

Table 4.23   Results of the Fractional Polynomial Analysis of TBSA

	df	Deviance	Dev. Dif.	p	Powers
Not in Model	0	532.483	203.409	<0.001	
Linear	1	339.785	10.711	0.013	1
$m = 1$	2	329.592	0.518	0.772	.5
$m = 2$	4	329.074	—	—	−2 .5

Table 4.24   Fit of the Model Using $TBSAFP1 = \sqrt{TBSA}$, the One-Term Fractional Polynomial Transformation, $n = 1000$

	Coeff.	Std. Err.	z	p	95% CI
TBSAFP1	0.922	0.0871	10.59	<0.001	0.751, 1.092
AGE	0.085	0.0086	9.84	<0.001	0.068, 0.101
RACE	−0.623	0.3031	−2.05	0.040	−1.217, −0.029
INH_INJ	1.595	0.3463	4.60	<0.001	0.916, 2.273
Constant	−9.526	0.7544	−12.63	<0.001	−11.005, −8.048

and 90th (34.45%) percentiles of the distribution of burn area perform better (i.e., smaller deviance and AIC) than from four knots.

The results of the fit of the model using the two spline variables are shown in Table 4.25. In Figure 4.11 we plot the lowess smoothed logit and the mean adjusted logit from the one-term fractional polynomial fit,

$$gfp1 = 0.922 \times \sqrt{TBSA} - 5.468$$

Table 4.25   Fit Modeling TBSA with Restricted Cubic Splines Formed from Three Knots at 1.0, 6.0 and 34.45 Percent Burn Area, $n = 1000$

	Coeff.	Std. Err.	z	p	95% CI
TBSASPL1	0.217	0.0441	4.90	<0.001	0.130, 0.302
TBSASPL2	−0.331	0.1103	−3.00	0.003	−0.549, −0.116
AGE	0.085	0.0086	9.82	<0.001	0.068, 0.102
RACE	−0.637	0.3033	−2.10	0.036	−1.232, −0.043
INH_INJ	1.610	0.3506	4.59	<0.001	0.923, 2.297
Constant	−8.592	0.7387	−11.63	<0.001	−10.039, −7.143

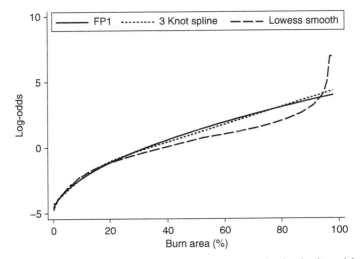

Figure 4.11   Plot of estimated logit from fits based on one-term (—) fractional polynomial, restricted cubic spline (···) and the lowess smooth (− − −) of TBSA. All fitted logistic regression models contain AGE, RACE, and INH_INJ.

and the spline fit in Table 4.25,

$$gspl = 0.217 \times TBSASPL1 - 0.331 \times TBSASPL2 - 4.331,$$

where the subtracted constants are the mean adjustments.

There is virtually no difference in the plot of the logit based on the square root of TBSA and the restricted cubic spline model. We note that the lowess smoothed logit departs from these two models above 40 percent burn area. While covering a large range there are fewer than 10% of the subjects with burns this severe. The deviance for the fractional polynomial model is $D = 329.589$ and, treating the power as an estimated parameter, yields AIC $= 329.589 + 2 \times (4 + 1 + 1) = 341.589$. The deviance for the spline model is $D = 330.299$ and AIC $= 330.299 + 2 \times (5 + 1) = 342.299$. Hence we choose the model containing AGE^2, the square root of TBSA, RACE and INH_INJ as our main effects model and its fit is shown in Table 4.26 where $AGEFP1 = (AGE/10)^2$, and $TBSAFP1 = \sqrt{TBSA}$.

Table 4.26   Main Effects Model for the Burn Injury Data, $n = 1000$

	Coeff.	Std. Err.	z	p	95% CI
AGEFP1	0.087	0.0082	10.53	<0.001	0.071, 0.103
TBSAFP1	0.936	0.0874	10.71	<0.001	0.765, 1.108
RACE	−0.609	0.3096	−1.97	0.049	−1.216, −0.002
INH_INJ	1.433	0.3421	4.19	<0.001	0.763, 2.104
Constant	−7.957	0.5967	−13.34	<0.001	−9.127, −6.788

Table 4.27   Preliminary Final Model With Interaction Term for the Burn Injury Data, $n = 1000$

	Coeff.	Std. Err.	z	p	95% CI
AGEFP1	0.096	0.0096	10.02	<0.001	0.077, 0.115
TBSAFP1	0.912	0.0878	10.39	<0.001	0.740, 1.084
RACE	−0.623	0.3100	−2.01	0.045	−1.231, −0.015
INH_INJ	2.420	0.5452	4.44	<0.001	1.351, 3.488
AFP1xINH	−0.034	0.0145	−2.35	0.019	−0.063, −0.006
Constant	−8.215	0.6314	−13.01	<0.001	−9.453, −6.978

The next step in the analysis is to select interactions. With only four main effects we examined all 6 possible interactions by adding one at a time to the model in Table 4.26. Two were significant at the 10 percent level: AGEFP1 by INH_INJ and TBSAFP1 by RACE. The interaction of TBSAFP1 by RACE did not make clinical sense to the burn surgeon and thus we excluded it from further consideration. The fit of the model with the interaction is shown in Table 4.27, where AFP1xINH denotes the interaction between AGEFP1 and INH_INJ.

Before leaving this example, let us revisit the goals of the analysis. The interaction term in Table 4.27 is highly significant, demonstrating that the presence or absence of inhalation involvement with the burn injury modifies the effect of age and, likewise, age modifies the effect of inhalation involvement. Clearly, if we were interested in estimating the effect of risk factors for death we would prefer the model in Table 4.27. However, it is not clear that inclusion of the interaction would improve estimation of the probability of death. Again, simpler is sometimes better, and so, for the time being, we are going to consider both models (the ones presented in Tables 4.26 and 4.27) as possible models until we evaluate their fit and performance in Chapter 5.

4.3   OTHER METHODS FOR SELECTING COVARIATES

In the previous section we discussed purposeful selection, a method that is completely controlled by the analyst, to select a subset of covariates from a larger collection. There are other commonly used methods where selection is more automated and statistically driven. Two approaches have a long history in statistical model building: stepwise selection and best subsets selection. A recent addition combines a version of stepwise selection with fractional polynomial modeling of continuous covariates. We consider each of these methods in this section and show how they are related to one another and compare them to purposeful selection in the context of modeling the GLOW data.

4.3.1 Stepwise Selection of Covariates

Stepwise selection of covariates has a long history in linear regression. All the major software packages have either a separate program or an option to perform this type of analysis. Currently, most, if not all, major software packages offer an option for stepwise logistic regression. At one time, stepwise regression was an extremely popular method for model building. Over the years there has been a shift away from deterministic methods for model building to methods like purposeful selection discussed in the previous section. However, we feel that stepwise methods may be useful as effective data analysis tools. In particular, there are times when the outcome being studied is relatively new and the important covariates may not be known and associations with the outcome not well understood. In these instances, most studies collect many possible covariates and screen them for significant associations. Employing a stepwise selection procedure can provide a fast and effective means to screen a large number of variables, and to fit a number of logistic regression equations simultaneously.

Any stepwise procedure for selection or deletion of variables from a model is based on a statistical algorithm that checks for the "importance" of variables, and either includes or excludes them on the basis of a fixed decision rule. The "importance" of a variable is defined in terms of a measure of the statistical significance of the coefficient, or coefficients when multiple design variables are used, for the variable. The statistics used depend on the assumptions of the model. In stepwise linear regression an F-test is used, since the model assumes that the errors are normally distributed. In logistic regression the errors are assumed to follow a binomial distribution, and significance can be assessed using any one of the three equivalent tests discussed in Chapters 1 and 2: likelihood ratio, score, and Wald test. A particular software package may or may not offer the user a choice of which of the three tests to use. We use the likelihood ratio test, in what follows, to describe the methods. The other two tests could be used equally well. In practice, we have not seen important differences in models identified when the three tests are used on the same set of data. Given a choice we prefer to use the likelihood ratio test but use of one of the other tests by a statistical package does not present a problem or disadvantage.

We discussed in Chapter 3 that a polychotomous variable with k levels is appropriately modeled through its $k - 1$ design variables. Since the magnitude of the likelihood ratio test, G, depends on its degrees of freedom, any procedure based on the likelihood ratio test, or one of the other two tests, must account for possible differences in degrees of freedom between variables. This is done by assessing significance through the p-value for G.

We describe and illustrate the algorithm for forward selection followed by backward elimination in stepwise logistic regression. Any variants of this algorithm are simple modifications of this procedure. The method is described by considering the statistical computations that the computer must perform at each step.

Step (0): Assume that we have available a total of p possible independent variables, all of which are judged to be of plausible "clinical" importance in studying the outcome variable. Step (0) begins by fitting the "intercept only model" and evaluating its log-likelihood, L_0. Next, each of the p possible univariable logistic regression models is fit and its corresponding log-likelihood computed. Let the value of the log-likelihood for the model containing variable x_j at step zero be denoted by $L_j^{(0)}$. The subscript j refers to the variable that has been added to the model, and the superscript (0) refers to the step. This notation is used throughout the discussion of stepwise logistic regression to keep track of both step number and variables in the model.

Let the value of the likelihood ratio test for the model containing x_j versus the intercept only model, be denoted by $G_j^{(0)} = -2(L_0 - L_j^{(0)})$, and its p-value be denoted by $p_j^{(0)}$. This p-value is equal to the probability $\Pr[\chi^2(\nu) > G_j^{(0)}] = p_j^{(0)}$, where $\nu = 1$ if x_j is continuous or dichotomous, and $\nu = k - 1$ if x_j is polychotomous with k categories.

The "most important" variable is the one with the smallest p-value. If we denote this variable by x_{e_1}, then $p_{e_1}^{(0)} = \min(p_j^{(0)})$, where "min" stands for selecting the minimum of the quantities enclosed in the brackets. The subscript "e_1" is used to denote that the variable is a candidate for entry at step 1. For example, if variable x_2 had the smallest p-value, then $p_2^{(0)} = \min(p_j^{(0)})$, and $e_1 = 2$. The fact that x_{e_1} is the most important variable does not guarantee that it is "statistically significant". For example, if $p_{e_1}^{(0)} = 0.83$, we would probably conclude that there is little point in continuing this analysis because the most important variable is not related to the outcome. On the other hand, if $p_{e_1}^{(0)} = 0.003$, we would examine the logistic regression containing this variable and then determine whether there are other variables that are important given that x_{e_1} is in the model.

A crucial factor when using stepwise logistic regression is the choice of an "alpha" level to judge the importance of variables. Let p_E denote our choice where the "E" stands for entry. The choice for p_E determines how many variables eventually are included in the model. Bendel and Afifi (1977) studied the choice of p_E for stepwise linear regression, and Costanza and Afifi (1979) studied the choice for stepwise discriminant analysis. Lee and Koval (1997) examined the issue of significance level for forward stepwise logistic regression. The results of this research have shown that the choice of $p_E = 0.05$ is too stringent, often excluding important variables from the model. Choosing a value for p_E in the range from 0.15 to 0.20 is highly recommended.

Sometimes the goal of the analysis may be to provide a more complete set of possible predictors of the response variable. In these cases, use of $p_E = 0.25$ (or even larger) might be a reasonable choice. Whatever the choice for p_E, a variable is judged important enough to include in the model if the p-value for G

is less than p_E. Thus, the program proceeds to step (1) if $p_{e_1}^{(0)} < p_E$; otherwise, it stops.

Step (1): This step begins with a fit of the logistic regression model containing x_{e_1}. Let $L_{e_1}^{(1)}$ denote the log-likelihood of this model. To determine whether any of the remaining $p - 1$ variables are important once the variable x_{e_1} is in the model, we fit the $p - 1$ logistic regression models containing x_{e_1} and $x_j, j = 1, 2, 3, \ldots, p$ and $j \neq e_1$. For the model containing x_{e_1} and x_j let the log-likelihood be denoted by $L_{e_1 j}^{(1)}$, and let the likelihood ratio chi-square statistic of this model versus the model containing only x_{e_1} be denoted by $G_j^{(1)} = -2(L_{e_1}^{(1)} - L_{e_1 j}^{(1)})$. The p-value for this statistic is denoted by $p_j^{(1)}$. Let the variable with the smallest p-value at step (1) be x_{e_2} where $p_{e_2}^{(1)} = \min(p_j^{(1)})$. If this value is less than p_E then we proceed to Step (2); otherwise we stop.

Step (2): The step begins with a fit of the model containing both x_{e_1} and x_{e_2}. It is possible that once x_{e_2} has been added to the model, x_{e_1} is no longer important. Thus, Step (2) includes a check for backward elimination. In general, this check is done by fitting models that delete one of the variables added in the previous steps to assess the continued importance of the variable removed. At Step (2) let $L_{-e_j}^{(2)}$ denote the log-likelihood of the model with x_{e_j} removed. In similar fashion let the likelihood ratio test of this model versus the full model at Step (2) be $G_{-e_j}^{(2)} = -2(L_{-e_j}^{(2)} - L_{e_1 e_2}^{(2)})$ and $p_{-e_j}^{(2)}$ be its p-value.

To ascertain whether a variable should be deleted from the model the program selects that variable, which when removed, yields the maximum p-value. Denoting this variable as x_{r_2}, then $p_{r_2}^{(2)} = \max(p_{-e_1}^{(2)}, p_{-e_2}^{(2)})$. To decide whether x_{r_2} should be removed, the program compares $p_{r_2}^{(2)}$ to a second pre-chosen "alpha" level p_R, which indicates some minimal level of continued contribution to the model where "R" stands for remove. Whatever value we choose for p_R, it must exceed the value of p_E to guard against the possibility of having the program enter and remove the same variable at successive steps.

If we do not wish to exclude many variables once they have entered, then we might use $p_R = 0.9$. A more stringent value would be used if a continued "significant" contribution were required. For example, if we used $p_E = 0.15$, then we might choose $p_R = 0.20$. If the maximum p-value to remove $p_{r_2}^{(2)}$, exceeds p_R, then x_{r_2} is removed from the model. If $p_{r_2}^{(2)}$ is less than p_R then x_{r_2} remains in the model. In either case the program proceeds to the variable selection phase.

At the forward selection step each of the $p - 2$ logistic regression models are fit containing x_{e_1}, x_{e_2} and x_j for $j = 1, 2, 3, \ldots p, j \neq e_1, e_2$. The program evaluates the log-likelihood for each model, computes the likelihood ratio test versus the model containing only x_{e_1} and x_{e_2} and determines the corresponding p-value. Let x_{e_3} denote the variable with the minimum p-value, that is, $p_{e_3}^{(2)} = \min(p_j^{(2)})$. If this p-value is smaller than p_E, $p_{e_3}^{(2)} < p_E$, then the program proceeds to Step (3); otherwise, it stops.

Step (3): The procedure for Step (3) is identical to that of Step (2). The program fits the model including the variable selected during the previous step, performs a check for backward elimination followed by forward selection. The process continues in this manner until the program stops at Step (S).

Step (S): This step occurs when: (i) all p variables have entered the model or (ii) all variables in the model have p-values to remove that are less than p_R, and the variables not included in the model have p-values to enter that exceed p_E. The model at this step contains those variables that are important relative to the criteria of p_E and p_R. These may or may not be the variables reported in a final model. For instance, if the chosen values of p_E and p_R correspond to our preferred levels for statistical significance, then the model at step S may well contain the significant variables. However, if we have used values for p_E and p_R that are less stringent, then we should select the variables for a final model from a table that summarizes the results of the stepwise procedure.

There are two methods that may be used to select variables from a summary table; these are comparable to methods commonly used in stepwise linear regression. The first method is based on the p-value for entry at each step, while the second is based on a likelihood ratio test of the model at the current step versus the model at the last step. In most cases we prefer to use the first method as it can be performed with the output provided by statistical packages.

Let "q" denote an arbitrary step in the procedure. In the first method we compare $p_{e_q}^{(q-1)}$ to a pre-chosen significance level such as $\alpha = 0.15$. If the value $p_{e_q}^{(q-1)}$ is less than α, then we move to Step (q). We stop at the step when $p_{e_q}^{(q-1)}$ exceeds α. We consider the model at the previous step for further analysis. In this method the criterion for entry is based on a test of the significance of the coefficient for x_{e_q} conditional on $x_{e_1}, x_{e_2}, \ldots, x_{e_{q-1}}$ being in the model. The degrees of freedom for the test are 1 or $k - 1$ depending on whether x_{e_q} is continuous or polychotomous with k categories.

In the second method, rather than comparing the model at the current step [Step (q)] to the model at the previous step [Step ($q - 1$)] we compare it to the model at the last step [Step (S)]. We evaluate the p-value for the likelihood ratio test of these two models and proceed in this fashion until this p-value exceeds α. This tests that the coefficients for the variables added to the model from Step (q) to Step (S) are all equal to zero. At any given step it has more degrees of freedom than the test employed in the first method. For this reason the second method, on occasion, may select a larger number of variables than the first method, but only when rather liberal, large, values are used for the entry and removal criteria.

It is well known that the p-values calculated in stepwise selection procedures are not p-values in the traditional hypothesis testing context. Instead, they should be thought of as indicators of relative importance among variables. We recommend that one err in the direction of selecting a relatively rich model following stepwise selection. The variables so identified should then be subjected to the more intensive analysis described in the previous section.

A common modification of the stepwise selection procedure just described is to begin with a model at step zero that contains known important covariates. Selection is then performed from among the other available variables. One instance when this approach may be useful is to select interactions from among those possible from a main effects model.

Freedman (1983) urges caution when considering a model with many variables, noting that significant linear regressions may be obtained from "noise" variables, completely unrelated to the outcome variable. Flack and Chang (1987) have shown similar results regarding the frequency of selection of "noise" variables. Thus, a thorough analysis that examines statistical and clinical significance is especially important following any stepwise method.

Other versions of stepwise selection are possible. One might choose to use the previously described method but only enter variables, allowing no option for removal at each step. This is called forward selection. Another popular method is to begin at Step (0) with all p variables in the model and then proceed to sequentially eliminate nonstatistically significant variables. This is called backward elimination. We illustrate backward elimination in Section 4.3.2 as a way to approximate best subset selection.

As an example, we apply the stepwise variable selection procedure to the GLOW data analyzed using purposeful selection in Section 4.2. The reader is reminded that this procedure should be viewed as a first step in the model building process—basic variable selection. Subsequent steps such as determination of scale, as described in Section 4.2, would follow. The calculations were performed in SAS, which uses the Score Test for entry and the Wald test for removal of variables. The results are presented in Table 4.28 in terms of the p-values to enter and remove calculated at each step. The order of the variables given column-wise in the table is the order in which they were selected. In each column the values below the horizontal line are p_E values and values above the horizontal line are p_R values. The program was run using $p_E = 0.15$ and $p_R = 0.20$.

We choose to use SAS as it has the option to display the step-by-step details required for Table 4.28. One disadvantage of SAS is that it does not allow one to group the design variables formed from a categorical covariate with more than two levels for entry or removal. STATA does have this feature but has not provided step-by-step detail. However the models selected by both SAS and STATA are the same at Step (S).

Step (0): At Step (0) the program selects as a candidate for entry at Step (1) the variable with the smallest p-value in the first column of Table 4.28. The variable is history of prior fracture (PRIORFRAC). As seen in the table the p-values of both PRIORFRAC and AGE are <0.0001, but the value of the Score test (not shown) for PRIORFRAC is 23.8 while that for AGE is 21.6, each with one degree of freedom. Hence PRIORFRAC was selected for entry at Step (1).

Step (1): The program begins by fitting the model containing PRIORFRAC. The program does not remove the variable just entered since we choose the criterion such that $p_R > p_E$. This is true for the variable entered at any step—not just the first step. The variable with the smallest p-value to enter

Table 4.28 Results of Applying Stepwise Variable Selection Using the Score Test to Select Variables and the Wald Test for Removal of Variables in the GLOW Data

Variable/Step	0	1	2	3	4	5	6	7
PRIORFRAC	<0.001	<0.001	<0.001	0.002	0.003	0.003	0.007	0.009
AGE	<0.001	<0.001	<0.001*	<0.001	0.001	0.002	0.010	0.009
RATERISK3	0.006	0.046	0.017	0.018*	0.016	0.028	0.054*	0.016
HEIGHT	0.002	0.009	0.0336	0.032	0.033*	0.022	0.011	0.016
MOMFRAC	0.017	0.021	0.027	0.051	0.032	0.034*	0.030	0.043
ARMASSIST	0.001	0.011	0.053	0.099	0.046	0.040	0.041	0.056
RATERISK2	0.749	0.607	0.649	0.045	0.065	0.094	0.129	0.131*
BMI	0.738	0.745	0.217	0.110	0.128	0.091	0.342	0.333
WEIGHT	0.418	0.482	0.770	0.545	0.166	0.120	0.420	0.412
SMOKE	0.479	0.320	0.533	0.525	0.501	0.512	0.437	0.453
PREMENO	0.845	0.866	0.361	0.389	0.439	0.413	0.586	0.669

At each step the p-values to enter are presented below the horizontal line, and the p-value to remove are presented above the horizontal line in each column. The asterisk denotes the maximum p-value to remove at each step.

at step (1) is age at entry in the study (AGE) with $p < 0.001$, which is less than 0.15 so the program moves to Step (2).

Step (2): The p-values to remove appear above the solid line in each column of Table 4.28. We denote the largest p-value to remove with an "*". The model containing both PRIORFRAC and AGE is fit and we see that both p-values to remove are <0.001. Since neither exceeds 0.20, the program moves to the variable selection phase. The smallest p-value to enter among the remaining variables not in the model is $p = 0.017$, for the design variable comparing level 3 to level 1 of self-reported risk of fracture. Since the value is less than 0.15 the program proceeds to Step (3).

Step (3): At Step (3) Table 4.28 shows that the largest p-value to remove is for the variable that just entered the model, RATERISK3 and, since this does not exceed 0.20, the program moves to the variable selection phase. The smallest p-value to enter among the remaining variables not in the model is for height at enrollment in the study (HEIGHT) with $p = 0.032$. This value is less than 0.15 so the program proceeds to Step (4).

Step (4): At Step (4) the program finds that the maximum p-value to remove is HEIGHT, which just entered the model. Hence it is not removed from the model. In the selection phase the program finds that the minimum p-value for entry is 0.032 for the variable mother had a fracture, MOMFRAC. Since this value is less than 0.15, the program proceeds to Step (5).

Step (5): At Step (5) the largest p-value to remove is for MOMFRAC, which just entered the model, so it is not removed. Next the program selects for entry the variable "arms are needed to stand from a chair" (ARMASSIST).

Since the p-value for entry of 0.040 is less than p_E it enters the model at Step (6).

Step (6): At Step (6) the variable with the largest p-value to remove is RATERISK3 with p-value less than 0.20, so none are removed. The variable with the smallest p-value to enter is the design variable for self-reported rate of risk at level 2 versus level 1, RATERISK2, with $p = 0.129$. Since this value is less than 0.15 it enters the model at Step (7).

Step (7): The variable with the largest p-value to remove is RATERISK2, which just entered the model so no variables are removed. At the selection for entry phase we see that body mass index, BMI, has the smallest p-value, but its value, 0.333, exceeds the criterion for entry of 0.15. The program stops at Step (7) as no variables can be removed and none can enter using our chosen criteria of $p_E = 0.15$ and $p_R = 0.20$.

If, for some reason, we wanted to see every variable enter the model then we would have to rerun the program with much larger values. For example, at Step (7) we see that the largest p-value for entry is 0.669 for early menopause, PREMENO. So choosing $p_E = 0.80$ and $p_R = 0.85$ would probably allow all variables to enter the model. Having said this, it would be highly unusual to choose a p-value for entry that exceeds 0.50. The idea behind letting in variables that are unlikely to be in the final model is to check for the possible confounding effect of marginally significant variables. We know from practical experience that it is rare for a variable to be a confounder if its estimated coefficient(s) in a multivariable model are significant at 0.15 or higher.

Before moving on, we note that the model selected by stepwise methods in Table 4.28 contains the same seven covariates identified by purposeful selection in Table 4.8. This is often, though not always, the case. The purposeful selection model was further simplified by excluding RATERISK2, since it was not a confounder and subject matter experts felt it was reasonable to pool "same risk" and "less risk" into a single reference category, thus using only RATERISK3. For the time being we are going to use the model at Step (7) that includes both design variables.

We noted that there are two methods to select the final model from a table summarizing the steps. In our example, the program was run with $p_E = 0.15$, a value that, we believe, selects variables with significant coefficients; thus, it is not necessary to go to the summary table to select the variables to be used in a final model. The second method is based on comparing the model at each step to the last step that–in work not shown–also selects the model at Step (7). We leave performing stepwise selection on the GLOW data using $p_E = 0.80$ and $p_R = 0.85$, with final model selection based on the second method as an exercise.

At the conclusion of the stepwise selection process we have only identified a collection of variables that seem to be statistically important. If there were known clinically important variables then these should have been added before proceeding with stepwise selection of other covariates. If at the end of stepwise selection there are continuous covariates in the model, then at this point, one should determine their appropriate scale in the logit. The model contains age and height, both of which were shown to be linear in the logit in Section 4.2.

Once the scale of the continuous covariates has been examined, and corrected if necessary, we may consider applying stepwise selection to identify interactions. The candidate interaction terms are those that seem clinically reasonable given the main effect variables in the model. We begin at Step (0) with the main effects model, including any clinically significant covariates, and sequentially select from among the possible interactions. We can use either method 1 or method 2 to select the significant interactions. The final model contains previously identified main effects and significant interaction terms.

The same software may be used for stepwise selection of interactions as was used for the selection of main effects. The difference is that all main effect variables are forced into the model at Step (0) and selection is restricted to interactions. In total there are 15 possible interactions listed in Table 4.29 where they are inverse rank ordered by the p-values at the last step. We again use SAS to select the interactions stepwise. We remind the reader that, in SAS, selection for entry is based on the Score test, and the test for removal is based on the Wald test.

Before proceeding with stepwise selection of interactions we decided to remove RATERISK2 from the model and keep RATERISK3. Thus, we have chosen to use the recoded version of the self-reported risk variable from purposeful selection in the previous section. There are 15 interactions that can be formed from the six main effects and subject matter experts considered all 15 to be clinically reasonable.

Table 4.29 Results of Applying Stepwise Variable Selection to Interactions from the Main Effects Model from the GLOW Study Using the Score Test to Select Variables and the Wald Test to Remove Variables

Variable/Step	0	1	2
AGE*PRIORFRAC	0.024	0.025*	0.033
MOMFRAC*ARMASSIST	0.028	0.038	0.040*
HEIGHT*MOMFRAC	0.112	0.110	0.162
ARMASSIST*RATERISK3	0.135	0.123	0.174
PRIORFRAC*MOMFRAC	0.092	0.123	0.188
HEIGHT*ARMASSIST	0.206	0.184	0.252
HEIGHT*RATERISK3	0.319	0.308	0.0386
PRIORFRAC*ARMASSIST	0.636	0.399	0.423
AGE*RATERISK3	0.304	0.446	0.435
AGE*MOMFRAC	0.708	0.753	0.463
MOMFRAC*RATERISK3	0.465	0.468	0.580
AGE*HEIGHT	0.716	0.803	0.795
HEIGHT*PRIORFRAC	0.644	0.815	0.904
PRIORFRAC*RATERISK3	0.726	0.843	0.959
AGE*ARMASSIST	0.702	0.968	0.999

At each step the p-values to enter are presented below the horizontal line, and the p-value to remove are presented above the horizontal line in each column. The asterisk denotes the maximum p-value to remove at each step.

The results in Table 4.29 show that only two of the interactions were selected. At Step (1) the interaction of age and history of prior fracture (PRIORFRAC) entered and at Step (2) the interaction of mother having had a fracture (MOMFRAC) and need arms to rise from a chair (ARMASSIST) entered. The most significant interaction among those not selected at Step (2) is that of HEIGHT and MOMFRAC with $p = 0.162$, which is not less than the criterion for entry of 0.15 and hence does not enter the model.

It is worthwhile to point out that the p-values for Step (0) in Table 4.29, which are based on the Score test, are quite similar to those in the last column of Table 4.14 that are based on the likelihood ratio test.

Adding the two selected interactions to the main effects (all of which were selected stepwise) yields the same model obtained by purposeful selection shown in Table 4.16. This may not always be the case. In our experience, models obtained by these two approaches rarely differ by more than a couple of variables. In a situation where different approaches yield different models, we recommend proceeding with a combined larger model via purposeful selection using both confounding and statistical significance as criteria for model simplification.

Since the stepwise model is shown in Table 4.16 we do not repeat the results in another table in this section.

In conclusion, we emphasize that stepwise selection identifies variables as candidates for a model solely on statistical grounds. Thus, following stepwise selection of main effects all variables should be carefully scrutinized for clinical plausibility. In general, interactions must attain statistical significance to alter the point and interval estimates from a main effects model. Thus, stepwise selection of interactions using statistical significance can provide a valuable contribution to model identification, especially when there are large numbers of clinically plausible interactions generated from the main effects.

4.3.2 Best Subsets Logistic Regression

An alternative to stepwise selection of variables for a model is best subset selection. This approach to model building has been available for linear regression for many years and makes use of the branch and bound algorithm of Furnival and Wilson (1974). Typical software implementing this method for linear regression identifies a specified number of "best" models containing one, two, three variables, and so on, up to the single model containing all p variables. Lawless and Singhal (1978, 1987a, 1987b) proposed an extension that may be used with any nonnormal errors model. The crux of their method involves application of the Furnival-Wilson algorithm to a linear approximation of the cross-product sum-of-squares matrix that yields approximations to the maximum likelihood estimates. Selected models are then compared to the model containing all variables using a likelihood ratio test. Hosmer et al. (1989) show that, for logistic regression, the full generality of the Lawless and Singhal approach is not needed. Best subsets logistic regression may be performed in a straightforward manner using any program capable of best subsets linear regression. Also, some packages, including SAS, have implemented the Lawless and Singhal method in their logistic regression modules. The advantage of these two approaches is that one may examine, and hence compare, several different models selected by some criterion. If, however, one is merely interested in obtaining the best model from the best subsets method, then a quick route to this end is to employ a method described in Royston and Sauerbrei (2008, Chapter 2). They discuss results showing that the model selected using stepwise backward elimination with $p_R = 0.157$ yields a model that agrees, in content, quite closely with the best of the best subset selected models using a criterion such as AIC from equation (4.4). The disadvantage of this quicker approach is that one is not able to see the content of other best models. We illustrate best subsets selection using the GLOW data. An important caveat to using best subsets selection is that, as described, it only identifies a collection of main effects. As described in the previous two sections, there is considerable work remaining in the model building process after main effects are selected.

Applying best subsets linear regression software to perform best subsets logistic regression is most easily explained using vector and matrix notation. In this regard, we let $\mathbf{X}$ denote the $n \times (p + 1)$ matrix containing the values of all p independent variables for each subject, with the first column containing 1 to represent the constant term. Here the p variables may represent the total number of variables, or those selected at the univariable stage of model building. We let $\mathbf{V}$ denote an $n \times n$ diagonal matrix with general element $v_i = \hat{\pi}_i(1 - \hat{\pi}_i)$ where $\hat{\pi}_i$ is the estimated logistic probability computed using the maximum likelihood estimate, $\hat{\boldsymbol{\beta}}$, and the data for the ith case, $\mathbf{x}_i$.

For the sake of clarity of presentation in this section, we repeat the expression for $\mathbf{X}$ and $\mathbf{V}$ given in Chapter 2. They are as follows:

$$\mathbf{X} = \begin{bmatrix} 1 & x_{11} & x_{12} & \cdots & x_{1p} \\ 1 & x_{21} & x_{22} & \cdots & x_{2p} \\ \vdots & \vdots & \vdots & \ddots & \vdots \\ 1 & x_{n1} & x_{n2} & \cdots & x_{np} \end{bmatrix}$$

and

$$\mathbf{V} = \begin{bmatrix} \hat{\pi}_1(1 - \hat{\pi}_1) & 0 & \cdots & 0 \\ 0 & \hat{\pi}_2(1 - \hat{\pi}_2) & \cdots & 0 \\ \vdots & 0 & \ddots & \vdots \\ 0 & \cdots & 0 & \hat{\pi}_n(1 - \hat{\pi}_n) \end{bmatrix}.$$

As noted in Chapter 2, the maximum likelihood estimate is determined iteratively. It may be shown [see Pregibon (1981)] that $\hat{\boldsymbol{\beta}} = (\mathbf{X}'\mathbf{VX})^{-1}\mathbf{X}'\mathbf{Vz}$, where $\mathbf{z} = \mathbf{X}\hat{\boldsymbol{\beta}} + \mathbf{V}^{-1}\mathbf{r}$ and r is the vector of residuals, $\mathbf{r} = (\mathbf{y} - \hat{\pi})$. This representation of $\hat{\boldsymbol{\beta}}$ provides the basis for use of linear regression software. It is easy to verify that any linear regression package that allows weights produces coefficient estimates identical to $\hat{\boldsymbol{\beta}}$ when used with z_i as the dependent variable and case weights, v_i, equal to the diagonal elements of $\mathbf{V}$.

If we wanted to replicate the results of the maximum likelihood fit from a logistic regression package using a linear regression package, for each case we would first calculate the value of a dependent variable as follows:

$$
\begin{aligned}
z_i &= \hat{\beta}_0 + \sum_{j=1}^{p} \hat{\beta}_j x_{ij} + \frac{(y_i - \hat{\pi}_i)}{\hat{\pi}_i(1 - \hat{\pi}_i)} \\
&= \ln\left(\frac{\hat{\pi}_i}{1 - \hat{\pi}_i}\right) + \frac{(y_i - \hat{\pi}_i)}{\hat{\pi}_i(1 - \hat{\pi}_i)}
\end{aligned}
\tag{4.5}
$$

and a case weight

$$
v_i = \hat{\pi}_i(1 - \hat{\pi}_i).
\tag{4.6}
$$

Note that all we need is access to the fitted values, $\hat{\pi}_i$, to compute the values of z_i and v_i. Next, we would run a linear regression program using the values of z_i for the dependent variable, the values of $\mathbf{x}_i$ for our vector of independent variables, and the values of v_i for our case weights.

Proceeding further with the linear regression, it can be shown that the residuals from this fit are

$$
(z_i - \hat{z}_i) = \frac{(y_i - \hat{\pi}_i)}{\hat{\pi}_i(1 - \hat{\pi}_i)}
$$

and the weighted residual sum-of-squares produced by the program is

$$
\sum_{i=1}^{n} v_i(z_i - \hat{z}_i)^2 = \sum_{i=1}^{n} \frac{(y_i - \hat{\pi}_i)^2}{\hat{\pi}_i(1 - \hat{\pi}_i)},
$$

which is X^2, the Pearson chi-square statistic from a maximum likelihood logistic regression program. It follows that the mean residual sum-of-squares is $s^2 = X^2/(n - p - 1)$. The estimates of the standard error of the estimated coefficients produced by the linear regression program are s times the square root of the diagonal elements of the matrix $(\mathbf{X}'\mathbf{VX})^{-1}$. Thus, to obtain the correct values given in equation (2.5) we would have to divide the estimates of the standard error produced by the linear regression program by s, the square root of the mean square error (or standard error of the estimate).

The ability to duplicate the maximum likelihood fit in a linear regression package forms the foundation of the suggested method for performing best subsets logistic regression. In particular, Hosmer et al. (1989) show that use of any best subsets linear regression program with values of z_i in equation (4.5) for the dependent variable, case weights v_i shown in equation (4.6), and covariates $\mathbf{x}_i$, produces for any subset of q variables, the approximate coefficient estimates of Lawless and Singhal (1978). Hence, we may use any best subsets linear regression program to execute the computations for best subsets logistic regression. One practical difficulty is that there is not much software available that actually implements the traditional best subsets linear regression. A recent user-supplied contribution to the STATA package by Lindsey and Sheather (2010) does perform this analysis but only provides the content of the best model of each size.

The subsets of variables selected for "best" models depend on the criterion chosen for "best." In best subsets linear regression a number of different criteria have been used to select variables. Two are based on the concept of the proportion of the total variation explained by the model. These are R^2, the ratio of the regression sum-of-squares to the total sum-of-squares, and adjusted R^2 (or AR^2), the ratio of the regression mean squares to the total mean squares. Since the adjusted R^2 is based on mean squares rather than sums-of-squares, it provides a correction for the number of variables in the model. This is important, as we must be able to compare models containing different variables and different numbers of variables. If we use R^2, the best model is always the model containing all p variables, a result that is not at all helpful. An obvious extension for best subsets logistic regression is to base the R^2 measures, in a manner similar to that shown in Chapter 5, on deviance rather than Pearson chi-square. However, we do not recommend the use of the R^2 measures for best subsets logistic regression. Instead, we prefer to use C_q, a measure developed by Mallows (1973) or the Akaike Information Criterion (AIC) developed by Akaike (1974) and defined in equation (4.4).

Mallows' C_q is a measure of predictive squared error. We note that the measure is denoted as C_p by other authors. We chose to use "q" instead of "p" in this text since we use p to refer to the total number of possible variables, while q refers to some subset of variables.

A summary of the development of the criterion C_q in linear regression may be found in many texts on this subject, for example, Ryan (1997). Hosmer et al. (1989) show that when best subsets logistic regression is performed via a best subsets linear regression package in the manner described previously in this section, Mallows' C_q has the same intuitive appeal as it does in linear regression. In particular they show that for a subset of q of the p variables

$$C_q = \frac{X^2 + \lambda^*}{X^2/(n - p - 1)} + 2(q + 1) - n,$$

where

$$X^2 = \sum \{(y_i - \hat{\pi}_i)^2 / [\hat{\pi}_i(1 - \hat{\pi}_i)]\},$$

the Pearson chi-square statistic for the model with p variables and λ^* is the multivariable Wald test statistic for the hypothesis that the coefficients for the $p - q$ variables not in the model are equal to zero. Under the assumption that the model fit is the correct one, the approximate expected values of X^2 and λ^* are $(n - p - 1)$ and $p - q$, respectively. Substitution of these approximate expected values into the expression for C_q yields $C_q = q + 1$. Hence, models with C_q near $q + 1$ are candidates for a best model. The best subsets linear regression program selects as best that subset with the smallest value of C_q.

The Akaike Information Criterion (AIC) does not have a reference standard based on the number of variables, in or out of the model. The best model is simply the one with the smallest value of

$$\text{AIC}_q = -2 \times L_q + 2 \times (q + 1). \tag{4.7}$$

We modified the definition in equation (4.6) by adding the subscript "q" to denote the fact that AIC is being computed over models of different sizes.

Some programs, for example, SAS's PROC LOGISTIC, provide a best subsets selection of covariates based on the Score test for the variables in the model. For example, the best two variable model is the one with the largest Score test among all two variable models. The output lists the covariates and Score test for a user specified number of best models of each size. The difficulty one faces when presented with this output is that the Score test increases with the number of variables in the model. Hosmer et al. (2008) show how an approximation to Mallows' C_q can be obtained from Score test output in a survival time analysis. A similar approximation can be obtained from C_q for logistic regression. First, we assume that the Pearson chi-square statistic is equal to its mean, that is $X^2 \approx (n - p - 1)$. Next we assume that the Wald statistic for the $p - q$ excluded covariates may be approximated by the difference between the values of the Score test for all p covariates and the Score test for q covariates, namely $\lambda_q^* \approx S_p - S_q$. This results in the following approximation

$$
\begin{aligned}
C_q &= \frac{X^2 + \lambda^*}{X^2/(n - p - 1)} + 2(q + 1) - n \\
&\approx \frac{(n - p - 1) + (S_p - S_q)}{1} + 2(q + 1) - n \\
&\approx S_p - S_q + 2q - p + 1.
\end{aligned}
\tag{4.8}
$$

The value of S_p is the Score test for the model containing all p covariates and is obtained from the computer output. The value of S_q is the Score test for the particular subset of q covariates and its value is also obtained from the output. Use of a best subsets logistic regression package should help identify, in the same way its application in linear regression does, a core of important covariates from the p possible covariates. After identifying the important variables, we suggest that further modeling proceed in the manner described in Section 4.2 for purposeful selection of covariates. Users should not be lured into accepting the variables suggested by a best subset strategy without considerable critical evaluation.

We illustrate best subsets selection using the Score test method implemented in SAS with the GLOW data. The variables used were the 10 indicated in Table 1.7, with the exception of the fracture risk score, since it is a composite formed from many individual covariates. Self-reported rate of risk is modeled using two design variables RATERISK2 and RATERISK3. In Table 4.30 we present the results of the five best models selected using C_q in (4.8) as the criterion. In addition to the variables selected, we show the values of C_q and the values of S_q for each model and the value of AIC$_q$ from (4.7).

Using only the summary statistics, we would select Model 1 as the best model since it has the smallest values of both C_q and AIC$_q$. It is interesting to note that this model is different from the model selected by purposeful selection (Model 5), and stepwise (Model 4), in that height is not in the model, but weight and BMI are included. The differences in the values of both C_q and AIC$_q$ over the five models

Table 4.30   Five Best Models Identified Using the Score Test Approximation of Mallow's C_q, Table Lists Model Covariates, Approximate C_q, S_q, and AIC_q ($S_{11} = 59.1672$)

Model	Model Covariates	S_q	C_q	AIC_q
1	PRIORFRAC, AGE, WEIGHT, BMI, MOMFRAC, ARMASSIST, RATERISK2, RATERISK3	57.4602	7.707	523.1954
2	PRIORFRAC, AGE, WEIGHT, BMI, MOMFRAC, ARMASSIST, RATERISK3	55.4424	7.724	523.5289
3	PRIORFRAC, AGE, WEIGHT, BMI, MOMFRAC, RATERISK2, RATERISK3	55.2662	7.901	523.1987
4[a]	PRIORFRAC, AGE, HEIGHT, MOMFRAC, ARMASSIST, RATERISK2, RATERISK3	55.2657	7.902	523.5004
5[b]	PRIORFRAC, AGE, HEIGHT, MOMFRAC, ARMASSIST, RATERISK3	53.2400	7.927	523.8178

[a] Main effects model identified by stepwise selection.
[b] Main effects model identified by purposeful selection.

are negligible. Thus choice among the five models comes down, as it should, to subject matter considerations.

Note that all five models contain PRIORFRAC, AGE, and MOMFRAC. Four of the five contain ARMASSIST. Three models contain WEIGHT and BMI and two contain HEIGHT. Three models contain both RATERISK2 and RATERISK3 and two contain only RATERISK3. Hence, we conclude that the core of important variables in these five models is PRIORFRAC, AGE, MOMFRAC, ARMASSIST, RATERISK2, and RATERISK3, with body composition modeled either by WEIGHT and BMI or by HEIGHT.

In using purposeful selection in Section 4.2 we found that the estimated coefficient for RATERISK2 was not significant and, in consultation with experts, decided to only use RATERISK3, which is a design variable for level 3 versus 1 and 2. Now the choice is between model 2 and model 5. Further analysis showed that the estimated coefficient for ARMASSIST is not significant, $p = 0.125$, in model 2. Deleting it yields a sixth best model (not shown) with $C_q = 8.182$ and $AIC_q = 523.87$. Thus, the choice is now between two models, each with six covariates. The more important difference between the two models is that one contains HEIGHT and the other contains WEIGHT and BMI. We leave further comparison of these two models as an exercise.

In practice, once we have finalized the main effects model, we could employ best subsets selection to decide on possible interactions. We leave this as an exercise.

Application of the backwards elimination approach described by Royston and Sauerbrei (2008, Sections 2.6.3 and 2.9.3) with $p_R = 0.157$ to the GLOW data yields the same best subsets model, Model 1 in table 4.30. This is not always going to be the case, but this easy to use approach should always identify a reasonable set of model covariates for further evaluation.

The advantage of the proposed method of best subsets logistic regression is that more models can be quickly screened than is possible with the other variable selection methods. There is, however, one potential disadvantage with the best subsets approach: we must be able to fit the model containing all of the possible covariates. In analyses that include a large number of variables this may not be possible. Numerical problems can occur when we overfit a logistic regression model. If the model has many variables, we run the risk that the data are too thin to be able to estimate all the parameters. If the full model proves to be too rich, then some selective weeding out of obviously unimportant variables with univariable tests may remedy this problem. Another approach is to perform the best subsets analysis using several smaller "full" models. Numerical problems are discussed in more detail in the next section.

In summary, the ability to use weighted least squares best subsets linear regression software or the Score test approximation method to identify variables for logistic regression should be kept in mind as a possible aid to variable selection. As is the case with any statistical selection method, the clinical basis of all variables should be addressed before any model is accepted as the final model.

4.3.3 Selecting Covariates and Checking their Scale Using Multivariable Fractional Polynomials

Sauerbrei et al. (2006) describe software for SAS, STATA and R that implements a multivariable fractional polynomial method. Royston and Sauerbrei (2008, Chapter 6) describe the method in detail and it is now available in distributed STATA. The method combines elements of backward elimination of nonsignificant covariates with an iterative examination of the scale of all continuous covariates and can be used with either the closed or sequential test procedures described in Section 4.2.

The multivariable fractional polynomial procedure requires that two significance levels be specified: the first, α_1, for the test for exclusion from or addition to, the model and the second, α_2, to assess the significance of the fractional polynomial transforms of a continuous covariate. We use the same notation as Royston and Sauerbrei (2008) to denote the method and its significance levels, namely $mfp(\alpha_1, \alpha_2)$.

The method begins, cycle 1, by fitting a multivariable model that contains the user-specified covariates. This initial collection, ideally, would include all study covariates. However, we may have a setting where this is not possible, for any one of a number of numerical problems. If this occurs, a reasonable solution is to choose a subset of covariates that includes the clinically important covariates and those significant at, say, the 25 percent level on univariable analysis. This is, basically, the starting point of purposeful selection.

The initial fit at cycle 1 includes all covariates as linear terms in the logit. In subsequent fits, each covariate is modeled according to a specified number of degrees of freedom. All dichotomous and design variables have one degree of freedom, meaning they are not candidates for fractional polynomial transformation. Continuous covariates may be forced to be modeled linearly by specifying one degree of freedom, or may be candidates for a one- or two-term fractional polynomial by specifying 2 or 4 degrees of freedom, respectively.

Following the initial multivariable linear fit, variables are considered in descending order of their Wald statistics. For covariates modeled with one degree of freedom, a partial likelihood ratio test is used to assess their contribution to the model, and its significance relative to the chosen level of significance, α_1, is noted. Continuous covariates are modeled using either the closed or sequential test method, noting whether the covariate should be removed using α_1, kept linear, or transformed using α_2. In keeping with our approach to stepwise selection and best subsets we set the level of significance for staying in the model at $\alpha_1 = 0.15$. We use the five percent level of significance, $\alpha_2 = 0.05$, for testing the need to transform. In the example, we use the closed test procedure, which is the default method in STATA. This completes the first cycle.

The second cycle begins with a fit of a multivariable model containing the significant covariates from cycle one (i.e., the model with significant continuous covariates, that may be transformed and significant dichotomous covariates). All covariates, examined in descending order of significance, are considered again for possible transformation, inclusion or exclusion from the model. Continuous covariates with a significant fractional polynomial transformation are entered transformed, which becomes their null model. The point of this step is twofold: (1) does the transformation "linearize" the covariate in the logit? and (2) does the transformation affect scaling of other covariates? Each covariate's level of significance is noted as well as the need to transform. This completes the second cycle.

The procedure stops when the results of two consecutive cycles are the same. The minimum number is two. More than two cycles occur if additional transformations of continuous covariates are suggested in cycle two and beyond, or if the level of significance of the partial likelihood ratio test for contribution to the model, changes the decision to include or exclude a covariate.

We use mfp(0.15, 0.05) on the GLOW500 data from the GLOW Study with the same 10 covariates used in the previous three sections and model self-reported risk of fracture with two design variables. We note that in STATA one may consider design variables formed from a categorical covariate with more than two levels as a group or separately. In the example, we consider the two design variables for self-reported risk of fracture separately, as that is how they were modeled in stepwise and best subsets. The method took two cycles to converge. We present the results from cycle 1 in Table 4.31, and cycle 2 in Table 4.32.

The cycle begins by fitting the model containing all 11 covariates. In Table 4.31, the first covariate processed is having had a prior fracture, PRIORFRAC, so we know it had the largest Wald statistic. Because PRIORFRAC is dichotomous the first test, line* 1, compares the 10 covariate model not containing PRIORFRAC to the 11 covariate model containing PRIORFRAC. This is indicated in the last two

---

*The STATA output does not include line numbers. We included them in Table 4.31 and Table 4.32 to help in discussing the results.

Table 4.31 Results from the Cycle 1 Fit of MFP Applied to the GLOW500 Data

Line	Variable	Model	(vs.)	Deviance	G	p	Powers	(vs.)
1	PRIORFRAC	null	lin.	511.004	7.167	0.007*	.	1
2		Final		503.837			1	
3	AGE	null	FP2	510.869	7.629	0.106*	.	3 3
4		lin.		503.837	0.598	0.897	1	
5		Final		503.837			1	
6	RATERISK3	null	lin.	510.335	6.498	0.011*	.	1
7		Final		503.837			1	
8	MOMFRAC	null	lin.	507.944	4.107	0.043*	.	1
9		Final		503.837			1	
10	RATERISK2	null	lin.	506.123	2.286	0.131*	.	1
11		Final		503.837			1	
12	BMI	null	FP2	506.098	4.524	0.340	.	−2 1
13		Final		506.098			.	
14	ARMASSIST	null	lin.	508.155	2.058	0.151	.	1
15		Final		508.155			.	
16	WEIGHT	null	FP2	510.209	6.103	0.192	.	−2 −2
17		Final		510.209			.	
18	HEIGHT	null	FP2	514.905	6.689	0.153	.	−2 −2
19		Final		514.905			.	
20	SMOKE	null	lin.	515.296	0.391	0.532	.	1
21		Final		515.296			.	
22	PREMENO	null	lin.	515.844	0.547	0.459	.	1
23		Final		515.844			.	

*$p <$ chosen significance level for inclusion.

†$p <$ chosen significance level for transformation.

columns of line 1 where "." denotes that the covariate is not in the model and "1" denotes that it is modeled linearly in the logit. The value in the Deviance column, 511.004, in line 1 is for the model that excludes PRIORFRAC. The value in the G column of line 1, 7.167, is the difference between 511.004 and the Deviance for the model containing PRIORFRAC. The value in the p column in line 1 is the significance level using one degree of freedom, $\Pr[\chi^2(1) \geq 7.167] = 0.007$. The "*" denotes that the test is significant at the specified significance level for inclusion in the model, $\alpha_1 = 0.15$. Because the test is significant and since PRIORFRAC is dichotomous the final model in line 2 is the one that includes PRIORFRAC. Hence, in this case, the value of the Deviance in line 1 is the sum of the Deviance in line 2 and G in line 1 and the "1" in the "Powers" column means it enters as a single-term (i.e., linear in the logit).

The second covariate processed is age, AGE, as it had the second largest Wald statistic. This variable is continuous and, as such, it is first modeled using the best two-term fractional polynomial transformation with the powers shown in the last column of line 3, (3, 3), that is $[AGE^3, AGE^3 \times \ln(AGE)]$. The partial likelihood ratio test comparing this best two-term fractional polynomial modeling of age to the 10 covariate model that excludes age is, from line 3, $G = 7.269$ which, with 4

Table 4.32   Results from the Cycle 2 Fit of MFP Applied to the GLOW500 Data

Line	Variable	Model	(vs.)	Deviance	G	p	Powers	(vs.)
1	PRIORFRAC	null	lin.	524.264	8.42	0.004*	.	1
2		Final		515.844			1	
3	AGE	null	FP2	529.003	13.744	0.008*	.	3 3
4		lin.		515.844	0.584	0.9	1	
5		Final		515.844			1	
6	RATERISK3	null	lin.	523.740	7.897	0.005*	.	1
7		Final		515.844			1	
8	MOMFRAC	null	lin.	518.899	3.055	0.080*	.	1
9		Final		515.844			1	
10	RATERISK2	null	lin.	519.360	3.517	0.061*	.	1
11		Final		515.844			1	
12	BMI	null	FP2	515.844	4.433	0.351	.	−2 −2
13		Final		515.844			.	
14	ARMASSIST	null	lin.	515.844	2.41	0.121*	.	1
15		Final		513.434			1	
16	WEIGHT	null	FP2	513.434	3.611	0.461	.	−2 −2
17		Final		513.434			.	
18	HEIGHT	null	FP2	513.434	7.749	0.101*	.	−2 −2
19		lin.		507.500	1.816	0.612	1	
20		Final		507.500			1	
21	SMOKE	null	lin.	507.500	0.587	0.444	.	1
22		Final		507.500			.	
23	PREMENO	null	lin.	507.500	0.181	0.67	.	1

*p < chosen significance level for inclusion.
$^{†}p$ < chosen significance level for transformation.

degrees of freedom, yields $\Pr[\chi^2(4) \geq 7.629] = 0.106$. Since this is significant at the 0.15 level the two-term fractional polynomial model is compared to the linear model in line 4. The partial likelihood ratio test in line 4 is $G = 0.598$, which with 3 degrees of freedom, yields $p = 0.897$. Since two different parameterizations of age are being compared, the p-value is compared to $\alpha_2 = 0.05$ and the test is not significant. Hence, there is no further modeling of age with the final model, age linear, given in line 5. Had the two-term fractional polynomial model been significantly different from the linear model the best one-term fractional polynomial model would have been found and compared to the two-term model, again at the α_2 level of significance.

The next three variables examined are the dichotomous covariates RATERISK3, MOMFRAC and RATERISK2. Each is significant at the $\alpha_1 = 0.15$ level and thus will be retained in the model fit at cycle 2.

The covariate BMI is next examined in line 12. The partial likelihood ratio test comparing the best two-term fractional polynomial model, powers $(-2, 1)$, with the model that excludes BMI is $G = 4.524$ which, with four degrees of freedom, results in $p = 0.340$. This is not significant at the $\alpha_1 = 0.15$ level, so BMI is not included in the model fit in cycle 2. The remaining five covariates, ARMASSIST, WEIGHT, HEIGHT, SMOKE, and PREMENO, are individually not significant at the 0.15 level. However, the significance of the partial likelihood ratio tests for ARMASSIST and HEIGHT have p-values that are close to the threshold of 0.15. It is possible that these two could be selected for inclusion in cycle 2 when a smaller model is fit.

The model fit at cycle two contains the first five covariates in Table 4.31, namely PRIORFRAC, AGE, RATERISK3, MOMFRAC and RATERISK2. The results of cycle 2 are shown in Table 4.32.

The results in the first 13 lines of Table 4.32 are similar to those in Table 4.31 for these covariates. The difference between these tables is that the partial likelihood ratio tests in Table 4.32 are based now, not on the full 11 covariate model, but on a five covariate model. In line 14 we see that ARMASSIST contributes to the model at the 0.15 level with $p = 0.121$. In line 18 we see that HEIGHT also is significant ($p = 0.101$). Hence at the next cycle a seven covariate model is fit: the five in lines 1–10 plus ARMASSIST and HEIGHT. The decisions based on this fit are similar to those in Table 4.31. Hence the procedure converges at cycle 2.

We note that application of mfp(0.15, 0.05) to the GLOW500 data yields exactly the same model identified by purposeful selection and stepwise selection. The model obtained using best subsets was similar but selected BMI and WEIGHT in place of HEIGHT. Much of the congruence between the various methods can be attributed to the fact that, in this example, none of the continuous covariates had significant fractional polynomial transformations.

To provide an example when continuous covariates are transformed we apply mfp(0.15, 0.05) to the Burn Study data analyzed in Section 4.2. The covariates modeled (see Table 1.9) are total burn surface (TBSA), age (AGE), burn involving an inhalation injury (INH_INJ), race (RACE, $0 = $ non-white, $1 = $ white), burn involving a flame (FLAME) and gender (GENDER, $0 = $ female, $1 = $ male). The procedure converged in two cycles and we show the results from cycle 2 in Table 4.33.

The results for TBSA and AGE in Table 4.33 provide good examples of when fractional polynomial transformations are found to be significant with the mfp method.

The first variable processed is TBSA. The results in line 1 show that the two-term fractional polynomial model, powers $(-2, 0.5)$, is significant when compared to the model not containing TBSA with $p < 0.001$. Hence the procedure now compares the two-term fractional polynomial model to the model linear in TBSA in line 2. With $p = 0.001$, the test is significant at the $\alpha_2 = 0.05$ level, as indicated by the "+". Next, the two-term model is compared to the best one-term fractional polynomial model [power (0.5)]. The significance level, computed with 2 degrees of freedom is $p = 0.520$. Since this is not significant at the 0.05 level the process stops and the one-term fractional polynomial model is the final model for TBSA, shown in line 4.

The results for age in lines 5–8 are similar to those for TBSA in that the final model is the one-term fractional polynomial model with power (2). The results for

Table 4.33   Results from the Cycle 2 Fit of MFP Applied to the Burn Data

Line	Variable	Model	(vs.)	Deviance	G	p	Powers	(vs.)
1	TBSA	null	FP2	528.892	208.263	<0.001*	.	−2 .5
2		lin.		336.842	16.213	0.001†	1	
3		FP1		321.935	1.306	0.52	0.5	
4		Final		321.935			0.5	
5	AGE	null	FP2	505.022	184.862	<0.001*	.	1 1
6		lin.		329.589	9.429	0.024†	1	
7		FP1		321.935	1.775	0.412	2	
8		Final		321.935			2	
9	INH_INJ	null	lin.	339.521	17.586	0.000*	.	1
10		Final		321.935			1	
11	RACE	null	lin.	325.869	3.934	0.047*	.	1
12		Final		321.935			1	
13	FLAME	null	lin.	321.935	1.838	0.175	.	1
14		Final		321.935			.	
15	GENDER	null	lin.	321.935	0.129	0.719	.	1
16		Final		321.935			.	

*p < chosen significance level for inclusion.
†p < chosen significance level for transformation.

inhalation injury in lines 9 and 10 show it is significant as is race in lines 11 and 12. The last two covariates processed, FLAME and GENDER, do not contribute to the model with significance levels of $p = 0.175$ and $p = 0.719$ respectively. As noted the mfp procedure converged at two cycles. The resulting model with four covariates, $\sqrt{TBSA}$, AGE^2, INH_INJ and RACE, is the same model initially obtained using purposeful selection in Section 4.2. As we noted there, we added AGE to the model for purposes of ease of interpretation, even though its coefficient was not significant when added to the model containing AGE^2.

The mfp(α_1, α_2) method is clearly an extremely powerful analytic modeling tool, which on the surface, would appear to relieve the analyst of having to think too hard about model content. This is not the case, of course. We recommend that, if one uses this approach then its model be considered as a suggestion for a possible main effects model, much in the way that stepwise and best subsets identify possible models. The model needs a thorough evaluation to be sure all covariates and transformations make clinical sense, that transformations are not caused by a few extreme observations and, importantly, that excluded covariates are not confounders of model covariate estimates of effect. We highly recommend that you spend time with Royston and Sauerbrei (2008, Chapter 6), Sauerbrei et al. (2006) and the host of other excellent papers cited that describe in detail, the development and use of both fractional polynomials and the mfp(α_1, α_2) procedure.

In summary, stepwise, best subsets and multivariable fractional polynomials have their place as covariate selection methods, but it is always the responsibility of the user to choose the content and form of the final model.

4.4   NUMERICAL PROBLEMS

In previous chapters we have occasionally mentioned various numerical problems that can occur when fitting a logistic regression model. These problems are caused by certain structures in the data coupled with the lack of appropriate checks in some logistic regression software. The goal of this section is to illustrate these structures in certain simple situations and illustrate what can happen when the logistic regression model is fit to such data. The issue here is not one of model correctness or specification, but the effect certain data patterns have on the computation of parameter estimates. Some of these problems are due to "thin" data, namely not enough outcomes, usually $y = 1$, and/or small frequencies for a categorical covariate. In some settings use of exact logistic regression methods, discussed in Section 10.3 can provide correctly estimated coefficients and standard errors. In this section we present results from running various example data in several different packages.

For some of the examples we do not state which package produced the results. The reason is that packages are revised and the results we get in one version with these ill conditioned data might well change in the next release. Also different packages might provide different output from the same ill conditioned data. The point of the examples is to learn the numerical signs and symptoms that indicate a numerical problem in the data.

Perhaps the simplest and thus most obvious situation is when we have a frequency of zero in a contingency table. An example of such a contingency table is given in Table 4.34. The estimated odds ratios and log-odds ratios using the first level of the covariate as the reference group are given in the first two rows below the table. The point estimate of the odds ratios for level 3 versus level 1 is infinite since all subjects at level 3 responded. The results of fitting a logistic regression model to these data are given in the last two rows. The estimated coefficient in the first column is the intercept coefficient. The particular package used does not really matter as many, but not all, packages produce similar output. One program that does identify the problem is STATA. It provides an error message that $x = 3$ perfectly predicts the outcome and the design variable for $x = 3$ is not included

Table 4.34   A Contingency Table with a Zero Cell Count and the Results of Fitting a Logistic Regression Model to these Data

Outcome / x	1	2	3	Total
1	7	12	20	39
0	13	8	0	21
Total	20	20	20	60
$\widehat{OR}$	1	2.79	inf	
$\ln(\widehat{OR})$	0	1.03	inf	
$\hat{\beta}$	−0.62	1.03	11.7	
$\widehat{SE}$	0.47	0.65	34.9	

in the fit of the model. Other programs may or may not provide some sort of error message indicating that convergence was not obtained or that the maximum number of iterations was used. What is rather obvious, and the tip-off that there is a problem with the model, is the large estimated coefficient for the second design variable and especially its large estimated standard error.

A common practice to avoid having an undefined point estimate is to add one-half to each of the cell counts. Adding one-half may allow us to move forward with the analysis of a single contingency table, but such a simplistic remedy is rarely satisfactory with a more complex data set.

As a slightly more complex example we consider the stratified 2 by 2 tables shown in Table 4.35. The stratum-specific point estimates of the odds ratios are provided below each 2 by 2 table. The results of fitting a series of logistic regression models are provided in Table 4.36.

In the case of the data shown in Table 4.35 we do not encounter problems until we include the stratum z, by risk factor x, and interaction terms, $x \times z\_2$ and $x \times z\_3$ in the model. The addition of the interaction terms results in a model that is equivalent to fitting a model with a single categorical variable with six levels, one for each column in Table 4.35. Thus, in a sense, the problem encountered when we include the interaction is the same one illustrated in Table 4.34. As was the case when fitting a model to the data in Table 4.34, the presence of a zero cell count is manifested by an unbelievably large estimated coefficient and estimated standard error.

The presence of a zero cell count should be detected during the univariable screening of the data. Knowing that the zero cell count is going to cause problems

Table 4.35   Stratified 2 by 2 Contingency Tables with a Zero Cell Count Within One Stratum

Stratum (z)	1		2		3	
Outcome / x	1	0	1	0	1	0
1	5	2	10	2	15	1
0	5	8	2	6	0	4
Total	10	10	12	8	15	5
$\widehat{\text{OR}}$	4		15		inf	

Table 4.36   Results of Fitting Logistic Regression Models to the Data in Table 4.35

Model	1		2	
Variable	Coeff.	Std. Err.	Coeff.	Std. Err.
x	2.77	0.72	1.39	1.01
z_2	1.19	0.81	0.29	1.14
z_3	2.04	0.89	0.00	1.37
$x \times z\_2$			1.32	1.51
$x \times z\_3$			11.54	50.22
Constant	−2.32	0.77	−1.39	0.79

in the modeling stage of the analysis we could collapse the categories of the variable in a meaningful way to eliminate it, eliminate the category completely, or if the variable is at least ordinal scale, treat it as continuous.

The type of zero cell count illustrated in Table 4.35 results from spreading the data over too many cells. This problem is not likely to occur until we begin to include interactions in the model. When it does occur, we should examine the three-way contingency table equivalent to the one shown in Table 4.35. The unstable results prevent us from determining whether, in fact, the interaction is important. To assess the interaction we first need to eliminate the zero cell count. One way to do this is by collapsing categories of the stratification variable. For example, in Table 4.35 we might decide that values of $z = 2$ and $z = 3$ are similar enough to pool them. The stratified analysis would then have two 2 by 2 tables the second of which results from pooling the tables for $z = 2$ and $z = 3$. A second approach is to define a new variable equal to the combination of the stratification variable and the risk factor and to pool over levels of this variable and model it as a main effect variable. Using Table 4.35 as an example, we would have a variable with six levels corresponding to the six columns in the table. We could collapse levels five and six together. Another pooling strategy would be to pool levels three and five, and four and six. This pooling strategy is equivalent to collapsing over levels of the stratification variable. The net effect is the loss of degrees of freedom commensurate with the amount of pooling. Twice the difference in the log-likelihood for the main effects only model, and the model with the modified interaction term added, provides a statistic for the significance of the coefficients for the modified interaction term.

The fitted models shown in Tables 4.34 and 4.36 resulted in large estimated coefficients and estimated standard errors. In some examples we have encountered, the magnitude of the estimated coefficient was not large enough to suspect a numerical problem, but the estimated standard error always was. Hence, we believe that the best indicator of a numerical problem in logistic regression is the estimated standard error. In general, any time that the estimated standard error of an estimated coefficient is large relative to the point estimate, we should suspect the presence of one of the data structures described in this section.

A second type of numerical problem occurs when a collection of the covariates completely separates the outcome groups or, in the terminology of discriminant analysis, the covariates discriminate perfectly. For example, suppose that the age of every subject with the outcome present was greater than 50 and the age of all subjects with the outcome absent was less than 49. Thus, if we know the age of a subject we know with certainty the value of the outcome variable. In this situation there is no overlap in the distribution of the covariates between the two outcome groups. This type of data has been shown by Bryson and Johnson (1981) to have the property of monotone likelihood. The net result is that the maximum likelihood estimates do not exist [see Albert and Anderson (1984); Santner and Duffy (1986)]. In order to have finite maximum likelihood estimates we must have some overlap in the distribution of the covariates in the model.

Table 4.37   Estimated Slope ($\hat{\beta}_x$), Constant ($\hat{\beta}_0$), and Estimated Standard Errors ($\widehat{SE}$) when the Data Have Complete Separation, Quasicomplete Separation, and Overlap

Estimates/x_6	5.5	6.0	6.05	6.10	6.15	6.20	8.0
$\hat{\beta}_x$	20.3	7.5	3.7	3.0	2.6	2.3	0.2
$\widehat{SE}$	36.0	42.4	6.3	4.4	3.6	3.0	0.7
$\hat{\beta}_0$	−116.6	−44.0	−22.2	−17.9	−15.3	−13.5	−0.1
$\widehat{SE}$	208.1	254.3	38.2	27.1	22.1	189.1	5.8

A simple example illustrates the problem of complete separation and the results of fitting logistic regression models to such data. Suppose we have the following 12 pairs of covariate and outcome, (x, y) : (1,0), (2,0), (3,0), (4,0), (5,0), ($x_6 = 5.5$, or 6.0, or 6.05, or 6.1, or 6.2, or 8.0, $y_6 = 0$), (6,1), (7,1), (8,1), (9,1), (10,1), (11,1). The results of fitting logistic regression models when x_6 takes on one of the values 5.5, 6.0, 6.05, 6.1, 6.2, or 8, using SAS version 9.2 are given in Table 4.37. When we use $x_6 = 5.5$ we have complete separation and all estimated parameters are huge, since the maximum likelihood estimates do not exist. SAS provides a warning but at the same time provides the values of the estimates at the last iteration, leaving the ultimate decision about how to handle the output to the user. Similar behavior occurs when the value of $x_6 = 6.0$ is used. SAS notes this fact and again provides estimates. When overlap is at a single or a few tied values the configuration was termed by Albert and Anderson (1984) as quasi complete separation. As the value of x_6 takes on values greater than 6.0 the overlap becomes greater and the estimated parameters and standard errors begin to attain more reasonable values. The sensitivity of the fit to the overlap depends on the sample size and the range of the covariate. The tip-off that something is amiss is, as in the case of the zero cell count, the very large estimated coefficients and especially the large estimated standard errors. Other programs, including STATA, do not provide output when there is complete or quasicomplete separation, for example, $x_6 = 5.5$ or $x_6 = 6$. In the remaining cases STATA and SAS produce similar results.

The occurrence of complete separation in practice depends on the sample size, the number of subjects with the outcome present, and the number of variables included in the model. For example, suppose we have a sample of 25 subjects and only five have the outcome present. The chance that the main effects model demonstrates complete separation increases with the number of variables we include in the model. Thus, the modeling strategy that includes all variables in the model is particularly sensitive to complete separation. Albert and Anderson (1984) and Santner and Duffy (1986) provide rather complicated diagnostic procedures for determining whether a set of data displays complete or quasicomplete separation. Albert and Anderson (1984) recommend that in the absence of their diagnostic, if one looks at the estimated standard errors and if these tend to increase substantially with each iteration of the fit, then one can suspect the presence of complete separation. As

Table 4.38 Data Displaying Near Collinearity Among the
Independent Variables and Constant

Subject	x_1	x_2	x_3	y
1	0.225	0.231	1.026	0
2	0.487	0.489	1.022	1
3	−1.080	−1.070	1.074	0
4	−0.870	−0.870	1.091	0
5	−0.580	−0.570	1.095	0
6	−0.640	−0.640	1.010	0
7	1.614	1.619	1.087	0
8	0.352	0.355	1.095	1
9	−1.025	−1.018	1.008	0
10	0.929	0.937	1.057	1

noted in Chapter 3 the easiest way to address complete separation is to use some careful univariable analyses. The occurrence of complete separation is not likely to be of great clinical importance as it is usually a numerical coincidence rather than describing some important clinical phenomenon. It is a problem we must work around.

As is the case in linear regression, model fitting via logistic regression is also sensitive to collinearities among the independent variables in the model. Most software packages have some sort of diagnostic check, like the tolerance test employed in linear regression. Nevertheless it is possible for variables to pass these tests and have the program run, but yield output that is clearly nonsense. As a simple example, we fit logistic regression models using STATA to the data displayed in Table 4.20. In the table $x_1 \sim N(0, 1)$ and the outcome variable was generated by comparing a $U(0, 1)$ variate, u, to the true probability $\pi(x_1) = e^{x_1}/(1 + e^{x_1})$ as follows: if $u < \pi(x_1)$ then $y = 1$, otherwise $y = 0$. The notation $N(0, 1)$ indicates a random variable following the standard normal (mean $= 0$, variance $= 1$) distribution and $U(a, b)$ indicates a random variable following the uniform distribution on the interval $[a, b]$. The other variables were generated from x_1 and the constant as follows: $x_2 = x_1 + U(0, 0.1)$ and $x_3 = 1 + U(0, 0.01)$. Thus, x_1 and x_2 are highly correlated and x_3 is nearly collinear with the constant term. The results of fitting logistic regression models to various subsets of the variables shown in Table 4.38 are presented in Table 4.39.

The model that includes the highly correlated variables x_1 and x_2 has both very large estimated slope coefficients and estimated standard errors. For the model containing x_3 we see that the estimated coefficients are of reasonable magnitude but the estimated standard errors are much larger than we would expect. The model containing all variables is a composite of the results of the other models. In all cases the tip-off for a problem comes from the aberrantly large estimated standard errors.

In a more complicated data set, an analysis of the associations among the covariates using a collinearity analysis similar to that performed in linear regression should be helpful in identifying the dependencies among the covariates. Belsley

Table 4.39   Estimated Coefficients and Standard Errors from Fitting Logistic Regression Models to the Data in Table 4.38

Var.	Coeff.	Std. Err.	Coeff.	Std. Err.	Coeff.	Std. Err.	Coeff.	Std. Err.
x_1	1.4	1.0	104.2	256.2			79.8	272.6
x_2			−103.4	256.0			−78.3	272.5
x_3					1.8	20.0	−11.1	206.6
Cons.	−1.0	0.8	−0.3	1.3	−2.7	21.1	11.4	27.8

et al. (1980) discuss a number of methods that are implemented in many linear regression packages. One would normally not employ such an in-depth investigation of the covariates unless there was evidence of degradation in the fit similar to that shown in Table 4.39. An alternative is to use the ridge regression methods proposed by Schaefer (1986).

In general, the numerical problems of a zero cell count, complete separation, and collinearity, are manifested by extraordinarily large estimated standard errors and sometimes by a large estimated coefficient as well. New users and those without much computer experience are especially cautioned to look at their results carefully for evidence of numerical problems. In many settings all is not lost. Heinze and Schemper (2002) and Heinze (2006) discuss and illustrate the use of methods that can produce valid parameter estimates and confidence intervals with data containing zero frequency cells and/or separation. These methods include exact logistic regression and penalized likelihood methods, which we discuss and illustrate in Section 10.3.

EXERCISES

1. Show algebraically and with a numerical example of your choice that the restricted cubic spline functions in equation (4.3) meet at the three knots.

2. In the modeling of the GLOW500 data using purposeful selection age was modeled as linear in the logit. We noted that the estimated coefficients for the quartile design variables for age in Table 4.10 suggested an alternative parameterization: using the design variable for the fourth quartile AGE_4. This parameterization of age was not pursued further. Proceed with purposeful selection using AGE_4. To save time, assume that your main effects model is the one in Table 4.9 but with AGE replaced by AGE_4. Compare your model to the one in Table 4.15 that resulted when age was modeled as linear in the logit. Which model do you think is the better one for estimating risk factors for fracture?

3. In the modeling of the Burn Injury data questions came up as to how to model age. There were essentially three choices: linear (power 1), quadratic (powers 1 and 2) and the best fractional polynomial model (power 2). In the text we

proceeded with power 2. Perform selection of interactions for the other two parameterizations and save your work for an exercise on model evaluation in Chapter 5.

4. Demonstrate best subset selection of interactions by beginning with the main effects model from the GLOW500 data.

5. The restricted cubic spline analysis for age in the Burn Injury Study shown in Table 4.21 used four knots at the 5th, 35th, 65th, and 95th percentiles (see Table 4.1). Verify that spline functions formed from these four knots provide a better model than using three or five knots placed at the respective percentiles in Table 4.1.

6. Consider the data from the Myopia Study described in Section 1.6.6 whose variables are described in Table 1.10. The binary outcome variable is MYOPIC ($0 =$ Yes, $1 =$ No). Consider as independent variables all others in Table 1.10 except spherical equivalent refraction (SPHEQ) as it is used to define the outcome variable, the composite of near-work hours (DIOPTERHR) and study year (STUDYYEAR).

    (a) Use purposeful selection to obtain what you feel is the best model for estimating the effect of the risk factors on myopia. This analysis must include identification of the scale in the logit of all continuous covariates and selection of interactions. Assume that all possible interactions among your main effects are clinically reasonable.

    (b) Repeat problem 6(a) using stepwise selection of covariates (main effects and then interactions among main effects forcing in the main effects).

    (c) Repeat problem 6(a) using best subset selection of covariates with Mallows' C_q (main effects and then interactions among main effects forcing in the main effects).

    (d) Repeat problem 6(a) using multivariable fractional polynomial selection of main effects followed by purposeful selection of interactions.

CHAPTER 5

Assessing the Fit of the Model

5.1 INTRODUCTION

We begin our discussion of methods for assessing the fit of an estimated logistic regression model with the assumption that we are, at least preliminarily, satisfied with our efforts at the model building stage. By this we mean that, to the best of our knowledge, the model contains those variables (main effects as well as interactions) that should be in the model and that variables have been entered in the correct functional form. Now we would like to know whether the probabilities produced by the model accurately reflect the true outcome experience in the data. This is referred to as its *goodness of fit*.

If we intend to assess the goodness of fit of the model, then we should have some specific ideas about what it means to say that a model fits. Assume that we denote the observed sample values of the outcome variable, in vector form, as $\mathbf{y}$, where $\mathbf{y}' = (y_1, y_2, y_3, \ldots, y_n)$. We denote the values estimated by the model, or *fitted values*, as $\hat{\mathbf{y}}$, where $\hat{\mathbf{y}}' = (\hat{y}_1, \hat{y}_2, \hat{y}_3, \ldots, \hat{y}_n)$. We conclude that the model fits if: (1) summary measures of the distance between $\mathbf{y}$ and $\hat{\mathbf{y}}$ are small and (2) the contribution of each pair, $(y_i, \hat{y}_i)$, $i = 1, 2, 3, \ldots, n$, to these summary measures is unsystematic and small relative to the error structure of the model. Thus, a complete assessment of the fitted model involves both the calculation of summary measures and a thorough examination of the individual components of these measures.

Before getting into the details of assessing model fit we discuss some approaches that have been used that supposedly assess model fit, but actually do not. The model building techniques discussed in Chapter 4 compare competing fitted models that are based on hypothesis tests that one or more of the model coefficients are equal to zero. For example, does weight contribute to a model containing age and history of fracture? Stated in other words: Is the model with weight *better than* the model without weight? Thus, we are really comparing two sets of different fitted values. While we do not include references here, we have read numerous subject matter

Applied Logistic Regression, Third Edition.
David W. Hosmer, Jr., Stanley Lemeshow, and Rodney X. Sturdivant.

papers over the years where authors state something like "we added the square of age to the model and it was not significant so we conclude that the model fits". This test merely asserts that the model with age squared is not *better than* the model without age squared. Assessing goodness of fit is not a *relative* comparison, it is an *absolute* comparison. When we assess goodness of fit we are comparing the fitted values to the observed values, where we can think of the observed values as being from the best possible (saturated) model. Another way to describe this is to consider a sequence of progressively larger (more covariates) models. The smallest model contains only the constant term, β_0. The process of model building adds variables to the model and the significance of added covariates is assessed by referring backward, to a smaller model, one without the added covariates. In assessing goodness of fit we compare the fitted model to the largest possible model, the saturated model, not a smaller model.

In summary, the components of our proposed approach to assess model fit and adequacy are: (1) computation and evaluation of overall measures of fit, (2) examination of the individual components of the summary statistics, often graphically, and (3) examination of other measures of the difference or distance between the observed and fitted values.

5.2 SUMMARY MEASURES OF GOODNESS OF FIT

We begin with the summary measures of goodness of fit, as many are routinely provided as output by statistical software and give an indication of the overall fit of the model. Summary statistics, by nature, may not provide information about the individual model components. A small value for one of these statistics does not rule out the possibility of some substantial and thus interesting deviation from fit for a few subjects. On the other hand, a large value for one of these statistics is a clear indication of a substantial problem with the model.

Before discussing specific goodness of fit statistics, we consider the effect the fitted model has on the degrees of freedom available for the assessment of model performance. We use the term *covariate pattern* to describe a particular configuration of values for the covariates in a model. For example, in a data set containing values of age, race, sex and weight for each subject, the combination of these factors may result in as many different covariate patterns as there are subjects. On the other hand, if the model contains only race and sex, each coded at two levels, there are only four possible covariate patterns. We note that during model development it is not necessary to be concerned about the number of covariate patterns. The degrees of freedom for tests are based on the difference in the number of parameters in competing models, not on the number of covariate patterns. However, the number of covariate patterns may be an issue when the fit of a model is assessed.

Goodness of fit is assessed over the fitted values determined by the covariates in the model, not the total collection of available covariates. For instance, suppose that our fitted model contains p independent variables, $\mathbf{x}' = (x_1, x_2, x_3, \ldots, x_p)$, and let J denote the number of distinct values of $\mathbf{x}$ observed. If some subjects have the same value of $\mathbf{x}$ then $J < n$. We denote the number of subjects with $\mathbf{x} = \mathbf{x}_j$ by $m_j, j = 1, 2, 3, \ldots, J$. It follows that $\sum m_j = n$. Let y_j denote the number of responses, $y = 1$, among the m_j subjects with $\mathbf{x} = \mathbf{x}_j$. It follows that $\sum y_j = n_1$, the total number of subjects with $y = 1$. The statistical distributions of the summary goodness of fit statistics are obtained by letting n become large while holding the number of parameters, coefficients, in the model fixed. If the number of covariate patterns also increases with n then each value of m_j tends to be small. For example, if we have age in the model, then increasing n will likely increase the distinct ages in the sample. Distributional results obtained under the condition that only n becomes large are said to be based on n-asymptotics. If we fix $J < n$ and let n become large then each value of m_j also tends to become large. Distributional results based on each m_j becoming large are said to be based on m-asymptotics. The difference between these asymptotics and the need to distinguish between them should become clearer as we discuss summary statistics in greater detail.

Initially, we assume that $J \approx n$. This is the case most frequently encountered in practice when there is at least one continuous covariate in the model. It also presents the greatest challenge in developing distributions of goodness of fit statistics.

5.2.1 Pearson Chi-Square Statistic, Deviance, and Sum-of-Squares

In linear regression, summary measures of fit, as well as diagnostics for casewise effects on the fit, are functions of a residual defined as the difference between the observed and fitted value $(y - \hat{y})$. In logistic regression there are several possible ways to measure the difference between the observed and fitted values. To emphasize the fact that the fitted values in logistic regression are calculated for each covariate pattern and depend on the estimated probability for that covariate pattern, we denote the fitted value for the jth covariate pattern as $\hat{y}_j$ where

$$\hat{y}_j = m_j \hat{\pi}_j = m_j \left\{ \frac{e^{\hat{g}(\mathbf{x}_j)}}{1 + e^{\hat{g}(\mathbf{x}_j)}} \right\}$$

where $\hat{g}(\mathbf{x}_j) = \hat{\beta}_0 + \hat{\beta}_1 x_{j1} + \hat{\beta}_2 x_{j2} + \cdots + \hat{\beta}_p x_{jp}$ is the estimated logit.

We begin by considering three measures of the difference between the observed and the fitted values: the Pearson residual, the deviance residual and the residual used in linear regression. For a particular covariate pattern the Pearson residual is

$$r(y_j, \hat{\pi}_j) = \frac{(y_j - m_j \hat{\pi}_j)}{\sqrt{m_j \hat{\pi}_j (1 - \hat{\pi}_j)}}. \tag{5.1}$$

The summary statistic based on these residuals is the Pearson chi-square statistic

$$X^2 = \sum_{j=1}^{J} \left[r\left(y_j, \hat{\pi}_j\right) \right]^2. \tag{5.2}$$

The deviance residual is

$$d(y_j, \hat{\pi}_j) = \pm \left\{ 2 \left[y_j \ln \left(\frac{y_j}{m_j \hat{\pi}_j} \right) + (m_j - y_j) \ln \left(\frac{(m_j - y_j)}{m_j (1 - \hat{\pi}_j)} \right) \right] \right\}^{1/2}, \quad (5.3)$$

where the sign $+$ or $-$ is the same as the sign of $(y_j - m_j \hat{\pi}_j)$. For covariate patterns with $y_j = 0$ the deviance residual is

$$d(y_j, \hat{\pi}_j) = -\sqrt{2 m_j |\ln(1 - \hat{\pi}_j)|}$$

and the deviance residual when $y_j = m_j$ is

$$d(y_j, \hat{\pi}_j) = \sqrt{2 m_j |\ln(\hat{\pi}_j)|} .$$

The summary statistic based on the deviance residuals is the deviance

$$D = \sum_{j=1}^{J} d(y_j, \hat{\pi}_j)^2. \quad (5.4)$$

In a setting where $J = n$, this is the same quantity shown in equation (1.10).

The linear regression-like residual is defined as the difference between the observed and predicted outcome (as determined by the model), namely

$$s(y_j, \hat{\pi}_j) = (y_j - m_j \hat{\pi}_j) \quad (5.5)$$

and the fit statistic is the sum-of-squares

$$S = \sum_{j=1}^{J} s(y_j, \hat{\pi}_j)^2. \quad (5.6)$$

The distribution of the statistics X^2 and D under the assumption that the fitted model is correct in all aspects is supposed to be chi-square with degrees of freedom equal to $J - (p + 1)$. For the deviance this statement follows from the fact that D is the likelihood ratio test statistic of a saturated model with J parameters versus the fitted model with $p + 1$ parameters. Similar theory provides the null distribution of X^2. The problem is that when $J \approx n$, the distribution is obtained under n-asymptotics, and hence the number of parameters is increasing at the same rate as the sample size. Thus, p-values calculated for these two statistics when $J \approx n$, using the $\chi^2(J - p - 1)$ distribution, are incorrect. We describe below a method that centers and scales the Pearson chi-square statistic so that the standard normal distribution may be used to obtain a correct p-value. The distribution of S is a little more complex, but an approximation is discussed later in this section.

One way to avoid the above noted difficulties with the distributions of X^2 and D when $J \approx n$ is to group the data in such a way that m-asymptotics can be used. To understand the rationale behind the various grouping strategies that have been proposed, it is helpful to think of X^2 as the Pearson chi-square statistic and D as the log-likelihood chi-square statistic that result from a $2 \times J$ table. The rows of the table correspond to the two values of the outcome variable $y = 1, 0$. The J columns correspond to the J possible covariate patterns. The estimate of the expected value under the hypothesis that the logistic model in question is the correct model for the cell corresponding to the $y = 1$ row and jth column is $m_j \hat{\pi}_j$. It follows that the estimate of the expected value for the cell corresponding to the $y = 0$ row and jth column is $m_j (1 - \hat{\pi}_j)$. The statistics X^2 and D are calculated in the usual manner from this table.

Thinking of the statistics as arising from the $2 \times J$ table gives some intuitive insight as to why we cannot expect them to follow the $\chi^2(J - p - 1)$ distribution. When chi-square tests are computed from a contingency table the p-values are correct under the null hypothesis when the estimated expected values are "large" in each cell. This condition holds under m-asymptotics. In practice, minimum required expected frequencies have been proposed (e.g., among others, $m_j \hat{\pi}_j > 5$). Although this is an oversimplification of the situation, it is essentially correct. In the $2 \times J$ table described above the expected values are always quite small since the number of columns increases as n increases. One way to avoid this problem is to collapse the columns into a fixed number of groups g, and then calculate observed and expected frequencies. By fixing the number of columns, the estimated expected frequencies become large as n becomes large. Thus, m-asymptotics hold.

The theory required to derive the distribution of the statistics based on a collapsed table is not quite so straightforward, but the intuitive appeal of thinking in this manner is helpful. The relevant distribution theory presented in a series of papers by Moore (1971), and Moore and Spruill (1975), considers what happens to chi-square goodness of fit tests when the boundaries forming the cells are functions of random variables, namely the estimated coefficients.

5.2.2   The Hosmer–Lemeshow Tests

Hosmer and Lemeshow (1980) and Lemeshow and Hosmer (1982) proposed grouping based on the values of the estimated probabilities. Assume, for the sake of discussion, that $J = n$. In this case we think of the n columns as corresponding to the n values of the estimated probabilities, with the first column corresponding to the smallest value, and the nth column to the largest value. Two grouping strategies were proposed as follows: (i) collapse the table based on percentiles of the estimated probabilities and (ii) collapse the table based on fixed values of the estimated probability.

With the first method, use of $g = 10$ groups results in the first group containing the $n_1' = n/10$ subjects having the smallest estimated probabilities, and the last group containing the $n_{10}' = n/10$ subjects having the largest estimated probabilities. With the second method, use of $g = 10$ groups results in cutpoints defined at the values $k/10$, $k = 1, 2, \ldots, 9$ and the groups contain all subjects with estimated probabilities between adjacent cutpoints. For example, the first group contains all subjects whose estimated probability is less than or equal to 0.1, while the tenth group contains those subjects whose estimated probability is greater than 0.9. For the $y = 1$ row, estimates of the expected values are obtained by summing the estimated probabilities over all subjects in a group. For the $y = 0$ row, the estimated expected value is obtained by summing, over all subjects in the group, one minus the estimated probability. For either grouping strategy, the Hosmer-Lemeshow goodness of fit statistic, $\hat{C}$, is obtained by calculating the Pearson chi-square statistic from the $g \times 2$ table of observed and estimated expected frequencies. A formula defining the calculation of $\hat{C}$ is as follows:

$$\hat{C} = \sum_{k=1}^{g} \left[\frac{(o_{1k} - \hat{e}_{1k})^2}{\hat{e}_{1k}} + \frac{(o_{0k} - \hat{e}_{0k})^2}{\hat{e}_{0k}} \right], \tag{5.7}$$

where

$$o_{1k} = \sum_{j=1}^{c_k} y_j,$$

$$o_{0k} = \sum_{j=1}^{c_k} (m_j - y_j),$$

$$\hat{e}_{1k} = \sum_{j=1}^{c_k} m_j \hat{\pi}_j,$$

$$\hat{e}_{0k} = \sum_{j=1}^{c_k} m_j (1 - \hat{\pi}_j)$$

and c_k is the number of covariate patterns in the kth group. With a bit of algebra one may show that

$$\hat{C} = \sum_{k=1}^{g} \frac{(o_{1k} - n'_k \bar{\pi}_k)^2}{n'_k \bar{\pi}_k (1 - \bar{\pi}_k)}, \tag{5.8}$$

where $\bar{\pi}_k$ is the average estimated probability in the kth group,

$$\bar{\pi}_k = \frac{1}{n'_k} \sum_{j=1}^{c_k} m_j \hat{\pi}_j.$$

Using an extensive set of simulations, Hosmer and Lemeshow (1980) demonstrated that, when $J = n$ and the fitted logistic regression model is the correct model, the distribution of the statistic $\hat{C}$ is well approximated by the chi-square distribution with $g - 2$ degrees of freedom $\chi^2(g - 2)$. While not specifically examined, it is likely that $\chi^2(g - 2)$ also approximates the distribution when $J \approx n$.

An alternative to the denominator shown in equation (5.8) is obtained if we consider o_{1k} to be the sum of independent nonidentically distributed random variables. This suggests that we should standardize the squared difference between the observed and estimated expected frequency by

$$\sum_{j=1}^{c_k} m_j \hat{\pi}_j (1 - \hat{\pi}_j).$$

It is easy to show that

$$\sum_{j=1}^{c_k} m_j \hat{\pi}_j (1 - \hat{\pi}_j) = n'_k \overline{\pi}_k (1 - \overline{\pi}_k) - \sum_{j=1}^{c_k} m_j (\hat{\pi}_j - \overline{\pi}_k)^2.$$

In a series of simulations Xu (1996) showed that use of

$$\sum_{j=1}^{c_k} m_j \hat{\pi}_j (1 - \hat{\pi}_j)$$

results in a trivial increase in the value of the test statistic. Pigeon and Heyse (1999a, 1999b) proposed an adjustment that is the ratio of two estimators

$$\phi_k = \frac{\displaystyle\sum_{j=1}^{c_k} m_j \hat{\pi}_j (1 - \hat{\pi}_j)}{n'_k \overline{\pi}_k (1 - \overline{\pi}_k)}$$

yielding the statistic

$$\widehat{C}_p = \sum_{k=1}^{g} \frac{1}{\phi_k} \left[\frac{(o_{1k} - \hat{e}_{1k})^2}{\hat{e}_{1k}} + \frac{(o_{0k} - \hat{e}_{0k})^2}{\hat{e}_{0k}} \right]$$

$$= \sum_{k=1}^{g} \frac{1}{\phi_k} \frac{(o_{1k} - n'_k \overline{\pi}_k)^2}{n'_k \overline{\pi}_k (1 - \overline{\pi}_k)}$$

$$= \sum_{k=1}^{g} \left[\frac{(o_{1k} - n'_k \overline{\pi}_k)^2}{\displaystyle\sum_{j=1}^{c_k} m_j \hat{\pi}_j (1 - \hat{\pi}_j)} \right],$$

which is the statistic examined by Xu (1996). Pigeon and Heyse report in their simulations that the distribution of $\widehat{C}_p$, under the hypothesis that one has fit the correct model with a sufficiently large sample, is approximated by the $\chi^2(g-1)$ distribution. This appears to contradict Xu who showed in her simulations that the distribution of $\widehat{C}_p$ could be well approximated by $\chi^2(g-2)$. In a recent simulation study Canary (2012) showed that the distribution of $\widehat{C}_p$ was much closer to $\chi^2(g-2)$ than $\chi^2(g-1)$. Since the modified statistic $\widehat{C}_p$ is not readily available in software packages, we use $\widehat{C}$ calculated using equation (5.7) or (5.8).

Additional research by Hosmer et al. (1988) has shown that the grouping method based on percentiles of the estimated probabilities is preferable to the one based on fixed cutpoints in the sense of better adherence to the $\chi^2(g-2)$ distribution, especially when many of the estimated probabilities are small (i.e., less than 0.2). Thus, unless stated otherwise, $\widehat{C}$ is based on the percentile-type of grouping, usually with $g = 10$ groups. These groups are often referred to as the "deciles of risk". This term comes from health sciences research where the outcome $y = 1$ often represents the occurrence of some disease. Most if not all logistic regression software packages provide the capability to obtain $\widehat{C}$ and its p-value, usually based on 10 groups. In addition many packages provide or have the option to obtain a 10×2 table listing the observed and estimated expected frequencies in each decile.

The results of applying the decile of risk grouping strategy to the estimated probabilities computed from the model for the GLOW Study in Table 4.16 are shown in Table 5.1. For example, the observed frequency in the fracture group, (FRACTURE $= 1$), for the sixth decile of risk, $0.208 < \hat{\pi}_j \leq 0.249$, is 13. This value is obtained from the sum of the observed outcomes for the 50 subjects in this group. The corresponding estimated expected frequency for this decile is 11.4, which is the sum of the 50 estimated probabilities for these subjects. The observed frequency for the no fracture on follow up group (FRACTURE $= 0$) is $50 - 13 = 37$, and the estimated expected frequency is $50 - 11.4 = 38.6$.

The value of the Hosmer–Lemeshow goodness of fit statistic computed from the frequencies in Table 5.1 is $\widehat{C} = 6.39$ and the corresponding p-value computed from the chi-square distribution with 8 degrees of freedom is 0.603. This indicates that the model seems to fit quite well. A comparison of the observed and expected frequencies in each of the 20 cells in Table 5.1 shows close agreement within each decile of risk.

Since the distribution of $\widehat{C}$ depends on m-asymptotics, the appropriateness of the p-value depends on the validity of the assumption that the estimated expected

Table 5.1 Observed (Obs) and Estimated Expected (Exp) Frequencies Within Each Decile of Risk for FRACTURE = 1 and FRACTURE = 0 Using the Fitted Logistic Regression Model for the GLOW Study in Table 4.16

		FRACTURE $= 1$		FRACTURE $= 0$		
Decile	Cut Point	Obs	Exp	Obs	Exp	Total
1	0.085	3	3.3	47	46.7	50
2	0.111	4	4.9	46	45.1	50
3	0.141	7	6.3	43	43.7	50
4	0.176	11	8.1	40	42.9	51
5	0.208	7	9.4	42	39.6	49
6	0.249	13	11.4	37	38.6	50
7	0.323	9	14.3	41	35.7	50
8	0.389	19	17.6	31	32.4	50
9	0.483	25	21.8	25	28.2	50
10	0.747	27	28.0	23	22.0	50

frequencies are large. Examining Table 5.1 we see that only two of the estimated expected frequencies is less than five and none are less than one. In general, our point of view is a bit more liberal than those who maintain that with tables of this size (about 20 cells), all expected frequencies must be greater than 5. In this case, we feel that there is reason to believe that the calculation of the p-value is accurate enough to support the hypothesis that the model fits. If one is concerned about the magnitude of the expected frequencies, selected adjacent rows of the table may be combined to increase the size of the expected frequencies, while at the same time, reducing the number of degrees of freedom.

A few additional comments about the calculation of $\widehat{C}$ are needed. When the number of covariate patterns is less than n, we have the possibility that one or more of the empirical deciles will occur at a pattern with $m_j > 1$. If this happens then the value of $\widehat{C}$ will depend, to some extent, on how these ties are assigned to deciles. The fitted model in Table 4.16 has 457 covariate patterns, but only two deciles have frequencies that differ from 50. This indicates that the tied values did not occur exactly at a cut point. The results presented in Table 5.1 were obtained from STATA where ties are assigned to the same decile in such as way as to make the column totals as close to $n/10$ as possible. Other statistical packages may use different strategies to handle ties. For example, fitting the same model in SAS version 9.2 yielded the same fitted model shown in Table 4.16, but with $\widehat{C} = 5.658$ the corresponding p-value is 0.686. The use of different methods to handle ties by different packages is not likely to be an issue unless the number of covariate patterns is so small that assigning all tied values to one decile results in a huge imbalance in decile size, or worse, considerably fewer than 10 groups. In this case the computed value of $\widehat{C}$ may be quite different from one package to the next. In addition, when too few groups are used to calculate $\widehat{C}$, we run the risk that we do not have the sensitivity needed to distinguish observed from expected frequencies. It has been our experience that when $\widehat{C}$ is calculated from fewer than 6 groups, it almost always indicates that the model fits.

As a second example we evaluate the model fit to the Burn Study data shown in Table 4.27. The value of the goodness of fit statistic based on deciles of risk is $\widehat{C} = 8.630$ and, with 8 degrees of freedom yields $p = 0.374$, which supports model fit. The table of observed and estimated expected frequencies in each decile of risk is shown in Table 5.2.

Results similar to those in Table 5.2 are not unlike many others we have seen in practice and present an interesting question: Does a small value of $\widehat{C}$ and large p-value support model fit when so many (in this case seven) of the 20 cells have extremely small expected frequencies (in this case <5, and in five instances, <1)? We must remember that the goal of this analysis is to determine whether there is evidence of model fit, in the sense of agreement between the observed values of the outcome variable and the estimated probabilities of the outcome based on the model. While the estimated number of deaths in each of the first seven deciles of risk is small, the observed number is also small and agrees well with the estimated number. The largest difference between the two among the 20 cells is in the seventh decile. One measure of the difference that we use in practice comes from contingency

Table 5.2 Observed (Obs) and Estimated Expected (Exp) Frequencies Within Each Decile of Risk for DEATH = 1 and DEATH = 0 Using the Fitted Logistic Regression Model for the Burn Study in Table 4.27

Decile	Cut Point	DEATH = 1 Obs	DEATH = 1 Exp	DEATH = 0 Obs	DEATH = 0 Exp	Total
1	0.0007	0	0.1	100	99.9	100
2	0.0013	0	0.1	100	99.9	100
3	0.0023	0	0.2	100	99.8	100
4	0.0041	0	0.3	100	99.7	100
5	0.0080	0	0.6	100	99.4	100
6	0.0182	3	1.2	97	98.8	100
7	0.0535	0	3.3	100	96.7	100
8	0.2273	15	11.4	85	88.6	100
9	0.7122	43	43.5	57	56.5	100
10	0.9986	89	89.4	11	10.6	100

table analysis methods and is

$$\frac{|\hat{o} - \hat{e}|}{\sqrt{\hat{e}}} = \frac{|0 - 3.3|}{\sqrt{3.3}} = 1.82.$$

When the estimated expected frequency is large and we have fit the correct model the standardized difference should follow a standard normal distribution. Hence a number exceeding 1.96 might be used as evidence of a significant difference. (We typically use 2.0 in practice.) Hence our conclusion is that the data in Table 5.2 do support model fit. The actual p-value may not be 0.374, but it is highly unlikely that with such close agreement, it could be smaller than 0.05.

The advantage of any summary goodness of fit statistic, for example $\hat{C}$, is that it provides a single and easily interpretable number that can be used to assess fit. The disadvantage is that in the process of grouping we may miss an important deviation from fit due to a small number of individual data points. Hence we advocate that, before finally accepting that a model fits, an analysis of the individual residuals and relevant diagnostic statistics be performed. These methods are presented in the next section.

Our experience is that a table like the one presented in Table 5.1 or Table 5.2 contains valuable descriptive information for assessing the adequacy of the fitted model over the deciles of risk. Comparison of observed to expected frequencies within each cell may indicate regions where the model does not perform satisfactorily.

One frequently cited disadvantage of the decile of risk grouping is that subjects within each decile may have quite different values for the covariates. The only thing they may have in common is that their estimated probabilities are similar. For this reason Pigeon and Heyse (1999a) suggest that different groupings be used to assess the sensitivity of $\hat{C}$ to this choice. The magnitude of $\hat{C}$ is certain to vary. However, if the correct model is fit then there still should be agreement between the observed and estimated expected frequencies regardless of the grouping used and the test should support model fit.

Other grouping strategies have been proposed that lead to statistics similar to $\hat{C}$. Pulkstenis and Robinson (2002) suggest that, when the model contains one or more continuous covariates, groups be formed by first using the values of the categorical covariates in the model. Within each of these groups partitioning the observations at the median of the estimated probabilities forms two more subgroups. Then a two group table is formed and $\hat{C}$ is calculated as in equation (5.7). This strategy does provide better insights into how fit might change over the categorical covariates, but some of the same criticism holds unless all the continuous covariates have either positive or negative coefficients. When the signs of the coefficients are different one can have similar estimated probabilities, but widely different values for the continuous covariates. Since this grouping strategy is not readily available in software packages and, in our view, offers only a small advantage over the decile of risk grouping, we typically do not use it.

Tsiatis (1980) suggested a goodness of fit statistic based on an explicit partition of the covariates into g regions. This new categorical variable with g levels is introduced into the model. The goodness of fit test is the Score test of the coefficients for the new grouping variable. Tsiatis showed that the Score test for this variable is based on a comparison of the observed frequency to estimated expected frequency within each of the g groups. The test has $g - 1$ degrees of freedom. This test can be easily carried out in SAS and other packages with Score test capabilities. An alternative in packages not having the capability to perform the Score test is to use the maximum partial likelihood test for the coefficients for the addition of the $g - 1$ design variables to the model. With a complicated model like the one in Table 4.16 containing two continuous, four dichotomous covariates and two interactions, it is not a simple task to form groups. If we dichotomize at the median of age and height and use the four dichotomous covariates this would generate $g = 2^6 = 64$ groups. In settings like this where it is difficult or unclear how to partition the covariate space into meaningful groups, an alternative to explicit partitioning is to use deciles of risk. Application of the likelihood ratio test to assess the fit of the model in Table 4.16 using the deciles of risk shown in Table 5.1 yields a value of 4.56 which, with 9 degrees of freedom, gives a p-value of 0.871. Hence, this test also supports the fit of the model. One disadvantage of using the maximum partial likelihood or Score test is that actual values of the observed and estimated expected frequencies need not be obtained. These quantities may be useful, when there is evidence of lack of fit, in indicating those deciles where it is occurring. Canary (2011), using simulations, compares the Tsiatis statistic, $\hat{C}$ and $\hat{C}_P$, and concludes that the performance of the three was similar in that each attained the nominal alpha level when the correct model was fit and had about the same power to detect model misspecification.

Testing goodness of fit using the Pearson chi-square statistic with $J - (p + 1)$ degrees of freedom has generated quite a bit of work in recent years. Osius and Rojek (1992) extended the work by McCullagh (1985a, 1985b, 1986) and derived an easily computed large sample normal approximation to the distribution of the Pearson chi-square statistic. Farrington (1996) proposed a modification of the Pearson chi-square that has better sparse data properties. However, the value of the statistic is identically equal to n when $J = n$. Kuss (2002) simulated the performance of these two versions as well as $\widehat{C}$ and found that with sparse data Farrington's modification out performed $\widehat{C}$. From a practical stand point the Farrington test is not easy to use as it is not calculated by software packages and its moments are complex. Thus we do not consider it further.

Su and Wei (1991) propose a test based on cumulative sums of residuals whose p-value must be determined by complicated and time consuming simulations. Le Cessie and van Houwelingen (1991, 1995) propose tests based on sums-of-squares of smoothed residuals whose p-values may be evaluated using either a normal approximation or an easily computed scaled chi-square distribution. However, neither test is available in software packages at this time.

Stukel (1988) proposes a test that is not a goodness of fit test in the sense of explicitly comparing observed outcomes to predicted outcomes based on the model, but instead determines whether the basic form of the model is consistent with the shape and symmetry of the logistic function. The test statistic has 1 or 2 degrees of freedom, and tests whether a generalized logistic model is better than a standard model fit to the data. Hosmer et al. (1997) examined the distributional properties of these tests via simulations. They recommend that overall assessment of fit be examined using a combination of tests: the Hosmer-Lemeshow decile of risks test, the Osius and Rojek normal approximation to the distribution of the Pearson chi-square statistic, and Stukel's test.

A large sample normal approximation to the distribution of the Pearson chi-square statistic derived by Osius and Rojek (1992) may be easily computed in any package that has the option to save the fitted values from the logistic regression model and do a weighted linear regression. The essential steps in the procedure when we have J covariate patterns are as follows:

1. Save the fitted values from the model, denoted as $\hat{\pi}_j$, $j = 1, 2, 3, \ldots, J$.
2. Create the variable $v_j = m_j \hat{\pi}_j (1 - \hat{\pi}_j)$, $j = 1, 2, 3, \ldots, J$.
3. Create the variable $c_j = \frac{(1 - 2\hat{\pi}_j)}{v_j}$, $j = 1, 2, 3, \ldots, J$.
4. Compute the Pearson chi-square statistic shown in equation (5.2), namely,

$$X^2 = \sum_{j=1}^{J} \frac{(y_j - m_j \hat{\pi}_j)^2}{v_j}.$$

5. Perform a weighted linear regression of c, defined in step 3, on $\mathbf{x}$ the model covariates, using weights v defined in step 2. Note that the sample size for this regression is J, the number of covariate patterns. Let RSS denote the residual sum-of-squares from this regression. Some packages, for example STATA, scale the weights to sum to 1.0. In this case the reported residual sum-of-squares must be multiplied by the mean of the weights to obtain the correct RSS.

6. Compute the correction factor for the variance, denoted for convenience as A, as follows:

$$A = 2\left(J - \sum_{j=1}^{J}\frac{1}{m_j}\right).$$

7. Compute the standardized statistic

$$z_{X^2} = \frac{[X^2 - (J - p - 1)]}{\sqrt{A + RSS}} \tag{5.9}$$

8. Compute a two-tailed p-value using the standard normal distribution.

Application of the eight-step procedure using the model in Table 4.16 yields $X^2 = 442.3392$, $RSS = 170.7262$, $A = 39.6667$ and

$$z = \frac{442.3392 - (457 - 8 - 1)}{\sqrt{39.6667 + 170.7262}} = -0.3903.$$

The two-tailed p-value is $p = 0.6963$. Again, we cannot reject the null hypothesis that the model fits.

To carry out the above analysis it is necessary to form an aggregated data set. This is easy to do in some software packages and impossible in others. In these latter packages we suggest using a second package to create the aggregated data set and then returning to the logistic regression package with this new data set. The essential steps in any package are: (i) Define the main effects as aggregation variables in the model. This defines the covariate patterns. (ii) Calculate the sum of the outcome variable and the number of terms in the sum over the aggregation variables. This produces y_j and m_j for each covariate pattern. (iii) Output a new data set containing the values of the aggregation variables, covariate patterns, and the two calculated variables, y_j and m_j.

The same approach may be used to obtain a normal approximation to the distribution of S. The standardized statistic is

$$z_S = \frac{\left(S - \sum_{j=1}^{J} m_j \hat{\pi}_j \left(1 - \hat{\pi}_j\right)\right)}{\sqrt{A + RSS^*}}, \tag{5.10}$$

where A is defined in Step 6 above, and RSS^* is the residual sum-of-squares of the weighted linear regression of $d_j = (1 - 2\hat{\pi}_j)$ on the covariates in the model with weights $v_j = m_j \hat{\pi}_j (1 - \hat{\pi}_j)$.

Application of the procedure using the model in Table 4.16 yields $S = 82.2760$, $\sum m_j \hat{\pi}_j (1 - \hat{\pi}_j) = 82.0790$, $RSS^* = 0.2176$, $A = 39.6667$ and

$$z = \frac{82.2760 - 82.0790}{\sqrt{39.6667 + 0.2176}} = 0.0312.$$

The two-tailed p-value is $p = 0.975$. Again, we cannot reject the null hypothesis that the model fits.

Hosmer et al. (1997) compared the normalized Pearson chi-square, z_{X^2} and the normalized sum-of-squares z_S by simulation and showed that, in most settings, the two statistics performed similarly. The exception is in settings having extremely small and/or large estimated probabilities and when the outcome "went against the model" (i.e., $y = 0$ when $\hat{\pi}$ is large or $y = 1$ when $\hat{\pi}$ is small). In these cases, the Pearson residual in equation (5.1) can become extremely large resulting in an aberrantly large value of X^2. In fact, the value of a single squared Pearson residual can be large enough to reject fit. Another adverse affect is just the opposite. Namely, such pairs can inflate the variance to the point that even a quite large value of X^2 is declared to be not significant. In these settings we prefer to use S. In most other applied settings we have found little difference in the p-values computed from z_{X^2} and z_S.

Weesie (1998) has written a STATA program implementing a method proposed by Windmeijer (1990) for computing the significance of the Pearson chi-square statistic using the standard normal distribution. The approach is similar to the above eight-step procedure, but is only appropriate in settings when there are n covariate patterns. Thus it is less general than the above method.

Windmeijer (1990) points out that both the Pearson chi-square and the estimator of its variance used to form z in step 7 are quite sensitive, as noted above, to large or small estimated probabilities. Both values are inflated. He suggests that subjects with very small or large fitted values, near 0 or 1, be excluded when using the Pearson chi-square statistic. The default exclusion criteria in Weesie's STATA program are $\hat{\pi} < 1.0 \times 10^{-5}$ or $\hat{\pi} > (1 - 1.0 \times 10^{-5})$. In general, we think this is good advice, but urge considerable caution and complete honesty in reporting what is done so as to avoid possible criticism that the data have been tinkered with in order to obtain a good fitting model.

As described above, Stukel (1988) proposed a 1 or 2 degree of freedom statistic to test whether the parameters of a generalized logistic model are equal to zero. Briefly, the additional parameter(s) allow the tails of the logistic regression model (i.e., the small and large probabilities) to be either heavier/longer or lighter/shorter than the standard logistic regression model. It tests a basic logistic regression model assumption and in that sense we feel it is a useful adjunct to the Hosmer–Lemeshow and Osius–Rojek goodness of fit tests. The test has not been implemented in any package; but it can be easily obtained from the following procedure:

1. Save the fitted values from the model, denoted as $\hat{\pi}_j$, $j = 1, 2, 3, \ldots, J$.
2. Compute the estimated logits,

$$\hat{g}_j = \ln\left(\frac{\hat{\pi}_j}{1 - \hat{\pi}_j}\right) = \mathbf{x}'_j\hat{\boldsymbol{\beta}}, \quad j = 1, 2, 3 \ldots, J.$$

3. Compute two new covariates:

$$z_{1j} = 0.5 \times \hat{g}_j^2 \times I(\hat{\pi}_j \geq 0.5)$$

and

$$z_{2j} = -0.5 \times \hat{g}_j^2 \times I(\hat{\pi}_j < 0.5),$$

for $j = 1, 2, 3, \ldots, J$, where $I(\text{arg}) = 1$ if arg is true and zero if arg is false. Note that in a setting when all the fitted values are either less than or greater than 0.5 only one variable is created.

4. Perform the Score test for the addition of z_1 and/or z_2 to the model. If a package does not perform the Score test then the partial likelihood ratio test can be used.

Application of the four-step procedure to the fitted model in Table 4.16 yields a value for the partial likelihood ratio test of 5.202, and with 2 degrees of freedom, yields $p = 0.074$. Further examination of the results showed that the estimated coefficient for z_1 was large, negative, and marginally significant, Wald test $p = 0.045$. This indicates that the upper tail could possibly be longer than that of the fitted logistic model. However, there are only 41 subjects with estimated probabilities that exceed 0.5. For the moment, we choose not to modify the fitted model. This allows us to accommodate, for the time being, a longer upper tail, until we are able to examine in detail the case wise diagnostic statistics, as we do in the next section.

Application of the eight-step procedure for the Pearson chi-square to the model shown in Table 4.27 fit to the Burn Study data yielded $p = 0.443$. The likelihood ratio test version of Stukel's test also was not significant with $p = 0.311$. Hence we conclude that there is evidence that the model fits.

We leave further assessment of goodness of fit of the model fit to the Burn Study in Table 4.27 as an exercise.

Before moving on to consider other measures of model performance we conclude the discussion of summary tests of model fit with a few comments based on our experience using these tests in practice. When one uses one or more of these tests to assess model fit, the obvious, desirable outcome is to obtain small value(s) for the test statistic(s) and large p-value(s). In hypothesis testing terminology, our decision is "fail to reject that the model fits". In other words, we cannot say that the model does not fit. Hence, the hypothesis testing error that we could be making is the Type II error. Thus, the power of the test used becomes an issue. Unfortunately, as borne out in numerous simulations, none of the grouped decile of risk type tests have particularly high power with small to moderate sample sizes to detect small misspecifications of the model. For example, the simulation results reported in Hosmer et al. (1997) and Canary et al. (2012) indicate that none of the overall goodness of fit tests is especially powerful for sample sizes $n < 400$. For high power one needs both a large sample size as well as a frequently occurring outcome (e.g., $n \geq 500$ and $0.25 \leq n_1/n \leq 0.75$). The reason can be seen in Figure 1.1 where the relationship between age and the outcome is not at all obvious from the data. There is just too much variability for it to be seen. The ungrouped tests, such as the Pearson chi-square test, do have much higher power than the grouped tests to detect model misspecification, but they provide no visual evidence.

In practice, we typically begin by computing the decile of risk test and carefully examine the table of observed and expected frequencies to confirm that the p-value for the test statistic is supported by either their agreement or difference. In settings where the test is either significant or there are seemingly important departures in some deciles we go to the trouble to compute the standardized Pearson and sum-of-squares tests and their p-values. If the differences between observed and expected values are limited to upper and/or lower deciles we use Stukel's test to assess this departure. Note: We discuss alternatives to the logit link function in Chapter 10.

We noted the need for a large sample, and most applications with modeling problems we have seen generally fall into the "too small a sample" class. However, over the years users have contacted us with the opposite problem. They have such a large sample, usually thousands, if not hundreds of thousands of observations that fit is rejected by all tests for a model that seems quite reasonably and clinically plausible. The problem is too much power, enough so that even small differences between observed and expected values are judged to be statistically large. For example, the value of $\widehat{C}$ from Table 5.1 is 6.39 with $p = 0.603$. Assuming that we replicate each subject in the GLOW Study so that the sample size is now 1000 and then fit the model in Table 4.16, we obtain exactly the same estimated coefficients, but now $\widehat{C} = 12.78$ with $p = 0.120$. If we replicate each subject twice to increase the sample size to 1500 and fit the model, then $\widehat{C} = 19.18$ and $p = 0.014$. If we replicate each subject three times to obtain a sample size of 2000 and fit the model, then $\widehat{C} = 25.57$ and $p = 0.001$. In all cases the estimates of the coefficients are unchanged. The table of observed and expected frequencies in each setting is the appropriate multiple of the values in Table 5.1. All 20 cells still display good agreement and yet as n, n_1, and n_0 increase $\widehat{C}$ increases to the point where we reject the null hypothesis that the model fits.

In these cases we have suggested that the user consider partitioning their data into a developmental data set and a validation data set. The presumption is that the developmental data set will be smaller and thus not have extremely high power to detect trivial departures from fit. If this is not feasible then we suggest making an empirical assessment of fit. A modeling corollary to the "too large a sample" problem is that virtually every covariate may have a statistically significant coefficient. This can lead to a model that is too specific to the data (i.e., overfitting). Again, there is no one solution to the problem. In these settings we tend to exclude categorical covariates that have one or more values that are infrequent, less than 10%, and covariates whose estimated odds ratios are clinically small and uninteresting, for example, a 1% increase in the odds due to exposure.

Recently Paul et al. (2012) studied methods for specifying the number of groups so that the power would equal what one would have for a sample of size 1000. They suggest that, for samples sizes from 1000 to 25,000, the number of groups g should be equal to

$$ g = \max \left(10, \ \min \left\{ \frac{n_1}{2}, \frac{n - n_1}{2}, 2 + 8 \times \left(\frac{n}{1000} \right)^2 \right\} \right). \tag{5.11} $$

For example, if one has a sample with $n = 10,000$ and $n_1 = 1000$ then $g = 500$ groups are suggested. With an extremely large number of groups one is unable to visually examine the table of observed and estimated expected frequencies to find departures from model fit. In these cases a plot of observed versus the estimated expected frequencies is recommended, where departure from a line of slope 1 through the origin is the reference for lack of fit. Also as the number of groups gets large the decile test begins to approach the Pearson chi-square test. Hence one practical solution is to calculate the number of groups using equation (5.11), and if g seems unmanageably large use the standardized Pearson chi-square test in equation (5.9). Prabasaj et al. (2012) do not recommend the decile of risk type test for sample sizes exceeding 25,000, and for sample sizes less than 1000 they recommend using 10 groups.

At the end of the day one must use all the information available to make an informed decision about the fit of the model. If the decision is that the model fits, then one should still consider evaluating the model using the other measures and diagnostic statistics described in the sections following this chapter. If the decision is that the model does not fit and one has at least an inkling of the reason, then one might go back and revisit model building. If the reason for lack of fit is not clear then the other techniques in this chapter may help ferret out the reasons.

We want to emphasize that examining the observed and expected frequencies in each of the 20 cells of the 2×10 table is extremely important and may provide invaluable clues as to why the goodness of fit test is rejecting the fit of a model that seems to be good. Instances, where observed counts are small but expected counts are even smaller (i.e., 1 or less), can result in unreasonably large values of $\hat{C}$. For example, if $o_{ij} = 4$ while $\hat{e}_{ij} = 1$, then this cell contributes 9 to the value of $\hat{C}$, certainly enough to adversely influence a decision about the ability of the model to produce probabilities that accurately reflect the true outcome experience in the data.

Two final comments on goodness of fit tests: (1) We feel quite strongly that they should not be used to build models as the likelihood ratio tests for significance of coefficients are much more powerful and appropriate. (2) One should not use the p-value from goodness of fit tests of different models to decide that one is better than another. For example, suppose we have one model with $p = 0.5$ and a different model has $p = 0.7$, our conclusion would be that both models fit and that the choice between the two should be based on subject matter considerations. However, in a setting where $p = 0.02$ for one model and $p = 0.6$ for the other model, we would prefer the latter model. Even in this case, clinical considerations as to the plausibility of the competing models is an important factor.

Next we consider other summary measures of model performance that are often useful in their own right and can supplement the overall tests of fit just discussed.

5.2.3 Classification Tables

An intuitively appealing way to summarize the results of a fitted logistic regression model is via a classification table. This table is the result of cross-classifying the outcome variable, y, with a dichotomous variable whose values are derived from the estimated logistic probabilities. In this application the coefficients produced by the model are used for predicting the outcome (in a binary way) rather than for estimating the probability of the event.

To obtain the derived dichotomous variable we must define a cutpoint, c, and compare each estimated probability to c. If the estimated probability exceeds c then we let the derived variable be equal to 1; otherwise it is equal to 0. The most commonly used value for c is 0.5. The appeal of this type of approach to model assessment comes from the close relationship of logistic regression to discriminant analysis when the distribution of the covariates is multivariate normal within the two outcome groups. However, it is not limited to this model [e.g., see Efron (1975)].

In this approach, estimated probabilities are used to predict group membership. Presumably, if the model predicts group membership accurately according to some criterion, then this is thought to provide evidence that the model fits. Unfortunately, this may or may not be the case. For example, it is easy to construct a situation where the logistic regression model is, in fact, the correct model and thus fits, but classification is poor. Suppose that $\Pr(Y = 1) = \theta_1$ and that $X \sim N(0, 1)$ in the group with $Y = 0$ and $X \sim N(\mu, 1)$ in the group with $Y = 1$. In this discriminant analysis model the slope coefficient for the logistic regression model is (see equation (1.24)) $\beta_1 = \mu$ and the intercept is (see equation (1.23))

$$\beta_0 = \ln\left[\frac{\theta_1}{\left(1 - \theta_1\right)}\right] - \frac{\mu^2}{2}.$$

Under these assumptions, the probability of misclassification (PMC), may be shown to be

$$\text{PMC} = \theta_1 \Phi\left\{\frac{1}{\beta_1}\ln\left[\frac{\left(1 - \theta_1\right)}{\theta_1}\right] - \frac{\beta_1}{2}\right\}$$

$$+ (1 - \theta_1)\Phi\left\{\frac{1}{\beta_1}\ln\left[\frac{\theta_1}{\left(1 - \theta_1\right)}\right] - \frac{\beta_1}{2}\right\},$$

where Φ is the cumulative distribution function of the $N(0,1)$ distribution. Thus, the expected error rate is a function of the magnitude of the slope, not necessarily of the fit of the model. Accurate or inaccurate classification does not address our criteria for goodness of fit: that the distances between observed and expected values be unsystematic and small, relative to the variation of the model. However, the classification table may be a useful adjunct to other measures based more directly on residuals.

The results of classifying the observations of the GLOW Study using the fitted model given in Table 4.16 are presented in Table 5.3 and are fairly typical of those seen in many logistic regression applications. The overall rate of correct classification is estimated as $75.6\% = 100[(22 + 356)/500]\%$, with 94.93% (356/375) correct classification of the no fracture (i.e., FRACTURE = 0) group (specificity),

Table 5.3   Classification Table Based on the Logistic Regression Model for the GLOW Study in Table 4.16 Using a Cutpoint of 0.5

	Observed		
Classified	FRACTURE = 1	FRACTURE = 0	Total
FRACTURE = 1	22	19	41
FRACTURE = 0	103	356	459
Total	125	375	500

Sensitivity $= 22/125 = 17.6\%$; Specificity $= 356/375 = 94.93\%$.

but only 17.6% (22/125) correct classification in the group that actually experienced fracture (i.e., FRACTURE $= 1$) (sensitivity). Classification is sensitive to the relative sizes of the two component groups and always favors classification into the larger group, a fact that is also independent of the fit of the model. This is easily seen by considering the expression for PMC as a function of θ_1. The disadvantage of using PMC as a criterion is that it reduces a probabilistic model, where outcome is measured on a continuum, to a dichotomous model where predicted outcome is binary. For practical purposes there is little difference between the values of $\hat{\pi} = 0.48$ and $\hat{\pi} = 0.52$, yet use of a 0.5 cutpoint would establish these two individuals as markedly different.

An important reason why measures derived from a 2×2 classification table (such as sensitivity and specificity) should not be used as measures of model fit is that they depend heavily on the distribution of the estimated probabilities in the sample. Thus, if two models are being compared, differences between them with respect to sensitivity and specificity may depend entirely on "patient mix" rather than on the superiority of one model over another.

In the discussion that follows we must keep in mind the meaning of probability. Specifically, among n subjects, each having the same probability of the outcome of interest, $\hat{\pi}$, the number who are expected to develop the outcome is $n \times \hat{\pi}$ and the number expected to not develop the outcome is $n \times (1 - \hat{\pi})$. (This logic formed the basis of the discussion in Section 5.2.2 on goodness of fit testing.) Assume that 0.50 is the cutpoint being used for classification purposes and that 100 subjects had a probability $\hat{\pi} = 0.51$. All of these subjects would be predicted to have the outcome present, but assuming the model is well calibrated, only 51 of the subjects would actually develop the outcome. The remaining 49 subjects would not have developed the outcome. Thus 49 of the 100 patients would be misclassified.

Consider again the 2×2 classification table from the GLOW Study presented in Table 5.3. An examination of the estimated probabilities of fracture in the two classification groups reveals that among the 41 subjects predicted to have a fracture on follow up, probabilities ranged from 0.5002 to 0.746, with a mean of 0.574. Among the 459 subjects predicted not to have a fracture on follow up, probabilities ranged from 0.0208 to 0.49998, with a mean of 0.221. Clearly, because so many of the subjects in this study have probabilities close to the cutpoint, we expect a considerable amount of misclassification. In Table 5.3 we see that 356 of the 459 subjects predicted not to have a fracture on follow up actually did not have a fracture, whereas 19 of the 41 subjects predicted to have a fracture on follow up were misclassified. Thus, of the total 125 subjects who actually had a fracture on follow up, only 22 of them were correctly predicted (i.e., sensitivity $= 22/125 = 17.6\%$).

Assume now that we keep the prediction unchanged for each subject but alter the distribution of the estimated probabilities as follows:

$$\text{if } \hat{\pi} < 0.50, \text{ then let } \hat{\pi} = 0.05$$

$$\text{and if } \hat{\pi} \geq 0.50, \text{ then let } \hat{\pi} = 0.95.$$

Clearly, this modification would reflect a population that was very polarized with respect to their probability of having a fracture on follow up. If the model was *well calibrated* (i.e., probabilities reflecting the true outcome experience in the data), then only 5% of those predicted to have a fracture on follow up would actually be misclassified, that is, $2 \simeq 0.05 \times 41$, and similarly, only 5% of those predicted to not have a fracture on follow up would be misclassified, that is, $23 \simeq 0.05 \times 459$. The resulting 2×2 table would be as presented in Table 5.4. Note that both the sensitivity and specificity are considerably greater than they were for the actual population seen in Table 5.3, where there was a wide range of probabilities. The reason for the sensitivity being moderate even in this polarized population is that there were relatively few subjects whose probabilities of having a fracture on follow up were above 0.50.

Now consider a second hypothetical population where

$$\text{if } \hat{\pi} < 0.50, \text{ then let } \hat{\pi} = 0.45$$

$$\text{and if } \hat{\pi} \geq 0.50, \text{ then let } \hat{\pi} = 0.55.$$

This homogenous population is one where a great deal of misclassification would be expected. Assuming the probabilities accurately reflect the outcome experience in these data, the 2×2 table would be presented as in Table 5.5. Note that the sensitivity is much worse and specificity slightly worse than was the case with the actual, heterogeneous, population.

Table 5.4 **Expected Classification Table Based on the Logistic Regression Model for the GLOW Study in Table 4.16 Using a Cutpoint of 0.5, but All Probabilities $\hat{\pi} < 0.50$ Are Replaced with $\hat{\pi} = 0.05$ and All Probabilities $\hat{\pi} \geq 0.50$ Are Replaced with $\hat{\pi} = 0.95$**

Classified	Observed		Total
	FRACTURE $= 1$	FRACTURE $= 0$	
FRACTURE $= 1$	39	2	41
FRACTURE $= 0$	23	436	459
Total	62	438	500

Sensitivity $= 39/62 = 62.9\%$; Specificity $= 436/438 = 99.5\%$.

Table 5.5   Expected Classification Table Based on the Logistic Regression Model for the GLOW Study in Table 4.16 Using a Cutpoint of 0.5, but All Probabilities $\hat{\pi} < 0.50$ Are Replaced with $\hat{\pi} = 0.45$ and All Probabilities $\hat{\pi} \geq 0.50$ Are Replaced with $\hat{\pi} = 0.55$

	Observed		
Classified	FRACTURE = 1	FRACTURE = 0	Total
FRACTURE = 1	23	18	41
FRACTURE = 0	207	252	459
Total	230	270	500

Sensitivity = 23/230 = 10.0%; Specificity = 252/270 = 93.3%.

Table 5.6   Classification Table Based on the Logistic Regression Model for the Burn Study in Table 4.27 Using a Cutpoint of 0.5

	Observed		
Classified	DEATH = 1	DEATH = 0	Total
DEATH = 1	108	29	137
DEATH = 0	42	821	863
Total	150	850	1000

Sensitivity = 108/150 = 72.0%; Specificity = 821/850 = 96.66%.

For these reasons, one cannot compare models on the basis of measures derived from 2×2 classification tables since these measures are completely confounded by the distribution of probabilities in the samples upon which they are based. The same model, evaluated in two populations, could give very different impressions of performance if sensitivity or specificity was used as the measure of performance.

Classification is a goal for the model fit to the Burn Study data shown in Table 4.27. The model's classification table is given in Table 5.6. The specificity is, not unexpectedly, high at 96.66% and the sensitivity is surprisingly good at 72% and overall 92.9% correctly classified. This model, besides having good fit, classifies quite well.

In summary, the classification table is most appropriate when classification is a stated goal of the analysis; otherwise it should only supplement more rigorous methods of assessment of fit.

5.2.4   Area Under the Receiver Operating Characteristic Curve

Sensitivity and specificity as well as other measures of classification performance computed from a 2×2 table, like Table 5.3, depend on the single cutpoint used to classify a test result as positive. A better and more complete description of classification accuracy is the area under the Receiver Operating Characteristic (ROC) curve. This curve, originating from signal detection theory, shows how the receiver detects the existence of signal in the presence of noise. It plots the probability of detecting true signal (sensitivity) and false signal (1–specificity) for an entire range of possible cutpoints. This measure has now become the standard for evaluating a fitted model's ability to assign, in general, higher probabilities of the outcome to the subgroup who develop the outcome ($y = 1$) than it does to the subgroup who do not develop the outcome ($y = 0$).

The area under the ROC curve, which ranges from 0.5 to 1.0, provides a measure of the model's ability to *discriminate* between those subjects who experience the outcome of interest versus those who do not. As an example, consider the model for estimating the probability that a woman has a fracture on follow up in Table 4.16. Assuming that we were interested in *predicting* the outcome for each woman, one rule we might try is the one shown in Table 5.3, where we predict that the woman will have a fracture on follow up if $\Pr(y = 1) \geq 0.50$, and predict that the woman will not have a fracture on follow up if $\Pr(y = 1) < 0.50$. There are some statistical benefits associated with using 0.5, but we could consider what happens when we use other cutpoints. For example, assuming that we used a cutpoint of 0.6 instead, the resulting classification table is shown in Table 5.7, where the sensitivity is only 3.2% but the specificity is 98.13%. The same can be done for any possible choice of cutpoint. Table 5.8 summarizes the results of choosing cutpoints between 0.05 and 0.75 in increments of 0.05.

If our objective was to choose an optimal cutpoint for the purposes of classification, one might select a cutpoint that maximizes both sensitivity and specificity. This choice is facilitated through a graph such as the one shown in Figure 5.1, which plots sensitivity and specificity versus each possible cutpoint. The values in Table 5.8 provide plotting coordinates for 15 of the points on the two curves, the remainder of the plotted points come from other possible cutpoints. We see that an "optimal" choice for a cutpoint might be 0.24 as that is approximately where the sensitivity and specificity curves cross.

As we described above, the ability of a fitted model to discriminate between the two outcomes is more a function of the difference between the groups and magnitudes of the slope coefficients than the logistic model itself. Thus, as noted, we can have well fitting models that discriminate poorly, just as we could have models with poor fit that discriminate well. Illustrating how the values in Table 5.8 are obtained from a fitted model can emphasize these points. Histograms of the

Table 5.7   Classification Table Based on the Logistic Regression Model for the GLOW Study in Table 4.16 Using a Cutpoint of 0.60

Classified	Observed		Total
	FRACTURE $= 1$	FRACTURE $= 0$	
FRACTURE $= 1$	4	7	11
FRACTURE $= 0$	121	368	489
Total	125	375	500

Sensitivity $= 4/125 = 3.2\%$; Specificity $= 368/375 = 98.13\%$.

Table 5.8 Summary of Sensitivity, Specificity, and 1–Specificity for Classification Tables Based on the Logistic Regression Model for the GLOW Study in Table 4.16 Using a Cutpoint of 0.05 to 0.75 in Increments of 0.05

Cutpoint	Sensitivity	Specificity	1–Specificity
0.05	100.0	1.6	98.4
0.10	95.2	19.7	80.3
0.15	84.8	38.4	61.6
0.20	76.8	55.2	44.8
0.25	64.0	68.5	31.5
0.30	62.4	76.5	23.5
0.35	48.8	82.9	17.1
0.40	39.2	88.0	12.0
0.45	29.6	92.3	7.7
0.50	17.6	94.9	5.1
0.55	8.8	96.8	3.2
0.60	3.2	98.1	2.9
0.65	2.4	99.5	0.5
0.70	0.0	99.5	0.5
0.75	0.0	100.0	0.0

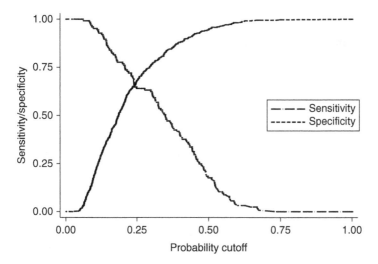

Figure 5.1 Plot of sensitivity and specificity versus all possible cutpoints in the GLOW Study.

estimated probabilities from the fitted model in Table 4.16 within the two outcome groups are shown in Figure 5.2. The cutpoints defining the rectangles in the histograms are the values in the cutpoint column of Table 5.8. The vertical line is drawn at 0.25.

The histograms have been constructed so that the sum of the areas of the rectangles is 1.0 for each outcome group. Using 0.25 cutpoint, as an example, to classify

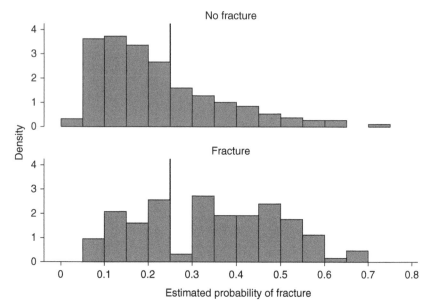

Figure 5.2 Histogram of the estimated probabilities from the GLOW model in Table 4.16 by fracture status on follow up with vertical line at 0.25.

women to fracture on follow up, the sensitivity is the sum of the areas of the nine rectangles above 0.25 in the lower histogram (patients experiencing facture). From Table 5.8 we see that this value is 0.64. The specificity of the model at this cutpoint is the sum of the areas of the five rectangles below 0.25 in the upper histogram (patients not experiencing facture), and from Table 5.8, we see that this value is 0.685. Thus, the sum of the areas of the rectangles above the cutpoint of 0.25 for the upper histogram is 0.315 and is 1−specificity. The values in each row of the Sensitivity and 1−Specificity columns of Table 5.8 are obtained in a similar manner using the stated cutpoints. Each value is equal to the sum of the areas of the rectangles lying to the right of the cutpoint in the respective histogram. Thus, as the cutpoint ranges from zero to one the values decrease from 100% to 0%.

We can see in Figure 5.2 that there is considerable overlap in the two histograms. The distributions of the estimated probabilities within the two outcome groups are rather similar. If the two distributions were identical then the areas to the right of any cutpoint would be identical (i.e., sensitivity = 1−specificity). If the two distributions had little overlap (i.e., the lower histogram was mostly to the right of the upper one) then, as 1−specificity decreased from 100% to 0.0% the sensitivity would remain at nearly 100%. Perfect discrimination occurs if there is no overlap at all in the two histograms.

A plot of sensitivity versus 1−specificity over all possible cutpoints (i.e., using each individual estimated probability rather than grouped data) is shown in Figure 5.3. The curve generated by these points is called the *ROC Curve* and the area under the curve provides a measure, whose calculation is described below,

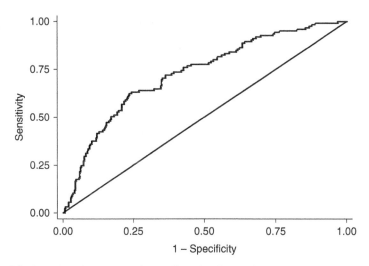

Figure 5.3 Plot of sensitivity versus 1–specificity for all possible cutpoints in the GLOW Study.

of discrimination that is the estimated probability that, under the fitted model, a woman who has a fracture on follow up will have a higher $\hat{\pi}(\mathbf{x})$ than a woman who does not have a fracture on follow up. As noted, if the distribution of the model estimated probabilities is the same in the two groups then the ROC curve would be identical to the straight line shown in Figure 5.3. Since this line bisects the one by one square the area under it would be 0.5, indicating that one might as well toss a coin as use the fitted model to predict outcome. As the distributions of the probabilities estimated by the model become more distinct the plot of the ROC curve rises more rapidly and the area under it increases from 0.5 to its theoretical maximum of 1.0.

So, what area under the ROC curve describes good discrimination? Unfortunately there is no "magic" number, only general guidelines. In general, we use the following rule of thumb:

$$
\text{If} \begin{cases}
ROC = 0.5 & \text{This suggests no discrimination, so we might as well flip a coin.} \\
0.5 < ROC < 0.7 & \text{We consider this poor discrimination, not much better than a coin toss.} \\
0.7 \leq ROC < 0.8 & \text{We consider this acceptable discrimination.} \\
0.8 \leq ROC < 0.9 & \text{We consider this excellent discrimination.} \\
ROC \geq 0.9 & \text{We consider this outstanding discrimination.}
\end{cases}
$$

The ROC curve for the fitted model in Table 4.16 for the GLOW Study is shown in Figure 5.3. The area under the ROC Curve is 0.7286, which is at the low end of acceptable discrimination.

Another perhaps more intuitive way to understand the meaning of the area under the ROC Curve is as follows: recall that we let n_1 denote the number of subjects with $y = 1$ and n_0 denote the number of subjects with $y = 0$. We then create $n_1 \times n_0$ pairs: each subject with $y = 1$, is paired with each subject with $y = 0$. Of these $n_1 \times n_0$ pairs, we determine the proportion of pairs where the subject with $y = 1$ had the higher of the two probabilities. This proportion may be shown to be equal to the area under the ROC Curve. For example, in the GLOW Study, there were 500 subjects. Of these, 125 had a fracture while 375 did not, yielding a total of $125 \times 375 = 46,875$ comparisons. We count the number of times that the probability of having a fracture is higher for the woman who had a fracture than for the woman who did not. (This assumes there are no ties.) For these data the count of the number of times that the subject with $y = 1$ had a higher probability than the subject with $y = 0$ was 34,153. (The reader may recognize that this count is the Mann–Whitney U statistic for these data.) The ratio $34,153/46,875 = 0.7286$ is the area under the ROC curve.

Royston and Altman (2010) investigate visual methods for assessing discrimination of fitted logistic regression models. They suggest using the plots in Figures 5.1–5.3 as well as a scatter plot of the outcome versus the estimated probabilities from the fitted model. Instead of plotting the y values at 0 or 1 we present jittered values. The jittered values of the outcome are $y_i^* = y_i + u_i$, where u_i is an independently generated value from the Uniform$(-0.05, 0.05)$ distribution. This plot is shown in Figure 5.4 for the fitted model from the GLOW Study in Table 4.16.

If the two groups were well separated then the points on the upper band $1 + u_i$, would tend to have larger estimated probabilities (the upper half of the scatter plot) while those on the lower band $0 + u_i$, would tend to have lower probabilities.

In order to illustrate the different levels of discrimination we show in Figure 5.5 to Figure 5.8 the four plots obtained from four hypothetical data sets. Each data

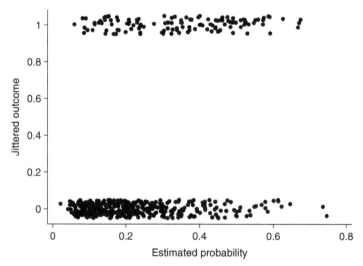

Figure 5.4 Plot of jittered outcome versus estimated probabilities from the fitted model for the GLOW Study in Table 4.16.

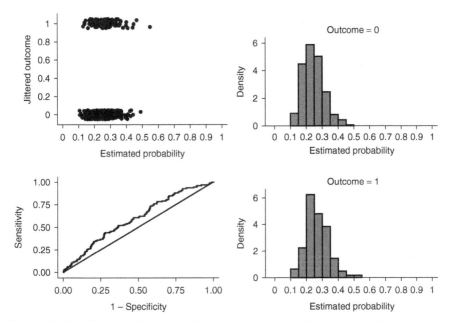

Figure 5.5 Four diagnostic plots to describe discrimination in a model fit to data with an area under the ROC of 0.6, $n = 500$.

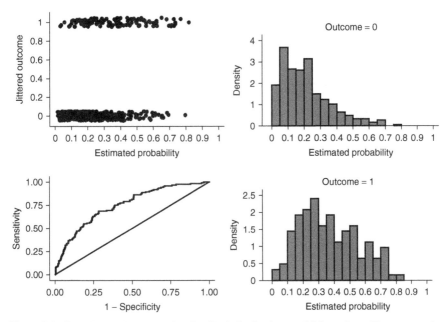

Figure 5.6 Four diagnostic plots to describe discrimination in a model fit to data with an area under the ROC of 0.75, $n = 500$.

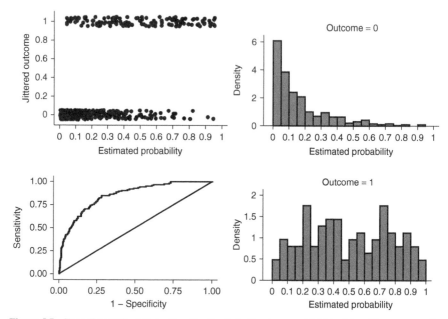

Figure 5.7 Four diagnostic plots to describe discrimination in a model fit to data with an area under the ROC of 0.85, $n = 500$.

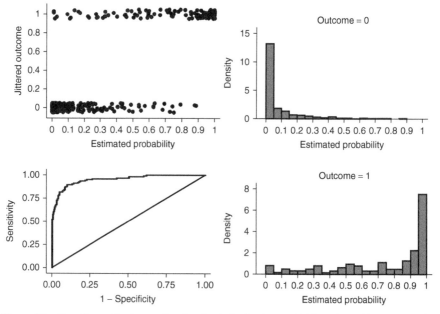

Figure 5.8 Four diagnostic plots to describe discrimination in a model fit to data with an area under the ROC of 0.95, $n = 500$.

set has 500 observations and exactly 125 with the outcome of interest. The data in the group with $y = 0$ are distributed as $N(0, 1)$ and the group with $y = 1$ as $N(\mu, 1)$. To obtain $ROC = 0.6$ we used $\mu = 0.4$ (Figure 5.5), for $ROC = 0.75$ $\mu = 0.95$ (Figure 5.6), for $ROC = 0.85$ $\mu = 1.5$ (Figure 5.7) and for $ROC = 0.95$ $\mu = 2.5$ (Figure 5.8). Actually, for each value of μ we kept generating data until we obtained an ROC close to the stated value, none were exact. One can see, by comparing the four figures, that in order to have excellent discrimination the estimated probabilities for the group with $y = 0$ need to be quite different from the values for those with $y = 1$ and for outstanding discrimination the two distributions are almost completely separated. In all cases the estimated logistic regression model had good fit.

Now we use the four plots, shown in Figure 5.9, to describe discrimination for the model fit to the Burn Study data in Table 4.27. The scatterplot of the jittered outcome versus the estimated probability, top left, shows that subjects who died tended to have much higher estimated probabilities than subjects who lived. Note the dense cluster above 0.9 for $y = 1$ and below 0.1 for $y = 0$. This is further supported in the separation seen in the two histograms of the estimated probabilities, top right and bottom right. The ROC curve is in the bottom left position and its area is 0.9683. All four graphs support the outstanding discrimination of this model.

We remind the reader that the data in the Burn Study were sampled from a much larger set of data and the results of model fitting in this text may not

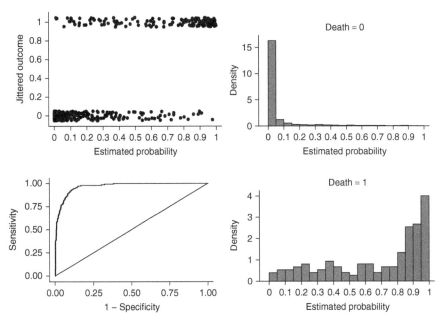

Figure 5.9 Four diagnostic plots to describe discrimination for the model fit to the Burn Study data in Table 4.27. Area under the ROC is 0.9683.

apply to the larger data set. That being said, the fitted model does display exceptional ability to discriminate between patients who died as compared to those who lived.

In Section 5.4 we use the Burn Study to illustrate methods for model validation in an external data set.

We recommend that one present the discrimination of the fitted model using the four plots shown in Figure 5.9, rather than simply reporting the area under the ROC curve.

5.2.5   Other Summary Measures

For sake of completeness we present a short discussion of R^2 measures that have been proposed for use with logistic regression models. In general, these measures are based on various comparisons of the predicted values from the fitted model to those from model(0), the no data or intercept only model and, as a result, do not assess goodness of fit. We think that a true measure of fit is one based strictly on a comparison of observed to expected values from the fitted model. However there may be settings where an R^2 like measure might provide useful information for comparing competing models fit to the same set of data. Mittlböck and Schemper (1996) study the properties of 12 different measures using the criteria: (i) the measure has an easily understood interpretation, (ii) the squared measure can attain a lower bound of 0 and an upper bound of 1 and (iii) the measure is consistent with the character of logistic regression (i.e., not being changed by a linear transformation of model covariates). They recommend two for routine use: the squared Pearson correlation coefficient of observed outcome with the estimated probability and a linear regression like sum-of-squares, R^2. All other measures, including some popular likelihood-based R^2 statistics are judged to be inadequate on at least one of their criteria.

In a setting with n covariate patterns the squared Pearson correlation coefficient is

$$r^2 = \frac{\left[\sum_{i=1}^{n} (y_i - \overline{y})(\hat{\pi}_i - \overline{\pi}) \right]^2}{\left[\sum_{i=1}^{n} (y_i - \overline{y})^2 \right] \times \left[\sum_{i=1}^{n} (\hat{\pi}_i - \overline{\pi})^2 \right]}, \tag{5.12}$$

where $\overline{y} = \overline{\pi} = n_1/n$. The linear regression-like measure is

$$R_{ss}^2 = 1 - \frac{\sum_{i=1}^{n} (y_i - \hat{\pi}_i)^2}{\sum_{i=1}^{n} (y_i - \overline{y})^2}. \tag{5.13}$$

Mittlböck and Schemper (1996) did not consider the case of $J < n$ covariate patterns. However, the extensions of the two measures to this setting are

$$
r_c^2 = \frac{\left[\sum_{j=1}^{J} (y_j - m_j \bar{y})(m_j \hat{\pi}_j - m_j \bar{\pi}) \right]^2}{\left[\sum_{j=1}^{J} (y_j - m_j \bar{y})^2 \right] \times \left[\sum_{j=1}^{J} (m_j \hat{\pi}_j - m_j \bar{\pi})^2 \right]}
\tag{5.14}
$$

and

$$
R_{ssc}^2 = 1 - \frac{\sum_{j=1}^{J} (y_j - m_j \hat{\pi}_j)^2}{\sum_{j=1}^{J} (y_j - m_j \bar{y})^2}.
\tag{5.15}
$$

Mittlböck and Schemper (2002) studied two modifications of R_{ss}^2 when the sample size is small and the model contains many covariates. The first is analogous to the adjusted R^2 from linear regression and is defined as

$$
R_{ss,adj}^2 = 1 - \frac{\dfrac{\sum_{j=1}^{J} (y_j - m_j \hat{\pi}_j)^2}{n-p-1}}{\dfrac{\sum_{j=1}^{J} (y_j - \bar{y})^2}{n-1}}.
\tag{5.16}
$$

The second adjusts for shrinkage in the estimates, a condition that is typically present when the model is fit with a small sample (see Section 10.3 for a discussion of shrinkage), and is defined as

$$
R_{ss,shr}^2 = R^2 \times \hat{\gamma},
\tag{5.17}
$$

where

$$
\hat{\gamma} = \frac{G - p}{G},
$$

and G is the value of the likelihood ratio test for the significance of the model.

Using the fitted model in Table 4.16 and evaluating the squared Pearson correlation coefficient defined in equation (5.12), we obtain $r^2 = 0.12355$. The value of the linear regression like sum-of-squares measure from equation (5.13) is

$$
R_{ss}^2 = 1 - \left(\frac{82.167267}{93.75} \right) = 0.12355.
$$

The value adjusted for the number of covariates from equation (5.16) is

$$R^2_{ss,adj} = 1 - \left(\frac{\dfrac{82.167267}{500 - 8 - 1}}{\dfrac{93.75}{500 - 1}} \right) = 0.1093.$$

The value adjusted for shrinkage is

$$R^2_{ss,shr} = 0.1235 \times \frac{61.838525 - 8}{61.838525} = 0.1075.$$

The fitted model has 521 covariate patterns. Evaluating the covariate pattern version of the Pearson correlation coefficient in equation (5.14) yields $r_c^2 = 0.1363$. The increase from the value of 0.1135 in the $J = n$ case is due to increased range of y_j (0–2) versus y_i (0–1) in the values being correlated. The sum-of-squares measure is

$$R^2_{ssc} = 1 - \left(\frac{82.2560}{95.25} \right) = 0.1083.$$

We obtain another version of R^2_{ss} when we use log-likelihoods in place of sums-of-squares. Mittlböck and Schemper (1996) do not recommend it for routine use, as it is not as intuitively easy to explain. However the measure is calculated in a number of packages under various names (e.g., pseudo R^2 in STATA). If we let L_0 and L_p denote the log-likelihoods for models containing only the intercept and the model containing the intercept plus the p covariates respectively, then the log-likelihood-based R^2 is

$$R^2_L = \frac{L_0 - L_p}{L_0} = 1 - \frac{L_p}{L_0}. \tag{5.18}$$

The maximum value for R^2_L is obtained when we fit the saturated model. If $J = n$ then the log-likelihood for the saturated model $= L_s = 0 = L_p$ and we see that R^2_L is equal to 1.0. However, if $J < n$ then $L_s = L_p > 0$ and the maximum is less than 1.0. A modification of the statistic that can attain 1.0 in the $J < n$ case is

$$R^2_{LS} = \frac{L_0 - L_p}{L_0 - L_S}. \tag{5.19}$$

The value of the log-likelihood from the saturated model, L_S, may be easily obtained from the deviance for the model with p covariates and its log-likelihood is computed as

$$L_S = L_P + 0.5D,$$

where D is defined in equation (5.4). Hence, it would seem prudent to calculate L_S whenever $J < n$ and to use R^2_{LS}.

As an example, we evaluate equation (5.18) using the fitted model in Table 4.16, and assuming $J = 500$, we obtain

$$R_L^2 = 1 - \frac{-250.24831}{-281.16757} = 0.1099.$$

In order to evaluate equation (5.19) we need the value of L_S using $J = 457$ covariate patterns. The value of the deviance from equation (5.4) is $D = 469.63124$ and from the above expression we obtain

$$L_S = (-250.24831) + 0.5 \times (469.63124) = -15.43269$$

and

$$R_{LS}^2 = \frac{[(-281.16757) - (-250.24831)]}{[(-281.16757) - (-15.43269)]} = 0.1164.$$

A recent addition to summary measures of model performance is the coefficient of discrimination proposed by Tjur (2009). It is a measure of the separation of the distribution of the estimated probabilities in the two outcome groups, namely

$$CD = \overline{\hat{\pi}}_1 - \overline{\hat{\pi}}_0. \tag{5.20}$$

Tjur shows that

$$CD = 0.5 \times (R_{ss}^2 + R_{mod}^2),$$

where

$$R_{mod}^2 = \frac{\sum_{i=1}^{n} (\hat{\pi}_i - \overline{y})^2}{\sum_{i=1}^{n} (y_i - \overline{y})^2},$$

which we leave as an exercise to demonstrate with the GLOW model in Table 4.16. The average of the fitted values in the two groups are $\overline{\hat{\pi}}_1 = 0.34301$ and $\overline{\hat{\pi}}_0 = 0.2190$, thus $CD = 0.12401$. Tjur recommends, as a descriptive analysis, plotting histograms in the manner shown in Figures 5.5 to 5.9, in which case CD provides a nice summary measure of their separation.

We leave computing the various R^2 measures for the Burn Study data in Table 4.27 as an exercise.

All the various R^2 values for this example are low when compared to R^2 values typically encountered with good linear regression models. Unfortunately low R^2 values in logistic regression are the norm and this presents a problem when reporting their values to an audience accustomed to seeing linear regression values. As we demonstrate throughout this chapter, the fitted model in Table 4.16 is well calibrated but does not discriminate well. We always recommend the performing of a goodness of fit analysis. If the fitted model is to be used to discriminate between the two outcome groups, then and only then, do we recommend looking at the *ROC* and summary measures of discrimination.

We note here that in some instances, it may not be important to assess the calibration or discrimination of the model. An example is a case control study where the number of cases and the number of controls is fixed by the investigator. In this case the $\Pr(y = 1)$ is fixed.

When the focus of the study is on the $\hat{\beta}$'s (or odds ratios), calibration is not important. It is important when the estimated probabilities are meaningful and of interest to the investigator.

The coefficients of a logistic regression analysis are always the log-odds ratios—whether the model fits or not. However, if the study's objective is to estimate the $\Pr(y = 1)$ then we need to assess calibration and discrimination.

5.3 LOGISTIC REGRESSION DIAGNOSTICS

Each of the summary statistics based on the Pearson chi-square residuals described in the previous section provide a single number that summarizes the agreement between observed and fitted values. The advantage (as well as the disadvantage) of these statistics is that a single number is used to summarize considerable information. Therefore, before concluding that the model "fits", it is crucial that other measures be examined to see if fit is supported over the entire set of covariate patterns. This is accomplished through a series of specialized measures falling under the general heading of *regression diagnostics*. We assume that the reader has had some experience with diagnostics for linear regression. For a brief introduction to linear regression diagnostics see Kleinbaum et al. (1998). A more detailed presentation may be found in Cook and Weisberg (1982) and Belsley et al. (1980). Pregibon (1981) provided the theoretical work that extended linear regression diagnostics to logistic regression. Since that key paper, work has been focused on refining the use of logistic regression diagnostics in assessing goodness of fit. We begin by briefly describing logistic regression diagnostics. In this development we assume that the fitted model contains p covariates and that they form J covariate patterns. Deriving the diagnostic statistics requires a higher mathematical level than most of the other material in this text. However, an understanding of the mathematical development is not required for the effective application of the diagnostics in practice. Thus, less sophisticated mathematical readers may want to focus on the applications to the fitted models from Chapter 4.

The key quantities for logistic regression diagnostics, as in linear regression, are the components of the "residual sum-of-squares". In linear regression a key assumption is that the error variance does not depend on the conditional mean $E(Y_j|\mathbf{x}_j)$. However, in logistic regression we have binomial errors, and as a result, the error variance is a function of the conditional mean:

$$\text{var}(Y_j|\mathbf{x}_j) = m_j E(Y_j|\mathbf{x}_j) \times [1 - E(Y_j|\mathbf{x}_j)]$$
$$= m_j \pi(\mathbf{x}_j)[1 - \pi(\mathbf{x}_j)].$$

Thus, we begin with residuals as defined in equations (5.1) and (5.3) that have been "divided" by estimates of their standard errors; this may not be entirely obvious in the case of the deviance residual. Let r_j and d_j denote the values of the expressions given in equations (5.1) and (5.3), respectively, for covariate pattern $\mathbf{x}_j$. Since each residual has been divided by an approximate estimate of its standard error, we expect that if the logistic regression model is correct, these quantities have a mean approximately equal to zero and a variance approximately equal to one. We discuss their distribution shortly.

In addition to the residuals for each covariate pattern, other quantities central to the formation and interpretation of linear regression diagnostics are the "hat" matrix and the leverage values derived from it. In linear regression the hat matrix is the matrix that provides the fitted values as the projection of the outcome variable onto the covariate space. Let $\mathbf{X}$ denote the $J \times (p+1)$ matrix containing the values for all J covariate patterns formed from the observed values of the p covariates, with the first column being one to reflect the presence of an intercept term in the model. The matrix $\mathbf{X}$ is often called the design matrix. In linear regression the hat matrix is $\mathbf{H} = \mathbf{X}(\mathbf{X}'\mathbf{X})^{-1}\mathbf{X}'$; clearly, $\hat{\mathbf{y}} = \mathbf{H}\mathbf{y}$. The linear regression residuals, $(\mathbf{y} - \hat{\mathbf{y}})$, expressed in terms of the hat matrix are $(\mathbf{I} - \mathbf{H})\mathbf{y}$ where $\mathbf{I}$ is the $J \times J$ identity matrix. Using weighted least squares linear regression as a model, Pregibon (1981) derived a linear approximation to the fitted values which yields a hat matrix for logistic regression. This matrix is

$$\mathbf{H} = \mathbf{V}^{1/2}\mathbf{X}(\mathbf{X}'\mathbf{V}\mathbf{X})^{-1}\mathbf{X}'\mathbf{V}^{1/2}, \tag{5.21}$$

where $\mathbf{V}$ is a $J \times J$ diagonal matrix with general element

$$v_j = m_j\hat{\pi}(\mathbf{x}_j)[1 - \hat{\pi}(\mathbf{x}_j)].$$

In linear regression the diagonal elements of the hat matrix are called the *leverage values* and are proportional to the distance of $\mathbf{x}_j$ to the mean of the data, $\bar{\mathbf{x}}$. This concept of distance to the mean is important in linear regression, as points that are far from the mean may have considerable influence on the values of the estimated parameters. The extension of the concept of leverage to logistic regression requires additional discussion and clarification.

Let the quantity h_j denote the jth diagonal element of the matrix $\mathbf{H}$ defined in equation (5.21). It may be shown that

$$h_j = m_j\hat{\pi}(\mathbf{x}_j)[1 - \hat{\pi}(\mathbf{x}_j)]\mathbf{x}_j'(\mathbf{X}'\mathbf{V}\mathbf{X})^{-1}\mathbf{x}_j$$
$$= v_j \times b_j \tag{5.22}$$

where

$$v_j = m_j\hat{\pi}(\mathbf{x}_j)[1 - \hat{\pi}(\mathbf{x}_j)]$$

is the model based estimator of the variance of y_j, and

$$b_j = \mathbf{x}_j'(\mathbf{X}'\mathbf{V}\mathbf{X})^{-1}\mathbf{x}_j$$

is the weighted distance of $\mathbf{x}_j$ from $\bar{\mathbf{x}}$, where $\mathbf{x}_j' = (1, x_{1j}, x_{2j}, \ldots x_{pj})$ is the vector of covariate values defining the jth covariate pattern and $\bar{\mathbf{x}}$ is the vector of means.

The sum of the diagonal elements of $\mathbf{H}$ is, as is the case in linear regression, $\sum_{j=1}^{J} h_j = (p+1)$, the number of parameters in the model. In linear regression the dimension of the hat matrix is usually $n \times n$ and thus ignores any common covariate patterns in the data. With this formulation, any diagonal element in the hat matrix has an upper bound of $1/k$ where k is the number of subjects with the same covariate pattern. If we formulate the hat matrix for logistic regression as an $n \times n$ matrix then each diagonal element is bounded from above by $1/m_j$, where m_j is the total number of subjects with the same covariate pattern. When the hat matrix is based upon data grouped by covariate pattern, the upper bound for any diagonal element is 1.

It is important to know whether the statistical package being used calculates the diagnostic statistics by covariate pattern. For example, STATA's logistic regression procedure uses individual subject data to fit models. Following estimation it computes all diagnostic statistics by covariate pattern but retains the size of the original data set. Thus all subjects in a particular covariate pattern have the same covariate values, fitted values and diagnostic statistics, but each subject has an individual outcome. On the other hand, SAS's logistic procedure computes diagnostic statistics based on the data structure in its model statement. If one assumes that there are n covariate patterns (and the outcome is either 0 or 1) then diagnostic statistics are based on individual subjects. However, if the data have been previously collapsed or grouped into covariate patterns and if binomial trials input (y_j/m_j) is used, then diagnostic statistics are by covariate pattern. In general, we recommend that diagnostic statistics be computed taking into account the covariate patterns. This is especially important when the number of covariate patterns, J, is much smaller than n, or if some values of m_j are larger than 5. For example, in the final model for the Glow Study shown in Table 4.16 we have $J = 457$ covariate patterns among the 500 subjects. There are 419 covariate patterns with $m = 1$, 33 with $m = 2$ and five with $m = 3$. In this situation we might not bother, in practice, to calculate the diagnostic statistics by covariate pattern. If, on the other hand, we had a model with $J = 300$ and $n = 500$ then we should definitely take the trouble of aggregating the data by covariate patterns.

When the number of covariate patterns is much smaller than n, there is the risk that we may fail to identify influential and/or poorly fit covariate patterns. Consider a covariate pattern with m_j subjects, $y_j = 0$ and estimated logistic probability $\hat{\pi}_j$. The Pearson residual defined in equation (5.1), computed individually for each subject with this covariate pattern is

$$r_i = \frac{(0 - \hat{\pi}_j)}{\sqrt{\hat{\pi}_j(1 - \hat{\pi}_j)}}$$

$$= -\sqrt{\frac{\hat{\pi}_j}{(1 - \hat{\pi}_j)}},$$

while the Pearson residual based on all subjects with this covariate pattern is

$$r_i = \frac{(0 - m_j\hat{\pi}_j)}{\sqrt{m_j\hat{\pi}_j(1 - \hat{\pi}_j)}}$$

$$= -\sqrt{m_j}\sqrt{\frac{\hat{\pi}_j}{(1 - \hat{\pi}_j)}},$$

which increases negatively as m_j increases. If $m_j = 1$ and $\hat{\pi}_j = 0.5$, then $r_j = -1$, which is not a large residual. On the other hand, if there were $m_j = 16$ subjects with this covariate pattern, then $r_j = -4.0$ which is quite large. If we performed the analysis in STATA then the Pearson residual would be -4.0 for each of the 16 subjects in the covariate pattern. If we performed the analysis in SAS with a sample of size n then the Pearson residual would be -1.0 for all 16 subjects. Thus the diagnostic statistics are different even though both packages produce the same fitted model.

A major point that must be kept in mind when interpreting the magnitude of the leverage is the combined effect in equation (5.22) of v_j and b_j, on the value of the leverage h_j. Pregibon (1981) notes that the fit determines the estimated coefficients, and since the estimated coefficients determine the estimated probabilities, points with large values of h_j are extreme in the covariate space and thus lie far from the mean. Lesaffre (1986, p.117) refutes this point, where he shows that the term v_j in the expression for h_j cannot be ignored. The following example demonstrates that, up to a point, both Pregibon and Lesaffre are correct.

In Figure 5.10 we plot the values of v_j and b_j versus the estimated probabilities for a sample of 100 observations from a logistic model with $g(x) = 0.8x$ and $x \sim N(0, 9)$. Recall that the notation $N(0, 9)$ describes a variable following a normal distribution with mean 0 and variance 9.

We see that the distance, b_j, increases as the estimated probability gets further from 0.5 (x gets further from its mean, nominally zero) while the variance term, v_j, decreases. The leverage is the product of these two factors and the exact effect of these opposing factors cannot be seen so we plot the leverage versus the estimated probabilities in Figure 5.11. In this figure we see that the most extreme points in the covariate space, ones with estimated probability less than 0.1 or greater then 0.9, do not have the highest leverage. The reason that the leverage goes to zero as the estimated probabilities approach zero or one is that v_j goes to zero exponentially, while b_j grows large at the slower rate of x^2. The practical consequence of this is that to interpret a particular value of the leverage in logistic regression correctly, one needs to know whether the estimated probability is small (<0.1) or large (>0.9). If the estimated probability lies between 0.1 and 0.9 then the leverage gives a value that may be thought of as distance. When the estimated probability lies outside the interval 0.1 to 0.9, then the value of the leverage may not measure distance, in the sense that, further from the mean implies a larger value. We discuss the effect of leverage on the fit of the model after considering residual-based diagnostics.

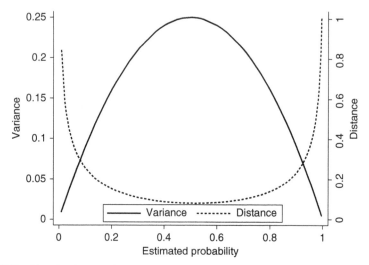

Figure 5.10 Plot of variance estimator (v, —) and the distance portion of leverage (b, - -) versus the estimated logistic probability ($\hat{\pi}$) for a hypothetical univariable logistic regression model.

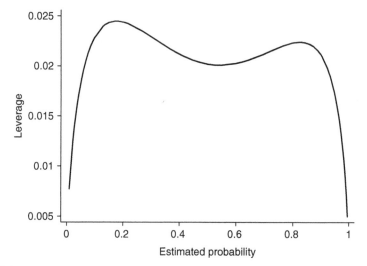

Figure 5.11 Plot of the leverage (h) versus the estimated logistic probability ($\hat{\pi}$) for a hypothetical univariable logistic regression model.

If we use the Pregibon (1981) linear regression-like approximation for the residual for the jth covariate pattern, $[y_j - m_j \hat{\pi}(\mathbf{x}_j)] \approx (1 - h_j) y_j$, then the estimator of the variance of the residual is approximately

$$m_j \hat{\pi}(\mathbf{x}_j)[1 - \hat{\pi}(\mathbf{x}_j)](1 - h_j),$$

which suggests that the Pearson residuals do not have variance equal to 1 unless they are further standardized. Recall that we denote by r_j the Pearson residual given in equation (5.1). The standardized Pearson residual for covariate pattern $\mathbf{x}_j$ is

$$r_{sj} = \frac{r_j}{\sqrt{1 - h_j}} \tag{5.23}$$

Another useful diagnostic statistic is one that examines the effect that deleting all subjects with a particular covariate pattern has on the value of the estimated coefficients and the overall summary measures of fit X^2 and D. The change in the value of the estimated coefficients is analogous to the measure proposed by Cook (1977, 1979) for linear regression. It is obtained as the standardized difference between $\hat{\boldsymbol{\beta}}$ and $\hat{\boldsymbol{\beta}}_{(-j)}$, where these represent the maximum likelihood estimates computed using all J covariate patterns and excluding the m_j subjects with pattern $\mathbf{x}_j$ respectively, and standardizing via the estimated covariance matrix of $\hat{\boldsymbol{\beta}}$. Pregibon (1981) showed, to a linear approximation, that this quantity for logistic regression is

$$\Delta\hat{\boldsymbol{\beta}}_j = (\hat{\boldsymbol{\beta}} - \hat{\boldsymbol{\beta}}_{(-j)})' (\mathbf{X}' \mathbf{V} \mathbf{X})(\hat{\boldsymbol{\beta}} - \hat{\boldsymbol{\beta}}_{(-j)})$$

$$= \frac{r_j^2 h_j}{(1 - h_j)^2}$$

$$= \frac{r_{sj}^2 h_j}{(1 - h_j)}. \tag{5.24}$$

Using similar linear approximations it can be shown that the decrease in the value of the Pearson chi-square statistic due to deletion of the subjects with covariate pattern $\mathbf{x}_j$ is

$$\Delta X_j^2 = \frac{r_j^2}{(1 - h_j)}$$

$$= r_{sj}^2. \tag{5.25}$$

A similar quantity may be obtained for the change in the deviance,

$$\Delta D_j = d_j^2 + \frac{r_j^2 h_j}{(1 - h_j)}.$$

If we replace r_j^2 by d_j^2 this yields the approximation

$$\Delta D_j = \frac{d_j^2}{(1 - h_j)}, \tag{5.26}$$

which is similar in form to the expression in equation (5.25).

These diagnostic statistics are conceptually quite appealing, as they allow us to identify those covariate patterns that are poorly fit (large values of ΔX_j^2 and/or ΔD_j), and those that have a great deal of influence on the values of the estimated parameters (large values of $\Delta\hat{\beta}_j$). After identifying these influential patterns (subjects), we can begin to address the role they play in the analysis.

Before proceeding to the use of the diagnostics in an example, we make a few summary comments on what we might expect their application to tell us. Consider first the measure of fit, ΔX_j^2. This measure is smallest when y_j and $m_j\hat{\pi}(\mathbf{x}_j)$ are close. This is most likely to happen when $y_j = 0$ and $\hat{\pi}(\mathbf{x}_j) < 0.1$ or $y_j = m_j$ and $\hat{\pi}(\mathbf{x}_j) > 0.9$. Similarly ΔX_j^2 is largest when y_j is furthest from $m_j\hat{\pi}(\mathbf{x}_j)$. This is most likely to occur if we have a value of $y_j = 0$ and $\hat{\pi}(\mathbf{x}_j) > 0.9$, or with $y_j = m_j$ and $\hat{\pi}(\mathbf{x}_j) < 0.1$. These same covariate patterns are not likely to have a large $\Delta\hat{\beta}_j$ as, when $\hat{\pi}(\mathbf{x}_j) < 0.1$ or $\hat{\pi}(\mathbf{x}_j) > 0.9$, $\Delta\hat{\beta}_j \approx \Delta X_j^2 h_j$ and the leverage h_j approaches zero. The influence diagnostic $\Delta\hat{\beta}_j$ is large when both ΔX_j^2 and h_j are at least moderate. This is most likely to occur when $0.1 < \hat{\pi}(\mathbf{x}_j) < 0.3$, or $0.7 < \hat{\pi}(\mathbf{x}_j) < 0.9$. As we know from Figure 5.11, these are the intervals where the leverage h_j is largest. In the region of fitted values between 0.3 and 0.7 the chances are not as great that either ΔX_j^2 or h_j is large. Table 5.9 summarizes these observations. This table reports what might be expected, not what may actually happen in any particular example. Therefore, it should only be used as a guide to further understanding and interpretation of the diagnostic statistics.

In linear regression essentially two approaches are used to interpret the value of the diagnostics, often in conjunction with each other. The first is graphical. The second employs the distribution theory of the linear regression model to develop the distribution of the diagnostics under the assumption that the fitted model is correct. In the graphical approach, large values of diagnostics either appear as spikes or reside in the extreme corners of plots. A value of the diagnostic statistic for a point appearing to lie away from the balance of the points is judged to be extreme if it exceeds some percentile of the relevant distribution. This may sound a little too hypothesis-testing oriented, but under the assumptions of linear regression with normal errors, there is a known statistical distribution whose percentiles provide some guidance as to what constitutes a large value. Presumably, if the model is correct and fits, then no values should be exceptionally large and the plots should appear as expected under the distribution of the diagnostic statistic.

In logistic regression we have to rely primarily on visual assessment, as the distribution of the diagnostics under the hypothesis that the model fits is known only in certain limited settings. For instance, consider the Pearson residual, r_j. It is

Table 5.9 Likely Values of Each of the Diagnostic Statistics ΔX^2, $\Delta\hat{\beta}$, and h Within Each of Five Regions Defined by the Value of the Estimated Logistic Probability ($\hat{\pi}$)

$\hat{\pi}$	ΔX^2	$\Delta\hat{\beta}$	h
<0.1	Large or Small	Small	Small
0.1–0.3	Moderate	Large	Large
0.3 − 0.7	Moderate to Small	Moderate	Moderate to Small
0.7 − 0.9	Moderate	Large	Large
>0.9	Large or Small	Small	Small

often stated that the distribution of this quantity is approximately $N(0, 1)$ when the model is correct. This statement is only true when m_j is sufficiently large to justify that the normal distribution provides an adequate approximation to the binomial distribution, a condition obtained under m-asymptotics. For example, if $m_j = 1$ then r_j has only two possible values and it can hardly be expected to be normally distributed. Jennings (1986) has stated this point clearly and with all the necessary technical details. All of the diagnostics are evaluated by covariate pattern; hence any approximations to their distributions based on the normal distribution, under binomial errors, depend on the number of subjects with that pattern. When a fitted model contains some continuous covariates then the number of covariate patterns J is of the same order as n, and m-asymptotic results cannot be relied upon. Thus, in practice, an assessment of "large" is of necessity, a judgment call based on experience and the particular set of data being analyzed. Using the $N(0, 1)$ or equivalently, the $\chi^2(1)$ distribution for squared quantities may provide some guidance as to what "large" is. However, we urge that these percentiles be used with extreme caution.

Recently Martin and Pardo (2009) derived the asymptotic distribution of Cook's Distance, $\Delta\hat{\beta}$. They suggest using $(2p/n)$ as the critical value for leverage, the $\chi^2_{0.50}(p+1)$ percentile for ΔX^2 and $\overline{hh} \times \chi^2_{0.95}(1)$ for $\Delta\hat{\beta}$, where $\overline{hh}$ is the average of the J values of $h_j/(1 - h_j)$. Our experience is that these values identify too many covariate patterns as being extreme. Instead, we prefer to focus on covariate patterns whose values for one or more of the diagnostic statistics fall well away from the rest of the values. We discuss this point further when we use the diagnostics to evaluate the fitted models from the Glow and Burn Injury studies. In the end, there is just no substitute for experience in the effective use of diagnostic statistics. The only way to gain this kind of experience is to begin by employing the methods described below, each time one develops a logistic regression model.

We have defined seven diagnostic statistics that may be divided into three categories: (i) the basic building blocks, which are of interest in themselves, but also are used to form other diagnostics, (r_j, d_j, h_j); (ii) derived measures of the effect of each covariate pattern on the fit of the model, $(r_{sj}, \Delta X_j^2, \Delta D_j)$; and (iii) a derived measure of the effect of each covariate pattern on the value of the estimated parameters, $(\Delta\hat{\beta}_j)$. Most logistic regression software packages provide the capability to obtain at least one of the measures within each group.

A number of different types of plots have been suggested for use, each directed at a particular aspect of fit. Some are formed from the seven diagnostics while others require additional computation. For example, see the methods based on grouping and smoothing in Landwehr et al. (1984) and Fowlkes (1987). It is impractical to consider all possible suggested plots, so we restrict attention to a few of the more easily obtained ones that are meaningful in most logistic regression analyses. We consider them to be the core of an analysis of diagnostics. These consist of the following:

1. Plot h_j versus $\hat{\pi}_j$.
2. Plot ΔX_j^2 versus $\hat{\pi}_j$.

3. Plot ΔD_j versus $\hat{\pi}_j$.
4. Plot $\Delta\hat{\beta}_j$ versus $\hat{\pi}_j$.

Other plots that are sometimes useful include:

5. Plot ΔX_j^2 versus h_j.
6. Plot ΔD_j versus h_j.
7. Plot $\Delta\hat{\beta}_j$ versus h_j.

These last three allow direct assessment of the contribution of leverage to the value of the diagnostic statistic. One additional plot that we have found especially useful is a plot of ΔX_j^2 versus $\hat{\pi}_j$ where the size of the plotting symbol is proportional to the size of $\Delta\hat{\beta}_j$. This plot is also used in the examples that follow.

To illustrate the use of the diagnostic statistics and their related plots, we consider the model for the GLOW Study given in Table 4.16. Recall that the summary statistics indicated that the model fits. Thus, we do not expect an analysis of diagnostics to show large numbers of covariate patterns being fit poorly. We might, however, uncover a few covariate patterns that do not fit, or that have considerable influence on the estimated parameters. The key plots are given in Figures 5.12–5.16. We discuss each plot in turn.

The diagnostics ΔX^2 and ΔD plotted versus the estimated logistic probabilities are shown in Figures 5.13 and 5.14, respectively. We prefer to use these plots instead of plots of r_j and d_j versus $\hat{\pi}_j$. The reasons for this choice are as follows: (i) When $J \approx n$, most positive residuals correspond to covariate patterns where

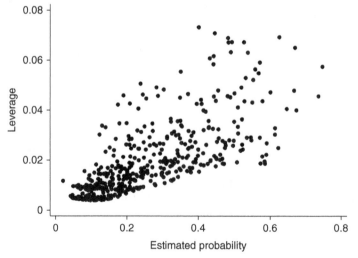

Figure 5.12 Plot of h versus the estimated probability from the fitted model from the GLOW Study in Table 4.16, $J = 547$ covariate patterns.

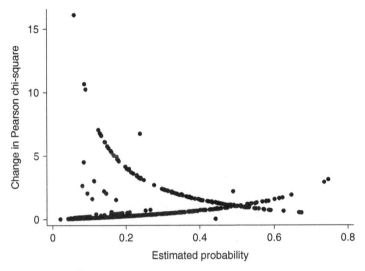

Figure 5.13 Plot of ΔX^2 versus the estimated probability from the fitted model from the GLOW Study in Table 4.16, $J = 547$ covariate patterns.

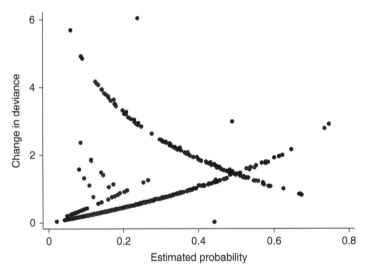

Figure 5.14 Plot of ΔD versus the estimated probability from the fitted model from the GLOW Study in Table 4.16, $J = 547$ covariate patterns.

$y_j = m_j$ (e.g., 1) and negative residuals to those with $y_j = 0$. Hence, the sign of the residual is not useful. (ii) Large residuals, regardless of sign, correspond to poorly fit points. Squaring these residuals further emphasizes the lack of fit and removes the issue of sign. (iii) The shape of the plot allows us to determine which patterns have $y_j = 0$ and which have $y_j \geq 1$.

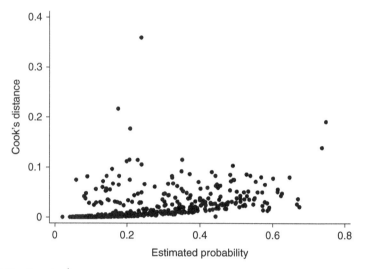

Figure 5.15 Plot of $\Delta\hat{\beta}$ versus the estimated probability from the fitted model from the GLOW Study in Table 4.16, $J = 547$ covariate patterns.

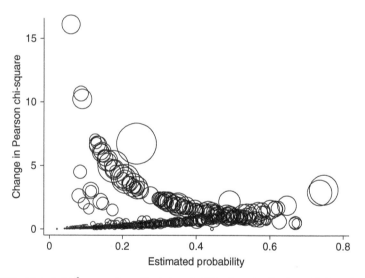

Figure 5.16 Plot of ΔX^2 versus the estimated probability from the fitted model from the GLOW Study in Table 4.16 with size of the plotting symbol proportional to $\Delta\hat{\beta}$, $J = 457$ covariate patterns.

The shapes of the plots in Figures 5.12 and 5.13 are similar and show quadratic like curves. The points on the curves going from the top left to bottom right corner correspond to covariate patterns with $y_j \geq 1$. The ordinate for these points is proportional to $(1 - \hat{\pi}_j)^2$ since $m_j = 1$ for most covariate patterns. The points on the other curves, going from the bottom left to top right corner, correspond to covariate patterns with $y_j = 0$. The ordinate for these points is proportional to $(0 - \hat{\pi}_j)^2$. Covariate patterns that are poorly fit generally are typically represented by points falling in the top left or top right corners of plots like those in Figures 5.12 and 5.13. We look for points that fall some distance from the balance of the data plotted. Assessment of this distance is partly based on numeric value and partly based on visual impression.

In Figure 5.13 we see three points (i.e., covariate patterns) that are poorly fit in the top left corner of the plot. In each case, $\Delta X^2 > 10$. There is one other point that lies a bit away from the others with $\Delta X^2 \approx 7$ and $\hat{\pi} \approx 0.23$. These same four points are seen in Figure 5.14 but note that the point with $\hat{\pi} \approx 0.23$ has the largest value of ΔD. The range of ΔX^2 is much greater than ΔD. This is a property of Pearson versus deviance residuals. Whenever possible we prefer to use plots of both ΔX^2 and ΔD versus $\hat{\pi}$.

Aside from the four points noted, the plots show that the model fits reasonably well. Most of the values of ΔX^2 are less than 6 and ΔD less than 4.5. We use 4 as a crude approximation to the upper ninety-fifth percentile of the distribution of ΔX^2 and ΔD as, under m-asymptotics, these quantities would be distributed approximately as $\chi^2(1)$ with $\chi^2_{0.95}(1) = 3.84$.

The influence diagnostic $\Delta\hat{\beta}$ is plotted versus $\hat{\pi}$ in Figure 5.15. We see five points that lie somewhat away from the rest of the data. The values themselves are not especially large, as all are less than 0.4. In our experience the influence diagnostic must be larger than 1.0 for an individual covariate pattern to have an effect on the estimated coefficients. However there are always exceptions and it is good practice to note outlying values of $\Delta\hat{\beta}$, regardless of the actual magnitude.

We noted in Table 5.9 that the largest values of $\Delta\hat{\beta}$ are most likely to occur when both ΔX^2 and leverage are at least moderately large. However large values can also occur when either component is large. In Figure 5.15 the covariate pattern with the largest influence diagnostic is the not the one with the largest value of ΔX^2. This covariate pattern is in the region of high leverage and moderate lack of fit. The other points in this same region of estimated probabilities would demonstrate lower values for leverage, but moderately large values of both ΔX^2 and ΔD.

In Figure 5.16 we plot ΔX^2 versus $\hat{\pi}$ with the size of the symbol proportional to $\Delta\hat{\beta}$. This plot allows us to more clearly ascertain the contributions of residual and leverage to $\Delta\hat{\beta}$. The largest circle in the left center of the plot corresponds to a moderately large value of ΔX^2, and as can be seen in Figure 5.12, moderately high leverage. Three other large circles are in the top left and correspond to the three covariate patterns with the largest values of ΔX^2. Two other large circles are seen in the lower right hand corner of the plot and have not especially large values of ΔX^2, hence we conclude that high leverage must be a contributing factor.

One problem with the influence diagnostic $\Delta\hat{\beta}$, is that it is a summary measure of change over all coefficients in the model simultaneously. For this reason it is important to examine the changes in the individual coefficients due to specific covariate patterns identified as influential.

Examination of Figures 5.12–5.16 identifies eight covariate patterns with outlying values on one or more of the diagnostics statistics. These include the patterns

Table 5.10   Covariate Values, Observed Outcome (y_j), Number (m_j), Estimated Logistic Probability ($\hat{\pi}$), and the Value of the Four Diagnostic Statistics $\Delta\hat{\beta}$, ΔX^2, ΔD, and Leverage (h) for the Eight Covariate Patterns (P#) with at Least One Large Value

P#	7	39	91	144	187	190	259	332
AGE	56	57	60	63	65	65	70	75
HEIGHT	155	166	162	153	167	168	142	175
PRIORFRAC	0	0	0	1	0	0	1	0
MOMFRAC	0	0	1	1	0	1	1	1
ARMASSIST	0	0	1	0	0	0	0	1
RATERISK3	0	0	1	1	0	0	0	0
y_j	1	1	1	0	1	2	0	1
m_j	1	1	1	1	1	2	1	1
$\hat{\pi}$	0.089	0.059	0.208	0.736	0.086	0.238	0.747	0.175
ΔX^2	10.23	16.10	3.97	2.91	10.67	6.74	3.13	4.93
ΔD	4.86	5.70	3.28	2.79	4.92	6.04	2.92	3.64
h	0.007	0.005	0.043	0.046	0.004	0.051	0.575	0.042
$\Delta\hat{\beta}$	0.081	0.075	0.177	0.139	0.048	0.359	0.191	0.217

with large values of ΔX^2 and/or ΔD, and four more with outlying values of $\Delta\hat{\beta}$. Information on these patterns is presented in Table 5.10. The quantity P# in Table 5.10 refers to the covariate pattern number. This number is somewhat arbitrary, as its value depends on how the data were aggregated. It should be noted that P# is not the original study identification code.

The next step in the analysis is to delete each covariate pattern identified (those in Table 5.10), one at a time, to assess their individual effect on the estimated coefficients. We leave the details of this step as an exercise. All deletions yielded percent changes less than 10% except for covariate pattern 190 where the coefficient for mother having had a fracture (MOMFRAC) changed by 18%. Covariate pattern 190 has two subjects, both had a fracture, a mother with a fracture, and not unexpectedly, their removal lowered the estimate. Following deletion of individual covariate patterns we usually delete all the patterns identified as poorly fit, then delete all those identified as being influential, and finally delete all covariate patterns identified. These results are presented in Table 5.11.

We see, in Table 5.11, that when we delete the four poorest fit patterns the maximum change is −15.9% for the dichotomous covariate self-reported risk greater than others (RATERISK3). Deleting the five most influential patterns produces greater than 20% changes in the coefficients for height and the "mother fracture by arm assist" interaction. Examining the data for these patterns, we see that the values of height for covariate patterns 259 and 332 are, respectively, among the shortest and tallest in the study. When we deleted just these two patterns we see that 17% of the 24% is accounted for by these two patterns. On examining the data for the interaction we find that two of the five patterns (91 and 332) when deleted account for 24% of the 26% change. These two patterns were among only 25 where both

Table 5.11   Estimated Coefficients from All Data (Table 4.16), the Percent Change when the Covariate Patterns Are Deleted, and Values of Model Statistics for Each Model

Variable	All Data Coefficients	Percent Change from All Data Coefficients when Covariate Patterns Are Deleted		
		Poorest Fit 7, 39, 187, 190	Largest Influence 91, 190, 144, 259, 332	All Eight
AGE	0.057	−12.6	−3.7	−15.4
HEIGHT	−0.047	−8.8	−24.3	−27.4
PRIORFRAC	4.612	−12.3	−8.3	−18.5
MOMFRAC	1.247	8.0	−5.3	−13.0
ARMASSIST	0.644	−8.5	−1.4	−10.1
RATERISK3	0.469	−15.9	−7.1	−16.4
AGE*PRIORFRAC	−0.055	−13.3	−7.2	−7.2
MOMFRAC*ARMASSIST	−1.281	5.8	−25.8	−31.5
Constant	1.717	−1.6	−56.1	−52.9
Model Statistics				
D	500.50	478.34	481.18	464.55
X^2	442.33	418.01	437.34	412.41
$\hat{C}$	6.39	5.81	5.23	9.68

"mother fracture" and "arm assist" were present. This is fully consistent with our experience modeling interactions of dichotomous covariates. Namely, the present-present cell tends to be least frequent of the four and thus deletion of any of these patterns tends to have the greatest effect on the estimate of the interaction coefficient, but not necessarily the main effect coefficients.

The percent changes, when all eight patterns (nine subjects) are deleted, are shown in the last column of Table 5.11. Three of the coefficients changed by greater than 25% and four more are greater than 15% (in absolute value). So, in aggregate, deleting these covariate patterns does have an affect on the estimated coefficients. We note that the signs are all negative indicating, from the definition of $\Delta\hat{\beta}\%$, and that the coefficients from the deleted model are all larger than the full data model. So we conclude that we have removed nine subjects whose pattern of data go against the model in the sense that the estimated probabilities are less than what would be expected based on the observed data.

The next step is to make a decision on the continued role in the analysis of the eight covariate patterns. This decision should always be made in conjunction with subject matter scientists. In this case all of the data were judged to be completely reasonable and should not be deleted. A phrase we often use when teaching about diagnostics is: "We use diagnostics statistics to identify subjects and subject matter considerations to decide on exclusion". One should not simply lift the rug and sweep potentially inconvenient data under it, no matter what affect deletion might have on a fitted model.

The model for the GLOW data in Table 4.16 is an example where the model fits well, and use of diagnostics identified only a few covariate patterns where the model did not fit, and/or the patterns were influential. Also, the model fit statistics at the bottom of Table 5.11 show that fit does not deteriorate when the stated covariate patterns are deleted and the model refit. Assume instead that we have a model where the summary statistics indicate that there is substantial deviation from fit. In this situation, we have evidence that for more than a few covariate patterns, y_j differs from $m_j \hat{\pi}_j$. One or more of three things has likely happened: (i) the logistic model does not provide a good approximation to the correct relationship between the conditional mean $E(Y|\mathbf{x}_j)$ and $\mathbf{x}_j$, (ii) we have not measured and/or not included an important covariate into the model, or (iii) at least one of the covariates in the model has not been entered in the correct scale. We discuss each of these in turn.

The logistic regression model is remarkably flexible. Unless we are dealing with a set of data where most of the probabilities are very small or very large, or where the fit is extremely poor in an identifiable systematic manner, it is unlikely that any alternative model will provide a better fit. Cox (1970) demonstrates that the logistic and other similar symmetric models are virtually identical in the region from 0.2 to 0.8. If one suspects, based on clinical or other reasons (such as graphical presentations, or Stukel's test, described in Section 5.2.2), that the logistic model is the wrong one, then careful thought should be given to the choice of the alternative model. Particular attention should be given to issues of interpretation. Are the coefficients clinically interpretable? The approach that tries all other possible models and selects the "best fitting" one is not recommended, as no thought is given to the clinical implications of the selected model. In some situations, inadequacy of a fitted logistic model can be corrected by returning to model building and rechecking variable selection and scale identification. Model fitting is an iterative procedure. We rarely obtain a final model on the first pass through the data. However, we must keep in mind the distinction between getting a model to fit and having the theoretically correct model.

Some interesting theoretical work has been done by White (1982, 1989) and Hjort (1988, 1999) on the use of maximum likelihood estimation with a misspecified model. These authors show that the fitted logistic regression model is the one that minimizes the Kullbeck–Leibler information distance between the theoretically correct model and the logistic model. In this sense the fitted logistic regression model is a best approximation to the true model. Maldonado and Greenland (1993) examine the interpretation of model coefficients in this setting and conclude that if one follows a thorough model building paradigm, similar to one presented in Chapter 4 and this chapter, then the estimated coefficients can provide useful estimates of effect even when the model is somewhat misspecified. Along these same lines Lin et al. (1998) present a method to quantify the sensitivity of estimates of effect to unmeasured confounders.

White (1982, 1989) provides a test for the hypothesis that the fitted model is the theoretically correct one. The test is elegant but is difficult to compute in practice, and its power has not been adequately studied. Hence, we recommend that assessment of the adequacy of the fitted logistic model be performed using the methods suggested in this chapter. When there is evidence that the logistic model does not fit the data an alternative model should be selected on the basis of clinical considerations.

When performing an analysis, we hope that the study was designed carefully so that data on all major covariates were collected. However, it is possible that the clinical factors associated with the outcome variable are not well known and, in this case, a key variable may not be present in the observed data. The potential biases and pitfalls of this oversight are enormous. Little can be done if this is the case, except to go back and collect these data. This approach of retroactive data collection is also impractical in most research situations.

Lack of fit may also occur if the variability in the outcome variable exceeds what would be predicted by the model and binomial variation. The early work on this problem is motivated by toxicological experiments where a dependence in the observations is present due to the outcome being measured on littermates having the same parentage, see Haseman and Hogan (1975), Haseman and Kupper (1979), Legler and Ryan (1997), Ryan (1992), and Williams (1975). In this context, source of lack of fit is often called extrabinomial variation. More recently work on this problem has focused on settings where the dependence is due to a general clustering of groups of responses (e.g., when a treatment is randomly assigned to a group of subjects such as a school or patients of a physician). The clustering can also be due to repeated observations on subjects over time. This continues to be quite an active area of methodological research and several software packages now incorporate the capability to fit appropriately modified logistic regression models. Because of its practical importance, models and methods for the analysis of clustered binary data are presented in detail in Chapter 9.

In summary, one should not proceed to presenting the results from a fitted model until the fit of model has been thoroughly assessed using both summary measures and diagnostic statistics.

Before leaving this section we report on the results of using diagnostic statistics to examine the effect of subjects on the fit of the model for the Burn Study data shown in Table 4.27. The overall fit of the model is shown in Table 5.2 where $\widehat{C} = 8.63$ with $p = 0.374$. Analyses (that we leave as an exercise to confirm, similar to that discussed above for the GLOW Study) yielded four poorly fit subjects ($m_j = 1$) with $\Delta X^2 > 40$. All had outcomes that went against the model: three of the subjects who died were middle aged with small burn areas, and the fourth, who lived,was older with a large burn area. When we refit the model excluding these four subjects only the estimated coefficients for RACE changed by more than 20%. The fit, as measured by $\widehat{C}$, was nearly identical to the fit shown in Table 5.2. Three subjects ($m_j = 1$) had values of $\Delta\widehat{\boldsymbol{\beta}}$ that stood out in the scatter plot versus the predicted probabilities. When we refit the model excluding these three we found the estimated coefficient for the interaction of age, fractional polynomial transformed, and inhalation injury (AGEFP1*INH_INJ) changed by over 50% and became nonsignificant. Most of this change was due to two older subjects who had inhalation injury complications and lived (i.e., their outcome went against the

Table 5.12 New Final Model for the Burn Injury Data, $n = 1000$

	Coeff.	Std. Err.	z	p	95% CI
AGEFP1	0.087	0.0082	10.52	<0.001	0.071, 0.103
TBSAFP1	0.936	0.0874	10.71	<0.001	0.765, 1.108
RACE	−0.609	0.3096	−1.97	0.049	−1.216, −0.002
INH_INJ	1.433	0.3422	4.19	<0.001	0.763, 2.104
Constant	−7.957	0.5967	−13.34	<0.001	−9.127, −6.788

model). The third was a younger subject with a small burn area and inhalation injury complications who died, again an outcome that goes against the model. The fit of the model deleting these three subjects is $\widehat{C} = 7.75$ with $p = 0.46$.

At this point we began to question the need for the interaction term in the model. Is it good statistical practice to have a model containing a covariate whose coefficient is largely determined by 3 of 1000 subjects? We think not and are thus inclined to remove the interaction from the model. In addition, recall that a major purpose of the model is to provide predicted probabilities of death for patients hospitalized for a burn injury at a burn treatment center. In this setting a simpler model is likely to perform better in an external data set (a topic considered in Section 5.4) than a more complicated model. Thus, for these two reasons, we removed the interaction term from the model, and did not delete the three influential subjects. Consultation with a burn surgeon confirmed this choice. The fit of the new and smaller Burn Study model is shown in Table 5.12.

Assessing the fit of the model in Table 5.12 yielded $\widehat{C} = 6.97$ with $p = 0.54$. We leave as an exercise further fit analysis using other goodness of fit tests and diagnostic statistics.

5.4 ASSESSMENT OF FIT VIA EXTERNAL VALIDATION

In some studies it may be possible to exclude a sub-sample of our observations, develop a model based on the remaining subjects, and then assess the model in the originally excluded subjects. In other situations it may be possible to obtain a new sample of data to assess the goodness of fit and discrimination of a previously developed model. This type of assessment is often called model validation, and may be especially important when the fitted model is to be used to predict the outcome for future subjects. The reason for considering this type of assessment of model performance is that the fitted model always performs in an optimistic manner on the developmental data set. Harrel et al. (1996) discuss this within a general model building context. The use of validation data amounts to an assessment where the fitted model is considered to be theoretically known, and no estimation is performed. Some of the diagnostics discussed in Section 5.3 (ΔX^2, ΔD, $\Delta\widehat{\boldsymbol{\beta}}$) mimic this idea by computing, for each covariate pattern, a quantity based on the exclusion of the particular covariate pattern. With a new data set a more thorough assessment is possible.

Obviously, we hope that the analysis supports that the model fits as there are many reasons why a model might not fit the validation data. Lack of fit could be due to an incorrectly specified systematic component, such as omitted covariates (e.g., interactions), incorrect specification of the parametric form for continuous covariates, the constant term is incorrect (too large or small) due to a large difference in the proportion of responses in the developmental and validation data and/or the logit transformation is the incorrect link function. As we demonstrate in this section, it is possible to repair a slightly broken model, but when this repair fails, one has little choice but to go back to square one and rebuild the model in the new data.

The methods for assessment of fit in the validation sample parallel those described in Sections 5.2 and 5.3 for the developmental sample. The major difference is that the values of the coefficients in the model are regarded as fixed constants rather than estimated values.

Assume that the validation sample consists of n_v observations $(y_i, \mathbf{x}_i)$, $i = 1, 2, \ldots, n_v$, which may be grouped into J_v covariate patterns. In keeping with previous notation, let y_j denote the number of positive responses among the m_j subjects with covariate pattern $\mathbf{x} = \mathbf{x}_j$ for $j = 1, 2, \ldots, J_v$. The logistic probability for the jth covariate pattern is π_j, the value of the previously estimated logistic model using the covariate pattern $\mathbf{x}_j$, from the validation sample. These quantities become the basis for the computation of the summary measures of fit, X^2, D, S, and C, from the validation sample. Each of these is considered in turn.

The computation of the Pearson chi-square statistic follows directly from equation (5.2), with obvious substitution of quantities from the validation sample. In this case X^2 is computed as the sum of J_v independent terms. If each $m_j\pi_j$ is large enough to use the normal approximation to the binomial distribution, then X^2 is distributed as $\chi^2(J_v)$ under the hypothesis that the model is correct. We expect that in practice the observed numbers of subjects within each covariate pattern is small, with most $m_j = 1$. Hence, we cannot employ m-asymptotics. In this case we can use results presented in Osius and Rojek (1992) to obtain a statistic that follows the standard normal distribution under the hypothesis that the model is correct and J_v is sufficiently large. The procedure is similar to the one presented in Section 5.2. Specifically one computes the standardized statistic

$$z_{X^2} = \frac{X^2 - J_v}{\sigma_v} \qquad (5.27)$$

where

$$\sigma_v^2 = 2J_v + \sum_{j=1}^{J_v} \frac{1}{m_j\pi_j(1-\pi_j)} - 6\sum_{j=1}^{J_v} \frac{1}{m_j}. \qquad (5.28)$$

The test uses a two-tailed p-value based on z_{X^2}. Note that when $m_j = 1$ the variance in equation (5.28) simplifies to

$$\sigma_v^2 = \sum_{i=1}^{n_v} \frac{1}{\pi_i(1-\pi_i)} - 4n_v. \qquad (5.29)$$

The adverse affect of pairs with small or large π and an outcome that is 1 or 0 is the same as that noted in Section 5.2, an aberrantly large value of X^2 and / or σ_v^2. As in Section 5.2 we prefer to use the sum-of-squares statistic

$$S = \sum_{j=1}^{J_v} (y_j - m_j \pi_j)^2$$

in these cases. The standardized version for assessing fit in the validation sample is

$$z_S = \frac{S - \sum_{j=1}^{J_v} m_j \pi_j (1 - \pi_j)}{\sigma_S}, \qquad (5.30)$$

where

$$\sigma_S^2 = \sum_{j=1}^{J_v} m_j \pi_j (1 - \pi_j)[1 + 2 m_j \pi_j (1 - \pi_j) - 6\pi_j (1 - \pi_j)] \qquad (5.31)$$

and we use a two tailed p-value. Under the assumption that $m_j = 1$ the expression in equation (5.31) simplifies to

$$\sigma_S^2 = \sum_{i=1}^{n} \pi_i (1 - \pi_i)(1 - 2\pi_i)^2. \qquad (5.32)$$

Stallard (2009) derives the same expressions for means and variances of X^2 and S under the assumption that $m_j = 1$.

The same line of reasoning discussed in Section 5.2.2 to develop the Hosmer–Lemeshow test may be used to obtain an equivalent statistic for the validation sample. Assume that we wish to use 10 groups composed of the deciles of risk. Any other grouping strategy could be used with obvious modifications in the calculations. Let n_k denote the approximately $n_v/10$ subjects in the kth decile of risk. Let $o_k = \sum y_j$ be the number of positive responses among the covariate patterns falling in the kth decile of risk. The estimate of the expected value of o_k under the assumption that the model is correct is $e_k = \sum m_j \pi_j$, where the sum is over the covariate patterns in the decile of risk. The Hosmer–Lemeshow statistic is obtained as the Pearson chi-square statistic computed from the observed and expected frequencies (see equations (5.7) and (5.8))

$$C_v = \sum_{k=1}^{g} \frac{(o_k - e_k)^2}{n_k \overline{\pi}_k (1 - \overline{\pi}_k)} \qquad (5.33)$$

where $\overline{\pi}_k = \sum m_j \pi_j / n_k$. The subscript v, has been added to C to emphasize that the statistic has been calculated from a validation sample. Under the hypothesis that the model is correct, and the assumption that each e_k is sufficiently large for each term in C_v to be distributed as $\chi^2(1)$, it follows that C_v is distributed as

$\chi^2(10)$. In general, if we use g groups then the distribution is $\chi^2(g)$. In addition to calculating a p-value to assess overall fit, we recommend that each term in C_v be examined to assess the fit within each decile of risk. The comments given in Section 5.2.2 regarding modification of the denominator of the test statistic $\hat{C}$, in equation (5.8) also apply to C_v in equation (5.33).

The classification table and area under the ROC curve are two other summary statistics that we are likely to use with the validation sample—but only in instances where classification is an important use of the model. These two measures are obtained in exactly the same manner as shown in Section 5.2.3, with the modification that probabilities are no longer thought of as being estimated. The resulting table can be used to compute statistics such as sensitivity, specificity, and positive and negative predictive values. Interpretation of these quantities depends on the particular situation.

We use two examples to illustrate model assessment in a validation sample. In Section 5.2 we developed a prediction model for the Burn Study (shown in Table 4.27) and assessed its fit in Section 5.2. We used diagnostic statistics in Section 5.3 to further examine the model where we found that the significance of an interaction term was largely due to 3–4 subjects. As a result, we excluded the interaction term and refit the main effects only model (shown in Table 5.12). Now we would like to see how this model works in a different set of burn injury data. Using a method similar to the one used to select the Burn Study data described in Section 1.6.5 we selected two additional data sets of size 500—one where the model in Table 5.12 fits and one where it does not. We feel that it is important to see both as one cannot assume that any statistical model, no matter how carefully built, will perform comparably in a new set of data.

The first data set (we call this BURN_EVAL_1) is available electronically in the same locations as the data described in Section 1.6. A total of 14.4% of the 500 subjects died. The first step in the evaluation is to compute the fractional polynomial transformations of age, $AGEFP1 = (AGE/10)^2$, and total burn surface area, $TBSAFP1 = \sqrt{TBSA}$. Next we calculate logistic probabilities for all 500 subjects using the estimated coefficients in Table 5.12. The ten by two decile of risk table of observed and expected frequencies is shown in Table 5.13. The value of the decile of risk test is $C_v = 5.78$, which with 10 degrees of freedom gives $p = 0.833$. Thus we cannot conclude that the previously developed model for the Burn Study does not fit the new data. In short, the decile of risk test suggests that the observed outcomes of mortality agree with the estimated probabilities from the logistic model. A few things should be noted about the frequencies in Table 5.13. First the sums of the expected frequencies within each outcome group are not equal to the observed. This is due to the fact that the coefficients used to compute the probabilities were not from a model fit to these data. Second, the estimated expected frequencies are less than 5 in 8 of the 20 cells. Thus the actual p-value may not be quite equal to the stated value. Regardless, there is close agreement between observed and expected frequencies in all 20 cells of Table 5.13. Hence the overall picture is that of a model that produces estimated probabilities that reflect the true outcome experience in these data (i.e., fits the data).

Table 5.13 Observed (Obs) and Estimated Expected (Exp) Frequencies Within Each Decile of Risk for DEATH = 1 and DEATH = 0 from BURN_EVAL_1 Using the Estimated Coefficients from the Fitted Model in Table 5.12

	Death = 1		Death = 0		
Decile	Obs	Exp	Obs	Exp	N
1	0	0.00	50	49.97	50
2	0	0.07	50	49.93	50
3	0	0.12	50	49.88	50
4	0	0.20	50	49.80	50
5	0	0.35	50	49.65	50
6	0	0.66	50	49.34	50
7	2	1.76	48	48.24	50
8	7	7.45	43	42.55	50
9	20	25.32	30	24.68	50
10	43	45.78	7	4.22	50
Total	72	81.71	428	418.26	500

To further examine fit we evaluate the standardized Pearson chi-square statistic in equation (5.27) and the standardized sum-of-squares statistic in equation (5.30). There are 497 covariate patterns in the BURN_EVAL_1 data so we did not form the covariate pattern data, instead computing the statistic using $m_j = 1$. The value of the Pearson chi-square statisitic is $X^2 = 257.6541$. The estimate of the variance of X^2 from equation (5.29) is $\sigma_v^2 = 168428.05$ and the value of the standardized statistic is

$$z_{X^2} = \frac{(257.6541 - 500)}{\sqrt{168428.05}} = -0.5905,$$

yielding a two-tailed $p = 0.555$. The large variance estimate is due to the fact that 50% of the predicted probabilities are less than 0.01, which contributes 160097.83 to the estimate.

The value of the sum-of-squares statistic is $S = 25.1747$. The estimate of the variance from equation (5.31) is $\sigma_S^2 = 8.4626$ and the value of the standardized statistic is

$$z_S = \frac{(25.1747 - 24.3620)}{\sqrt{8.4626}} = 0.279$$

and the two-tailed $p = 0.780$.

All three goodness of fit tests support the fit of the model in Table 5.12 to the validation data set BURN_EVAL_1. The next step is to check and see how well the model discriminates between those subjects who died and lived through the area under the ROC curve. Computing the area under the ROC curve using probabilities estimated using the model in Table 5.12 yields the value 0.966, excellent discrimination. Hence by all measures the model in Table 5.12 has excellent fit and discrimination in the BURN_EVAL_1 data. One reason for the good performance is that the distribution of the outcome and also model covariates in BURN_EVAL_1

Table 5.14 Observed (Obs) and Estimated Expected (Exp) Frequencies Within Each Decile of Risk for DEATH = 1 and DEATH = 0 from BURN_EVAL_2 Using the Estimated Coefficients from the Fitted Model in Table 5.12

Decile	Death = 1		Death = 0		N
	Obs	Exp	Obs	Exp	
1	0	0.03	50	49.97	50
2	1	0.06	49	49.94	50
3	2	0.12	48	49.88	50
4	2	0.21	48	49.79	50
5	0	0.37	50	49.63	50
6	6	0.78	44	49.22	50
7	9	2.52	41	47.47	50
8	17	11.47	33	38.53	50
9	38	31.06	12	18.94	50
10	46	46.33	4	3.67	50
Total	121	92.95	379	407.04	500

are quite similar to the Burn Study data. We leave the details of showing this as an exercise.

Next we apply the model in Table 5.12 to the BURN_EVAL_2 data. In this sample of 500 patients with a burn injury 24% died, compared to only 15% in the Burn Study data. The value of the decile of risk test is $\widehat{C} = 120.19$, which with 10 degrees of freedom, yields $p < 0.001$. We conclude that the model in Table 5.12 does not fit the data in BURN_EVAL_2. The observed and estimated expected frequencies are given in Table 5.14. In general the model underestimates the number of deaths in all deciles of risk. The estimated expected values are small in eight of the 20 cells, and thus the p-value may not be accurate, but there is compelling evidence of poor model fit.

Evaluating the standardized Pearson chi-square statistic in equation (5.27) using the estimator of the variance when $m_j = 1$ in equation (5.29) yields

$$z_{\chi^2} = \frac{(2800.1072 - 500)}{\sqrt{181702.76}} = 5.396,$$

corresponding to $p < 0.001$. The standardized sum-of-squares statistic using the variance estimator in equation (5.32) is

$$z_S = \frac{(43.2009 - 26.7685)}{\sqrt{8.6153}} = 5.598,$$

yielding $p < 0.001$. We see that all three goodness of fit tests reject model fit. From our point of view, since the model does not fit, there is no compelling need to evaluate the model's discrimination. However, for sake of comparison, we report the area under the ROC curve as 0.928. Hence the evaluation shows that while the model can distinguish between patients who die from those who live, the estimated probabilities do not accurately describe the true outcome experience in these patients.

Two questions emerge at this point: (i) What is the problem with the model in Table 5.12? and (ii) Can the model be easily modified to fit the BURN_EVAL_2 data?

At this point we have to make some assumptions about our access to the new data, BURN_EVAL_2. In the previous analyses we assumed that the researcher who constructed the two EVAL data sets provided us with a data set containing only the outcome variable and the estimated probabilities (as calculated from the model in Table 5.12) for the 500 patients. This is typical information provided when an investigator is trying to determine whether a new model can be tested on their data. Alternatively, the data could come from another setting in our own study. The former case is the more difficult case to deal with, as we do not have full information. When we do have access to all the data we have the option of fitting the model to the new data and making direct comparisons of the estimated coefficients from the two (i.e., old and new) models. Since this is essentially another model building exercise we do not consider it further; instead we focus on the more difficult case. As Miller et al. (1991) note, before embarking on a detailed look one should make sure that the range of covariates in the validation sample is contained within the range to the developmental sample to avoid inappropriate model extrapolation. This condition holds for both burn validation data sets.

Question 1: We know, from a frequency table of the outcome, that 24.2% of the patients in the BURN_EVAL_2 data died, but only 15% of the patients in the original Burn Study died. Hence, we can be reasonably certain that the intercept coefficient in Table 5.12 is too small. This observation is further supported by the fact that the sum of the expected frequencies in Table 5.14 is 93 not 121. As noted, without access to the BURN_EVAL_ 2 data we cannot make any specific evaluations of the other individual coefficients in the Table 5.12 model.

Question 2: Under the assumption that we are provided outcome data and the estimated probabilities from the model based on Table 5.12, it is possible to adjust the model so that the sum of the expected values is 121; but this is no guarantee that the adjusted model will fit. Miller et al. (1991) fully develop this approach, which was first suggested by Cox (1958). The procedure to adjust the model is as follows:

1. Denote the Table 5.12 model estimated probabilities as $\hat{\pi}_i^M$. Compute the logit for each subject in the validation data set,

$$\hat{g}_i^M = \ln\left(\frac{\hat{\pi}_i^M}{1 - \hat{\pi}_i^M}\right), i = 1, \ldots, n_v. \tag{5.34}$$

2. Fit the logistic regression model with $\hat{g}_i^M$ as the only covariate.

Let $\hat{\alpha}_0$ denote the estimate of the intercept and $\hat{\alpha}_1$ denote the estimate of the regression coefficient for $\hat{g}^M$. The estimated probabilities from this fit are

$$\hat{\theta}_i = \frac{\exp(\hat{\alpha}_0 + \hat{\alpha}_1 \hat{g}_i^M)}{1 + \exp(\hat{\alpha}_0 + \hat{\alpha}_1 \hat{g}_i^M)} \tag{5.35}$$

and it follows from the results in Chapter 1 that $\sum_{i=1}^{n_v} \hat{\theta}_i = n_{v1}$, for example, the sum of estimated probabilities equals the sum of the observed outcomes, $\sum_{i=1}^{n_v} y_i = n_{v1}$. If the fitted model described by the logit $\hat{g}^M$, is identical to within sampling error of the same model fit to the new data set in 2, then $\hat{\alpha}_0$ should be within sampling variation of 0.0 and $\hat{\alpha}_1$ should be within sampling variation of 1.0. This can be easily checked by seeing if 0.0 is contained in the confidence interval for the constant term and 1.0 in the confidence interval for the regression coefficient. A Wald test of the joint hypothesis is also not difficult to calculate, although likely not necessary. Miller et al. (1991) also describe two conditional tests: $H_0 : \alpha_1 = 1|\alpha_0$ and $H_0 : \alpha_0 = 0|\alpha_1$. Cox (1958) notes that if $\hat{\alpha}_1 > 1$, the probabilities $\hat{\pi}^M$ are reasonably positively correlated with the outcome, but have too little variation (i.e., the range of $\hat{g}^M$ may not be wide enough to yield small and large enough values of $\hat{\pi}^M$). If the estimate $\hat{\alpha}_1 < 1$, then there is too much variability in $\hat{\pi}^M$ (i.e., the range of $\hat{g}^M$ is too wide yielding too small and too large values of $\hat{\pi}^M$). If the estimate of the slope is such that $\hat{\alpha}_1 < 0$ then the probabilities, $\hat{\pi}^M$, go in the wrong direction. (Note: This is likely to occur only if, by mistake, one reverses the outcome to $y = 0$). If the estimate of the constant term $\hat{\alpha}_0$ is positive, then the probabilities are consistently too small. The opposite is the case when the constant is negative.

Operationally, we suggest that, following the fit in 2, one examines the confidence intervals to see if they contain the respective null values. If we have rejected the hypothesis that the model fits the new data, as we have done with the model in Table 5.12, then we fully expect that at least one of the confidence intervals will not contain the null value. Next we perform the usual goodness of fit tests using the model fit in 2. This step checks to see if this simple adjustment $\hat{\alpha}_0 + \hat{\alpha}_1 \hat{g}_i^M$, provides a model that fits. If the adjusted model fits, then we can apply the corrections to the model coefficients and proceed with the adjusted model. If the adjusted model does not fit then there is little more we can do as the lack of fit is more complex, as discussed at the beginning of this section, and cannot be resolved by the simple regression adjustment.

The results of the fit described in 2 above to the BURN_EVAL_2 data where $\hat{g}^M$ is based on the coefficients in Table 5.12 are shown in Table 5.15.

Table 5.15 Results of the Adjusted Fit to the BURN_EVAL_2 Data

	Coeff.	Std. Err.	z	p	95% CI
$\hat{g}^M$	0.730	0.0650	11.22	<0.001	0.602, 0.857
Constant	0.571	0.1908	2.99	0.003	0.196, 0.945

We see that neither one nor zero is contained in the respective confidence intervals. The fact that estimate of the slope is less than one $\hat{\alpha}_1 = 0.73$, implies that there is too much variability in the $\hat{\pi}^M$. The fact that the estimate of the constant is positive ($\hat{\alpha}_0 = 0.571$) implies, as noted above, that the probabilities $\hat{\pi}^M$ are too small. Testing goodness of fit using the adjusted probabilities computed using the results in Table 5.15 in equation (5.35), we obtain $\hat{C} = 6.85$ with $p = 0.552$, computed with 8 degrees of freedom as the model is estimated. We do not present the results, but both the standardized Pearson chi-square and the standardized sum-of-squares statistics are not significant. Hence, in this example, the adjusted model fits the BURN_EVAL_2 data. The area under the ROC curve using the adjusted probabilities is 0.928.

Miller et al. (1991) provide expressions to compute casewise diagnostic statistics of the effect each pair $(1, \hat{g}^M)$ has on the departure of $\hat{\alpha}_0$ from zero and $\hat{\alpha}_1$ from 1. The computations, while not complex, do require matrix manipulations and are not programmed into STATA or other packages. An alternative is to use the diagnostic statistics discussed in Section 5.3 computed from the fit in 2 above. The differences being that these measures have an effect on the estimate and not on the departure from the null values. Regardless, aberrant and influential values can be identified.

We conclude that the model using the estimates in Table 5.12 does not fit the BURN_EVAL_2 data, but a simple adjustment of the estimated probabilities, provides estimates that do fit the data and have good discrimination.

Before concluding this section we present some comparisons in Table 5.16 of the individual coefficients from three fitted models. The first column repeats the results from Table 5.12. The second column presents the value of the adjusted estimates based on the estimated coefficients in Table 5.15. The third column presents the estimated probabilities from an actual fit to the data in BURN_EVAL_2. In practice this fit is possible only if we have access to the data. In the fourth column we show the percent difference between the adjusted estimate and the one from the fit to the data.

Table 5.16 Comparison of the Estimated Coefficients in Table 5.12 to Adjusted Coefficients and those from a Model Fit to the BURN_EVAL_2 Data

	Table 5.12 Coeff.	Adjusted[a] Coeff.	Fit to Data Coeff.	$\Delta\hat{\beta}\%$[b] Adjusted vs. Fit
AGEFP1	0.087	0.064	0.059	7.64
TBSAFP1	0.936	0.683	0.753	−9.26
RACE	−0.609	−0.445	0.277[c]	−260.49
INH_INJ	1.433	1.046	0.743	40.79
Constant	−7.957	−5.238	−5.813	−9.90

[a] Adjusted slope = 0.73 × Slope Coeff. from Table 5.12; adjusted Intercept = 0.73 × Constant Coeff. from Table 5.12 + 0.571.

[b] $\Delta\hat{\beta}\% = \dfrac{100(\hat{\beta}_{Adjusted} - \hat{\beta}_{Fit})}{\hat{\beta}_{Fit}}$.

[c] Estimate is no longer significant, $p = 0.48$.

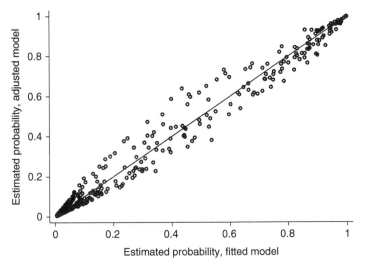

Figure 5.17   Plot of the estimated probabilities from the adjusted model versus those from the fitted model.

What is interesting is that despite some large differences between the adjusted and newly fit coefficients, the adjusted model, in aggregate, performs well in the BURN_EVAL_2 data. To see why this is the case we show in Figure 5.17, a scatter plot of the predicted probabilities computed from the adjusted and fitted models.

The plot shows that there is a high level of agreement between the two estimates, especially in the tails. The largest differences, departure from the solid line of equality, are the approximately 60 (12%) values between 0.3 and 0.7.

Based on the above analyses, our conclusions are: (1) the model based on the coefficients in Table 5.12 is not appropriate for use in the new setting, (2) the adjusted model in Table 5.15 performs well enough to be used in the new setting for prediction purposes, and (3) we do not recommend using the adjusted model to estimate the effects of model covariates in the new setting. This conclusion is not based on the results in Table 5.16, but rather on taking a more conservative view that the adjustment is really to the logit as a whole rather than to its individual coefficients.

In summary, model validation on an external data set should consist of an evaluation of its fit and an ROC analysis if the model fits. When the model fits the validation data set one can have some confidence that the values of the individual coefficients in the model approximate to a good degree the covariate effect in the validation setting. When the model does not fit, we recommend trying the simple adjustment procedure described in this section as it can often yield a good fitting model that can be used for prediction purposes. We do not recommend using the adjusted model to estimate effects in the validation setting. If the simple adjustment procedure does not yield a good fitting model the differences between the developmental and validation settings are more complex and a new custom fit model is needed.

5.5 INTERPRETATION AND PRESENTATION OF THE RESULTS FROM A FITTED LOGISTIC REGRESSION MODEL

Once we are satisfied that the fit of the model is adequate, we are ready to use the model to address the inferential goals of the particular study. In our experience this almost always involves using the estimates of model coefficients to obtain estimates of the adjusted odds ratios for model covariates. For our first example, we use the model fit to the GLOW Study data presented in Table 4.16, whose fit was checked earlier in this chapter. After presenting the results of the GLOW Study model we consider a second example using the model fit to the Burn Study data shown in Table 5.12.

For convenience we reproduce the fitted model of Table 4.16 in Table 5.17. The model is fairly typical of models reported in the subject matter literature in that it contains two continuous covariates (AGE and HEIGHT) that are scaled linearly in the logit, four dichotomous covariates (PRIORFRAC, MOMFRAC, ARMASSIST and RATERISK3), an interaction between a continuous and dichotomous covariate (AGE*PRIORFRAC) and an interaction between two dichotomous covariates (MOMFRAC*ARMASSIST).

As shown in Section 3.2 we obtain estimates of the odds ratios and their confidence intervals for dichotomous covariates (coded zero or one), and polychotomous covariates not involved in any interactions, with 0/1 reference cell design variables, by exponentiating their respective coefficients and the end points of their respective confidence intervals. The odds ratio and confidence interval for RATERISK3 and HEIGHT, obtained by exponentiating the results in Table 5.17, are given in Table 5.18. As shown in Section 3.4, we obtain the results for height in Table 5.18 by multiplying the estimated coefficient and the end points of the 95% confidence interval by 5 and then exponentiating.

In the first column of Table 5.18, for self-reported risk of fracture, we indicate the covariate and each of its levels. The reference level, less or same level of risk, is indicated by an odds ratio equal to 1.0. Some readers may question the need to include all levels, preferring instead to indicate the reference level by exclusion.

Table 5.17 Final Model Fit to the Glow Study Data, $n = 500$

	Coeff.	Std. Err.	z	p	95% CI
AGE	0.057	0.0165	3.47	0.001	0.025, 0.090
HEIGHT	−0.047	0.0183	−2.55	0.011	−0.083, −0.011
PRIORFRAC	4.612	1.8802	2.45	0.014	0.927, 8.297
MOMFRAC	1.247	0.3930	3.17	0.002	0.476, 2.017
ARMASSIST	0.644	0.2519	2.56	0.011	0.150, 1.138
RATERISK3	0.469	0.2408	1.95	0.051	−0.003, 0.941
AGE*PRIORFRAC	−0.055	0.0259	−2.13	0.033	−0.106, −0.004
MOMFRAC*ARMASSIST	−1.281	0.6230	−2.06	0.040	−2.502, −0.059
Constant	1.717	3.3218	0.52	0.605	−4.793, 8.228

Table 5.18   Estimated Odds Ratios and 95% Confidence Intervals for
Self-Reported Risk of Fracture and Height in the GLOW Study, $n = 1000$

Self-Reported Risk of Fracture Compared to Others	Odds Ratio	95% CI
Less or Same	1.00	
Greater	1.60	1.00, 2.56
Height	0.79[a]	0.66, 0.95

[a]Increase of 5 cm.

Either approach is acceptable; however, we feel the explicit method shown in Table 5.18 can be clearer and may make the discussion easier to follow.

The estimate of the odds ratio for self-reported risk is 1.60. The correct interpretation is that the odds of fracture on follow-up for a woman who perceives her risk as being greater than others is 1.6 times greater than the odds for a similar woman (with respect to the other covariates in the model) whose self-reported risk is less or same as others. In many, if not most subject matter journals, this interpretation would be stated more concisely, but incorrectly, as the risk of fracture among women whose self-reported risk is greater than others is 1.6 times larger than women who rate their risk as the same or less than others.

The second interpretation relies on the "odds ratio approximates relative risk" argument. We go into this in more detail in Chapter 6 where we discuss case–control studies, but it is sufficient at this point to indicate that this is only true when the outcome is "rare". As a rule of thumb, this argument is likely to be true when the outcome occurs less than 10% of the time. In our example, this means that the probability of fracture should be small. This is not true, since, overall 25% of the women in this data set experienced a fracture and the estimated probabilities of fracture from the fitted model range from 0.02 to 0.75. Zhang and Yu (1998) examine the extent to which the odds ratio overestimates the relative risk when the outcome is not rare. Their results show that the overestimation can be quite pronounced for odds ratios greater than 2.5 or less than 0.5. How important their results are, in practice, depends on how the estimated odds ratio is going to be used. In our model, both interpretations of the estimated odds ratio provide a reasonable statement of the fact that the odds of fracture is higher among women who rate their risk as greater than others. On the other hand, if it is vitally important to accurately describe the relative risk from the fit of a logistic regression model, then one should present the odds ratio results using the correct interpretation and then attempt to correct the overestimation. One can obtain a crude correction of the odds ratio from Zhang and Yu (1998). For example, an odds ratio of 1.6 with an "incidence among the unexposed" of 33% corrects to a relative risk of about 1.25. Zhang and Yu (1998) proposed this correction method before relative risk regression models, binary outcome with a log-link function, could be fit in many packages. We present a short discussion of fitting the log-link model to binary outcome data in Section 10.7.

The confidence interval estimate for the odds ratio for self-reported risk in Table 5.18 suggests that the increase in the "odds for greater risk than others" could range from no increase (1.0) to as much as 2.56 times the increase with 95% confidence.

The other main effect not involved in an interaction is height (cm) at enrollment in the study. A careful analysis of the scale of this covariate in Section 4.2 showed that it is linear in the logit in these data. We show in Table 5.18 that the estimated odds ratio for a positive difference of five centimeters is 0.79 with a 95% confidence interval from 0.66 to 0.95. The interpretation is that for every 5 cm increase in height there is a 0.79-fold decrease in the odds of fracture and the decrease could be as much as a 0.66-fold or as little as a 0.95-fold decrease. While this interpretation is correct, subject matter scientists usually find the percent change from one interpretation easier to understand when the odds ratio is less than one. Thus the alternative interpretation is: for every increase of 5 cm in height there is a 21% decrease in the odds of fracture and this decrease could be as much as 34% or as little as 5% with 95% confidence.

Next we estimate the odds ratios for a mother having had a fracture (MOM-FRAC) and reports that her arms are needed to stand from a chair (ARMASSIST). Since there is a significant interaction we must estimate the odds ratio for one covariate at each of the two levels of the other covariate. We presented and illustrated the four step procedure to estimate an odds ratio whose purpose is to yield exactly the correct function of estimated coefficients and covariate values required to estimate an odds ratio in Chapter 3. There we noted that, in the presence of interactions or non-linearity in continuous covariates, it may be the only way one could obtain the correct estimator. With this in mind, we use the four step method to estimate the odds ratio for mother having had a fracture. Denote the logit of the model in Table 5.17, in terms of the two covariates of interest, as

$$\hat{g}(x_1, x_2) = \hat{\beta}_0 + \hat{\beta}_1 x_1 + \hat{\beta}_2 x_2 + \hat{\beta}_3 x_1 \times x_2 + \hat{\boldsymbol{\theta}}' \mathbf{z},$$

where x_1 denotes MOMFRAC, x_2 denotes ARMASSIST and $\hat{\boldsymbol{\theta}}' \mathbf{z}$ denotes the contribution of the other covariates.

Step 1. Specify the values of the covariates to be compared: women whose mother had a history of fracture and who do not need arms to rise from a chair ($x_1 = 1, x_2 = 0$), versus women whose mother did not have a history of fracture and who do not need arms to rise from a chair ($x_1 = 0, x_2 = 0$).

Step 2. Substitute these values into the equation for the logit:

$$\hat{g}(x_1 = 1, x_2 = 0) = \hat{\beta}_0 + \hat{\beta}_1 \times 1 + \hat{\beta}_2 \times 0 + \hat{\beta}_3 \times 1 \times 0 + \hat{\boldsymbol{\theta}}' \mathbf{z}$$
$$= \hat{\beta}_0 + \hat{\beta}_1 + \hat{\boldsymbol{\theta}}' \mathbf{z}$$

and

$$\hat{g}(x_1 = 0, x_2 = 0) = \hat{\beta}_0 + \hat{\beta}_1 \times 0 + \hat{\beta}_2 \times 0 + \hat{\beta}_3 \times 0 \times 0 + \hat{\boldsymbol{\theta}}' \mathbf{z}$$
$$= \hat{\beta}_0 + \hat{\boldsymbol{\theta}}' \mathbf{z}.$$

Step 3. Take the difference between the two logits and algebraically simplify.

$$\hat{g}(x_1 = 1, x_2 = 0) - \hat{g}(x_1 = 0, x_2 = 0) = \hat{\beta}_0 + \hat{\beta}_1 + \hat{\boldsymbol{\theta}}'\mathbf{z} - \hat{\beta}_0 - \hat{\boldsymbol{\theta}}'\mathbf{z}$$
$$= \hat{\beta}_1.$$

Step 4. Exponentiate the value of the simplified expression in Step 3, yielding

$$\widehat{OR}(MOMFRAC = 1, MOMFRAC = 0| \ ARMASSIST = 0) = e^{\hat{\beta}_1}.$$

In this case the estimator is simply the exponentiation of the main effect coefficient for MOMFRAC in Table 5.17. Hence, we obtain the confidence interval estimate by exponentiating the ends points of the confidence interval estimate of the coefficient. These results are shown in the second row of Table 5.19.

Now we repeat the four step procedure for women who do need to use arms to rise from a chair [i.e., Step 1 with $(x_1 = 1, x_2 = 1)$ and $(x_1 = 0, x_2 = 1)$].

Step 2. Substitute these values into the equation for the logit:

$$\hat{g}(x_1 = 1, x_2 = 1) = \hat{\beta}_0 + \hat{\beta}_1 \times 1 + \hat{\beta}_2 \times 1 + \hat{\beta}_3 \times 1 \times 1 + \hat{\boldsymbol{\theta}}'\mathbf{z}$$

and

$$\hat{g}(x_1 = 0, x_2 = 1) = \hat{\beta}_0 + \hat{\beta}_1 \times 0 + \hat{\beta}_2 \times 1 + \hat{\beta}_3 \times 0 \times 1 + \hat{\boldsymbol{\theta}}'\mathbf{z}$$
$$= \hat{\beta}_0 + \hat{\beta}_2 + \hat{\boldsymbol{\theta}}'\mathbf{z}.$$

Step 3. Take the difference between the two logits and algebraically simplify:

$$\hat{g}(x_1 = 1, x_2 = 1) - \hat{g}(x_1 = 0, x_2 = 1) = \hat{\beta}_0 + \hat{\beta}_1 + \hat{\beta}_2 + \hat{\beta}_3 + \hat{\boldsymbol{\theta}}'\mathbf{z}$$
$$- (\hat{\beta}_0 + \hat{\beta}_2 + + \hat{\boldsymbol{\theta}}'\mathbf{z})$$
$$= \hat{\beta}_1 + \hat{\beta}_3.$$

Table 5.19 Estimated Odds Ratios and 95% Confidence Intervals for History of Mother Fracture and Needs Arms to Rise from a Chair in the GLOW Study, $n = 1000$

Variable	Subgroup	Odds Ratio	95% CI
History of mother having had a fracture	Does not need arms to rise	3.50	1.61, 7.51
	Does need arms to rise	0.97	0.38, 2.49
Need arms to rise from a chair	Mother does not have a history of fracture	1.90	1.16, 3.12
	Mother does have a history of fracture	0.53	0.17, 1.64

Step 4. Exponentiate the value of the simplified expression in Step 3, yielding

$$\widehat{OR}(MOMFRAC = 1, MOMFRAC = 0 \mid ARMASSIST = 1) = e^{\hat{\beta}_1 + \hat{\beta}_3}.$$

Now the expression involves two estimated coefficients. Using the estimates in Table 5.17 the estimate of the odds ratio is

$$\widehat{OR}(MOMFRAC = 1, MOMFRAC = 0 \mid ARMASSIST = 1) = e^{1.247 - 1.281}$$
$$= 0.97.$$

The estimator of the standard error of the sum of the two coefficients is

$$\widehat{SE}(\hat{\beta}_1 + \hat{\beta}_3) = [\widehat{Var}(\hat{\beta}_1) + \widehat{Var}(\hat{\beta}_3) + 2\widehat{Cov}(\hat{\beta}_1, \hat{\beta}_3)]^{0.5}.$$

Values of the estimated variances and the covariance term may be easily obtained from all packages and are: $\widehat{Var}(\hat{\beta}_1) = 0.1544$, $\widehat{Var}(\hat{\beta}_3) = 0.3881$, $\widehat{Cov}(\hat{\beta}_1, \hat{\beta}_3) = -0.1549$ and thus, the estimated standard error is $\widehat{SE}(\hat{\beta}_1 + \hat{\beta}_3) = 0.4824$. The endpoints of the 95% confidence interval for the estimator of the odds ratio are

$$\exp(-0.034 \pm 1.96 \times 0.4824) = (0.38, 2.49)$$

and are given in Table 5.19.

The calculations for the estimates and for the odds ratios for need arms for the two levels of mother fracture history are identical to those shown in detail for mother fracture history, just substitute $\hat{\beta}_2$ for $\hat{\beta}_1$ in the above expressions. As such, we do not present the details and present the results in the last two rows of Table 5.19.

The results in Table 5.19 show that both mother's history and needing arms to rise from a chair increase the odds of fracture significantly in the absence of the other factor, with the odds ratio for mother's history being slightly less than twice that for needing arms to rise (i.e., 3.5 vs. 1.9). In the presence of the other factor the odds ratios for mother's history and needing arms are no longer significant.

The remaining two variables to estimate odds ratios for are age (AGE) and history of a fracture (PRIORFRAC). We used a model containing just these two covariates in Section 3.5 as an example of estimating odds ratios in the presence of interaction. We refer the reader to that section for the relevant expressions that result from applying the four step procedure. The difference between what we are doing here and what we did in Section 3.5 is that here we use estimates based on the model in Table 5.17. A graph illustrating the odds ratio of prior fracture as a function of age was given in Figure 3.5. In Figure 5.18 we present a comparable result basing all calculations on the multivariable model in Table 5.17. Tabulated results similar to those in Table 3.13 are also easily calculated using the expressions in Section 3.5, but are not shown here.

The results in Figure 5.18 show that history of a prior fracture is increasingly important to the odds of a current fracture the younger the woman is. The effect

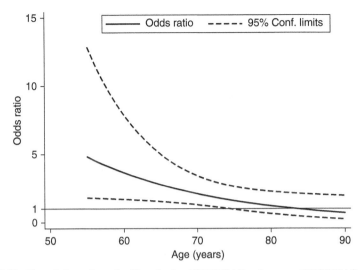

Figure 5.18 Plot of the estimated odds ratio for *PRIORFRAC* = 1 versus *PRIORFRAC* = 0 as a function of age, with 95% confidence bands.

Table 5.20 **Estimated Odds Ratios and 95% CI for Ten Year Positive Difference in Age for Two Subgroups of Women: Those Without and Those With a History of a Prior Fracture in the GLOW Study, *n* = 1000**

Variable	Subgroup	Odds Ratio	95% CI
Age	No history of prior fracture	3.47	1.13, 1.57
	With history of prior fracture	1.01	0.82, 1.23

of history of prior fracture becomes not significant after about age 75, as this is where the $\widehat{OR} = 1$ line becomes contained in the confidence interval.

The estimated odds ratios for a 10 year increase in age among women without and with a history of fracture are given in Table 5.20. Among women without a history of fracture a 10 year difference in age increases the odds of fracture by almost 3.5 times, while there is effectively no increase among those with a history. The conclusion is that history may be more important than age as a risk factor for fracture.

Since the main purpose of the GLOW Study is to assess risk factors for fracture as opposed to estimating the probability of fracture we do not present graphs or plots of estimated probabilities.

The goal of the Burn Injury Study is primarily, to develop a model to estimate the probability of death following admission to a burn treatment center. Estimation of effects of risk factors is of secondary importance. However, since the model contains two nonlinearly scaled covariates it provides the opportunity to illustrate how to estimate odds ratios in this situation. For convenience, we show the fitted model in Table 5.21.

Table 5.21   New Final Model for the Burn Injury Data, $n = 1000$

	Coeff.	Std. Err.	z	p	95% CI
AGEFP1	0.087	0.0082	10.52	<0.001	0.071, 0.103
TBSAFP1	0.936	0.0874	10.71	<0.001	0.765, 1.108
RACE	−0.609	0.3096	−1.97	0.049	−1.216, −0.002
INH_INJ	1.433	0.3422	4.19	<0.001	0.763, 2.104
Constant	−7.957	0.5967	−13.34	<0.001	−9.127, −6.788

Table 5.22   Estimated Odds Ratios and 95% Confidence Intervals for Nonwhite Race and Inhalation Injury Involved in the Burn

Variable	Odds Ratio	95% CI
Race	0.544	0.30, 1.00
Inhalation Injury	4.119	2.14, 8.20

Estimating the odds ratios for the dichotomous covariates race (RACE; $0 =$ White, $1 =$ Nonwhite) and inhalation injury (INH_INJ; $0 =$ No, $1 =$ Yes) should be routine for most readers by this point, so we only present the results in Table 5.22.

The results in Table 5.22 are in the abbreviated form where the reference and exposed categories have either been stated earlier, are assumed known, or are clear from the definition of the variable. We see that there is an estimated 46% reduction in the odds of death among whites compared to nonwhites, while involvement of an inhalation injury results in an estimated 4.1-fold increase in the odds of death. Since the Wald test p-value for RACE in Table 5.21 is 0.049 it is not surprising that, to two decimal places, the null value of one is contained in the confidence interval. The lower endpoint suggests that the decrease could be as much as 70% with 95% confidence. The increase in the odds of death for inhalation injury involvement could be as little as 2.1-fold or as much as 8.2-fold with 95% confidence.

Age and total burn surface area are continuous and each is modeled with a one term fractional polynomial transformation in the logit. For both of these covariates subject matter scientists are likely to be more interested in an overall description of the effect as opposed to accurate estimates of the effect of an increase in the covariate from a specific covariate value. Hence we choose to provide a graph with 95 percent confidence bands for positive differences of 10 years of age and 10% in the total burn area. The algebra required to obtain the appropriate expressions is identical for the two covariates, so we provide the details only for age. Each is obtained by applying the four step method.

Denote the equation for the four covariate model in Table 5.21 as

$$\hat{g}(\mathbf{x}, \hat{\boldsymbol{\beta}}) = \hat{\beta}_0 + \hat{\beta}_1 AGEFP1 + \hat{\beta}_2 TBSAFP1 + \hat{\beta}_3 RACE + \hat{\beta}_4 INH\_INJ.$$

The details of the four step method are:

Step 1: The two covariate values are $AGE = a$ and $AGE = a + 10$, holding the values of the other three covariates constant.

Step 2: Substitute the values into the equation for the logit:

$$\hat{g}(a, \hat{\beta}) = \hat{\beta}_0 + \hat{\beta}_1 \times \left(\frac{a}{10}\right)^2 + \hat{\beta}_2 TBSAFP1 + \hat{\beta}_3 RACE + \hat{\beta}_4 INH\_INJ$$

and

$$\hat{g}(a + 10, \hat{\beta}) = \hat{\beta}_0 + \hat{\beta}_1 \times \left(\frac{a + 10}{10}\right)^2 + \hat{\beta}_2 TBSAFP1$$
$$+ \hat{\beta}_3 RACE + \hat{\beta}_4 INH\_INJ.$$

Step 3: Take the difference in the two logits and simplify:

$$\hat{g}(a + 10, \hat{\beta}) - \hat{g}(a, \hat{\beta})$$

$$= \left\{ \hat{\beta}_0 + \hat{\beta}_1 \times \left(\frac{a + 10}{10}\right)^2 + \hat{\beta}_2 TBSAFP1 + \hat{\beta}_3 RACE + \hat{\beta}_4 INH\_INJ \right\}$$

$$- \left\{ \hat{\beta}_0 + \hat{\beta}_1 \times \left(\frac{a}{10}\right)^2 + \hat{\beta}_2 TBSAFP1 + \hat{\beta}_3 RACE + \hat{\beta}_4 INH\_INJ \right\}$$

$$= \hat{\beta}_1 \times \left[\left(\frac{a + 10}{10}\right)^2 - \left(\frac{a}{10}\right)^2 \right]$$

$$= \hat{\beta}_1 \times (0.2a + 1).$$

Step 4: Exponentiate the simplified difference from Step 3:

$$\widehat{OR}(a + 10, a) = \exp[\hat{\beta}_1 \times (0.2a + 1)].$$

Since we wish to graph the estimated odds ratio we would compute this expression for each value of age in the Burn Study. The endpoints of the 95% confidence interval for a change of 10 years of age at $AGE = a$ are

$$\widehat{OR}(a + 10, a) = \exp\{\hat{\beta}_1 \times (0.2a + 1) \pm 1.96 \times \widehat{SE}(\hat{\beta}_1 \times (0.2a + 1))\},$$

where

$$\widehat{SE}(\hat{\beta}_1 \times (0.2a + 1)) = \widehat{SE}(\hat{\beta}_1) \times (0.2a + 1).$$

The plot of the estimated odds ratio for a difference of 10 years of age and the 95% confidence bands is shown in Figure 5.19.

The plot in Figure 5.19 shows that the odds increase significantly, since the value 1.0 is always below the lower confidence bound, for a 10-year increase in age at all ages. The increase in the odds is less than twofold for subjects younger

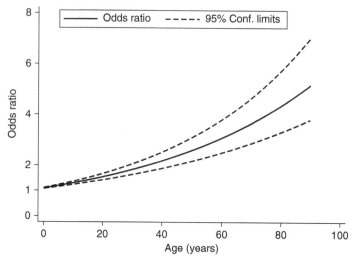

Figure 5.19 Plot of the estimated odds ratio for a 10 year difference in age at the plotted value of age with 95% confidence bands.

than 35 years and increases rapidly after age 35, reaching a maximum of about a five-fold increase for subjects in their 80s.

The calculations for a 10% increase in the size of the burn area are identical to those shown for age, but using $TBSAFP1 = \sqrt{TBSA}$. If we denote the reference burn area size as b then the equation to compute the estimated odds ratio is

$$\widehat{OR}(b + 10, b) = \exp[\hat{\beta}_2 \times (\sqrt{TBSA + 10} - \sqrt{TBSA})]$$

and the equation for the standard error to compute the confidence bands is

$$\widehat{SE}(\hat{\beta}_2 \times (\sqrt{TBSA + 10} - \sqrt{TBSA})) = \widehat{SE}(\hat{\beta}_2) \times (\sqrt{TBSA + 10} - \sqrt{TBSA}).$$

The plot of the estimated odds ratio and confidence bands is shown in Figure 5.20. At first glance one might think that something is incorrect as the odds ratio approaches one as burn size increases. However, what we are estimating is the odds ratio for a 10% larger burn. What the plot shows is that increasing the burn size increases the odds of death, but the multiplicative increase in the odds decreases with size of the burn. The plot essentially shows that once a burn reaches a certain size, increasing a bit more does not greatly increase the odds of dying.

Since an important objective of the modeling of the Burn Study data is to obtain a model to estimate the probability of death, it is natural to display some plots of the model. Here we present two figures with each containing four plots. The four lines in each plot correspond to the four possible levels of race and inhalation injury involvement. In Figure 5.21 we plot over age setting total burn surface area at its median value of 6%. The equations defining the logit functions and estimated

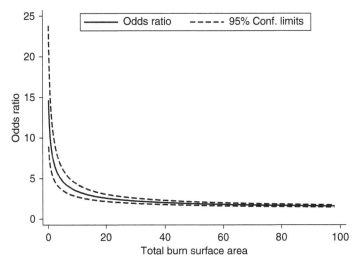

Figure 5.20 Plot of the estimated odds ratio for a 10% increase in the size of the burn area at the plotted value of burn area with 95% confidence bands.

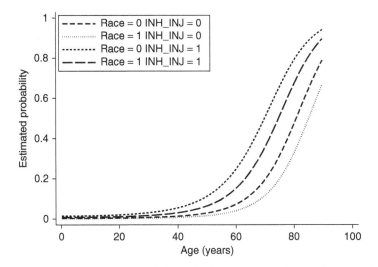

Figure 5.21 Plot of the estimated probability of dying versus age at burn surface area of 6%.

probabilities based on the values of the estimated coefficients in Table 5.21 are

$$\hat{g}(AGE)_{ij} = -7.957 + 0.87 \times AGEFP1 + 0.936 \times \sqrt{6} - 0.069 \times i + 1.433 \times j$$

and

$$\hat{\pi}(AGE)_{ij} = \frac{\exp[\hat{g}(AGE)_{ij}]}{1 + \exp[\hat{g}(AGE)_{ij}]}$$

where $AGEFP1 = (AGE/10)^2$, $i = 0, 1$, and $j = 0, 1$.

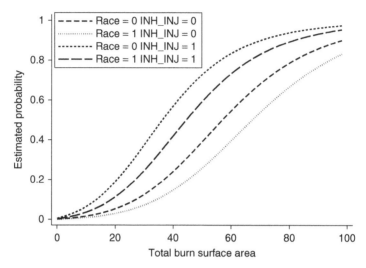

Figure 5.22 Plot of the estimated probability of dying versus total burn surface area at age 32 years.

In Figure 5.22 we plot over total burn surface area setting age at its median value of 32 years. The equations for the logit and estimated probabilities are similar to those shown and plotted in Figure 5.21. Since each line plotted in both Figures 5.21 and 5.22 is a known function of the four covariates we could easily calculate the 95% confidence bands, but chose not to do so as inclusion of these would hopelessly clutter the figures.

The lower two lines in Figure 5.21 correspond to whites and nonwhites with no inhalation injury. The upper two are for the same racial groups, but with an inhalation injury. We see that, at the median burn size (6%), it is not until age 65 that any of the estimated probabilities exceed 0.5, but the four lines rise rapidly after age 50. Similar lines could be calculated or even tabulated for other values of total burn surface area. The effect of a larger area would be to move all four curves higher up in the figure, but retaining the same basic shape plotted over age.

As in Figure 5.21, the lower two lines in Figure 5.22 correspond to whites and nonwhites with no inhalation injury. The upper two are for the same racial groups, but with an inhalation injury. We see the rather dramatic effect of increasing burn size as all four lines rise rapidly after about 10%. Again, similar lines could be calculated or even tabulated for other values of age with the effect that increasing age would move all four curves higher up in the figure, but retaining the same basic shape plotted over total burn surface area.

The plots used in Figures 5.21 and 5.22 to describe the estimated probability of death following a burn injury should be viewed as just two examples. In any setting, the choice of plots should be dictated by what would be most informative to the subject matter scientists.

Before concluding this Chapter we end with a few comments on model building. Comparatively speaking the models we developed for the GLOW and Burn Study data may be a bit more complicated than some logistic regression models we have encountered in the health sciences literature. The typical model in the literature has a few continuous covariates modeled linearly, a few design variables, and in rare instances, an interaction. There seems to be some reluctance on the part of subject matter scientists to consider more complicated models. We think that the reason is a lack of confidence in being able to determine when more complicated non-linear terms are needed, and if they are included, insecurity on how to interpret the results. What we hope to have accomplished in Chapters 4 and 5 is to provide a set of methods that can serve as a basic paradigm for model building, model evaluation, and model presentation that will allow the reader to feel confident that he/she has developed the best possible model within the constraints of the data, and to feel secure in his/her ability to present and interpret the results of the model, regardless of how complicated it may appear to be. In particular, we hope that through the discussion in this section the reader has developed a firm grasp of the fundamental principal that the estimate of an odds ratio comes from exponentiating a logit difference.

EXERCISES

1. Evaluate the goodness of fit for the Burn Study model in Table 4.27 using the standardized sum-of-squares statistic.

2. Using the diagnostic statistics verify that the significance of the interaction term in the fitted model for the Burn Study in Table 4.27 is due to only three covariate patterns.

3. Perform a full evaluation of model assessment for the smaller Burn Study Model in Table 5.12. This should include all goodness of fit tests, diagnostic statistics and an ROC analysis.

4. As is the case in linear regression, effective use of diagnostic statistics depends on our ability to interpret and understand the values of the statistics. The purpose of this problem is to provide a few structured examples to examine the effect on the fitted logistic regression model and diagnostic statistics when data are moved away from the model (i.e., poorer fit), and also toward the model (i.e., better fit). Table 5.23 lists values of the independent variable x, and seven different columns of the outcome variable y, labeled "Model". All models fit in this problem use the given values of x for the covariate. Different models are fit using the seven different columns for the outcome variable. The data for the column labeled "Model 0" are constructed to represent a "typical" realization when the logistic regression model is correct. In the columns labeled " Model 1" to "Model 3" we have changed some of the y values away from the original model. Namely some cases with small values of x have had y changed from 0 to 1 and others with large values of x have had the y values changed from 1 to 0. For models labeled "Model −1" and "Model −2" we have

Table 5.23 Hypothetical Data to Illustrate the Use of Diagnostic Statistics to Detect Poorly Fit and Influential Subjects and Complete Separation

				Model			
x	$-i$	-2	-1	0	1	2	3
-5.65	0	0	0	0	0	0	0
-4.75	0	0	0	0	0	1	1
-3.89	0	0	0	0	0	0	0
-3.12	0	0	0	0	0	0	0
-2.93	0	0	0	0	0	0	0
-2.87	0	0	0	0	0	0	0
-1.85	0	0	0	0	1	1	1
-1.25	0	1	1	1	1	1	1
-0.97	0	0	0	0	0	0	0
-0.19	1	1	1	1	1	1	1
-0.15	1	1	1	1	1	1	1
0.69	1	1	1	1	1	1	1
1.07	1	1	1	1	1	1	1
1.18	1	1	1	1	1	1	1
1.45	1	1	0	0	0	0	0
2.33	1	1	1	0	0	0	0
3.57	1	1	1	1	1	1	1
4.41	1	1	1	1	1	1	1
4.57	1	1	1	1	1	1	0
5.85	1	1	1	1	1	1	1

moved the y values in the direction of the model. That is, we have changed y from 1 to 0 for some small values of x and have changed y from 0 to 1 for some large values of x. Fit the six logistic regression models for the data in columns "Model -2" to "Model 3". Compute for each fitted model the values of the leverage, h, the change in chi-square, ΔX^2, and the influence diagnostic, $\Delta \hat{b}$. Plot each of these versus the fitted values, predicted logistic probabilities. Compare the plots over the various models. Do the statistics pick out poorly fit and influential cases? How do the estimated coefficients change relative to Model 0? Fit "Model $-i$". What happens and why? Refer to the discussion in Section 4.5 on complete separation.

5. When we built the model for the Burn Study data in Chapter 4 we used the one-term fractional transformation for age, $AGEFP1 = (AGE/10)^2$. One could argue, and we often do, that the lower order term, AGE, should also be included in the model. Perform a full model assessment of the model that adds AGE to the model in Table 4.27. That is, keep all the other terms and just add age. Which model, with or without age, would you prefer to present to a panel of burn surgeons.

6. Based on the analysis in exercise 5 is there evidence that the interaction is due to the same three covariate patterns? Would you recommend a model that excludes the interaction? If so, evaluate its fit.

7. Present and interpret the results of the final model for the Burn Study that includes AGE and AGEFP1.

CHAPTER 6

Application of Logistic Regression with Different Sampling Models

6.1 INTRODUCTION

Up to this point we have assumed that our data have come from a simple random sample. Considerable progress has been made in recent years to extend the use of the logistic regression model to other types of sampling. In this chapter we begin with a review of the classic cohort study. Next we consider the case-control study and the stratified case-control study. We conclude with a section that deals with fitting models when data come from a complex sample survey. The goals are to briefly describe some of the mathematics involved in fitting the model, to indicate how the model can be fit using available software and to discuss the interpretation of the estimated parameters. References to the literature for more detailed treatment of these topics are provided.

Throughout this chapter we assume that the outcome variable is dichotomous, coded as 0 or 1, and that its conditional probability given a vector of covariates is the logistic regression model. In addition, we assume that the number of covariate patterns is equal to the sample size. Modifications to allow for replication at covariate patterns are a notational detail, not a conceptual problem.

6.2 COHORT STUDIES

Several variations of the cohort (or prospective) study are in common use. In the simplest design, a simple random sample of subjects is chosen and the values of the covariates are determined. These subjects are then followed for a fixed period of time and the outcome variable is measured. This type of sample is identical to what is often referred to as the *regression sampling model*, in which we assume that

Applied Logistic Regression, Third Edition.
David W. Hosmer, Jr., Stanley Lemeshow, and Rodney X. Sturdivant.
© 2013 John Wiley & Sons, Inc. Published 2013 by John Wiley & Sons, Inc.

the values of the covariates are fixed and measured without error and the outcome is measured conditionally on the observed values of the covariates. Under these assumptions and independence of the observations, the likelihood function for a sample of size n is simply

$$l_1(\boldsymbol{\beta}) = \prod_{i=1}^{n} \Pr(Y_i = y_i | \mathbf{x}_i). \tag{6.1}$$

When the observed values of y and the logistic regression model are substituted into the expression for the conditional probability, $l_1(\boldsymbol{\beta})$ simplifies to the likelihood function in equation (1.3).

A modification of this situation is a randomized trial where subjects are first chosen via a simple random sample and then allocated independently and with known probabilities into "treatment" groups. Subjects are followed over time and the outcome variable is measured for each subject. If the responses are such that a normal errors model is appropriate we would be naturally led to consider a normal theory analysis of covariance model which would contain appropriate design variables for treatment, relevant covariates, and any interactions between treatment and covariates deemed necessary. The extension of the likelihood function in equation (6.1) to incorporate treatment and covariate information when the outcome is dichotomous is obtained by including these variables in the logistic regression model.

Another modification is for the design to incorporate a stratification variable such as location or clinic. In this situation the likelihood function is the product of the stratum-specific likelihood functions, each of which is similar in form to $l_1(\boldsymbol{\beta})$. We would perhaps add terms to the model to account for stratum-specific responses. These might include a design variable for stratum and interactions between this design variable and other covariates.

In each of these designs we use the likelihood function $l_1(\boldsymbol{\beta})$ as a basis for determining the maximum likelihood estimates of the unknown parameters in the vector $\boldsymbol{\beta}$. Tests and confidence intervals for the parameters follow from well-developed theory for maximum likelihood estimation [see Cox and Hinkley (1974)]. The estimated parameters may be used in the logistic regression model to estimate the conditional probability of response for each subject. The fact that the estimated logistic probability provides a model-based estimate of the probability of response permits the development of methods for assessment of goodness of fit such as those discussed in Chapter 5. Chambless and Boyle (1985) extend $l_1(\boldsymbol{\beta})$ to the setting where the data come from a stratified simple random sample.

In some prospective studies the outcome variable of interest is the time to the occurrence of some event. In these studies the time to event nowadays is most often modeled using the proportional hazards model or another regression model [see Hosmer et al. (2008)]. In these situations a method of analysis that is sometimes used is to ignore the actual failure time and model the occurrence or nonoccurrence of the event via logistic regression. This method of analysis was popular before easily used software became available in the major software packages to model time-to-event data. However, now such software is just as available and just as easy to use, and as such we see no need to use logistic regression analysis to model time to event data.

6.3   CASE-CONTROL STUDIES

One of the major reasons the logistic regression model has seen such wide use, especially in epidemiologic research, is the ease of obtaining adjusted odds ratios from the estimated slope coefficients when sampling is performed conditional on the outcome variables, as in a case-control study. Breslow (1996) has written an excellent review paper. Besides tracing the development of the case-control study he describes the statistical issues and controversies surrounding some famous studies such as the first Surgeon General's report on smoking and health [Surgeon General (1964)]. He presents some of the newer innovative applications involving nesting and matching as well as some of the current limitations of this study design. We encourage any reader not familiar with this powerful and frequently employed study design to read this paper. We only consider the use of logistic regression in the simplest case-control designs in this section. More advanced applications may be found in Breslow (1996) and cited references.

As noted by Breslow (1996), Cornfield (1951) is generally given credit for first observing that the odds ratio is invariant under study design (cohort or case-control). However, it was not until the work of Farewell (1979) and Prentice and Pyke (1979) that the mathematical details justifying the common practice of analyzing case-control data as if they were cohort data were worked out.

In contrast to cohort studies, the binary outcome variable in a case-control study is fixed by stratification. The dependent variables in this setting are one or more primary covariates, exposure variables in $\mathbf{x}$. In this type of study design, samples of fixed size are chosen from the two strata defined by the outcome variable. The values of the primary exposure variables and the relevant covariates are then measured for each subject selected. The covariates are assumed to include all relevant exposure, confounding, and interaction terms. The likelihood function is the product of the stratum-specific likelihood functions and depends on the probability that the subject was selected for the sample, and the probability distribution of the covariates.

It is not difficult algebraically to manipulate the case-control likelihood function to obtain a logistic regression model in which the dependent variable is the outcome variable of interest to the investigator. The key steps in this development are two applications of Bayes' theorem. As the likelihood function is based on subjects selected, we need to define a variable that records the selection status for each subject in the population. Let the variable s denote the selection ($s = 1$) or nonselection ($s = 0$) of a subject. The full likelihood for a sample of size n_1 cases ($y = 1$) and n_0 controls ($y = 0$) is

$$\prod_{i=1}^{n_1} \Pr(\mathbf{x}_i | y_i = 1, s_i = 1) \prod_{i=1}^{n_0} \Pr(\mathbf{x}_i | y_i = 0, s_i = 1). \tag{6.2}$$

For an individual term in the likelihood function shown in equation (6.2) the first application of Bayes' theorem yields

$$\Pr(\mathbf{x}|y, s = 1) = \frac{\Pr(y|\mathbf{x}, s = 1) \, \Pr(\mathbf{x}|s = 1)}{\Pr(y|s = 1)}. \tag{6.3}$$

The second application of Bayes' theorem is to the first term in the numerator of equation (6.3). This yields, when $y = 1$,

$$\Pr(y = 1|\mathbf{x}, s = 1)$$

$$= \frac{\Pr(y = 1|\mathbf{x}) \, \Pr(s = 1|\mathbf{x}, y = 1)}{\Pr(y = 0|\mathbf{x}) \, \Pr(s = 1|\mathbf{x}, y = 0) + \Pr(y = 1|\mathbf{x}) \, \Pr(s = 1|\mathbf{x}, y = 1)}. \tag{6.4}$$

Assume that the selection of cases and controls is independent of the covariates with respective probabilities τ_1 and τ_0; then

$$\tau_1 = \Pr(s = 1|y = 1, \mathbf{x}) = \Pr(s = 1|y = 1),$$

and

$$\tau_0 = \Pr(s = 1|y = 0, \mathbf{x}) = \Pr(s = 1|y = 0).$$

Substitution of τ_1, τ_0 and the logistic regression model, $\pi(\mathbf{x})$, for $\Pr(y = 1|\mathbf{x})$, into equation (6.4) yields

$$\Pr(y = 1|\mathbf{x}, s = 1) = \frac{\tau_1 \pi(\mathbf{x})}{\tau_0[1 - \pi(\mathbf{x})] + \tau_1 \pi(\mathbf{x})}. \tag{6.5}$$

If we divide the numerator and denominator of the expression on the right-hand side of equation (6.5) by $\tau_0[1 - \pi(\mathbf{x})]$, the result is a logistic regression model with intercept term $\beta_0^* = \ln(\tau_1/\tau_0) + \beta_0$. To simplify the notation, let $\pi^*(\mathbf{x})$ denote the right-hand side of equation (6.5). As we assume that sampling is carried out independent of covariate values, $\Pr(\mathbf{x}|s = 1) = \Pr(\mathbf{x})$, where $\Pr(\mathbf{x})$ denotes the probability distribution of the covariates. The general term in the likelihood shown in equation (6.3) then becomes, for $y = 1$,

$$\Pr(\mathbf{x}|y = 1, s = 1) = \frac{\pi^*(\mathbf{x}) \, \Pr(\mathbf{x})}{\Pr(y = 1|s = 1)}. \tag{6.6}$$

A similar term for $y = 0$ is obtained by replacing $\pi^*(\mathbf{x})$ by $[1 - \pi^*(\mathbf{x})]$ in the numerator and $\Pr(y = 1|s = 1)$ by $\Pr(y = 0|s = 1)$ in the denominator of equation (6.6). If we let

$$l^*(\boldsymbol{\beta}) = \prod_{i=1}^{n} \pi^*(\mathbf{x}_i)^{y_i} [1 - \pi^*(\mathbf{x}_i)]^{1-y_i},$$

the likelihood function shown in equation (6.2) becomes

$$l^*(\beta) \prod_{i=1}^{n} \left[\frac{\Pr(\mathbf{x}_i)}{\Pr(y_i|s_i = 1)} \right]. \tag{6.7}$$

The first term in equation (6.7), $l^*(\boldsymbol{\beta})$, is the likelihood obtained when we pretend the case-control data were collected in a cohort study, with the outcome of interest modeled as the dependent variable. If we assume that the probability distribution of $\mathbf{x}$, $\Pr(\mathbf{x})$, contains no information about the coefficients in the logistic regression model, then maximization of the full likelihood with respect to the parameters in the logistic model, $\pi^*(\mathbf{x})$, is only subject to the restriction that $\Pr(y_i = 1 | s_i = 1) = n_1/n$ and $\Pr(y_i = 0 | s_i = 1) = n_0/n$. The likelihood equation obtained by differentiating with respect to the parameter β_0^* assures that this condition is satisfied. Thus, maximization of the full likelihood with respect to the parameters in $\pi^*(\mathbf{x})$ need only consider that portion of the likelihood which looks like a cohort study. The implication of this is that *analysis of data from case-control studies via logistic regression may proceed in the same way and using the same computer programs as cohort studies.* Nevertheless, inferences about the intercept parameter β_0 are not possible without knowledge of the sampling fractions within cases and controls, τ_0 and τ_1.

The assumption that the marginal distribution of $\mathbf{x}$ contains no information about the parameters in the logistic regression model requires additional discussion, as it is not true in one historically important situation, the normal theory discriminant function model. This model was discussed briefly in Chapters 1 and 2. When the assumptions for the normal discriminant function model hold, the maximum likelihood estimators of the coefficients for the logistic regression model obtained from conditional likelihoods such as those in equations (6.2) and (6.7) are less efficient than the discriminant function estimator shown in equation (2.11) [see Efron (1975)]. However, the assumptions for the normal theory discriminant function model are rarely, if ever, attained in practice. Application of the normal discriminant function when its assumptions do not hold may result in substantial bias, especially when some of the covariates are dichotomous variables. As a general rule, estimation should be based on equations (6.2) and (6.7), unless there is considerable evidence in favor of the normal theory discriminant function model.

Prentice and Pyke (1979) have shown that the maximum likelihood estimators obtained by pretending that the case-control data resulted from a cohort sample have the usual properties associated with maximum likelihood estimators. Specifically, they are asymptotically normally distributed, with covariance matrix obtained from the inverse of the information matrix. Thus, percentiles from the $N(0, 1)$ distribution may be used in conjunction with estimated standard errors produced from standard logistic regression software to form Wald statistics and confidence interval estimates. The theory of likelihood ratio tests may be employed to compare models via the difference in the deviance of the two models, assuming of course that the models are nested. Scott and Wild (1991) have shown that inferences based on this approach are sensitive to incorrect specifications of the logit function. They show that failure to include necessary higher order terms in the logit produces a model with estimated standard errors that are too small. These results are special cases of more general results obtained by White (1982).

Modification of the likelihood function to incorporate additional levels of stratification beyond case-control status follows in the same manner as described for cohort data (i.e., inclusion of relevant design variables and interaction terms). Thus, model building and inferences from fitted models for case-control data may proceed using the methods developed for cohort data, as described in Chapters 4 and 5. However, this approach is not valid for matched or highly stratified data. Appropriate methods for the analysis of the latter are presented in detail in Chapter 7.

Fears and Brown (1986) proposed a method for the analysis of stratified case-control data that arise from a two-stage sample. Breslow and Cain (1988) and Scott and Wild (1991) provide further discussion and refinement of the method. This approach requires that we know the sampling rates for the first stage and the total number of subjects in each stratum. This information is used to define the relative sampling rates for cases and controls within each stratum. The ratio of these is included in the model in the form of an additional known constant added to the stratum-specific logit. Specifically, suppose we let n_j be the total number of subjects with $y = j$ observed out of a possible N_j and let the kth stratum-specific quantities be n_{jk} and N_{jk}, $j = 0, 1$, and $k = 1, 2, \ldots, K$. The relative stratum-specific sampling rates are $w_{1k} = (n_{1k}/N_{1k})/(n_1/N_1)$ and $w_{0k} = (n_{0k}/N_{0k})/(n_0/N_0)$. The Fears and Brown model uses stratum-specific logits of

$$g_k(\mathbf{x}) = \ln \left(\frac{w_{1k}}{w_{0k}} \right) + \beta_0 + \boldsymbol{\beta}'\mathbf{x},$$

$k = 1, 2, \ldots, K$. This model may be handled with standard logistic regression software by defining a new variable, typically referred to as an offset, which takes on the value $\ln(w_{1k}/w_{0k})$ and forcing it into the model with a coefficient equal to 1.0.

Breslow and Cain (1988) show that the estimator proposed by Brown and Fears is asymptotically normally distributed and derive an estimator of the covariance matrix. Breslow and Zhao (1988) and Scott and Wild (1991) point out that the estimated standard errors produced when standard logistic regression software is used to implement the Brown and Fears method overestimate the true standard errors. They provide expressions for a covariance matrix that yields consistent estimates of the variances and covariances of the estimated regression coefficients. The matrix is complicated to compute, as it requires a special purpose program or a high degree of skill in using a package allowing matrix calculations such as SAS, STATA, or R [R Development Core Team (2010)]. For these reasons we do not present the variance estimator in detail. We note that Breslow and Zhao use a slightly different offset, $\ln[(n_{1k}/N_{1k})/(n_{0k}/N_{0k})]$, which yields the same estimates of the regression coefficients but a different intercept.

Before leaving our discussion of logistic regression in the case-control setting, we briefly consider the application of the chi-square goodness of fit tests for the logistic regression model presented in Section 5.2. The essential feature of these tests is that for a particular covariate pattern, the number of subjects with the response of interest among m sampled is distributed binomially with parameters m and response probability given by the hypothesized logistic regression model. Recall that for cohort data, the likelihood function was parameterized directly in terms of the logistic probability. For case-control data, the function $\pi^*(\mathbf{x})$ is the probability $P(y = 1|\mathbf{x}, s = 1)$. For a particular covariate pattern, conditioning on the number of subjects m observed to have a given covariate pattern is equivalent to conditioning on the event, $(\mathbf{x}, s = 1)$. Thus, for case-control studies in which the logistic regression model assumption is correct, the conditional distribution of the number of subjects responding among the m observed to have a particular covariate pattern is binomial with parameters m and $\pi^*(\mathbf{x})$. Hence, the results developed in Chapter 5 based on m-asymptotics also apply. Nagelkerke et al. (2005) propose a test based on the effect on the estimated coefficients of weighting the observed outcomes. This test is focused specifically on model misspecification in the covariates and thus has, in simulations, higher power than the decile of risk test discussed in Chapter 5 when this is the source of lack of fit. The test is modestly complicated to calculate and as yet has not found its way into software packages. As such, we do not consider it further.

It is often the case that data from case-control studies do not arise from simple random samples within each stratum. For example, the design may call for the inclusion of all subjects with $y = 1$ and a sample of subjects with $y = 0$. For these designs there is an obvious dependency among the observations. If this dependency is not too great, or if we appeal to a super-population model [see Prentice (1986)], then employing a theory that ignores it should not bias the results significantly.

6.4 FITTING LOGISTIC REGRESSION MODELS TO DATA FROM COMPLEX SAMPLE SURVEYS

Some of the more recent improvements in logistic regression statistical software include routines to perform analyses with data obtained from complex sample surveys. These routines may be found in STATA, SAS, SUDAAN [Shah et al. (2002)], and other less well-known special-purpose packages. Our goal in this section is to provide a brief introduction to these methods and to illustrate them with an example data set. The reader who needs more detail is encouraged to see Korn and Graubard (1990), Roberts et al. (1987), Skinner et al. (1989), and Thomas and Rao (1987).

The essential idea, as discussed in Roberts et al. (1987), is to set up a function that approximates the likelihood function in the finite sampled population with a likelihood function formed from the observed sample and known sampling weights. Suppose we assume that the population may be broken into $k = 1, 2, \ldots, K$ strata, $j = 1, 2, \ldots, M_k$ primary sampling units in each stratum and $i = 1, 2, \ldots, N_{kj}$ elements in the kj^{th} primary sampling unit. Suppose our observed data consist of n_{kj} elements from m_k primary sampling units from stratum k. Denote the total number of observations as $n = \sum_{k=1}^{K} \sum_{j=1}^{m_k} n_{kj}$. Denote the known sampling weight for the kji^{th} observation as w_{kji}, the vector of covariates as $\mathbf{x}_{kji}$ and the dichotomous outcome as y_{kji}. The approximate log-likelihood function is

$$\sum_{k=1}^{K} \sum_{j=1}^{m_k} \sum_{i=1}^{n_{kj}} [w_{kji} \times y_{kji}] \times \ln[\pi(\mathbf{x}_{kji})] + [w_{kji} \times (1 - y_{kji})] \times \ln[1 - \pi(\mathbf{x}_{kji})].$$

$$(6.8)$$

Differentiating this equation with respect to the unknown regression coefficients yields the vector of $p + 1$ score equations

$$\mathbf{X}'\mathbf{W}(\mathbf{y} - \boldsymbol{\pi}) = \mathbf{0}, \tag{6.9}$$

where $\mathbf{X}$ is the $n \times (p + 1)$ matrix of covariate values, $\mathbf{W}$ is an $n \times n$ diagonal matrix containing the weights, $\mathbf{y}$ is the $n \times 1$ vector of observed outcomes, and $\boldsymbol{\pi} = [\pi(\mathbf{x}_{111}), \ldots, \pi(\mathbf{x}_{Km_K n_{Kj}})]'$ is the $n \times 1$ vector of logistic probabilities. In theory, any logistic regression package that allows weights could be used to obtain the solutions to equation (6.9). The problem comes in obtaining the correct estimator of the covariance matrix of the estimator of the coefficients. Naive use of a standard logistic regression package with weight matrix $\mathbf{W}$ would yield estimates on the matrix $(\mathbf{X}'\mathbf{D}\mathbf{X})^{-1}$ where $\mathbf{D} = \mathbf{W}\mathbf{V}$ is an $n \times n$ diagonal matrix with general element $w_{kji} \times \hat{\pi}(\mathbf{x}_{kji})[1 - \hat{\pi}(\mathbf{x}_{kji})]$. The correct estimator is

$$\widehat{\mathrm{Var}}(\hat{\boldsymbol{\beta}}) = (\mathbf{X}'\mathbf{D}\mathbf{X})^{-1}\mathbf{S}(\mathbf{X}'\mathbf{D}\mathbf{X})^{-1}, \tag{6.10}$$

where $\mathbf{S}$ is a pooled within-stratum estimator of the covariance matrix of the left-hand side of equation (6.9). Denote a general element in the vector in equation (6.9) as $\mathbf{z}'_{kji} = \mathbf{x}'_{kji} w_{kji}(y_{kji} - \pi(\mathbf{x}_{kji}))$, the sum over the n_{kj} sampled units in the jth primary sampling unit in the kth stratum as $\mathbf{z}_{kj} = \sum_{i=1}^{n_{kj}} \mathbf{z}_{kji}$ and their stratum-specific mean as $\bar{\mathbf{z}}_k = 1/m_k \sum_{j=1}^{m_k} \mathbf{z}_{kj}$. The within-stratum estimator for the kth stratum is

$$\mathbf{S}_k = \frac{m_k}{m_k - 1} \sum_{j=1}^{m_k} (\mathbf{z}_{kj} - \bar{\mathbf{z}}_k)(\mathbf{z}_{kj} - \bar{\mathbf{z}}_k)'.$$

The pooled estimator is $\mathbf{S} = \sum_{k=1}^{K} (1 - f_k)\mathbf{S}_k$. The quantity $(1 - f_k)$ is called the *finite population correction factor*, where $f_k = m_k/M_k$ is the ratio of the number of observed primary sampling units to the total number of primary sampling units in stratum k. In settings where M_k is unknown it is common practice to assume it is large enough that f_k is quite small and the correction factor is equal to 1.

The likelihood function in equation (6.8) is only an approximation to the true likelihood. Thus, inferences about model parameters should be based on univariable and multivariable Wald statistics rather than likelihood ratio tests. Wald tests are formed by comparing an estimated coefficient to an estimate of its standard error, or variance, computed from specific elements of equation (6.10) in the same manner as described in Chapter 2. However, simulations in Korn and Graubard (1990) as well as Thomas and Rao (1987) show that when data come from a complex sample survey from a finite population, use of a modified Wald statistic and the F distribution, described below, yield tests with better adherence to the stated alpha level. STATA and SUDAAN report results from these modified Wald tests. The problem is that none of the simulations referred to actually examines logistic regression models fit using continuous and categorical covariates with estimates obtained from equation (6.9) and variances from equation (6.10). Korn and Graubard appear to use a linear regression with normal errors model and refer to theoretical results in Anderson (1984) that depend on rather stringent assumptions of multivariate normality. Thomas and Rao examine models with a dichotomous or polychotomous outcome and a few categorical covariates. Another problem, in our opinion, is the fact that software packages, for example STATA, use the t distribution to assess significance of Wald statistics for individual coefficients. Given the paucity of appropriate simulations and theory we are not convinced that there is sufficient evidence to support the use of the modified Wald statistic with the F distribution with logistic regression models. One possible justification is that the use of the modified Wald statistic with the F distribution is conservative in that significance levels using this approach are, in general, larger than those obtained from treating the Wald statistics as being multivariate normal for sufficiently large samples (as is assumed in previous chapters). We present results based on both tests in the example.

The relationship between the Wald test and the modified Wald test is as follows. Let W denote the Wald statistic for testing that all p slope coefficients in a fitted model are equal to 0, that is

$$W = \hat{\boldsymbol{\beta}}'[\widehat{\text{Var}}(\hat{\boldsymbol{\beta}})_{p \times p}]^{-1}\hat{\boldsymbol{\beta}}, \tag{6.11}$$

where $\hat{\boldsymbol{\beta}}$ denotes the vector of p slope coefficients and $\widehat{\text{Var}}(\hat{\boldsymbol{\beta}})_{p \times p}$ is the $p \times p$ submatrix obtained from the full $(p + 1) \times (p + 1)$ matrix in equation (6.10). That is, one leaves out the row and column for the constant term. The p-value is computed using a chi-square distribution with p degrees of freedom as $\Pr[\chi^2(p) \geq W]$.

The adjusted Wald statistic is

$$F = \frac{(s - p + 1)}{sp} W, \tag{6.12}$$

where $s = \left(\sum_{k=1}^{K} m_k\right) - K$ is the total number of sampled primary sampling units minus the number of strata. The p-value is computed using an F distribution with p and $(s - p + 1)$ degrees of freedom as $\Pr[F(p, s - p + 1) \geq F]$.

For purposes of illustration we use selected variables (see Table 1.11) from the 2009–2010 cycle of the National Health and Nutrition Examination Study [NHANES III Reference Manuals and Reports (2012)]. We describe the data in Section 1.6.7. It should be noted that the NHANES, like just about any other large survey, suffers from the fact that complete data are not available for every subject. This problem is exacerbated in complex sample surveys because every subject carries along a unique statistical weight based on the number of individuals in the population he or she represents. Hence, if that subject is missing a measurement on just one of the variables involved in a multivariable problem, then that subject will be eliminated from the analysis and the sum of the statistical weights of the subjects remaining will not equal the size of the population for which inference is to be made.

Survey statisticians have studied this problem extensively. Solutions to it range from redistributing the statistical weights of the dropped subjects among the subjects remaining, to imputing every missing value so that the weights will be preserved. Another, perhaps simplistic, approach is simply to run the analyses with the subjects having complete data and assume that the relationships would not change had all subjects been used. Because it is our intention in this book to demonstrate the use of logistic regression analysis with complex survey data rather than to obtain precise population parameter estimates, we will follow this simple approach. (NHANES actually advocates this approach if the number of missing observations is small, less than 10%.)

For purposes of illustrating fitting logistic models to sample survey data in Section 6.4 we chose selected variables, see Table 1.11, from the 2009–2010 cycle of the NHANES III Reference Manuals and Reports (2012) and made some modifications to the data. This is a stratified multistage probability sample of the civilian noninstitutionalized population of the United States.

As an example we fit a logistic regression model to data from the 2009–2010 cycle of the National Health and Nutrition Examination Study [NHANES III Reference Manuals and Reports (2012)] described in Section 1.6.7. The model, shown in Table 6.1, contains age in decades (AGE10), diastolic blood pressure (DBP), gender (GENDER), walk or bike to work (WLKBIK), participates in vigorous recreational activities (VIGRECEXR), moderate work activity (MODWRK), and participates in moderate recreational activities (MODRECEXR). The 5858 subjects used in the analysis represent 204,203,191 individuals between 16 and 80 years of age living in the United States in 2009–2010.

We assessed the overall significance of the model via the multivariable Wald test and adjusted Wald test for the significance of the seven regression coefficients in the model. For the model in Table 6.1 the value of the Wald test in equation (6.11) is

$$W = \hat{\beta}'[\widehat{\text{Var}}(\hat{\beta})_{7 \times 7}]^{-1}\hat{\beta} = 179.0189,$$

where $\hat{\beta}$ is the vector of the seven estimated slope coefficients and $\widehat{\text{Var}}(\hat{\beta})_{7 \times 7}$ is the 7×7 sub-matrix computed using equation (6.10). The significance level of the test is $\Pr[\chi^2(7) \geq 179.0189] < 0.001$. The value of s for the adjusted Wald

Table 6.1 Estimated Coefficients, Standard Errors, z-Scores, Two-Tailed p-Values, and 95% Confidence Intervals for a Logistic Regression Model for the Modified NHANES Study with Dependent Variable OBESE, $n = 5858$

	Coeff.	Std. Err.	t	p	95% CI	
AGE10[a]	0.001	0.0258	0.05	0.962	−0.054,	0.056
DBP	0.019	0.0046	4.09	0.001	0.009,	0.029
GENDER	0.467	0.1240	3.76	0.002	0.202,	0.731
WLKBIK	0.489	0.0920	5.32	<0.001	0.293,	0.685
VIGRECEXR	0.801	0.1100	7.29	<0.001	0.567,	1.036
MODWRK	−0.027	0.0923	−0.29	0.773	−0.224,	0.170
MODECEXR	0.330	0.1721	1.92	0.074	−0.037,	0.697
Constant	−4.610	0.4237	−10.88	<0.001	−5.513,	−3.707

[a] $\text{AGE10} = \frac{\text{AGE}}{10}$.

test is $30 - 15 = 15$ and the adjusted Wald test from equation (6.12) is

$$F = \frac{(15 - 7 + 1)}{15 \times 7} \times 179.0189 = 15.3444,$$

and $p = \Pr[F(7, 9) \geq 15.3444] < 0.001$. Both tests indicate that at least one of the coefficients may be different from 0.

The results in Table 6.1 indicate, on the basis of the individual p-values for the Wald statistics, that age, moderate work activity and moderate recreation may not be significant at the 5% level. As age ranges from 16 to 80 and there is evidence that obesity is most prevalent in middle age we suspect that the logit may be nonlinear in age. Hence, for subject matter reasons we do not consider age for exclusion from the model at this time. As we noted, the function in equation (6.8) is not a true likelihood function. Thus, we cannot use the partial likelihood ratio test to compare a smaller model to a larger model. In this case we must test for the significance of the coefficients of excluded covariates using a multivariable Wald test based on the estimated coefficients and estimated covariance matrix from the 8×8 larger model.

Application of the Wald test to assess the significance of the coefficients for MODWRK and MODRECEXR from the model in Table 6.1 uses the vector of estimated coefficients

$$\hat{\boldsymbol{\beta}}' = (-0.027088, 0.329987),$$

and the 2×2 sub-matrix of estimated variances and covariances obtained from the full matrix (not shown) computed using equation (6.10)

$$\widehat{\text{Var}}(\hat{\boldsymbol{\beta}})_{2 \times 2} = \begin{bmatrix} 0.00852197 & -0.00873523 \\ -0.00873523 & 0.02962245 \end{bmatrix}.$$

The Wald test statistic is

$$W = \hat{\boldsymbol{\beta}}'[\widehat{\text{Var}}(\hat{\boldsymbol{\beta}})_{2 \times 2}]^{-1}\hat{\boldsymbol{\beta}} = 4.5052,$$

with a p-value obtained as $P[\chi^2(2) \geq 4.5052] = 0.1051$. The adjusted Wald test is

$$F = \frac{(15 - 2 + 1)}{15 \times 2} \times 4.5052 = 2.1024,$$

and $p = \Pr[F(2, 14) \geq 2.1024] = 0.1591$. We note that the p-value for the adjusted Wald test is slightly larger than that of the Wald test; however, neither is significant. Thus, both tests indicate that we do not have sufficient evidence to conclude that the coefficients for MODWRKL and MODRECEXR are significantly different from 0. We now fit the reduced model.

The results of fitting the model deleting MODEXR and MODREXEXR are shown in Table 6.2. The first thing we do is to compare the magnitude of the coefficients in Table 6.2 to those in Table 6.1 to check for confounding due to the excluded covariates. As can be seen there is virtually no difference in the two sets of coefficients suggesting that neither covariate removed is a confounder of the relationship between any of the remaining covariates and obesity (BMI > 35).

Table 6.2   Estimated Coefficients, Standard Errors, z-Scores, Two-Tailed p-Values, and 95% Confidence Intervals for a Logistic Regression Model for the Modified NHANES Study with Dependent Variable OBESE, $n = 5859$

	Coeff.	Std. Err.	t	p	95% CI
AGE10[a]	0.001	0.0254	0.03	0.980	−0.054, 0.055
DBP	0.019	0.0045	4.09	0.001	0.009, 0.028
GENDER	0.458	0.1221	3.75	0.002	0.198, 0.718
WLKBIK	0.477	0.0898	5.32	<0.001	0.286, 0.669
VIGRECEXR	0.894	0.1040	8.59	<0.001	0.672, 1.115
Constant	−4.474	0.4471	−10.01	<0.001	−5.427, −3.521

[a] $\text{AGE}10 = \frac{\text{AGE}}{10}$.

Following the guidelines we established in previous chapters, at this point in the analysis we would:

- Determine whether the continuous covariates in the model are linear in the logit.
- Determine whether there are any significant interactions among the independent variables in the model.
- Assess model calibration and discrimination through goodness of fit tests and area under the ROC curve.
- Examine the case-wise diagnostic statistics to identify poorly fit and influential covariate patterns.

Unfortunately, most of these procedures are not easily performed when modeling data from complex sample surveys. However, there is much that can be done to approximate the correct analysis by using a weighted ordinary logistic regression.

We can check for nonlinearity in the logit by using fractional polynomials with weights equal to the sampling weights within the ordinary logistic regression program. If a significant nonlinear transformation is found then we can fit the model accounting for the sample weights and with the correct standard error estimates to see if the coefficients remain significant. In any case, any nonlinear transformation must make clinical sense. We applied a weighted fractional polynomial analysis to age and diastolic blood pressure. We found that the $(3, 3)$ transformation for age was significantly better than the linear and one term transformation, (3), using the closed test procedure. There was no evidence for nonlinearity in the logit for diastolic blood pressure. The fit of the model using the $m = 2$ fractional polynomial transformation for age is shown in Table 6.3.

We leave as an exercise demonstrating, using methods illustrated in Chapter 4, that the shape of the logit in the two-term fractional polynomial in age rises gradually from age 16 to its maximum at age 55 and then descends to its minimum at age 80. We also include in this exercise a demonstration that this transformation is better statistically and makes more clinical sense than a model quadratic in age (i.e., one with age and age^2).

Table 6.3 Estimated Coefficients, Standard Errors, z-Scores, Two-Tailed p-Values, and 95% Confidence Intervals for a Logistic Regression Model for the Modified NHANES Study with Dependent Variable OBESE, $n = 5859$

	Coeff.	Std. Err.	t	p	95% CI
AGEFP1[a]	0.019	0.0061	3.12	0.007	0.006, 0.032
AGEFP2[a]	−0.009	0.0029	−3.21	0.006	−0.016, −0.003
DBP	0.014	0.0051	2.66	0.018	0.003, 0.025
GENDER	0.457	0.1224	3.73	0.002	0.196, 0.718
WLKBIK	0.480	0.0928	5.17	<0.001	0.282, 0.677
VIGRECEXR	0.878	0.1014	8.66	<0.001	0.662, 1.094
Constant	−4.419	0.4526	−9.76	<0.001	−5.384, −3.454

[a] $AGE10 = \frac{AGE}{10}$, $AGEFP1 = (AGE10)^3$, $AGEFP2 = (AGE10)^3 \times \ln(AGE10)$.

It was decided that the only interactions that made clinical sense were those involving gender. None of these were found to be significant at the 5% level when added to the model in Table 6.3. Thus, our preliminary final model is the one shown in Table 6.3.

We noted earlier that one is able to obtain the correct value of the estimator of the coefficients by using a weighted ordinary logistic regression program. Some programs (e.g., STATA) can perform the decile of risk test following this weighted fit. The problem is that it does not test for fit of the model in the correct way. When it uses weights, the ordinary logistic regression program assumes that the value of the weights corresponds to actual observations on subjects, rather than what they really are: statistical weights. Hence the test statistic has an enormously large value and the values of the observed and expected frequencies in the 2×10 table have no relationship to the actual sample values.

Archer et al. (2007) describe an extension of the decile of risk test to sample survey data that correctly tests for model fit. Its implementation in STATA's survey commands is described in Archer and Lemeshow (2006). The test is calculated as follows:

1. Ten groups are formed from the sorted estimated probabilities from the fitted model in such a way that the sum of the sample weights in each group is approximately 10% of the total sum of the sample weights. Thus, the 10 groups are not deciles of risk in the sense used in Chapter 5.

2. Using the sample weights, calculate the weighted mean of the model's residuals, $(y - \hat{\pi})$, within each of the 10 groups. Denote these means as $\widehat{M}_k$, $k = 1, 2, \ldots, 10$. If the model does not fit then we expect the weighted means of the residuals to be different from 0.

3. A linearized estimator of the covariance matrix derived by Archer (2001), $\widehat{\mathbf{V}}(\widehat{\mathbf{M}})$, of the $\widehat{M}'s$ is then used to calculate the Wald test of the hypothesis that the means are equal to 0:

$$\widehat{W}_{\widehat{M}} = \widehat{\mathbf{M}}'[\widehat{\mathbf{V}}(\widehat{\mathbf{M}})]^{-1}\widehat{\mathbf{M}}.$$

4. The Wald statistic is modified to form an F-corrected test statistic

$$F_{\widehat{M}} = \frac{(s - 10 + 2)}{s \times 10} \widehat{W}_{\widehat{M}},$$

and the associated p-value is calculated as

$$p = \Pr[F(10 - 1, s - 10 + 2,) > F_{\widehat{M}}].$$

We note that this test can be used with any number of groups. It is described here with 10 groups because that is the default number in STATA. The number of groups used must be less than $s + 2$. One disadvantage of this test is that when the test rejects fit, we do not have a 2×10 table of observed and estimated expected frequencies to assist us in finding areas where the model does not fit.

Evaluating the test for the fitted model in Table 6.3 yields $F_{\widehat{M}} = 1.6984$ and $p = 0.2487$ (i.e., $\Pr[F(9, 7) > 1.6984] = 0.2487$). Hence the test supports model fit.

Roberts et al. (1987) extend the diagnostics discussed in Chapter 5 to the survey sampling setting. However, the diagnostic statistics have not, as yet, been implemented into any of the commonly available packages. The computations required to obtain the measures of leverage and the contribution to fit are not trivial and require considerable skill in programming matrix calculations. In addition, the version of Cook's distance is not an easily computed function of leverage and contribution to fit.

A "better than doing nothing at all" diagnostics evaluation can be based on fitting the model using an ordinary logistic regression program and obtaining the diagnostic statistics described in Chapter 5. An improvement on the values of the diagnostic statistics can be obtained from the ordinary logistic regression model using, as an initial guess, the values of the coefficients from Table 6.3 and setting the number of iterations to 0. This forces the fit to yield the coefficients in Table 6.3. Options to set the initial guess and control the number of iterations are available in most logistic regression packages. Diagnostic statistics are then calculated, saved and plotted as described in Chapter 5. We leave the details of this as an exercise. The reader might want to take a quick look at Table 6.4 where we show that the differences between the two possible sets of coefficients that one could use to calculate the diagnostics statistics differ by 10% or more for five of the seven values. We did evaluate the diagnostic statistics and found that a few observations are poorly fit but their deletion did not produce important changes in the coefficients. Thus we use the model in Table 6.3 as our final model.

Statistical analyses of survey data that take the survey design (stratification and clustering) and statistical weights into consideration are generally called *design-based*. When such features are ignored and the data are handled as if they arose from a simple random sample, the resulting statistical analyses are termed *model-based*. One approach that analysts have used when dealing with survey data is to estimate parameters using design-based methods but to use model-based methods to perform other functions. For example, in this analysis, determination of linearity of

Table 6.4   Coefficients and 95% Confidence Intervals for Covariates in Table 6.3 Using "Design-Based" versus "Model-Based" Analysis

Variable	"Design-Based" Analysis		"Model-Based" Analysis		Pct. Diff.[a]
	Coeff.	95% CI	Coeff.	95% CI	
AGEFP1	0.019	0.006, 0.032	0.021	0.013, 0.029	11.4
AGEFP2	−0.009	−0.016, −0.003	−0.010	−0.015, −0.006	11.7
DBP	0.014	0.003, 0.025	0.012	0.006, 0.019	−9.0
GENDER	0.457	0.196, 0.718	0.519	0.367, 0.671	13.7
WLKBIK	0.480	0.282, 0.677	0.412	0.233, 0.591	−14.1
VIGRECEXR	0.878	0.662, 1.094	0.665	0.440, 0.890	−24.3
Constant	−4.419	−5.384, −3.454	−4.066	−4.583, −3.549	8.0

[a] $\text{Pct.Diff.} = 100 \times \dfrac{(\hat{\beta}_{\text{Model}} - \hat{\beta}_{\text{Design}})}{\hat{\beta}_{\text{Design}}}$.

the logit for the continuous covariates in the model, assessment of model calibration and examination of diagnostic statistics could be carried out by treating the data as if they resulted from a simple random sample. Any discoveries made in those analyses would then be implemented in the final design-based analysis. For example, we used fractional polynomial analysis to find that the logit was not linear in age. This knowledge, obtained from the model-based analysis may then be implemented into the more appropriate design-based analysis to obtain the slope coefficients and estimated odds ratios.

It should also be noted that for *linear estimates* such as means, totals and proportions, design-based standard errors are typically much larger than model-based standard errors. In fact, for linear estimates, the design effect (defined as the ratio of the variance under design-based analysis to the variance under simple random sampling) is typically much larger than 1. This measure reflects the inflation in variance that occurs due to homogeneity within clusters and can be expressed as $1 + (n - 1)\rho_y$, where ρ_y is the intracluster correlation coefficient (ICC) and n is the average number of units in the sampled cluster. These ICCs can range from small negative values (when the data within clusters are highly heterogeneous) to unity (when the data in clusters are highly correlated). Only when the data are highly heterogeneous within clusters will the design effect be less than 1. However, as described by Neuhaus and Segal (1993), design effects for *regression coefficients* can be expressed as $1 + (n - 1)\rho_x\rho_y$. Note that in this expression the ICC for the independent variable is multiplied by the ICC for the dependent variable. Both of these quantities are, by definition, less than 1. As a result, the design effect will be smaller than what would be observed for means, totals, or proportions. We also note that because ρ_x and ρ_y are not necessarily in the same direction, the product of the intracluster correlation coefficients could be negative and the resulting design effect could be smaller than 1.

The estimated coefficients and their 95% confidence intervals under both design-based and model-based scenarios and the percentage difference in the two sets of coefficients are presented in Table 6.4. In this example, both modeling approaches produce coefficients of the same order of magnitude but they do differ by anywhere from 8% to 24%.

In summary, we fit logistic regression models to data obtained from complex sample surveys via an approximate likelihood that incorporates the known sampling weights. We assess the overall model significance as well as tests of subsets of coefficients using multivariable F-adjusted Wald tests. However, the interpretation of odds ratios from a fitted model is the same as for models fit to less complicated sampling plans. We note that work needs to be done to make available the case-wise diagnostics obtained from complex sample surveys to the typical user of logistic regression software.

EXERCISES

1. Fit the model in Table 6.4 using a model quadratic in AGE10. Graph the logit functions for the (3, 3) model and (1, 2) model using the method shown in Chapter 5. Which model do you prefer and why? Estimate the odds ratio, with 95% confidence intervals, using the estimated coefficients from the model you prefer.

2. Using all of the covariates in Table 6.1 build, using purposeful selection, a model assessing risk factors for obesity, BMI > 35.

3. Assess the fit and evaluate the diagnostics for the model developed in Problem 2.

4. Estimate the odds ratios and confidence intervals for obesity using your final model from Problem 2 and interpret them in context.

CHAPTER 7

Logistic Regression for Matched Case-Control Studies

7.1 INTRODUCTION

An important special case of the stratified case-control study discussed in Chapter 6 is the matched case-control study. A discussion of the rationale for matched studies may be found in epidemiology texts such as Breslow and Day (1980), Kleinbaum et al. (1982), Schlesselman (1985), Kelsey et al. (1986), and Rothman et al. (2008). In this study design, subjects are stratified on the basis of variables believed to be associated with the outcome. Age and gender are examples of commonly used stratification variables. Within each stratum, samples of cases ($y = 1$) and controls ($y = 0$) are chosen. The number of cases and controls need not be constant across strata, but the most common matched designs include one case and from 1–5 controls per stratum and are thus referred to as $1-M$ matched studies.

In this chapter we develop the methods for analyzing general matched studies. We illustrate the methods for both the $1-1$ matched study and a $1-3$ matched study (as an example of the more general $1-M$ design).

We begin by providing some motivation and rationale for the need for special methods for the matched study. In Chapter 6, it was noted that we could handle the stratified sample by including the design variables created from the stratification variable in the model. This approach works well when the number of subjects in each stratum is large. However, in a typical matched study we are likely to have few subjects per stratum. For example, in the $1-1$ matched design with n case-control pairs we have only two subjects per stratum. Thus, in a fully stratified analysis with p covariates, we would be required to estimate $n + p$ parameters consisting of the constant term, the p slope coefficients for the covariates, and the $n - 1$ coefficients for the stratum-specific design variables using a sample of size $2n$. The optimality properties of the method of maximum likelihood, derived by letting the

Applied Logistic Regression, Third Edition.
David W. Hosmer, Jr., Stanley Lemeshow, and Rodney X. Sturdivant.
© 2013 John Wiley & Sons, Inc. Published 2013 by John Wiley & Sons, Inc.

sample size become large, hold only when the number of parameters remains fixed. This is clearly not the case in any $1-M$ matched study. With the fully stratified analysis, the number of parameters increases at the same rate as the sample size. For example, with a model containing one dichotomous covariate it can be shown [see Breslow and Day (1980)] that the bias in the estimate of the coefficient is 100% when analyzing a matched $1-1$ design via a fully stratified likelihood. If we regard the stratum-specific parameters as nuisance parameters, and if we are willing to forgo their estimation, then we can use methods for conditional inference to create a likelihood function that yields maximum likelihood estimators of the slope coefficients in the logistic regression model that are consistent and asymptotically normally distributed. The mathematical details of conditional likelihood analysis may be found in Cox and Hinkley (1974).

Suppose that there are K strata with n_{1k} cases and n_{0k} controls in stratum $k, k = 1, 2, \ldots, K$. We begin with the stratum-specific logistic regression model

$$\pi_k(\mathbf{x}) = \frac{e^{\alpha_k + \boldsymbol{\beta}' \mathbf{x}}}{1 + e^{\alpha_k + \boldsymbol{\beta}' \mathbf{x}}}, \tag{7.1}$$

where α_k denotes the contribution to the logit of all terms constant within the kth stratum (i.e., the matching or stratification variable(s)). In this chapter, the vector of coefficients, $\boldsymbol{\beta}$, contains only the p slope coefficients, $\boldsymbol{\beta}' = (\beta_1, \beta_2, \ldots, \beta_p)$. It follows from the results in Chapter 3 that each slope coefficient gives the change in the log-odds for a one unit increase in the covariate holding all other covariates constant in every stratum. This is important to keep in mind as the steps, to be described, in developing a conditional likelihood result in a model that does not look like a logistic regression model, yet it contains the coefficient vector, $\boldsymbol{\beta}$. The fact that the model does not look like a logistic regression model leads new users to think that estimated coefficients must be modified in some way before they can be used to estimate odds ratios. This is not the case, and we pay particular attention in this chapter to estimation and interpretation of odds ratios.

The conditional likelihood for the kth stratum is obtained as the probability of the observed data conditional on the stratum total and the total number of cases observed, the sufficient statistic for the nuisance parameter. In this setting, it is the probability of the observed data relative to the probability of the data for all possible assignments of n_{1k} cases and n_{0k} controls to $n_k = n_{1k} + n_{0k}$ subjects. The number of possible assignments of case status to n_{1k} subjects among the n_k subjects, denoted here as c_k, is given by the mathematical expression

$$c_k = \binom{n_k}{n_{1k}} = \frac{n_k!}{n_{1k}!(n_k - n_{1k})!}.$$

Let the subscript j denote any one of these c_k assignments. For any assignment we let subjects 1 to n_{1k} correspond to the cases and subjects $n_{1k} + 1$ to n_k to the controls. This is indexed by i for the observed data and by i_j for the jth possible assignment. The conditional likelihood is

$$
l_k(\boldsymbol{\beta}) = \frac{\displaystyle\prod_{i=1}^{n_{1k}} P(\mathbf{x}_i | y_i = 1) \prod_{i=n_{1k}+1}^{n_k} P(\mathbf{x}_i | y_i = 0)}{\displaystyle\sum_{j=1}^{c_k} \left\{ \prod_{i_j=1}^{n_{1k}} P\left(\mathbf{x}_{ji_j} | y_{i_j} = 1\right) \prod_{i_j=n_{1k}+1}^{n_k} P(\mathbf{x}_{ji_j} | y_{i_j} = 0) \right\}}. \tag{7.2}
$$

The full conditional likelihood is the product of the $l_k(\boldsymbol{\beta})$ in equation (7.2) over the K strata, namely,

$$
l(\boldsymbol{\beta}) = \prod_{k=1}^{K} l_k(\boldsymbol{\beta}). \tag{7.3}
$$

If we assume that the stratum-specific logistic regression model in equation (7.1) is correct then application of Bayes' theorem to each $\Pr(\mathbf{x}|y)$ term in equation (7.2) yields

$$
l_k(\boldsymbol{\beta}) = \frac{\displaystyle\prod_{i=1}^{n_{1k}} e^{\boldsymbol{\beta}'\mathbf{x}_i}}{\displaystyle\sum_{j=1}^{c_k} \prod_{i_j=1}^{n_{1k}} e^{\boldsymbol{\beta}'\mathbf{x}_{ji_j}}}. \tag{7.4}
$$

Note that when we apply Bayes' theorem all terms of the form

$$
\frac{\exp(\alpha_k)}{1 + \exp(\alpha_k + \boldsymbol{\beta}'\mathbf{x})}
$$

appear equally in both the numerator and denominator of equation (7.2) and thus cancel out. Algebraic simplification yields the function shown in equation (7.4) where $\boldsymbol{\beta}$ is the only unknown parameter. The conditional maximum likelihood estimator for $\boldsymbol{\beta}$ is that value that maximizes equation (7.3) when $l_k(\boldsymbol{\beta})$ is as shown in equation (7.4). Except in one special case it is not possible to express the likelihood in equation (7.4) in a form similar to the unconditional likelihood in equation (1.3). However, as we noted earlier, the coefficients have not been modified, and thus have the same interpretation as those in equation (7.1).

The most frequently used matched design is one in which each case is matched to a single control; thus, there are two subjects in each stratum. It is helpful to consider this design, not only because it is used frequently in practice, but also because it helps illustrate some key differences in the effect covariate values have on the likelihood function in equations (1.3) and (7.4). To simplify the notation, let $\mathbf{x}_{1k}$ denote the data vector for the case and $\mathbf{x}_{0k}$ the data vector for the control in the kth stratum or pair. Using this notation, the conditional likelihood for the kth stratum from equation (7.4) is

$$
l_k(\boldsymbol{\beta}) = \frac{e^{\boldsymbol{\beta}'\mathbf{x}_{1k}}}{e^{\boldsymbol{\beta}'\mathbf{x}_{1k}} + e^{\boldsymbol{\beta}'\mathbf{x}_{0k}}}. \tag{7.5}
$$

Given specific values for β, $\mathbf{x}_{1k}$, and $\mathbf{x}_{0k}$, equation (7.5) is the probability that, within stratum k, the subject identified as the case is in fact the case under the assumptions that: (i) we have two subjects, one of whom is the case and (ii) the logistic regression model in equation (7.1) is the correct model. For example, suppose we have a model with a single dichotomous covariate and $\beta = 0.8$ and the observed data are $x_{1k} = 1$ and $x_{0k} = 0$ then the value of equation (7.5) is

$$l_k(\beta = 0.8) = \frac{e^{0.8 \times 1}}{e^{0.8 \times 1} + e^{0.8 \times 0}} = 0.690.$$

Thus, the probability is 0.69 that a subject with $x = 1$ is the case compared to a subject with $x = 0$. On the other hand, if $x_{1k} = 0$ and $x_{0k} = 1$ then

$$l_k(\beta = 0.8) = \frac{e^{0.8 \times 0}}{e^{0.8 \times 0} + e^{0.8 \times 1}} = 0.310$$

and the probability is 0.31 that a subject with $x = 0$ is the case compared to a subject with $x = 1$. Thus, we see that the affect of a covariate value is measured relative to the values in its matched set rather than relative to all values of the covariate, which is the case with the likelihood in equation (1.3) or its log-likelihood in equation (1.4).

It also follows from equation (7.5) that if the data for the case and the control are identical, $\mathbf{x}_{1k} = \mathbf{x}_{0k}$, then $l_k(\boldsymbol{\beta}) = 0.5$ for any value of $\boldsymbol{\beta}$ (i.e., the data for the case and control are equally likely under the model). Thus, case-control pairs with the same value for any covariate are *uninformative* for estimation of that covariate's coefficient. We use the term *uninformative* to describe the fact that the value of the covariate does not help distinguish which subject is more likely to be the case. This tends to occur most frequently with dichotomous covariates where common values, often called *concordant pairs*, are most likely to occur. A fact not discussed in this chapter, which can be found in Breslow and Day (1980), is that the maximum likelihood estimator of the coefficient for a dichotomous covariate in a univariable conditional logistic regression model fit to 1–1 matched data is the log of the ratio of discordant pairs. The practical significance of this is that the estimator may be based on a small fraction of the total number of possible pairs. We feel it is good practice to form the 2×2 table cross-classifying case versus control for all dichotomous covariates in order to determine the number of discordant pairs. This is essentially a univariable logistic regression and, as we have stated previously, univariable analyses of all covariates should be among the first steps in any model building process. The reader should be aware that, if both types of pairs, $(x_{1k} = 1, x_{0k} = 0)$ and $(x_{1k} = 0, x_{0k} = 1)$, are not present in the data, then the estimator is undefined. In this case, software packages will either remove the covariate from the model or give an impractically large coefficient and standard error. This is the same zero cell problem discussed in Section 4.5. The same type of problem can occur for polychotomous covariates, but it involves more complex relationships than simply a zero frequency cell in the cross-classification of case versus control [Breslow and Day (1980)].

As a few software packages still do not have specific commands for maximizing the conditional log-likelihood, it is possible, with some data manipulation, to use a standard logistic regression package to maximize the full conditional log-likelihood for the $1-1$ design. We begin by re-expressing equation (7.5) by dividing its numerator and denominator by $e^{\beta'x_{0k}}$ yielding

$$l_k(\beta) = \frac{e^{\beta'(x_{1k}-x_{0k})}}{1 + e^{\beta'(x_{1k}-x_{0k})}}$$

$$= \frac{e^{\beta'x_k^*}}{1 + e^{\beta'x_k^*}}. \tag{7.6}$$

The expression on the right side of equation (7.6) is the usual logistic regression model with the constant term set equal to zero ($\beta_0 = 0$) and data vector equal to the data value of the case minus the data value of the control, $x_k^* = (x_{1k} - x_{0k})$. It follows that the full conditional likelihood may be expressed as

$$l(\beta) = \prod_{k=1}^{K} \frac{e^{\beta'x_k^*}}{1 + e^{\beta'x_k^*}}$$

$$= \prod_{k=1}^{K} \left[\frac{e^{\beta'x_k^*}}{1 + e^{\beta'x_k^*}}\right]^{y_k} \left[\frac{1}{1 + e^{\beta'x_k^*}}\right]^{1-y_k},$$

where $y_k = 1$ for all k.

This observation allows one to use standard logistic regression software to compute the conditional maximum likelihood estimates and obtain estimated standard errors of the estimated coefficients. To do this, one must define the sample size as the number of case-control pairs, use as covariates the differences x_k^*, set the values of the response variable equal to one ($y_k = 1$), and exclude the constant term from the model. Thus, from a computational point of view, the $1-1$ matched design may be fit using any logistic regression program.

Software to perform the necessary calculations using the log of the likelihood in equation (7.3) is now available in most statistical software packages. For example, STATA has a special conditional logistic regression command. With SAS and a few other packages, one must perform a simple modification of the data and perform the analysis using the package's proportional hazards regression command. The calculations for this chapter were performed in STATA.

In summary, the methods for model building for matched data are identical to those discussed and illustrated in detail for unmatched data in Chapter 4. Hence, we do not repeat them here, but illustrate them in the examples. There are, however, important differences when one assesses the fit of the model from matched data. The ideas are the same as those discussed in Chapter 5 for unmatched data, but the calculations of the diagnostic statistics are different. These are presented and discussed in the next section. We conclude the chapter with examples of using logistic regression to model data from a $1-1$ and a $1-3$ design.

7.2 METHODS FOR ASSESSMENT OF FIT IN A 1−M MATCHED STUDY

Our approach to assessment of fit in the 1−M matched study is based on extensions of regression diagnostics for the unconditional logistic regression model. The mathematics required to develop these statistics is at a higher level than other sections of the book. Hence, less sophisticated mathematical readers may wish to skip this section and proceed to examples where the use of the diagnostic statistics is explained and illustrated. Moolgavkar et al. (1985) and Pregibon (1984) derive these diagnostic statistics for a general matched design, but only illustrate their use in the 1−1 matched design. STATA currently provides access to the diagnostics following the fit of a logistic model using equation (7.3). To simplify the notation somewhat we present the results for the setting when $M = 3$ (i.e., $M + 1 = 4$ subjects per stratum).

There are no easily computed goodness of fit tests for the matched data setting. Zhang (1999) discusses a test but it is not available in any software package. Arbogast and Lin (2005) propose a method based on cumulative sums of residuals within matched sets with significance and visual assessment based on simulations. Again, the method is complicated to compute and is not available in software packages.

Since the diagnostics are not computed in all software packages we describe them as if one was going to compute them following the fit of a model. The first step is to transform the observed values of the covariate vector by centering them about a weighted stratum-specific mean. That is, we compute for each stratum, k, and each subject within each stratum, j,

$$\tilde{\mathbf{x}}_{kj} = \mathbf{x}_{kj} - \sum_{l=1}^{4} \mathbf{x}_{kl}\hat{\theta}_{kl},$$

where

$$\hat{\theta}_{kj} = \frac{e^{\mathbf{x}'_{kj}\hat{\boldsymbol{\beta}}}}{\sum_{l=1}^{4} e^{\mathbf{x}'_{kj}\hat{\boldsymbol{\beta}}}}$$

and note that $\sum_{j=1}^{4} \hat{\theta}_{kj} = 1$. Let $\tilde{\mathbf{X}}$ be the $n = 4K$ by p matrix whose rows are the values of $\tilde{\mathbf{x}}_{kj}$, $k = 1, 2, \ldots, K$ and $j = 1, 2, 3, 4$. Let $\mathbf{U}$ be an n by n diagonal matrix with general diagonal element $\hat{\theta}_{kj}$. It may be shown that the maximum likelihood estimator, $\hat{\boldsymbol{\beta}}$, once obtained can be re-computed via the equation

$$\hat{\boldsymbol{\beta}} = (\tilde{\mathbf{X}}'\mathbf{U}\tilde{\mathbf{X}})^{-1}\tilde{\mathbf{X}}'\mathbf{U}\mathbf{z},$$

where $\mathbf{z}$ is the vector $\mathbf{z} = \tilde{\mathbf{X}}'\hat{\boldsymbol{\beta}} + \mathbf{U}^{-1}(\mathbf{y} - \hat{\boldsymbol{\theta}})$, $\mathbf{y}$ is the vector of values of the outcome variable ($y = 1$ for the case and $y = 0$ for the controls), and $\hat{\boldsymbol{\theta}}$ is the vector whose components are $\hat{\theta}_{kj}$. Recall that $\hat{\theta}_{kj}$ is, under the assumption of a logistic regression model, the estimated conditional probability that subject j within stratum k is a case.

It follows from the above expression for $\hat{\beta}$ that we may re-compute the maximum likelihood estimate for the conditional logistic regression model using a linear regression program allowing case weights. We use the vector $\tilde{\mathbf{x}}_{kj}$ as values of the independent variables,

$$z_{kj} = \tilde{\mathbf{x}}_{kj}' \hat{\beta} + \frac{y_{kj} - \hat{\theta}_{kj}}{\hat{\theta}_{kj}}$$

as the values of the dependent variable, and case weight $\hat{\theta}_{kj}$, for $k = 1, 2, \ldots, K$, $j = 1, 2, 3, 4$. It follows that the diagonal elements of the hat matrix computed by the linear regression are the leverage values we need, namely

$$h_{kj} = \hat{\theta}_{kj} \tilde{\mathbf{x}}_{kj}' (\tilde{\mathbf{X}}' \mathbf{U} \tilde{\mathbf{X}})^{-1} \tilde{\mathbf{x}}_{kj}. \tag{7.7}$$

We note that the leverage values in equation (7.7) are of the same form as those in equation (5.22). Here, the "v" part is the conditional probability $\hat{\theta}_{kj}$ and the "b" part is $\tilde{\mathbf{x}}_{kj}' (\tilde{\mathbf{X}}' \mathbf{U} \tilde{\mathbf{X}})^{-1} \tilde{\mathbf{x}}_{kj}$. The "v" part is not an estimator of the variance as it is in equation (5.22). However, the leverage in equation (7.7) does go to zero as $\hat{\theta}_{kj}$ goes to zero. The "b" part will be large when the individual covariate values are different from the matched set weighted mean, as opposed to the overall mean in equation (5.21). Hence subjects with high leverage will be those whose covariate values differ from the matched set mean and have an estimated conditional probability between 0.3 and 0.7.

We note that one must pay close attention to how weights are handled in the statistical package used for the weighted linear regression. For example, SAS's regression procedure outputs the values as defined in equation (7.7). STATA users need to multiply the leverage values created following the weighted regression by $\hat{\theta}_{kj}/\bar{\theta}$ to obtain the leverage values defined in equation (7.7), where $\bar{\theta} = \sum_{k=1}^{K} \sum_{j=1}^{M+1} \hat{\theta}_{kj} / [K(M+1)]$ is the mean of the estimated logistic probabilities.

The Pearson residual is

$$r_{kj} = \frac{(y_{kj} - \hat{\theta}_{kj})}{\sqrt{\hat{\theta}_{kj}}},$$

and the Pearson chi-square is

$$X^2 = \sum_{k=1}^{K} \sum_{j=1}^{M+1} \frac{(y_{kj} - \hat{\theta}_{kj})^2}{\hat{\theta}_{kj}}.$$

Unfortunately, the large sample approach of Osius and Rojek (1992) cannot be used in this setting to obtain a standardized statistic and significance level.

The standardized Pearson residual is

$$r_{skj} = \frac{(y_{kj} - \hat{\theta}_{kj})}{[\hat{\theta}_{kj}(1 - h_{kj})]^{1/2}}.$$

In keeping with the diagnostics for the unmatched design we define the square of the standardized residual as the lack of fit diagnostic

$$\Delta X_{kj}^2 = r_{skj}^2 \qquad (7.8)$$

and the influence diagnostic as

$$\Delta \hat{\beta}_{kj} = \Delta X_{kj}^2 \frac{h_{kj}}{1 - h_{kj}}. \qquad (7.9)$$

We feel that the most informative way to view the diagnostic statistics is via a plot of their values versus the fitted values, $\hat{\theta}_{kj}$. These plots are similar to those used in Chapter 5 to assess graphically the fit of the unconditional logistic regression. Examples of these plots are presented in the next section.

Moolgavkar et al. (1985) and Pregibon (1984) suggest that one should use the stratum-specific totals of the two diagnostics, ΔX^2 and $\Delta \hat{\beta}$ to assess what affect the data in an entire stratum have on the fit of the model. These statistics are computed as quadratic forms involving not only the leverage values for the subjects in the stratum, but also those terms in the hat matrix that account for the correlation among the fitted values. An easily computed approximation to these statistics is obtained by ignoring the off diagonal elements in the hat matrix. We feel that the approximations are likely to be accurate enough for practical purposes. For the kth stratum these are

$$\Delta X_k^2 = r_{sk}^2 = \sum_{j=1}^{4} r_{skj}^2 \qquad (7.10)$$

and

$$\Delta \hat{\beta}_k = \sum_{j=1}^{4} \Delta \hat{\beta}_{kj}. \qquad (7.11)$$

Strata with large values of these statistics would be judged to be poorly fit and/or have large influence respectively. One can use a boxplot or a plot of their values versus stratum number to identify those strata with exceptionally large values. For these strata, the individual contributions to these quantities should be examined carefully to determine whether cases and/or controls are the cause of the large values.

The diagnostic statistics described in this section are similar to the diagnostics one would obtain in the 1–1 matched setting by fitting the model using the difference data and computing the diagnostics shown in Chapter 5. For this reason, some users may prefer the difference data approach to the 1–1 design. Specifically, the diagnostics based on the difference data are based on one value per stratum, while those computed from equations (7.7)–(7.9) yield two values per stratum. The mathematical relationships between the two diagnostic statistics are complex. For example, the stratum totals described in equations (7.10) and (7.11) are not arithmetically equal to the values of ΔX^2 and $\Delta \hat{\beta}$ from Chapter 5. While it may appear that we have two different sets of values of the diagnostic statistics they do identify the same strata as being poorly fit or influential. Thus from a practical point of view one may use either the difference data or the results in this section to assess model adequacy in the 1–1 design. In all other matched designs, one must use the diagnostics described in this section.

In identifying poorly fit or influential subjects deletion of the case in a stratum, assuming a $1-M$ design, is tantamount to deletion of all subjects in the stratum. Without a case, a stratum contributes no information to the likelihood function. If some, but not all, controls are deleted in a specific stratum then the stratum may still have enough information to contribute to the likelihood function. A final decision on exclusion or inclusion of cases (entire strata) or controls should be based on the clinical plausibility of the data.

7.3 AN EXAMPLE USING THE LOGISTIC REGRESSION MODEL IN A 1–1 MATCHED STUDY

For illustrative purposes we created a 1–1 matched data set from the GLOW Study data by randomly matching each woman who had a fracture to a woman of the same age who did not have a fracture. It was not possible to exactly match age for six of the women who had a fracture. Thus, there are 119 matched case-control pairs. The covariates are the same as those listed in Table 1.7 and are available from the web site as GLOW11M.

As we noted earlier in this chapter, all model building and evaluation is done using STATA's clogit command. Before fitting multivariable models we note that the "intercept only" model (or base model) for assessing significance with the likelihood ratio test in the 1–1 design is a model with log-likelihood

$$L(\beta = 0) = \sum_{k=1}^{K} \ln(0.5) = K \times \ln(0.5),$$

a value usually not presented in computer output, but easily computed by hand calculation. However, some packages, for example STATA, report this as the value of the log-likelihood at the "zero-th" iteration.

The results of fitting univariable models are displayed in Table 7.1. The covariates significant at the 25 percent level are: HEIGHT, PRIORFRAC, PREMENO, MOMFRAC, and RATERISK. Normally we would fit a multivariable model containing just these covariates. However, the height, weight, and body mass index are interrelated, and a multivariable model containing two of the three may be better than a model containing the single variable, HEIGHT, that is significant in a univariable model. Hence, we decided to include all three in the initial multivariable model.

Table 7.1   Univariable Conditional Logistic Regression Models for the 1–1 Matched Data from the GLOW Study, $n = 119$ Pairs

Variable	Coeff.	Std. Err.	p^a	$\widehat{OR}$	95% CI	Discordant Pairs $(n_{10}, n_{01})^b$
HEIGHT	−0.057	0.0238	0.016	0.56^c	(0.35, 0.90)	Not relevant
WEIGHT	−0.001	0.0084	0.870	0.99^c	(0.94, 1.05)	Not relevant
BMI	0.019	0.0229	0.405	1.06	(0.93, 1.21)	Not relevant
PRIORFRAC	0.838	0.2992	0.005	2.31	(1.29, 4.16)	(37, 16)
PREMENO	0.693	0.4629	0.134	2.00	(0.81, 4.96)	(14, 7)
MOMFRAC	0.511	0.3651	0.162	1.67	(0.81, 3.41)	(20, 12)
ARMASSIST	0.633	0.3001	0.035	1.88	(1.05, 3.39)	(32, 17)
SMOKE	−0.336	0.5855	0.566	0.71	(0.23, 2.25)	(5, 7)
RATERISK2	0.552	0.2909	0.012	1.74	(0.98, 3.07)	Not relevant
RATERISK3	1.025	0.3669		2.79	(1.36, 5.72)	Not relevant

$^a p$ from the likelihood ratio test, $-2L(\boldsymbol{\beta} = 0) = 164.969$.
^{b}Discordant exposures: n_{10} = frequency of pairs with case exposed and control not, n_{01} = frequency of pairs with case not exposed and control exposed and $\widehat{OR} = n_{10}/n_{01}$.
^{c}Odds ratio for a 10 cm increase in height, 3 kg increase in weight, 3 kg/m^2 in BMI.

Table 7.2   Estimated Coefficients, Estimated Standard Errors, Wald Statistics, and Two-Tailed p-Values for the Model Containing All Covariates Except SMOKE

Variable	Coeff.	Std. Err.	z	p
HEIGHT	0.063	0.1220	0.52	0.604
WEIGHT	−0.154	0.1310	−1.18	0.239
BMI	0.387	0.3417	1.13	0.258
PRIORFRAC	0.694	0.3538	1.96	0.050
PREMENO	0.218	0.5523	0.39	0.693
MOMFRAC	0.725	0.4326	1.68	0.094
ARMASSIST	0.818	0.3824	2.14	0.032
RATERISK2	0.152	0.3412	0.44	0.657
RATERISK3	0.589	0.4256	1.38	0.166

The results of fitting the initial multivariable model are shown in Table 7.2. The fitted model is significant at the 0.1 percent level, but several of the covariates are not significant by the Wald test. Before sorting out height, weight, and body mass index we remove early menopause (PREMENO) and the two design variables for self-reported rate of fracture risk (RATERISK2 and RATERISK3). The partial likelihood ratio test for the removal of the three variables was not significant with $p = 0.493$, and none of the coefficients for covariates remaining in the model changed by more than 20 percent. Hence, we continue with the reduced model.

We fit each of the three models containing two of the three covariates: HEIGHT, WEIGHT, and BMI. In work not shown, we found the model containing WEIGHT and BMI had the smallest log-likelihood and both covariates had Wald statistics

Table 7.3   Estimated Coefficients, Estimated Standard Errors, Wald Statistics, and Two-Tailed p-Values for the Reduced Multivariable Model

Variable	Coeff.	Std. Err.	z	p
WEIGHT	−0.095	0.0299	−3.16	0.002
BMI	0.222	0.0810	2.75	0.006
PRIORFRAC	0.835	0.3396	2.46	0.014
MOMFRAC	0.727	0.4093	1.78	0.076
ARMASSIST	0.889	0.3666	2.42	0.015

for their respective estimated coefficients that were significant at the five percent level. The results of this fit are shown in Table 7.3.

The model in Table 7.3 contains the continuous covariates WEIGHT and BMI. We checked for the scale in the logit using fractional polynomials. No fractional polynomial transformation of either WEIGHT or BMI was significantly better than the model linear in the logit. Thus, we consider possible interactions using the main effects model in Table 7.3.

The GLOW Study subject matter experts felt that an interaction between any pair of variables in the model in Table 7.3 was clinically plausible. The method we used here is identical to that used in Section 4.2 to select interactions; see Table 4.14 for presentation details. We began by fitting each of the 10 models by adding a single interaction to the model in Table 7.3 and evaluated the significance of the coefficient for the interaction term using the partial likelihood ratio test. No interaction was significant at the five percent level of significance. By matching on age we are assured that age cannot confound the main effect associations of the covariates in the model. However, the matching variable can still be an effect modifier. Hence, we examined the interaction of the matching variable, age, with each of the five covariates. Again, no interaction was significant at the five percent level. Hence we proceed to model evaluation using the model in Table 7.3 as our preliminary final model.

Casewise diagnostic measures of leverage, lack of fit, and influence were computed using the results in equations (7.7)–(7.9), and the pairwise sum of lack of fit and influence were computed using equations (7.10) and (7.11). As in Chapter 5, we think that the most informative way to examine the casewise diagnostic statistics is via a plot versus the estimated probabilities. In the matched pairs setting, the estimated probabilities within a pair sum up to one, and are estimates of the probability of being the case. Thus a well fitting pair would be one where the estimate for the subject that is the case is large, while that of the control is small.

We plot the 238 estimated leverage values in Figure 7.1 using an "x" to indicate the case and an "o" to indicate a control. There are two controls and two cases with leverage values that fall well away from the rest of the plotted values. We remind the reader that leverage in a matched data setting is "distance from the weighted match set mean". Once we have examined all the diagnostic statistics we present a table containing all identified observations and their data.

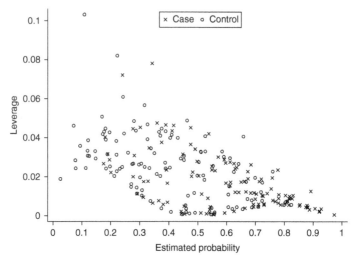

Figure 7.1 Plot of all 238 leverages versus the estimated probability from the fitted model from the GLOW 1–1 Matched Study in Table 7.3.

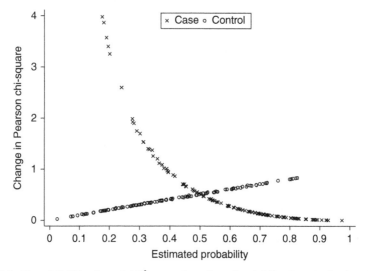

Figure 7.2 Plot of all 238 values of ΔX^2 versus the estimated probability from the fitted model from the GLOW 1–1 Matched Study in Table 7.3.

Next we examine the change in Pearson chi-square as a measure of lack of fit. We plot the 238 values in Figure 7.2. In the plot we see five values, all for cases, that are large relative to the other plotted values. In Chapter 5, we noted that we tend to define "large" as a value of $\Delta X^2 > 4$. Here the five values are all between 3 and 4. Regardless, we still think it is important to identify any and all subjects with potentially extreme values and examine their effect on the fitted model.

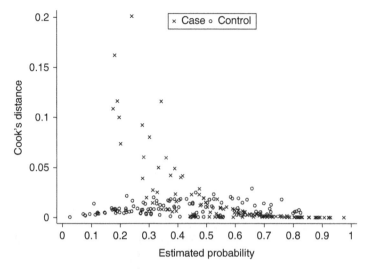

Figure 7.3   Plot of all 238 values of $\Delta\hat{\beta}\%$ versus the estimated probability from the fitted model from the GLOW 1–1 Matched Study in Table 7.3.

Next we examine the influence statistic $\Delta\hat{\beta}\%$ with all 238 values plotted in Figure 7.3. We see two values that lie well away from the remainder of the plotted points and each one corresponds to a case.

In the matched data setting we have two additional diagnostic statistics that estimate the effect of the matched set (pair here). These are the sum of the change in Pearson chi-square and influence over the subjects in each matched set. Here, we are interested in identifying the pair so plots are over the pair or matched set number rather than the estimated probability for one of the subjects in the matched set. The plot of the sum of the change in Pearson chi-square is shown in Figure 7.4 where we see 6 pairs with values that lie away from the other plotted values. Until we identify observations and pairs we cannot tell if these pairs correspond to the pairs whose individual cases were identified in any of the previous three plots.

We plot the pairwise sum of the Cook's distance diagnostic in Figure 7.5. We see only two values that seem to lie away from the rest of the plotted values. The next step is to identify subjects and pairs with extreme values in one or more of the figures.

Further examination of the values identified cases in pairs 37, 38, 67, 50, 100, and 117 as having a relatively large value of either or both ΔX^2 and $\Delta\hat{\beta}\%$. These same pairs corresponded to large pairwise sum statistics in Figure 7.4 and/or Figure 7.5. Of the four pairs with large leverage values in Figure 7.1 only one, the case in pair 50, was identified in another plot. The data and diagnostic statistics from the case and the control in the six identified pairs are listed in Table 7.4.

The first thing we notice in Table 7.4 is that the estimated probability of being the case is larger for the control than the case. There are 39 such pairs among the 119. When this occurs, it is not surprising that the summed measure of fit, sum

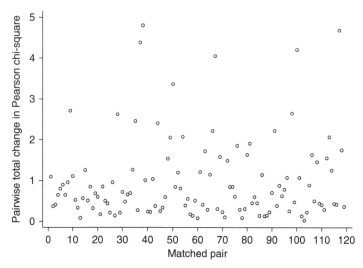

Figure 7.4   Plot of pairwise sum of ΔX^2 versus pair number from the fitted model from the GLOW 1–1 Matched Study in Table 7.3.

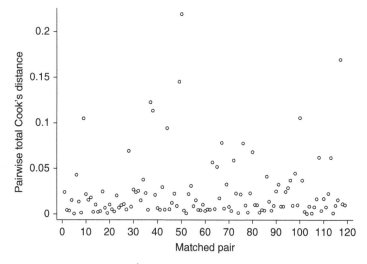

Figure 7.5   Plot of pairwise sum of $\Delta\hat{\boldsymbol{\beta}}\%$ versus pair number from the fitted model from the GLOW 1–1 Matched Study in Table 7.3.

ΔX^2, is large. The most influential of the six pairs is 50 with sum $\Delta\hat{\boldsymbol{\beta}}\% = 0.219$. In pair 50 the case weighs over 100 kg with a body mass index over 40 kg/m^2 while the control weighs 57 kg with a body mass index of 22 kg/m^2. Both sets of measurements are plausible, but with $\hat{\theta} = 0.76$ the control looks more like a case than the case with $\hat{\theta} = 0.26$.

Table 7.4 Pair, Status, Covariates, and Diagnostic Statistics for Six Extreme Pairs

Pair	Cont/Case	W^a	B	P	M	A	$\hat{\theta}$	ΔX^2	$\Delta\hat{\beta}\%$	h	SumΔX^2	Sum$\Delta\hat{\beta}\%$
37	Control	64.4	25.8	0	1	0	0.810	0.816	0.006	0.007	4.386	0.123
	Case	72.6	26.0	0	0	0	0.190	3.570	0.116	0.032		
38	Control	52.2	21.2	1	0	0	0.824	0.829	0.005	0.006	4.803	0.114
	Case	72.6	26.7	0	0	0	0.176	3.974	0.109	0.027		
50	Control	57.2	22.3	0	1	1	0.760	0.778	0.018	0.023	3.368	0.219
	Case	111.6	43.6	0	0	1	0.240	2.591	0.201	0.072		
67	Control	55.3	20.1	1	0	0	0.799	0.804	0.004	0.006	4.055	0.078
	Case	67.6	22.9	0	0	0	0.201	3.252	0.074	0.022		
100	Control	88.5	33.7	1	0	1	0.804	0.810	0.006	0.007	4.208	0.106
	Case	57.2	21.8	0	0	0	0.196	3.398	0.100	0.029		
117	Control	50.8	20.6	1	1	1	0.819	0.826	0.007	0.009	4.689	0.169
	Case	57.2	23.8	1	0	0	0.181	3.863	0.162	0.040		

^{a}Order of covariates: weight (W), body mass index (B), prior fracture (P), mother fracture (M), arm assist (A).

257

Table 7.5 Estimated Coefficients from Table 7.3 (All), Estimated Coefficients when Pair Is Deleted, and Percent Change from All

Data	WEIGHT	BMI	PRIORFRAC	MOMFRAC	ARMASSIST
All	−0.095	0.222	0.835	0.727	0.889
Delete 37	−0.103	0.243	0.842	0.887	0.925
Pct. change	−7.71	−8.38	−0.85	−18.06	−3.94
Delete 38	−0.101	0.231	0.956	0.737	0.925
Pct. change	−5.91	−3.62	−12.67	−1041.00	−3.89
Delete 50	−0.098	0.215	0.893	0.861	0.953
Pct. change	−2.87	3.50	−6.53	−15.63	−6.57
Delete 67	−0.099	0.230	0.943	0.735	0.913
Pct. change	−4.78	−3.27	−11.49	−1.19	−2.68
Delete 100	−0.098	0.234	0.904	0.742	0.976
Pct. change	−3.23	−4.94	−7.63	−2.03	−8.94
Delete 117	−0.099	0.228	0.845	0.882	1.022
Pct. Change	−4.09	−2.64	−1.21	−17.60	−13.01
Delete all 6	−0.133	0.283	1.334	1.362	1.401
Pct. Change	−28.58	−21.48	−37.39	−46.65	−36.55

Pct. Change $= 100 \times \dfrac{(\hat{\beta}_{All} - \hat{\beta}_{Deleted})}{\hat{\beta}_{Deleted}}$

The next step is to examine the sensitivity of the fit to these six pairs. In the one to one matched design, if one deletes either the case or the control then the pair is deleted. One must have at least one value of each outcome in a pair for it to be included in the analysis. The values of the estimated coefficients and the percent change from those in Table 7.3 are given in Table 7.5.

When pairs are deleted one at a time none of the estimated coefficients change by more than 20 percent from the estimates when data from all 119 pairs are used. The largest change is −18 percent in the estimate of the coefficient for mother having had a fracture (MOMFRAC). Recall that when the percent change is negative it means that the estimate, with the pair removed, is larger than the estimate when the pair is included. The percent changes in the coefficients when all six pairs are removed are shown in the last line of Table 7.5. Here changes exceed 20 percent for each of the coefficients and, for MOMFRAC, it is a −46 percent change. The magnitude of these changes is not totally unexpected since, in all six pairs, the control had the larger estimated probability. So, in a sense, all six pairs go against the effects of the covariates in the fitted model and, when removed, their effects increase. While collectively the six pairs have a substantial impact on the magnitude of the estimates of the coefficients the actual values of the covariates are not at all unusual or extreme. Hence, we cannot, in good conscience, exclude them just because they happen to go against the model. Thus we proceed with the model in Table 7.3 as our final model.

The estimated odds ratio for each of the model covariates is given in Table 7.6, along with its 95 percent confidence interval. The results show that history of prior fracture, mother having had a fracture, and the need to use arms to rise from a

**Table 7.6   Estimated Odds Ratios and 95 Percent Confidence
Intervals from the Fitted Model in Table 7.3**

Variable	Odds Ratio	95% CI
Weight	0.62^a	0.46, 0.84
Body mass index	3.04^b	1.38, 6.72
History of prior fracture	2.30	1.18, 4.48
Mother had a fracture	2.07	0.93, 4.61
Need to use arms to rise from a chair	2.43	1.18, 5.00

[a] Odds ratio for a 5 kg increase in weight.
[b] Odds ratio for a 5 kg/m^2 increase in body mass index.

chair each result in a more than twofold increase in the odds of fracture with the associated 95 percent confidence interval suggesting that the increase could be as little as a 1.2-fold or as much as a 4-fold increase for prior fracture and arm assist. Mother's history could be nonsignificant or result in as much as a 4.6-fold increase in the odds. There is an estimated 38 percent decrease in the odds of fracture for a 5 kg increase in weight and the decrease could be as small as 16 percent or as much as 54 percent with 95 percent confidence. Increasing body mass index by 5 kg/m^2 is associated with a 3-fold in the odds of fracture and the increase in the odds could be as little as 1.4-fold or as much as 6.7-fold with 95 percent confidence.

In summary, by following the purposeful selection method of main effects, factional polynomial analysis of continuous covariates and followed by purposeful selection of interactions, we obtained the relatively simple model shown in Table 7.3. One may also employ stepwise and best subsets selection of covariates described in Chapter 4 by obvious extensions of these methods. Extensions of the diagnostic statistics from Chapter 5 led us to identify six subjects that were either poorly fit or influential. The overall goodness of fit tests from Chapter 4 do not apply as the number of cases and controls are fixed by design. Clearly, once we account for the matching as a stratification variable and use conditional logistic regression, the modeling process proceeds as in the independent observation setting.

In closing this section, we note that many investigators break the matched pairs and proceed with the standard analysis as described in Chapters 4 and 5. Lynn and McCulloch (1992) provide some theoretical and simulation-based evidence for breaking the matches when the sample size is large. However, we believe that if data have been collected using a specific matched sampling design, then the analysis must have as its foundation the stratum-specific likelihood shown in equation (7.4) and the full likelihood in equation (7.3).

By ignoring the matching, we believe that investigators have used what is really an incorrect analysis for two basic reasons. First, the investigator probably is not comfortable with the conditional likelihood approach. He/she thinks that somehow the model has been changed and one cannot use estimated coefficients to estimate odds ratios in the usual manner. Second, until recently the analysis had to be performed using difference variables, a cumbersome and tedious data management task. We hope that the presentation of the example in this section convinces investigators that a matched analysis is no more difficult to carry out than an unmatched analysis.

7.4   AN EXAMPLE USING THE LOGISTIC REGRESSION MODEL IN A 1–M MATCHED STUDY

The general approach to the analysis of the 1–M matched design and, for that matter, any general matched or highly stratified design, is quite similar to that of the 1–1 matched design illustrated in the previous section. Again, we use STATA's clogit command, and associated diagnostic statistics to fit and analyze the model.

In the 1–1 matched design, the individual contribution of each matched pair to the likelihood in equation (7.4) is the conditional probability that the subject with $y = 1$ is the case among the two possible assignments of case status, the other being that the subject with $y = 0$ is the case. In a 1–M design, this same conditional probability is calculated (equation (7.4)) but there are now $M + 1$ possible assignments of case status to the matched subjects. Suppose, for example, that we consider a design where $M = 3$. Let the value of the covariates for the case in stratum k be denoted by $\mathbf{x}_{k1}$ and the values for the three controls be denoted $\mathbf{x}_{k2}$, $\mathbf{x}_{k3}$, and $\mathbf{x}_{k4}$. The contribution to the likelihood for this stratum of matched subjects from equation (7.4) is

$$l_k(\boldsymbol{\beta}) = \frac{e^{\boldsymbol{\beta}' \mathbf{x}_{k1}}}{e^{\boldsymbol{\beta}' \mathbf{x}_{k1}} + e^{\boldsymbol{\beta}' \mathbf{x}_{k2}} + e^{\boldsymbol{\beta}' \mathbf{x}_{k3}} + e^{\boldsymbol{\beta}' \mathbf{x}_{k4}}}. \tag{7.12}$$

The interpretation of equation (7.12), given the value of the coefficients, is the probability that the subject with data $\mathbf{x}_{k1}$ is the case relative to three controls with data $\mathbf{x}_{k2}$, $\mathbf{x}_{k3}$, and $\mathbf{x}_{k4}$. We note that if the covariates are identical for all four subjects then the stratum is uninformative for estimation of the coefficients as $l_k(\boldsymbol{\beta}) = 0.25$ for any value of $\boldsymbol{\beta}$. For an individual covariate, there must be at least one control that has a value different from the case or the stratum is uninformative for that specific coefficient. Unfortunately, there are no simple expressions involving discordant pairs for the estimator of the coefficient for a dichotomous covariate in a univariable model. One statistic that is helpful in assessing the potential for "thin data" for a dichotomous covariate is identifying how many of the matched sets have the sum of the covariates over the $M + 1$ subjects equal to 0 or $M + 1$. As always, we feel it is good practice to fit univariable models and use the estimated standard errors and confidence intervals as indirect evaluation for "thin data".

To provide a data set for an example and exercises we formed a 1–3 matched data set from the Burn Study data described in Section 1.6.5 and Table 1.9. We used these data in Chapter 4 for one of the examples of model building. There we found that increasing age is an important risk factor in surviving a burn injury. In Chapter 4, we included age in the model. An alternative approach to estimating the effects of covariates controlling for age is to match cases (subjects who die), to controls (subjects who live) on age. Unlike the example in Section 7.3 using the GLOW Study data we could not match exactly on age. Instead we categorized age into 5-year intervals and matched each case with three randomly selected controls from the same age group. For some age groups it was not possible to identify three controls for the case identified. For these age groups we used only as many cases as could be matched. This resulted in 97 matched sets or strata. In practice we likely would have used 1–1 or 1–2 matching in these age groups so as not to loose 28 cases. However, here the goal is to illustrate analyses with the conventional 1–*M* design. The covariates are listed in Table 1.9 and data are available at the web site as BURN13M and the covariate PAIR denotes the matched set.

We found that each of the four dichotomous covariates, race (RACE), gender (GENDER), inhalation injury (INH_INJ), and flame involved (FLAME) had a number of strata where the covariate was constant. These are described in Table 7.7. We felt that for all four covariates there were a sufficient number of strata with a nonconstant sum to retain the covariate for analysis.

Since there are only five covariates we began with a main effects model containing all five. The results of this fit are shown in Table 7.8. The Wald statistic *p*-values suggest that GENDER and FLAME are not significant. Since the *p*-value for FLAME is more than twice that of GENDER we next fit a model without FLAME. In results not shown, the likelihood ratio test comparing the model in Table 7.8 to one that excluded FLAME was not significant with $p = 0.695$. The Wald statistic for GENDER in the smaller model was not significant. We fit a model without GENDER and FLAME and confirmed that neither one contributed

Table 7.7 Distributions of Strata with Constant Covariate Sum

Covariate	Sum	Number of Strata
RACE	0	3
	4	10
GENDER	0	3
	4	25
INH_INJ	0	26
	4	0
FLAME	0	1
	4	17

Table 7.8 Estimated Coefficients, Estimated Standard Errors, Wald Statistics, and Two-Tailed *p*-Values for the Multivariable Model Containing All Covariates

Variable	Coeff.	Std. Err.	*z*	*p*
TBSA	0.133	0.0272	4.89	<0.001
GENDER	−0.670	0.5825	−1.15	0.250
RACE	−1.008	0.5269	−1.91	0.056
INH_INJ	1.500	0.6149	2.44	0.015
FLAME	−0.231	0.5869	−0.39	0.694

Table 7.9   Estimated Coefficients, Estimated Standard Errors, Wald Statistics, and Two-Tailed p-Values for the Preliminary Main Effects Model

Variable	Coeff.	Std. Err.	z	p
TBSA	0.124	0.0242	5.12	<0.001
RACE	−0.959	0.5137	−1.87	0.062
INH_INJ	1.366	0.5254	2.60	0.009

significantly to the model containing the remaining three covariates, nor was there any evidence of confounding. Hence our preliminary main effects model contains TBSA, RACE, and INH_INJ and is shown in Table 7.9.

The next step is to examine the scale of the continuous covariate total burn surface area (TBSA). In Chapter 4 using fractional polynomials we found that a model in ln(TBSA) was better than the linear model and not different from the best two term fractional polynomial model. However in this matched data set, fractional polynomial analysis using the closed test procedure did not yield a significant transformation. Further inspection of the results showed that the best one-term fractional polynomial model with power 0.5 did seem to offer some improvement over the linear model with $p = 0.057$. However, the simplicity of the linear model and the fact that the preferred closed test procedure was not significant lead us to choose modeling TBSA as linear in the logit. We leave modeling using $\sqrt{\text{TBSA}}$ as an exercise.

For interactions among model covariates, we only examined the interaction of TBSA with INH_INJ as a burn surgeon felt there was no clinical basis for any interactions with RACE. This interaction was not significant with $p = 0.167$ from the likelihood ratio test of the addition of the interaction to the model in Table 7.9. As noted in the previous section, the matching variable(s) can be effect modifiers, and thus it is good statistical practice to test for their interaction with model covariates. Rather than using the grouped age variable employed to create the matched case and three controls we used the actual value of age to form interactions with total burn surface area and inhalation injury. Neither interaction was significant at the five percent level. The AGE by TBSA interaction was significant at the 10 percent level. We leave as an exercise further analysis of a model with this interaction included. Hence, we continue using as our preliminary final model the one shown in Table 7.9.

The next step is to obtain the values of the casewise and stratum sum diagnostic statistics presented in Section 7.2 and plot them versus a relevant quantity. The plot shown in Figure 7.6 is of the leverage from equation (7.7) versus the estimated stratum specific probability, $\hat{\theta}_{kj}$. Recall that this probability estimates the stratum specific conditional probability that the subject is the case among the four subjects in the stratum. Hence, the sum of the four probabilities in each stratum is equal to one. In the figure, the controls are plotted using a small "o" and the cases are plotted using a small "x". We see that three controls have leverage values that exceed 0.06 and fall somewhat away from the rest of the data. As in the non-matched setting,

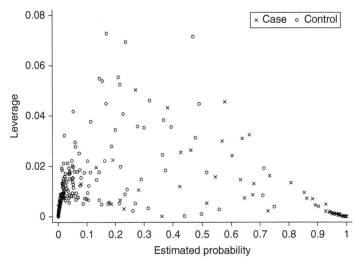

Figure 7.6 Plot of all 338 leverage values versus the estimated probability from the fitted model from the BURN 1–3 Matched Study in Table 7.9.

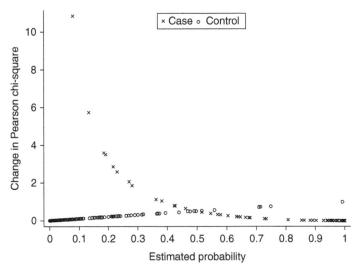

Figure 7.7 Plot of 336 values of $\Delta X^2 < 50$ versus the estimated probability from the fitted model from the BURN 1 – 3 Matched Study in Table 7.9.

we see that the leverage goes to zero as the estimated probability approaches zero or one.

Next, we plot the values of the lack of fit diagnostic, ΔX^2, from equation (7.8) versus the estimated probability. In doing so, we found that two extremely large values of 134 and 54, belonging to cases, totally distorted the plot. Hence, we excluded these two cases and plotted the diagnostic statistic in Figure 7.7. Here

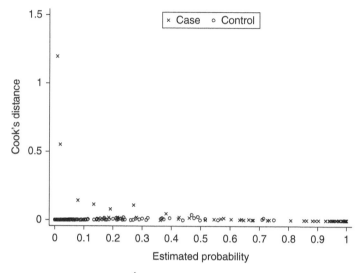

Figure 7.8   Plot of all 338 values of $\Delta\hat{\beta}\%$ versus the estimated probability from the fitted model from the BURN 1–3 Matched Study in Table 7.9.

we see that two cases have values exceeding 5 and lie away from the remainder of the data. So, in total, we found four cases with large values of the lack of fit diagnostic statistic.

The vales of the influence diagnostic statistic computed from equation (7.9) are plotted versus the estimated probability in Figure 7.8. The two values that lie well away from the rest of the data correspond to the two extremely poorly fit cases that we elected not to plot in Figure 7.7. No other values fall far enough from the rest of the data to cause concern.

The plot of the sum of the four values of ΔX^2 within 95 strata is shown in Figure 7.9. We excluded the two strata where the sum would exceed 50. The plot identifies the two strata containing the two cases identified in Figure 7.7.

Next we plot, for all 97 strata, the sum of the four values of $\Delta\hat{\beta}$ in Figure 7.10. The plot clearly identifies the two strata containing the cases that are poorly fit and excluded from Figure 7.9.

Use of the diagnostic statistics identified three controls with high leverage. When we refit the model, in work not shown, excluding these three subjects, none of the estimated coefficients changed by more than 20 percent. Hence, we do not delete these controls and consider the poorly fit and/or influential cases.

The data and values of the diagnostic statistics are shown in Table 7.10. Stratum 13 is the most poorly fit and influential. The reason is that the case's data are more like a control, moderate burn size with an inhalation injury, and the first control's data are more like that of a case, quite large burn size and an inhalation injury. The same is true, but to a lesser extent, in stratum 73 where the case had only a two percent burn area while two of the controls had areas greater than 20 percent. For strata 82 and 87, the case is also poorly fit, but less so than strata 13 and 73, and the data for the cases look more like those for controls.

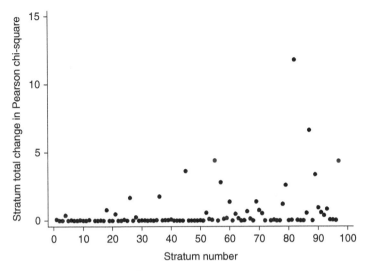

Figure 7.9   Plot of stratum sum of ΔX^2 for values less than 50 versus stratum number from the fitted model from the BURN 1–3 Matched Study in Table 7.9.

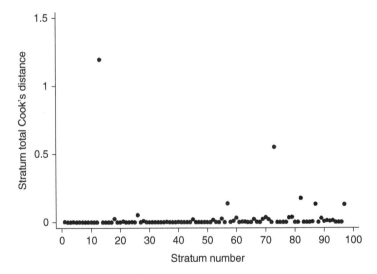

Figure 7.10   Plot of stratum sum of $\Delta\hat{\beta}\%$ versus stratum number from the fitted model from the BURN 1 – 3 Matched Study in Table 7.9.

   The next step is to sequentially delete each stratum, refit the model and compute the percent change in the coefficients from the estimates in Table 7.9. The results are shown in Table 7.11. When stratum 13 is deleted, the estimate of the coefficient for TBSA increases by 21 percent (see the definition of $\Delta\hat{\beta}$ at the bottom of Table 7.11). When we delete stratum 73 the coefficient for RACE increases by 27.8 percent.

Table 7.10 Stratum, Status, Covariates, and Diagnostic Statistics for Stratum with the Largest Values of the Diagnostic Statistics

STR	Death	T^a	R	I	$\hat{\theta}$	h	ΔX^2	$\Delta\hat{\beta}$	SumΔX^2	Sum$\Delta\hat{\beta}$
13	0	77.2	1	1	0.992	<0.001	0.992	<0.001	135.298	1.197
	0	6	1	0	0.000	<0.001	<0.001	<0.001		
	0	15	0	0	0.000	0.001	0.000	<0.001		
	1	30	0	1	0.007	0.009	134.305	1.197		
73	0	1.7	0	0	0.045	0.008	0.046	<0.001	54.977	0.553
	0	21	0	0	0.497	0.001	0.498	<0.001		
	0	20	0	0	0.439	<0.001	0.439	<0.001		
	1	2	1	0	0.018	0.010	53.994	0.552		
82	0	18	1	0	0.227	0.041	0.237	0.010	11.798	0.176
	0	2	0	1	0.319	0.046	0.335	0.016		
	0	11	1	1	0.374	0.018	0.381	0.007		
	1	9.5	1	0	0.079	0.013	10.845	0.143		
87	0	3	0	0	0.114	0.038	0.118	0.005	6.620	0.133
	0	14.5	1	1	0.714	0.019	0.728	0.014		
	0	2	1	0	0.039	0.009	0.039	<0.001		
	1	12	1	0	0.134	0.020	5.734	0.114		

^{a}Covariates: TBSA(T), RACE(R), and INH_INJ(I).

Table 7.11 Estimated Coefficients from Table 7.10 (All), Estimated Coefficients when Strata Are Deleted, and Percent Change from All

Data	TBSA	RACE	INH_INJ
All	0.124	−0.959	1.366
Delete stratum 13	0.157	−0.881	1.420
Pct. change	−21.0	8.8	−3.8
Delete stratum 73	0.141	−1.329	1.394
Pct. change	−12.1	−27.8	−2.0
Delete stratum 82	0.125	−1.065	1.583
Pct. change	−0.8	−9.9	−13.7
Delete stratum 87	0.126	−0.998	1.583
Pct. change	−1.6	−3.9	−13.7
Delete all four strata	0.216	−1.648	2.282
Pct. change	−42.6	−41.8	−40.1

Pct. change $= 100 \times \dfrac{(\hat{\beta}_{All} - \hat{\beta}_{Deleted})}{\hat{\beta}_{Deleted}}$

No coefficient changes by more than 20 percent when either stratum 82 or stratum 87 is deleted. When all four strata are deleted, a total of 16 observations, each estimate increases by more than 40 percent. Hence the diagnostic statistics have identified influential cases. The question now is: Are the data for these subjects clinically implausible or did the subject just die or survive when the model would have predicted otherwise? The only subject whose result could be suspect is the

Table 7.12   Estimated Odds Ratios and 95 Percent
Confidence Intervals from the Fitted Model in Table 7.9

Variable	Odds Ratio	95% CI
Total body surface area	3.5[a]	2.2, 5.6
Race: whites verses non-whites[a]	0.38	0.14, 1.05
Inhalation injury	3.9	1.4, 11.0

[a]Total burn surface area increase of 10%.

first control in stratum 13. On further examination, we find that this subject is quite young, 21 years old, and while all subjects in this stratum are between 20 and 24 it is unusual to survive when 77 percent of the body is burned. In the end, the burn surgeon felt that none of the data are implausible and none should be excluded. Hence, we use the fitted model in Table 7.9 as our final model.

We explore in the exercises alternative modeling of these data that compares the matched analysis to an unmatched analysis.

The estimated odds ratios and corresponding 95 percent confidence intervals for the three covariates are given in Table 7.12. Under the assumption that the logit is linear in burn area we see that for every 10 percent increase in the size of the burn the odds of dying increases 3.5-fold and the increase could be as little as 2.2 or as much as 5.6 with 95 percent confidence. The model estimates that the odds of whites dying is 62 percent less than non-whites and is not significant at the five percent level but is at the 10 percent level. The confidence interval suggests that the decrease could be as much as 86 percent. Having an inhalation injury involved in the burn increases the odds of dying by almost 4-fold and could be as little as a 1.4-fold increase or as much as an 11-fold increase.

The data used for the example in this section does not contain as many covariates as might be available in practice. However, the analysis presented certainly provides a template that could be followed for modeling in more complicated data sets.

In summary, we have shown in this chapter that modeling in the matched case-control study follows the same methods as for unmatched studies discussed in previous chapters. In particular, the diagnostic statistics are highly useful in identifying subjects and strata that have high leverage, are poorly fit and/or influential. However, at this time, there are no overall goodness of fit tests of the type discussed in Section 5.2.

EXERCISES

1. Using the first control and the case in each of the 97 strata of the BURN 1–3 matched data set, perform a complete 1–1 matched analysis.

2. Repeat the analysis in Section 7.4 using the covariate $\sqrt{TBSA}$ in place of TBSA.

3. Using the first and third controls and the case in each of the 97 strata of the Burn 1–3 matched study, perform the analysis in this 1–2 matched data.

4. Repeat the analysis in Section 7.4 as an unmatched case-control study including age as a covariate. Compare the results of this analysis to those in Section 7.4. Which analysis yields the more precise estimates of the odds ratios for TBSA, RACE, and INH_INJ?

5. Continue model building, evaluation, and presenting estimated odds ratios with the interaction between AGE and TBSA added to the model in Table 7.9.

CHAPTER 8

Logistic Regression Models for Multinomial and Ordinal Outcomes

8.1 THE MULTINOMIAL LOGISTIC REGRESSION MODEL

8.1.1 Introduction to the Model and Estimation of Model Parameters

In the previous chapters we focused on the use of the logistic regression model when the outcome variable is dichotomous or binary. This model can be easily modified to handle the case where the outcome variable is nominal with more than two levels. For example, consider a study of choice of a health plan from among three plans offered to the employees of a large corporation. The outcome variable has three levels indicating which plan, A, B or C is chosen. Possible covariates might include gender, age, income, family size, and others. The goal is to estimate the probability of choosing each of the three plans as well as to estimate the odds of plan choice as a function of the covariates and to express the results in terms of odds ratios for choice of different plans. McFadden (1974) proposed a modification of the logistic regression model and called it a *discrete choice model*. As a result, the model frequently goes by that name in the business and econometric literature while it is called the *multinomial*, *polychotomous*, or *polytomous* logistic regression model in the health and life sciences. We use the term *multinomial* in this text.

It would be possible to use an outcome variable with any number of levels to illustrate the extension of the model and methods. However, the details are most easily illustrated with three categories. Further generalization to more than three categories is a problem more of notation than of concept. Hence, in the remainder of this section, we restrict our attention to the situation where the outcome variable has three categories.

When one considers a regression model for a discrete outcome variable with more than two responses, one must pay attention to the measurement scale. In this section, we discuss the logistic regression model for the case in which the outcome

Applied Logistic Regression, Third Edition.
David W. Hosmer, Jr., Stanley Lemeshow, and Rodney X. Sturdivant.
© 2013 John Wiley & Sons, Inc. Published 2013 by John Wiley & Sons, Inc.

is nominal scale. We discuss logistic regression models for ordinal scale outcomes in the next section.

We assume that the categories of the outcome variable, Y, are coded 0, 1, or 2. In practice one should check that the software package that is going to be used allows a 0 code as we have used packages that require that the codes begin with 1. Recall that the logistic regression model we use for a binary outcome variable is parameterized in terms of the logit of $Y = 1$ versus $Y = 0$. In the three outcome category model we need two logit functions. We have to decide which outcome category to use as the referent value. The obvious extension is to use $Y = 0$ as the referent, or baseline, outcome and to form logit functions comparing each other category to it. We show later in this section that the logit function for $Y = 2$ versus $Y = 1$ is the difference between these two logit functions.

To develop the model, assume we have p covariates and a constant term, denoted by the vector $\mathbf{x}$, of length $p + 1$, where $x_0 = 1$. We denote the two logit functions as

$$
\begin{aligned}
g_1(\mathbf{x}) &= \ln \left[\frac{\Pr(Y = 1|\mathbf{x})}{\Pr(Y = 0|\mathbf{x})} \right] \\
&= \beta_{10} + \beta_{11} x_1 + \beta_{12} x_2 + \cdots + \beta_{1p} x_p \\
&= \mathbf{x}' \boldsymbol{\beta}_1
\end{aligned}
\tag{8.1}
$$

and

$$
\begin{aligned}
g_2(\mathbf{x}) &= \ln \left[\frac{\Pr(Y = 2|\mathbf{x})}{\Pr(Y = 0|\mathbf{x})} \right] \\
&= \beta_{20} + \beta_{21} x_1 + \beta_{22} x_2 + \cdots + \beta_{2p} x_p \\
&= \mathbf{x}' \boldsymbol{\beta}_2.
\end{aligned}
\tag{8.2}
$$

It follows that the conditional probabilities of each outcome category given the covariate vector are

$$
\Pr(Y = 0|\mathbf{x}) = \frac{1}{1 + e^{g_1(\mathbf{x})} + e^{g_2(\mathbf{x})}},
\tag{8.3}
$$

$$
\Pr(Y = 1|\mathbf{x}) = \frac{e^{g_1(\mathbf{x})}}{1 + e^{g_1(\mathbf{x})} + e^{g_2(\mathbf{x})}},
\tag{8.4}
$$

and

$$
\Pr(Y = 2|\mathbf{x}) = \frac{e^{g_2(\mathbf{x})}}{1 + e^{g_1(\mathbf{x})} + e^{g_2(\mathbf{x})}}.
\tag{8.5}
$$

Following the convention for the binary model, we let $\pi_j(\mathbf{x}) = \Pr(Y = j|\mathbf{x})$ for $j = 0, 1, 2$. Each probability is a function of the vector of $2(p + 1)$ parameters $\boldsymbol{\beta}' = (\boldsymbol{\beta}_1', \boldsymbol{\beta}_2')$.

A general expression for the conditional probability in the three category model is

$$\pi_j(\mathbf{x}) = \Pr(Y = j|\mathbf{x}) = \frac{e^{g_j(\mathbf{x})}}{\sum\limits_{k=0}^{2} e^{g_k(\mathbf{x})}},$$

where the vector $\boldsymbol{\beta}_0 = 0$ and $g_0(\mathbf{x}) = 0$.

To construct the likelihood function we create three binary variables coded 0 or 1 to indicate the group membership of an observation. We note that these variables are introduced only to clarify the likelihood function and are not used in the actual multinomial logistic regression analysis. The variables are coded as follows: if $Y = 0$ then $Y_0 = 1$, $Y_1 = 0$, and $Y_2 = 0$; if $Y = 1$ then $Y_0 = 0$, $Y_1 = 1$, and $Y_2 = 0$; and if $Y = 2$ then $Y_0 = 0$, $Y_1 = 0$, and $Y_2 = 1$. We note that no matter what value Y takes on, the sum of these variables is $\sum_{j=0}^{2} Y_j = 1$. Using this notation it follows that the conditional likelihood function for a sample of n independent observations is

$$l(\boldsymbol{\beta}) = \prod_{i=1}^{n} [\pi_0(\mathbf{x}_i)^{y_{0i}} \pi_1(\mathbf{x}_i)^{y_{1i}} \pi_2(\mathbf{x}_i)^{y_{2i}}].$$

Taking the log and using the fact that $\sum y_{ji} = 1$ for each i, the log-likelihood function is

$$L(\boldsymbol{\beta}) = \sum_{i=1}^{n} y_{1i} g_1(\mathbf{x}_i) + y_{2i} g_2(\mathbf{x}_i) - \ln(1 + e^{g_1(\mathbf{x}_i)} + e^{g_2(\mathbf{x}_i)}). \tag{8.6}$$

The likelihood equations are found by taking the first partial derivatives of $L(\boldsymbol{\beta})$ with respect to each of the $2(p + 1)$ unknown parameters. To simplify the notation somewhat, we let $\pi_{ji} = \pi_j(\mathbf{x}_i)$. The general form of these equations is:

$$\frac{\partial L(\boldsymbol{\beta})}{\partial \beta_{jk}} = \sum_{i=1}^{n} x_{ki}(y_{ji} - \pi_{ji}) \tag{8.7}$$

for $j = 1, 2$ and $k = 0, 1, 2, \ldots, p$, with $x_{0i} = 1$ for each subject.

The maximum likelihood estimator, $\hat{\boldsymbol{\beta}}$, is obtained by setting these equations equal to 0 and solving for $\hat{\boldsymbol{\beta}}$. The solution requires the same type of iterative computation that is used to obtain the estimate in the binary outcome case.

The matrix of second partial derivatives is required to obtain the information matrix and, from it, the estimator of the covariance matrix of the maximum likelihood estimator. The general form of the elements in the matrix of second partial derivatives is as follows:

$$\frac{\partial^2 L(\beta)}{\partial \beta_{jk} \partial \beta_{jk'}} = -\sum_{i=1}^{n} x_{k'i} x_{ki} \pi_{ji}(1 - \pi_{ji}) \tag{8.8}$$

and

$$\frac{\partial^2 L(\beta)}{\partial \beta_{jk} \partial \beta_{j'k'}} = \sum_{i=1}^{n} x_{k'i} x_{ki} \pi_{ji} \pi_{j'i} \tag{8.9}$$

for j and $j' = 1, 2$ and k and $k' = 0, 1, 2, \ldots, p$. The observed information matrix, $\hat{\mathbf{I}}(\hat{\boldsymbol{\beta}})$, is the $2(p+1)$ by $2(p+1)$ matrix whose elements are the negatives of the values in equations (8.8) and (8.9) evaluated at $\hat{\boldsymbol{\beta}}$. The estimator of the covariance matrix of the maximum likelihood estimator is the inverse of the observed information matrix,

$$\widehat{\text{Var}}(\hat{\boldsymbol{\beta}}) = [\hat{\mathbf{I}}(\hat{\boldsymbol{\beta}})]^{-1}.$$

A more concise representation for the estimator of the information matrix may be obtained by using a form similar to the binary outcome case. Let the matrix $\mathbf{X}$ be the n by $p+1$ matrix containing the values of the covariates for each subject; let the matrix $\mathbf{V}_j$ be the n by n diagonal matrix with general element $\hat{\pi}_{ji}(1 - \hat{\pi}_{ji})$ for $j = 1, 2$ and $i = 1, 2, 3, \ldots, n$; and let $\mathbf{V}_3$ be the n by n diagonal matrix with general element $\hat{\pi}_{1i}\hat{\pi}_{2i}$. The estimator of the information matrix may be expressed as

$$\hat{\mathbf{I}}(\hat{\boldsymbol{\beta}}) = \begin{bmatrix} \hat{\mathbf{I}}(\hat{\boldsymbol{\beta}})_{11} & \hat{\mathbf{I}}(\hat{\boldsymbol{\beta}})_{12} \\ \hat{\mathbf{I}}(\hat{\boldsymbol{\beta}})_{21} & \hat{\mathbf{I}}(\hat{\boldsymbol{\beta}})_{22} \end{bmatrix} \tag{8.10}$$

where

$$\hat{\mathbf{I}}(\hat{\boldsymbol{\beta}})_{11} = (\mathbf{X}'\mathbf{V}_1\mathbf{X}),$$

$$\hat{\mathbf{I}}(\hat{\boldsymbol{\beta}})_{22} = (\mathbf{X}'\mathbf{V}_2\mathbf{X}),$$

and

$$\hat{\mathbf{I}}(\hat{\boldsymbol{\beta}})_{12} = \hat{\mathbf{I}}(\hat{\boldsymbol{\beta}})_{21} = -(\mathbf{X}'\mathbf{V}_3\mathbf{X}).$$

8.1.2   Interpreting and Assessing the Significance of the Estimated Coefficients

To illustrate the methods and models in this chapter we use data from a study described in Fontanella et al. (2008) on determinants of aftercare placement for psychiatrically hospitalized adolescents. A subset of the data, suitably modified to protect confidentiality, has been made available to us by the authors. It is not our intent to repeat the detailed analyses reported in their paper, but rather to use the data to motivate and describe methods for modeling multinomial and ordinal scaled outcomes using logistic regression models. Fontanella et al. (2008) model a four-category outcome variable, PLACE, with the following values/categories: $0 =$ Outpatient, $1 =$ Day Treatment, $2 =$ Intermediate Residential and $3 =$ Residential. To simplify the presentation in this section we combined the first two placement categories, Outpatient and Day Treatment* to form a new outcome variable,

---

*We performed preliminary analyses, not shown here, that justify pooling these two outcome categories. We use the four category outcome in the exercises.

PLACE3, with values/categories as follows: $0 =$ Outpatient or Day Treatment, $1 =$ Intermediate Residential and $2 =$ Residential. The subset of variables from the main study that we use is described in Table 1.8. The data are available from the website in the file ALR3_APS.

To simplify the discussion of the estimation and interpretation of odds ratios in other multinomial outcome settings we need to generalize the notation used in the binary outcome case to include the outcomes being compared as well as the values of the covariate. We assume that the outcome labeled with $Y = 0$ is the reference outcome. The subscript on the odds ratio indicates which outcome is being compared to the reference outcome. The odds ratio of outcome $Y = j$ versus outcome $Y = 0$ for covariate values of $x = a$ versus $x = b$ is

$$OR_j(a, b) = \frac{Pr(Y = j|x = a)/Pr(Y = 0|x = a)}{Pr(Y = j|x = b)/Pr(Y = 0|x = b)}.$$

In the special case when the covariate is binary, coded 0 or 1, we simplify the notation to $OR_j = OR_j(1, 0)$.

We begin by considering a model containing a single dichotomous covariate coded 0 or 1. In the binary outcome model the estimated slope coefficient is identical to the log-odds ratio obtained from the 2×2 table cross-classifying the outcome and the covariate. As we noted, when the outcome has three levels there are two logit functions. We define these functions in such a way that the two estimated coefficients, one from each logit function are, respectively, equal to the log-odds ratios from the pair of 2×2 tables obtained by cross-classifying the $y = j$ and $y = 0$ outcomes by the covariate, with $y = 0$ as the reference outcome value.

As a specific example, consider the cross-classification of PLACE3 versus history of violence (VIOL) displayed in Table 8.1. When we use PLACE3 $= 0$ as the reference outcome the two odds ratios calculated from Table 8.1 are

$$\widehat{OR}_1 = \frac{104 \times 80}{179 \times 26} = 1.79$$

and

$$\widehat{OR}_2 = \frac{104 \times 80}{179 \times 15} = 3.10.$$

Table 8.1 Cross-Classification of Placement (PLACE3) by History of Violence (VIOL) and Estimated Odds Ratios Using Day or Outpatient as the Reference Outcome Value

PLACE3	History of Violence		Total	$\widehat{OR}$
	No (0)	Yes (1)		
Day or Outpatient (0)	80	179	259	1.00
Intermediate residential (1)	26	104	130	1.79
Residential (2)	15	104	119	3.10
Total	121	387	508	

The results of fitting a three-category logistic regression model, using STATA's mlogit command, to these data are presented in Table 8.2. In this table, the values labeled $\widehat{OR}$ are obtained by exponentiating the estimated slope coefficients, and they are identical to the odds ratios calculated directly from the cell counts given in Table 8.1.

As is the case in the binary outcome setting with a dichotomous covariate, the estimated standard error of the coefficient [i.e., the ln(OR)] is the square root of the sum of the inverse of the cell frequencies. For example, the estimated standard error of the coefficient for VIOL in the first logit is

$$\widehat{SE}(\hat{\beta}_{11}) = \left[\frac{1}{80} + \frac{1}{179} + \frac{1}{26} + \frac{1}{104}\right]^{0.5} = 0.2572,$$

which is identical to the value in Table 8.2.

The endpoints of the confidence interval for the odds ratio are obtained in exactly the same manner as for the binary outcome case. First we obtain the confidence interval for the coefficient and then exponentiate the endpoints of the interval to obtain the confidence interval for the odds ratio. For example, the 95% confidence interval for the odds ratio of PLACE3 = 1 versus PLACE3 = 0 shown in Table 8.2 is calculated as follows:

$$\exp(0.581 \pm 1.96 \times 0.2572) = (1.08, 2.96).$$

The endpoints for the confidence interval for PLACE3 = 2 versus PLACE3 = 0 in Table 8.2 are obtained in a similar manner.

We interpret each estimated odds ratio and its corresponding confidence interval as if it came from a binary outcome setting. In some cases it may further support the analysis to compare the magnitude of the two estimated odds ratios. This can be done with or without tests of equality.

The interpretation of the effect of history of violence is as follows: (i) The odds among adolescents with a history of violence of being placed in an intermediate residential facility is 1.79 times greater than the odds among adolescents without a history of violence. The confidence interval indicates that the odds could be a little as 1.1 times or as much as 3 times larger with 95% confidence. (ii) The odds among adolescents with a history of violence of being placed in a residential facility is 3.1 times greater than the odds among adolescents without a history of violence. The odds could be a little as 1.7 times or as much as 5.7 times larger with 95%

Table 8.2   Results of Fitting the Logistic Regression Model to the Data in Table 8.1

Logit	Variable	Coeff.	Std. Err.	$\widehat{OR}$	95% CI
1	VIOL	0.581	0.2572	1.79	1.08, 2.96
	Constant	−1.124	0.2257		
2	VIOL	1.131	0.3072	3.10	1.70, 5.66
	Constant	−1.674	0.2814		

confidence. Thus we see that having a history of violence is a significant factor for being placed in some type of residential facility.

Although the odds ratio for placement in a residential facility is roughly twice that for an intermediate facility, the two values may be within sampling variation of each other. We note that the test of the equality of the two odds ratios, $OR_1 = OR_2$, is equivalent to a test that the log-odds for PLACE3 $= 2$ versus PLACE3 $= 1$ is equal to 0. The simplest way to obtain the point and interval estimate is from the difference between the two estimated slope coefficients in the logistic regression model. For example, using the frequencies in Table 8.1 and the estimated coefficients from Table 8.2 we have

$$\hat{\beta}_{21} - \hat{\beta}_{11} = 1.131 - 0.581$$

$$= 0.550$$

$$= \ln\left(\frac{104/119}{15/119}\right) - \ln\left(\frac{104/130}{26/130}\right)$$

$$= \ln\left(\frac{26}{15}\right).$$

The estimator of the variance of the difference between the two coefficients, $\hat{\beta}_{21} - \hat{\beta}_{11}$, is

$$\widehat{\text{Var}}(\hat{\beta}_{21} - \hat{\beta}_{11}) = \widehat{\text{Var}}(\hat{\beta}_{21}) + \widehat{\text{Var}}(\hat{\beta}_{11}) - 2 \times \widehat{\text{Cov}}(\hat{\beta}_{21}, \hat{\beta}_{11}).$$

We obtain values for the estimates of the variances and covariances from a listing of the estimated covariance matrix, which is an option in most, if not all, packages. As described in Section 8.1.1 the form of this matrix is a little different from the covariance matrix in the binary setting. There are two matrices containing the estimates of the variances and covariances of the estimated coefficients in each logit and a third matrix containing the estimated covariances of the estimated coefficients from the different logits. The matrix for the model in Table 8.2 is shown in Table 8.3, where Logit 1 is the logit function for PLACE3 $= 1$ versus PLACE3 $= 0$ and Logit 2 is the logit function for PLACE3 $= 2$ versus PLACE3 $= 0$.

Using the results in Table 8.3 we obtain the estimate of the variance of the difference in the two estimated coefficients as

$$\widehat{\text{Var}}(\hat{\beta}_{21} - \hat{\beta}_{11}) = 0.09437 + 0.06616 - 2 \times 0.01809 = 0.12435.$$

Table 8.3   Estimated Covariance Matrix for the Fitted Model in Table 8.2

		Logit 1		Logit 2	
		VIOL	Constant	VIOL	Constant
Logit 1	VIOL	0.06616			
	Constant	−0.05096	0.05096		
Logit 2	VIOL	0.01809	−0.01250	0.09437	
	Constant	−0.01250	0.01250	−0.07917	0.07917

The endpoints of a 95% confidence interval for this difference are

$$0.550 \pm 1.96 \times \sqrt{0.12435} = (-0.1412, 1.2412).$$

As the confidence interval includes 0 we cannot conclude that the log-odds ratio for PLACE3 = 1 is different from the log-odds ratio for PLACE3 = 2. Equivalently, we can express these results in terms of odds ratios by exponentiating the point and interval estimates. This yields the odds ratio for PLACE3 = 2 versus PLACE3 = 1 as $\widehat{OR} = 1.73$ and a confidence interval of $(0.868, 3.460)$. The interpretation of this odds ratio is that the odds of residential placement is 1.73 times larger than the odds for intermediate residential placement among adolescents with a history of violence.

In practice, if there was no difference in the separate odds ratios over all model covariates then we might consider pooling outcome categories 1 and 2 to obtain the binary outcome: 0 = Outpatient or day treatment and 1 = Residential, intermediate or full time. We return to this question following model development in the next section.

We note that in a model with many covariates the extra computations required for these auxiliary comparisons could become a burden. In this setting, procedures like STATA's *test* or *lincom* commands are quite helpful.

A preliminary indication of the importance of the variable may be obtained from the two Wald statistics; however, as is the case with any multi degree of freedom variable, we should use the likelihood ratio test to assess the significance. For example, to test for the significance of the coefficients for VIOL we compare the log-likelihood from the model containing VIOL to the log-likelihood for the model containing only the two constant terms, one for each logit function. Under the null hypothesis that the coefficients are 0, minus twice the change in the log-likelihood follows a chi-square distribution with 2 degrees of freedom. In this example, the log-likelihood for the constant only model is $L_0 = -524.37093$ and the log-likelihood of the fitted model is $L_1 = -515.73225$. The value of the statistic is

$$G = -2 \times [-524.37093 - (-515.73225)] = 17.2774,$$

which yields a p-value of 0.0002. Thus, from a statistical point of view, the variable VIOL is significantly associated with adolescent placement.

In general, the likelihood ratio test for the significance of the coefficients for a variable has degrees of freedom equal to the number of outcome categories minus one times the degrees of freedom for the variable in each logit. For example, if we were using the four category outcome variable, PLACE, and the four category covariate danger to others (DANGER) then the degrees of freedom are $(4 - 1) \times (4 - 1) = 9$. This is easy to keep track of if we remember that we are modeling separate logits for comparing the reference outcome category to each other outcome category.

For a categorical covariate with more than two levels we expand the number of odds ratios to include comparisons of each level of the covariate to a reference level for each possible logit function. To illustrate this we consider the danger to others

(DANGER) modeled via three design variables using the value of 0 (Unlikely) as the reference covariate value. The cross-classification of PLACE3 by DANGER is given in Table 8.4.

Using the value of PLACE3 $= 0$ as the reference outcome category and DANGER $= 0$ as the reference covariate value, the six odds ratios are as follows:

$$\widehat{OR}_1(1, 0) = \frac{32 \times 42}{7 \times 46} = 4.174,$$

$$\widehat{OR}_1(2, 0) = \frac{48 \times 42}{7 \times 62} = 4.645,$$

$$\widehat{OR}_1(3, 0) = \frac{43 \times 42}{7 \times 109} = 2.367,$$

$$\widehat{OR}_2(1, 0) = \frac{23 \times 42}{5 \times 46} = 4.2,$$

$$\widehat{OR}_2(2, 0) = \frac{31 \times 42}{5 \times 62} = 4.2$$

and

$$\widehat{OR}_2(3, 0) = \frac{60 \times 42}{5 \times 109} = 4.624.$$

The results of fitting the logistic regression model to the data in Table 8.4 are presented in Table 8.5.

Table 8.4   Cross-Classification of Placement (PLACE3) by Danger to Others (DANGER)

| PLACE3 | DANGER | | | | |
	Unlikely (0)	Possibly (1)	Probably (2)	Likely (3)	Total
Day or Outpatient (0)	42	46	62	109	259
Intermediate Residential (1)	7	32	48	43	130
Residential (2)	5	23	31	60	119
Total	54	101	141	212	508

Table 8.5   Results of Fitting the Logistic Regression Model to the Data in Table 8.4

	Variable	Coeff.	Std. Err.	$\widehat{OR}$	95% CI
Logit 1	DANGER_1	1.429	0.4687	4.174	1.666, 10.459
	DANGER_2	1.536	0.4513	4.645	1.918, 11.249
	DANGER_3	0.862	0.4462	2.367	0.987, 5.675
	Constant	−1.792	0.4082		
Logit 2	DANGER_1	1.435	0.5376	4.200	1.464, 12.047
	DANGER_2	1.435	0.5217	4.200	1.511, 11.677
	DANGER_3	1.531	0.4997	4.624	1.737, 12.311
	Constant	−2.128	0.4731		

We see that exponentiation of the estimated logistic regression coefficients yields precisely the same odds ratios as were obtained from the cell counts of the 2×2 tables formed from the original 3×4 contingency table. The odds ratios for logit 1 are obtained from the 2×4 table containing the rows corresponding to PLACE3 $= 0$ and PLACE3 $= 1$ and the four columns. The odds ratios for logit 2 are obtained from the 2×4 table containing the rows corresponding to PLACE3 $= 0$ and PLACE3 $= 2$ and the four columns.

To assess the significance of the variable DANGER, we calculate minus twice the change in the log-likelihood relative to the constant only model. The value of the test statistic is

$$G = -2 \times [-524.37093 - (-510.21286)] = 28.3161,$$

and, with 6 degrees of freedom, yields a p-value of < 0.001.

Thus, we conclude that an adolescent's danger to others is significantly associated with placement. Before proceeding with further analyses of DANGER it is worth noting that the estimated standard error of a coefficient is the square root of the sum of the inverse of the cell frequencies. For example, the standard error of the log-odds of DANGER $= 3$ versus DANGER $= 0$ in the first logit is

$$\widehat{SE}(\hat{\beta}_{13}) = \left[\frac{1}{7} + \frac{1}{109} + \frac{1}{43} + \frac{1}{42} \right]^{0.5} = 0.4462.$$

We note that the frequencies in the last two rows of the "Unlikely" response column in Table 8.4 are small relative to rest of the table (i.e., 7 and 5). As "Unlikely" is the referent exposure value all standard error estimates contain the inverse of either 7 or 5. A question we are frequently asked is: "If I change the reference exposure to the one with the largest frequencies, 'Likely' in this case, will the estimated log-odds ratios have smaller estimated standard errors?" The answer is not a simple yes or no as the two sets of results are not comparable as they estimate entirely different odds ratios. Also, the value of the likelihood ratio test is exactly the same for all parameterizations of the six design variables. We leave examples showing this as an exercise. In our view, one should define the design variables to yield estimates of odds ratios that are most clinically meaningful. In the case of the covariate DANGER we feel that comparisons to "Unlikely" are most meaningful and are the simplest to interpret.

Any continuous covariate that is modeled as linear in the logit has a single estimated coefficient for each logit function. Hence exponentiation of the estimated coefficient gives the estimated odds ratio for a change of one unit in the variable. Thus, remarks in Chapter 3 about knowing what a single unit is and estimation of odds ratios for a clinically meaningful change apply directly to each logit function in the multinomial logistic regression model as well.

8.1.3 Model-Building Strategies for Multinomial Logistic Regression

In principle, the strategies and methods for multivariable modeling with a multinomial outcome variable are identical to those for the binary outcome variable discussed in Chapter 4. The theory for stepwise selection of variables has been worked out and is available in some packages. However, the method is not currently available in many of the other widely distributed statistical software packages, such as STATA. To illustrate modeling and interpretation of the results, we proceed with an analysis of the data from the Adolescent Placement Study.

The data we use for the Adolescent Placement Study has 11 independent variables and 508 subjects. We could begin model building with a model containing all 11 variables. However two covariates, NEURO and DANGER, have four response levels and this generates six coefficients each. Thus a model with all 11 covariates would have 32 estimated coefficients. With only 508 subjects we would almost certainly risk numeric instability. Hence, we begin by fitting the 11 individual univariable models with results summarized in Table 8.6.

The variable neuropsychiatric disturbance (NEURO) is not significant at the 0.25 level. Also, none of the Wald tests for the six coefficients are significant. Hence this variable is not a candidate for inclusion in the multivariable model.

The variable danger to others (DANGER) is highly significant but, as we saw from the calculations of the six odds ratios in Table 8.5, the values are not especially different from each other. The multivariable Wald test of the equality of the three coefficients in the second logit function in Table 8.5 is not significant with $p = 0.917$. This suggests that one could pool the three categories "Possible", "Probably", and "Likely" into a single category. The 2 degrees of freedom, multivariable Wald test for the first logit is significant ($p = 0.024$), but the one degree of freedom Wald test for the equality of the first two coefficients is not significant ($p = 0.721$). Hence there are several options available for pooling categories: (i) Form a dichotomous covariate with 0 = "Unlikely" and 1 = "Not Unlikely" or (ii) Form a three category variable with 0 = "Unlikely", 1 = "Possible", or "Probable", and 2 = "Likely". We choose option (i) as it results in a much simpler model with little difference in the first logit function. Thus we proceed using the dichotomous coding and call

Table 8.6 Results of Fitting Univariable Models with Three Levels of Placement (PLACE3) as the Outcome

Variable	Likelihood Ratio Test	DF	p
AGE	7.52	2	0.023
RACE	4.01	2	0.135
GENDER	3.70	2	0.157
NEURO	3.12	6	0.794
EMOT	7.37	2	0.025
DANGER	28.32	6	<0.001
ELOPE	10.57	2	0.005
LOS	165.85	2	<0.001
BEHAV	60.17	2	<0.001
CUSTD	225.15	2	<0.001
VIOL	17.28	2	<0.001
DANGER_D	18.53	2	<0.001

Table 8.7   Estimated Coefficients, Estimated Standard Errors, Wald Statistics, and Two-Tailed p-Values for the Multivariable Model

	Variable	Coeff.	Std. Err.	z	p
Logit 1	AGE	0.177	0.0938	1.89	0.058
	RACE	0.671	0.3111	2.16	0.031
	GENDER	0.493	0.3416	1.44	0.149
	EMOT	0.515	0.3613	1.42	0.154
	DANGER_D	1.226	0.6801	1.80	0.071
	ELOPE	−0.247	0.3356	−0.73	0.462
	LOS	0.055	0.0144	3.81	<0.001
	BEHAV	0.056	0.1018	0.55	0.582
	CUSTD	4.038	0.3459	11.67	<0.001
	VIOL	−0.208	0.4922	−0.42	0.673
	Constant	−7.500	1.6235	−4.62	<0.001
Logit 2	AGE	0.198	0.0981	2.02	0.043
	RACE	0.657	0.3232	2.03	0.042
	GENDER	0.406	0.3491	1.16	0.245
	EMOT	0.431	0.3824	1.13	0.260
	DANGER_D	0.208	0.8438	0.25	0.805
	ELOPE	0.389	0.3401	1.15	0.252
	LOS	0.087	0.0140	6.20	<0.001
	BEHAV	0.414	0.1144	3.62	<0.001
	CUSTD	2.515	0.3615	6.96	<0.001
	VIOL	−0.009	0.6049	−0.02	0.988
	Constant	−9.398	1.7796	−5.28	<0.001

it DANGER_D. Results for the fit of this model containing only DANGER_D are shown in the last row of Table 8.6.

Hence our first multivariable model is one containing 10 covariates with DANGER recoded. The results of the fit are presented in Table 8.7.

Since the fitted model contains 10 covariates each with two coefficients we must proceed cautiously with model simplification. We use the p-values from the Wald tests to identify possible variables to eliminate and then use the two degree of freedom likelihood ratio test to confirm our decision. Following the fit of the reduced model we must check that the coefficients for the remaining covariates have not changed by more than 20–25%.

The least significant variable in Table 8.7 is history of violence (VIOL). The significance level of the likelihood ratio test for its removal from the model is $p = 0.898$ and none of the coefficients changed by more than 20%. In a similar manner we eliminated ELOPE, EMOT and GENDER. The results for the fit of the six variable models are shown in Table 8.8.

We see that in this six-covariate model the estimated coefficient for the dichotomized version of danger to others (DANGER_D) is nearly significant in the first but not the second logit and the reverse is true for behavioral score (BEHAV). The two variables confound each other's association with placement

Table 8.8   Estimated Coefficients, Estimated Standard Errors, Wald Statistics, and Two-Tailed p-Values for the Six Variable Multivariable Model

	Variable	Coeff.	Std. Err.	z	p
Logit 1	AGE	0.174	0.0920	1.89	0.058
	RACE	0.623	0.3067	2.03	0.042
	DANGER_D	1.135	0.6235	1.82	0.069
	LOS	0.055	0.0142	3.87	<0.001
	BEHAV	0.058	0.0879	0.66	0.506
	CUSTD	3.956	0.3337	11.86	<0.001
	Constant	−7.229	1.5955	−4.53	<0.001
Logit 2	AGE	0.202	0.0962	2.10	0.036
	RACE	0.650	0.3193	2.04	0.042
	DANGER_D	0.210	0.7286	0.29	0.773
	LOS	0.086	0.0138	6.23	<0.001
	BEHAV	0.425	0.1009	4.21	<0.001
	CUSTD	2.528	0.3512	7.20	<0.001
	Constant	−9.070	1.7408	−5.21	<0.001

as the mean behavioral score at level unlikely (DANGER_D $= 0$) is 3 whereas the mean is 6 in the not unlikely group (DANGER_D $= 1$) and the difference is significant. When we delete one of the variables and perform the likelihood ratio test we find that it is not significant for deleting DANGER_D with $p = 0.15$ and is significant for BEHAV with $p < 0.001$. After evaluating the role that either of these variables may play as a confounder we find that none of the coefficients for AGE, RACE, LOS or CUSTD changed by more than 20% comparing the six to either five variable model. However, as expected, the coefficients for DANGER_D and BEHAV did change when the other was deleted. After considering these details we decided that we need both behavioral score and danger to others in the model. Hence we consider the model in Table 8.8 as our preliminary main effects model.

The model in Table 8.8 contains continuous covariates: age, length of stay and behavioral score. We checked for the scale of each of these covariates using fractional polynomials. This analysis showed that there was no evidence of nonlinearity in either logit function for both age and behavioral score. For length of stay the best one-term fractional polynomial transformation, the square root, was significantly better than the linear model and the best two-term fractional polynomial model was not better than the square root transformation. The log transformation was the second-best transformation. Hence our main effects model contains square root of length of stay, denoted by LOS_5.

The next step in model building is to consider possible interactions between the main effects. In work not shown, we found that the only significant interaction was between LOS_5 and CUSTD. The effect of the interactions on the model is to reduce the slope in the square root of LOS to the point of nonsignificance in the first logit but not in the second logit function. Since this interaction is clinically

Table 8.9   Estimated Coefficients, Estimated Standard Errors, Wald Statistics, and Two-Tailed p-Values for the Preliminary Final Multivariable Model

	Variable	Coeff.	Std. Err.	z	p
Logit 1	AGE	0.182	0.0942	1.93	0.053
	RACE	0.652	0.3144	2.07	0.038
	DANGER_D	1.073	0.6369	1.69	0.092
	BEHAV	0.080	0.0906	0.89	0.375
	LOS_5	0.634	0.1357	4.67	<0.001
	CUSTD	6.068	0.8365	7.25	<0.001
	LxC[a]	−0.639	0.2293	−2.79	0.005
	Constant	−8.956	1.7042	−5.26	<0.001
Logit 2	AGE	0.194	0.0968	2.00	0.045
	RACE	0.625	0.3211	1.94	0.052
	DANGER_D	0.248	0.7408	0.33	0.738
	BEHAV	0.410	0.1019	4.03	<0.001
	LOS_5	0.834	0.1272	6.56	<0.001
	CUSTD	3.086	0.8812	3.50	<0.001
	LxC[a]	−0.254	0.2281	−1.11	0.266
	Constant	−10.546	1.8145	−5.81	<0.001

[a]LxC = LOS_5 × CUSTD and LOS_5 = $\sqrt{LOS}$.

plausible our preliminary final model includes it, yielding the fitted model shown in Table 8.9.

The model in Table 8.9 contains two logit functions, each with seven covariates and a constant term. Each logit function is not overly complicated but the fact that there are two functions complicates presentation of results. However, the model in Table 8.9 is the *preliminary* final model. As in the examples in previous chapters, any model selected by purposeful selection is "preliminary" until we evaluate its fit and check for influential and poorly fit subjects.

In packages that do not support the full range of methods for assessing the fit of multinomial logistic models an alternative is to approximate the fit by fitting separate binary models. Begg and Gray (1984) proposed this approach. For example, in a three group problem we would fit a model for $Y = 1$ versus $Y = 0$ (ignoring the $Y = 2$ data) using a standard logistic regression package for a binary outcome variable and then fit separately a model for $Y = 2$ versus $Y = 0$ (ignoring the $Y = 1$ data). Begg and Gray show that the estimates of the logistic regression coefficients obtained in this manner are consistent, and under many circumstances the loss in efficiency is not too great. It has been our experience that the coefficients obtained from separately fit logistic models are, in general, close to those from the multinomial fit. This suggests that the individualized fitting approach can be useful for scale selection for continuous covariates in packages that do not support fractional polynomial analysis when fitting the multinomial model and for diagnostic statistics. We use this approach in the next section to examine the diagnostic statistics. We compare the estimated coefficients from the multinomial logistic fit in Table 8.9 to estimates obtained from the two separate binary fits in Table 8.10. Out of the

Table 8.10 Comparison of the Estimated Coefficients from a Multinomial Logistic Fit and Independent Logistic Regression Fit (ILR)

	Variable	Coeff. Multinomial Logistic	ILR	Pct. Difference[a]
Logit 1	AGE	0.182	0.137	−24.5
	RACE	0.652	0.646	−0.9
	DANGER_D	1.073	0.919	−14.4
	BEHAV	0.080	0.115	42.7
	LOS_5	0.634	0.589	−7.0
	CUSTD	6.068	5.899	−2.8
	LxC[b]	−0.639	−0.591	−7.5
	Constant	−8.956	−8.217	−8.2
Logit 2	AGE	0.194	0.200	3.1
	RACE	0.625	0.496	−20.5
	DANGER_D	0.248	0.203	−18.2
	BEHAV	0.410	0.459	11.8
	LOS_5	0.834	0.911	9.2
	CUSTD	3.086	3.219	4.3
	LxC[b]	−0.254	−0.277	9.0
	Constant	−10.546	−11.120	5.4

[a] $\Delta\hat{\beta}\% = 100 \times \frac{(\hat{\beta}_{ILR} - \hat{\beta}_{Mult})}{\hat{\beta}_{Mult}}$.

[b] $LxC = LOS\_5 \times CUSTD$ and $LOS\_5 = \sqrt{LOS}$.

16 coefficients, 4 differ by more than 18%. The largest difference, 42%, is between the estimates of the coefficient for BEHAV.

8.1.4 Assessment of Fit and Diagnostic Statistics for the Multinomial Logistic Regression Model

As with any fitted model, before it can be used to make inferences, the overall fit and the contribution of each subject to the fit must be assessed. In multinomial logistic regression, the multiple outcome categories make this a more difficult problem than was the case with a model for a binary outcome variable. When we model a binary outcome variable we have a single fitted value, the estimated logistic probability of the outcome being present, $\Pr(Y = 1|\mathbf{x})$. When the outcome variable has three categories we have two estimated logistic probabilities, the estimated probabilities of categories 1 and 2, $\Pr(Y = 1|\mathbf{x})$ and $\Pr(Y = 2|\mathbf{x})$.

Fagerland (2009) and Fagerland et al. (2008) developed an extension, for the multinomial logistic regression model, of the decile of risk goodness of fit test discussed in Chapter 5 for the binary case. Fagerland and Hosmer (2012a) presented a STATA program to calculate the test. Other work includes Goeman and le Cessie (2006), who developed a smoothed residual based test of goodness of fit, but this test has not been implemented in commonly available software packages. Fagerland (2009) extended the normalized Pearson chi-square test discussed in Chapter 5 to the multinomial setting. The computations are somewhat complex and the test is not yet available in current software.

Fagerland's extension of the decile of risk test forms g groups using the ranked values of $1 - \hat{\pi}_0$, the complement of the estimate of the probability $\Pr(Y = 0|\mathbf{x})$. One forms a table of observed and expected frequencies over the K levels of the outcome variable and g groups. The test statistic is calculated as

$$\widehat{C}_M = \sum_{i=1}^{g} \sum_{j=0}^{K-1} \frac{(O_{ij} - \hat{E}_{ij})^2}{\hat{E}_{ij}}, \tag{8.11}$$

where $O_{ij} = \sum_{l \in \Omega_i} y_{lj}$, $\hat{E}_{ij} = \sum_{l \in \Omega_i} \hat{\pi}_{lj}$, and Ω_i denote the subjects in the ith group. Fagerland (2009) and Fagerland et al. (2008) show by simulations that when the sample is sufficiently large and the correct model has been fit that $\widehat{C}_M$ follows a chi-square distribution with $(g - 2) \times (K - 1)$ degrees of freedom. In the binary outcome setting, $K = 2$, this test is identical to $\widehat{C}$ described in Chapter 5. In settings where the number of covariate patterns is appreciably less than the sample size $\widehat{C}_M$ should be calculated by covariate patterns, as shown in Chapter 5.

Lesaffre (1986), Lesaffre and Albert (1989) have proposed extensions of the logistic regression diagnostics to the multinomial logistic regression model. However, these methods are not easily calculated using the available software. This is somewhat surprising given that programs to fit the multinomial logistic regression model are now widespread. Thus, until software developers add these methods to their packages we recommend calculating multinomial logistic regression diagnostics using the individual logistic regressions approach of Begg and Gray. An alternative to using the coefficients from the separate logistic regression fit, see Table 8.10, is to employ the "trick" illustrated in Section 6.4 where one forces the iterative estimation process to begin using the coefficients from the multinomial logistic fit in Table 8.9 and the iterations are set to 0. This effectively forces calculation of the diagnostic statistics in Chapter 5 using the multinomial fit. If it is not possible to use the "trick" in a software package then we recommend using the separate logistic fit and its diagnostics statistics.

We illustrate the methods by considering assessment of fit of the multinomial logistic regression model shown in Table 8.9 for the Adolescent Placement Study. The results are shown in Table 8.11. In this example the number of covariate patterns is equal to the sample size so we calculate $\widehat{C}_M$ using equation (8.11). The value of the goodness of fit test is $\widehat{C}_M = 8.523$ and, with $16 = (10 - 8) \times (3 - 1)$ degrees of freedom, yields $p = 0.932$, which supports model fit. We note that there is quite good agreement between the observed and estimated expected frequencies. By way of explanation, the observed frequency of 23 in the "Place3 = 0" column and Group = 6 row is the number of subjects with PLACE_3 = 0 and estimated logistic probability $\hat{\pi}_0$ such that $0.4281 < 1 - \hat{\pi}_0 \le 0.7746$. The observed frequency is $23 = \sum_{l \in \Omega_6} y_{l0}$ and the estimated expected frequency is $19.12 = \sum_{l \in \Omega_6} \hat{\pi}_{l0}$. Other observed and expected values are calculated in a similar manner.

Table 8.11   Observed (Obs) and Estimated Expected (Exp) Frequencies Within Each Group for PLACE_3 = 1, PLACE_3 = 2, and PLACE_3 = 0 Using the Fitted Logistic Regression Model for the Adolescent Placement Study in Table 8.9

Group	Cut Point	Place_3 = 1		Place_3 = 2		Place_3 = 0		Total
		Obs	Exp	Obs	Exp	Obs	Exp	
1	0.0476	0	0.74	0	0.89	51	49.37	51
2	0.092	2	1.77	2	1.81	47	47.41	51
3	0.1389	3	3.22	4	2.8	44	44.99	51
4	0.2042	5	5.33	3	3.3	43	42.37	51
5	0.4281	11	9.08	7	5.08	32	35.84	50
6	0.7746	13	14.1	15	17.78	23	19.12	51
7	0.8606	12	10.09	28	31.59	11	9.32	51
8	0.9003	12	11.74	36	33.22	3	6.05	51
9	0.9536	19	19.33	28	27.9	4	3.78	51
10	1.0	42	43.61	7	5.63	1	0.76	50

The next step is to calculate and examine the diagnostic statistics to check for poorly fit and influential subjects. In this example we were able, using STATA, to obtain diagnostics based on the estimates of the coefficients in Table 8.9. We realize that some readers will not be able to obtain diagnostic statistics based on the coefficients in Table 8.9, as a result we also calculated diagnostics using the independent logistic fit (ILR) shown in Table 8.10. The same subjects were identified using either set of diagnostic statistics. We leave the plots as an exercise and summarize our findings.

For each plot (see Section 5.3 for our suggestions of plots to assess the diagnostic statistics) we selected, for further examination, all subjects with one or more diagnostic statistics that fell well away from the bulk of the plotted values. These are summarized in Table 8.12.

The standard procedure at this point is to successively delete each one of these subjects, refit the model and use $\Delta\hat{\beta}\%$ to evaluate their effect on the magnitude of the estimated coefficients. The results of the deletions are summarized in the last column of Table 8.12. There we see that five of the eight identified subjects have an undue influence on the estimate of the dichotomized version of danger to others, DANGER_D. The results agree with the diagnostic, except for subject 144 where the effect should have been on logit 1, not logit 2. The diagnostic statistics are not infallible predictors of effect and that is why it is always a good idea to delete and refit.

When we delete the five subjects with influence on the coefficient for DANGER_D in the second logit the estimate decreases by 178%. The magnitude of the change is not totally unexpected as two of the six frequencies in the 3×2 table of PLACE3 by DANGER_D are 7 and 5. In addition, the estimate of BEHAV increases by 51% in logit 1.

When we examined the data for the eight subjects in Table 8.12 no values seemed clinically implausible. Thus, based on our assessment of model fit and the

Table 8.12   **Subjects with Large Values for One or More Diagnostic Statistic from Either or Both Logit 1 or Logit 2 and their Effect on the Fitted Logistic Regression Model for the Adolescent Placement Study in Table 8.9**

Subject	Diagnostic	Deletion Effect on Estimated Parameters
76	Large ΔX^2 logit 1	No major effect on the estimates
85	Large $\Delta \hat{\beta}$ logit 1 and logit 2	Estimate of the coefficient of $L \times C$ decreases by 45%
109	Large $\Delta \hat{\beta}$ logit 2	Estimate of the coefficient of DANGER_D in logit 2 decreases by 105%
144	High leverage and large $\Delta \hat{\beta}$ logit 1	Estimate of the coefficient of DANGER_D in logit 2 decreases by 112%
220	Large ΔX^2 logit 2	Estimate of the coefficient of DANGER_D in logit 2 decreases by 52%
266	Large ΔX^2 and large $\Delta \hat{\beta}$ logit 2	Estimate of the coefficient of DANGER_D in logit 2 increases by 189%
288	Large ΔX^2 logit 1	No major effect on the estimates
421	Large ΔX^2 logit 2	Estimate of the coefficient of DANGER_D in logit 2 decreases by 46%

Table 8.13   **Estimated Odds Ratios and 95% Confidence Intervals for Age, Race, and Behavioral Symptoms Score**

Variable	Intermediate versus Outpatient or Day		Residential versus Outpatient or Day	
	Odds Ratio	95% CI	Odds Ratio	95% CI
AGE	1.44[a]	0.99, 2.08	1.47	1.01, 2.15
RACE	1.92	1.03, 3.55	1.87	0.99, 3.50
BEHAV	1.17[a]	0.82, 1.67	2.27	1.52, 3.39

[a]Odds ratio for a 2-year increase in age or 2-point increase in behavioral symptoms score.

diagnostic statistics we conclude that the final model is the one in presented in Table 8.9. Estimated odds ratios and 95% confidence intervals for covariates not involved in an interaction are shown in Table 8.13.

The estimated odds ratios in Table 8.13 show that with a 2-year increase in age there is a 1.4-fold increase in the odds of being placed in an intermediate or residential facility. Nonwhites have an approximately 1.9-fold increase in the odds of an intermediate or residential placement compared to whites. A two-point increase in the behavioral index score increases the odds of a residential placement 2.3-fold and is significant. However, the increase in the odds of an intermediate facility placement is not significant.

Length of stay transformed (LOS_5) and state custody (CUSTD) have a significant overall interaction using the 2 degrees of freedom likelihood ratio test, but the Wald test for the coefficient is significant only in logit 1. When we compare the results for these two covariates we see that, in the main effects model in Table 8.8, both are significant in each logit function. The fact that the interaction term is significant in only one logit function in Table 8.9 makes their combined effect difficult to discern by simply examining the coefficients. Hence we used the four-step procedure described in Chapter 4 and the coefficients in Table 8.9 to obtain the following equations for the log-odds ratio for each logit function:

$$\ln\{\widehat{OR}(CUSTD = 1, CUSTD = 0|LOS, Logit\ 1)\} = 6.068 - 0.639 \times LOS\_5$$

and

$$\ln\{\widehat{OR}(CUSTD = 1, CUSTD = 0|LOS, Logit\ 2)\} = 3.086 - 0.254 \times LOS\_5.$$

These two functions and their 95% confidence bands are plotted in Figure 8.1. We choose to show the two plots side by side on the same scale for the log-odds ratio to allow a better comparison. We added a line at 0 to aid in assessing the range of LOS where the log-odds ratio and hence odds ratio is significant. The general picture that emerges is: (i) The log-odds ratio decreases as length of stay increases. (ii) Being in state custody significantly increases the odds of placement in an intermediate residential facility compared to outpatient or day treatment when the length of stay is less than about 50 days. (iii) The log-odds ratio for state custody in the logit for residential placement versus outpatient or day treatment is significant only for LOS less than 10 days. Note that this is an entirely different conclusion than would have

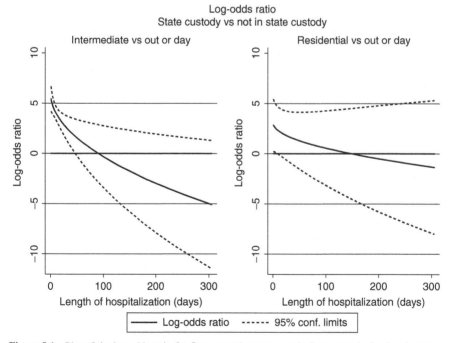

Figure 8.1 Plot of the log-odds ratio for State custody versus not in State custody for the placement in an intermediate residential facility versus outpatient or day treatment and residential facility versus outpatient or day treatment.

been reached had we, incorrectly, used the main effects model in Table 8.8. This is a good opportunity for the reader to reflect back on the differences, discussed in Chapter 4, between a covariate being a confounder and an effect modifier.

The next step is to estimate the odds ratio for increasing length of stay within levels of state custody for the two logit functions. The calculations are similar to those required for Figure 8.1 and we present the results for the log-odds ratio for a 5-day increase in length of stay in Figure 8.2. In each subfigure there are two curves each with confidence bands. One set of lines is for subjects in state custody (CUSTD = 1) and the other set is for subjects not in state custody (CUSTD = 0). Some of the confidence limit lines are so similar that they cannot be differentiated in the figure.

Looking at the left sub-figure in Figure 8.2 (intermediate versus outpatient or day treatment) we see that the log-odds ratio for subjects not in state custody is significantly different from 0, for example, OR > 1, but the effect of an additional 5 days decreases as the reference length of stay increases. The log-odds ratio for subjects in state custody is not significant. In fact, the log-odds ratio is nearly equal to 0 for all values of length of stay.

For the right sub-figure in Figure 8.2 (residential versus outpatient or day treatment) we see that the log-odds ratios at both levels of state custody are quite similar, as there is little separation between the solid and long dashed lines. At all

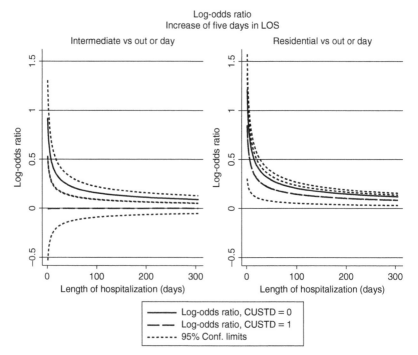

Figure 8.2 Plot of the log-odds ratio for an increase of 5 days in length of stay for subjects in State custody and subjects not in State custody in logit functions for placement in an intermediate residential facility versus outpatient or day treatment and residential facility versus outpatient or day treatment.

values of length of stay the lower confidence limits exceed 0 (i.e., OR > 1), hence the log-odds ratios are significant. The estimate of the effect of a 5-day increase decreases as the reference length of stay increases.

The main goal of the Adolescent Placement Study is to assess the effect of various subject characteristics on aftercare placement with little or no interest in estimation of probabilities. Thus an ROC analysis of the type described and illustrated in Chapter 5 would not be appropriate. However, if estimation of probabilities of placement were of interest then the ROC analyses would have to be performed using separate binary regressions as methods in Chapter 5 have not been extended to the multinomial logistic regression model.

As the discussion of the results shows, the real challenge when fitting a multinomial logistic regression model is the fact that there are multiple odds ratios for each model covariate. This certainly complicates the discussion. On the other hand, using a multinomial outcome can provide a more complete description of the process being studied. For example, if we had combined the two residential placements into a single outcome category "not outpatient or day treatment", we would have missed the differences in covariates effects in the two logits. From a statistical point of view, one should not pool the outcome categories unless the estimated coefficients in the logits are not significantly different from each other. In the case of the model in Table 8.9 the multivariable Wald test of the equality of the seven coefficients in the two logits is $W = 66.63$ which, with 7 degrees of freedom, yields $p < 0.001$. Thus we feel that there is strong statistical evidence that creating a pooled outcome category would not be appropriate.

In summary, fitting and interpreting the results from a multinomial logistic regression model follow the same basic paradigm as was followed for a binary model. The difference is that the user should be aware of the possibility that informative comparative statements may be required for the multiple odds ratios for each covariate.

8.2 ORDINAL LOGISTIC REGRESSION MODELS

8.2.1 Introduction to the Models, Methods for Fitting, and Interpretation of Model Parameters

There are occasions when the scale of a multiple category outcome is not nominal but ordinal. Common examples of ordinal outcomes include variables such as extent of disease (none, some, severe), job performance (inadequate, satisfactory, outstanding), and opinion on a political candidate's position on some issue (strongly disagree, disagree, agree, strongly agree). In such a setting one could use the multinomial logistic model described in Section 8.1. This analysis, however, would not take into account the ordinal nature of the outcome and hence the estimated odds ratios may not address the questions asked of the analysis. In this section we consider a number of different logistic regression models that do take the rank ordering of the outcomes into account. Each model we discuss can be fit either directly or with some slight modification of existing statistical software.

It has been our experience that a problem many users have with ordinal logistic regression models is that there is more than one model to choose from. In the next section we describe and then compare through an example three of the most commonly used models: the adjacent-category, the continuation-ratio and the proportional odds models. There is a fairly large literature considering various aspects of ordinal logistic regression models. A few of the more general references include the texts Agresti (2002) and Agresti (2010), which discuss the three models we consider as well as other more specialized models, and the text by McCullagh and Nelder (1989). Ananth and Kleinbaum (1997), in a review paper, consider the continuation-ratio and the proportional odds models as well as three other less frequently used models: the unconstrained partial-proportional odds model, the constrained partial-proportional odds model and the stereotype logistic model. Greenland (1994) also considers the continuation-ratio, the proportional odds models and the stereotype logistic model.

Assume that the ordinal outcome variable, Y, can take on $K + 1$ values coded $0, 1, 2, \ldots, K$. We denote a general expression for the probability that the outcome is equal to k conditional on a vector, $\mathbf{x}$, of p covariates as $\Pr[Y = k \mid \mathbf{x}] = \phi_k(\mathbf{x})$. If we assume that the model is the multinomial logistic model in Section 8.1 then $\phi_k(\mathbf{x}) = \pi_k(\mathbf{x})$ where, for $K = 2$, the model is given in equations (8.3)–(8.5). In the context of ordinal logistic regression models the multinomial model is frequently called the *baseline logit model*. This term arises from the fact that the model is usually parameterized so that the coefficients are log-odds ratios comparing category $Y = k$ to a "baseline" category, $Y = 0$. As shown in Section 8.1 the fully parameterized baseline logistic regression model has $K \times (p + 1)$ coefficients. Under this model the logits, as shown in Section 8.1, are

$$g_k(\mathbf{x}) = \ln \left[\frac{\pi_k(\mathbf{x})}{\pi_0(\mathbf{x})} \right] = \beta_{k0} + \mathbf{x}'\boldsymbol{\beta}_k \qquad (8.12)$$

for $k = 1, 2, \ldots, K$.

When we move to an ordinal model we have to decide what outcomes to compare and what the most reasonable model is for the logit. For example, suppose that we wish to compare each response to the next larger response. This model is called the *adjacent-category logistic model*. If we assume that the log-odds does not depend on the response and the log-odds is linear in the coefficients then the adjacent category logits are as follows:

$$a_k(\mathbf{x}) = \ln \left[\frac{\phi_k(\mathbf{x})}{\phi_{k-1}(\mathbf{x})} \right] = \alpha_k + \mathbf{x}'\boldsymbol{\beta} \qquad (8.13)$$

for $k = 1, 2, \ldots, K$. The adjacent-category logits are a constrained version of the baseline logits. To see this we express the baseline logits in terms of the adjacent-category logits as follows:

$$\frac{\phi_k(\mathbf{x})}{\phi_0(\mathbf{x})} = \frac{\phi_1(\mathbf{x})}{\phi_0(\mathbf{x})} \times \frac{\phi_2(\mathbf{x})}{\phi_1(\mathbf{x})} \times \cdots \times \frac{\phi_k(\mathbf{x})}{\phi_{k-1}(\mathbf{x})},$$

thus

$$\ln\left[\frac{\phi_k(\mathbf{x})}{\phi_0(\mathbf{x})}\right] = \ln\left[\frac{\phi_1(\mathbf{x})}{\phi_0(\mathbf{x})}\right] + \ln\left[\frac{\phi_2(\mathbf{x})}{\phi_1(\mathbf{x})}\right] + \cdots + \ln\left[\frac{\phi_k(\mathbf{x})}{\phi_{k-1}(\mathbf{x})}\right]$$

$$= a_1(\mathbf{x}) + a_2(\mathbf{x}) + \cdots + a_k(\mathbf{x})$$

$$= (\alpha_1 + \mathbf{x}'\boldsymbol{\beta}) + (\alpha_2 + \mathbf{x}'\boldsymbol{\beta}) + \cdots + (\alpha_k + \mathbf{x}'\boldsymbol{\beta})$$

$$= (\alpha_1 + \alpha_2 + \cdots + \alpha_k) + k\mathbf{x}'\boldsymbol{\beta}. \tag{8.14}$$

Thus we see that the model in equation (8.14) is a version of the baseline model in equation (8.12) with intercept $\beta_{k0} = (\alpha_1 + \alpha_2 + \cdots + \alpha_k)$ and slope coefficients $\boldsymbol{\beta}_k = k\boldsymbol{\beta}$. As we show shortly in an example, an easy way to fit the adjacent-category model is via a constrained baseline logistic model.

Suppose instead of comparing each response to the next larger response we compare each response to all lower responses that is $Y = k$ versus $Y < k$ for $k = 1, 2, \ldots, K$. This model is called the *continuation-ratio logistic model*. We define the logit for this model as follows:

$$r_k(\mathbf{x}) = \ln\left[\frac{\Pr(Y = k|\mathbf{x})}{\Pr(Y < k|\mathbf{x})}\right]$$

$$= \ln\left[\frac{\phi_k(\mathbf{x})}{\phi_0(\mathbf{x}) + \phi_1(\mathbf{x}) + \cdots + \phi_{k-1}(\mathbf{x})}\right]$$

$$= \theta_k + \mathbf{x}'\boldsymbol{\beta}_k \tag{8.15}$$

for $k = 1, 2, \ldots, K$. Under the parameterization in equation (8.15) the continuation-ratio logits have different constant terms and slopes for each logit. The advantage of this unconstrained parameterization is that the model can be fit via K ordinary binary logistic regression models. We demonstrate this fact via an example shortly. We can also constrain the model in equation (8.15) to have a common vector of slope coefficients and different intercepts, namely

$$r_k(\mathbf{x}) = \theta_k + \mathbf{x}'\boldsymbol{\beta}. \tag{8.16}$$

Special software is required to fit the model in equation (8.16). For example, Wolfe (1998) has developed a command for use with STATA. We note that it is also possible to define the continuation ratio in terms of $Y = k$ versus $Y > k$ for $k = 0, 1, \ldots, K - 1$. Unfortunately the results one obtains from the two parameterizations are not equivalent. We prefer the formulation given in equations (8.15) and (8.16) because, if $K = 1$, each of the models in equations (8.12)–(8.16) simplifies to the usual logistic regression model where the odds ratios compare response $Y = 1$ to response $Y = 0$.

The third ordinal logistic regression model we consider is the proportional odds model. With this model we compare the probability of an equal or smaller response,

$Y \le k$, to the probability of a larger response, $Y > k$,

$$c_k(\mathbf{x}) = \ln \left[\frac{\Pr(Y \le k | \mathbf{x})}{\Pr(Y > k | \mathbf{x})} \right]$$

$$= \ln \left[\frac{\phi_0(\mathbf{x}) + \phi_1(\mathbf{x}) + \cdots + \phi_k(\mathbf{x})}{\phi_{k+1}(\mathbf{x}) + \phi_{k+2}(\mathbf{x}) + \cdots + \phi_K(\mathbf{x})} \right]$$

$$= \tau_k - \mathbf{x}'\boldsymbol{\beta} \tag{8.17}$$

for $k = 0, 1, \ldots, K - 1$. We note that in the case when $K = 1$ the model as defined in equation (8.17) simplifies to the complement of the usual logistic regression model in that it yields odds ratios of $Y = 0$ versus $Y = 1$. We negate the coefficient vector in equation (8.17) to be consistent with software packages such as STATA and other references discussing this model.

The method used to fit each of the models, except the unconstrained continuation-ratio model, is based on an adaptation of the multinomial likelihood and its log shown in equation (8.6) for $K = 2$. The basic procedure involves the following steps: (i) the expressions defining the model-specific logits are used to create an equation defining $\phi_k(\mathbf{x})$ as a function of the unknown parameters. (ii) The values of a $K + 1$ dimensional multinomial outcome, $\mathbf{z}' = (z_0, z_1, \ldots, z_K)$, are created from the ordinal outcome as $z_k = 1$ if $y = k$ and $z_k = 0$ otherwise. It follows that only one value of z is equal to 1. The general form of the likelihood for a sample of n independent observations, $(y_i, \mathbf{x}_i)$, $i = 1, 2, \ldots, n$, is

$$l(\boldsymbol{\beta}) = \prod_{i=1}^{n} [\phi_0(\mathbf{x}_i)^{z_{0i}} \phi_1(\mathbf{x}_i)^{z_{1i}} \times \cdots \times \phi_K(\mathbf{x}_i)^{z_{Ki}}],$$

where we use "$\boldsymbol{\beta}$" somewhat imprecisely to denote both the p slope coefficients and the K model-specific intercept coefficients. It follows that the log-likelihood function is

$$L(\boldsymbol{\beta}) = \sum_{i=1}^{n} z_{0i} \ln[\phi_0(\mathbf{x}_i)] + z_{1i} \ln[\phi_1(\mathbf{x}_i)] + \cdots + z_{Ki} \ln[\phi_K(\mathbf{x}_i)]. \tag{8.18}$$

We obtain the MLEs of the parameters by differentiating equation (8.18) with respect to each of the unknown parameters, setting each of the $K + p$ equations equal to 0 and solving for "$\hat{\boldsymbol{\beta}}$". We obtain the estimator of the covariance matrix of the estimated coefficients in the usual manner by evaluating the inverse of the negative of the matrix of second order partial derivatives at "$\hat{\boldsymbol{\beta}}$".

At this point in the discussion it is not especially worthwhile to show the specific form of $\phi_k(\mathbf{x})$ for each model, the details of the likelihood equations or the matrix of second order partial derivatives. Instead, we focus on a simple example to illustrate the use of the models and to aid in the interpretation of the odds ratios that result from each of them. As we noted earlier, an ordinal scale outcome can arise in a number of different ways. For example, we can create an ordinal outcome by categorizing an observed continuous outcome variable. Alternatively, we may observe categories that we hypothesize have come from categorizing a hypothetical and unobserved continuous outcome. This is often a useful way to envision outcome scales in categories ranging from strongly disagree to strongly agree. Another possibility is that the outcome is a composite of a number of other scored variables. Common examples are health status or extent of disease, which arise from many individual clinical indicators such as the Apgar score of a baby at birth. The Apgar score ranges between 0 and 10 and is the sum of 5 variables, each scored as 0, 1, or 2.

The example we use to initially illustrate each of the models comes from the Low Birth Weight Study (see Section 1.6.2) where we form a four category outcome from birth weight (BWT) using cutpoints: 2500g, 3000g, and 3500g. This example is not typical of many ordinal outcomes that use loosely defined "low," "medium," or "high" categorizations of some measurable quantity. Instead, here we explicitly derived this variable from a measured continuous variable. We make use of this fact when we show how the proportional odds model can be derived from the categorization of a continuous variable. In addition some of the exercises are designed to extend this discussion. First, we need to give some thought to the assignment of codes to the outcome variable, as this has implications on the definition of the odds ratio calculated by the various ordinal models. The obvious choice is to use the naturally increasing sequence of codes: 0 if $BWT \leq 2500$, 1 if $2500 < BWT \leq 3000$, 2 if $3000 < BWT \leq 3500$, and 3 if $BWT > 3500$. This coding is appropriate if we want low or lower weight as the reference outcome. However this is in the opposite direction of how we modeled low birth weight in earlier chapters. Thus a decreasing sequence of codes might make more sense to use for some ordinal models namely: 3 if $BWT \leq 2500$, 2 if $2500 < BWT \leq 3000$, 1 if $3000 < BWT \leq 3500$, and 0 when $BWT > 3500$. With this coding, the heaviest births are the reference outcome. This is the coding we use for the outcome variable BWT4 in this section. In truth, the actual coding, for the most part, does not make much of a difference, as long as one is able to figure out how to correct the signs of the coefficients obtained by software packages. We illustrate this with examples.

As a starting point consider the crossclassification of BWT4 versus smoking status of the mother during the pregnancy shown in Table 8.14.

Table 8.14 Cross-Classification of the Four Category Ordinal Scale Birth Weight Outcome versus Smoking Status of the Mother

Birth Weight Category	Smoking Status		Total
	No (0)	Yes (1)	
0: BWT > 3500	35	11	46
1: 3000 < BWT ≤ 3500	29	17	46
2: 2500 < BWT ≤ 3000	22	16	38
3: BWT ≤ 2500	29	30	59
Total	115	74	189

The odds ratios for the multinomial or baseline logit model defined in equation (8.12) are

$$\widehat{OR}(1, 0) = \frac{17 \times 35}{29 \times 11} = 1.87,$$

$$\widehat{OR}(2, 0) = \frac{16 \times 35}{22 \times 11} = 2.31$$

and

$$\widehat{OR}(3, 0) = \frac{30 \times 35}{29 \times 11} = 3.29,$$

where we use $\widehat{OR}(k, 0)$ to denote the odds ratio of maternal smoking for BWT4 $= k$ versus BWT4 $= 0$. The increase in the odds ratio demonstrates an increase in odds of a progressively lower weight baby among women who smoke during pregnancy. The adjacent-category model postulates that the log-odds of each successively higher category compared to the baseline is a constant multiple of the log-odds of $Y = 1$ versus $Y = 0$.

Under the adjacent-category model, the relationship we require is $\ln[OR(k, 0)] = k \times \ln[OR(1, 0)]$. The results of fitting the adjacent-category model via a constrained baseline model are shown in Table 8.15.

We obtain the equations for the adjacent-category logits by using the algebraic relationship between the constrained baseline and adjacent-category models shown in equation (8.14). It follows that the first estimated adjacent-category logit is identical to the first estimated baseline logit, namely

$$\hat{a}_1(\text{SMOKE}) = -0.110 + 0.370 \times \text{SMOKE}.$$

The estimated coefficient for SMOKE in the second adjacent-category logit is the same as in the first. The estimated coefficient for logit 2 in Table 8.15 is twice the value in logit 1 and reflects the constraint placed on the fitted baseline logit model. It follows from equation (8.14) that the estimate of the constant term for the second adjacent-category logit is equal to the difference between the two estimated constant terms in Table 8.15,

$$\hat{\alpha}_2 = \hat{\beta}_{20} - \hat{\beta}_{10} = -0.441 - (-0.110) = -0.331.$$

Table 8.15   Estimated Coefficients, Standard Errors, z-Scores, and Two-Tailed p-Values for the Fitted Constrained Baseline Model

Logit	Variable	Coeff.	Std. Err.	z	p
1	SMOKE	0.370	0.1332	2.77	0.006
	Constant	−0.110	0.2106	−0.52	0.602
2	SMOKE	0.739	0.2664	2.77	0.006
	Constant	−0.441	0.2333	−1.89	0.059
3	SMOKE	1.109	0.3996	2.77	0.006
	Constant	−0.175	0.2495	−0.70	0.483

Log-likelihood = −255.6528

Hence the equation for the second adjacent-category logit is

$$\hat{a}_2(\text{SMOKE}) = -0.331 + 0.370 \times \text{SMOKE}.$$

The equation for the third adjacent-category logit is obtained in a similar manner. In particular the estimated coefficient for SMOKE shown in the third logit in Table 8.15 is three times the estimated coefficient for the first logit. It follows from equation (8.14) that the estimate of constant term is $\hat{\alpha}_3 = \hat{\beta}_{30} - \hat{\beta}_{20} = -0.175 - (-0.441) = 0.266$. Hence the third estimated adjacent-category logit is

$$\hat{a}_3(\text{SMOKE}) = 0.266 + 0.370 \times \text{SMOKE}.$$

Under the adjacent-category model the estimate of the odds ratio for smoking status during pregnancy of the mother is

$$\widehat{\text{OR}}(k, k-1) = \exp(0.370) = 1.45$$

for $k = 1, 2, 3$. The interpretation of this estimate is that the odds of a birth in the next lower weight category among women who smoke during pregnancy are 1.45 times the odds among women who do not smoke.

Since the adjacent-category model is a constrained baseline model we can test that the two models are not different from each other via a likelihood ratio test or multivariable Wald test. The log-likelihood for the fitted baseline model (output not shown) based on the data in Table 8.14 is -255.4859. Thus, the likelihood ratio test is

$$G = -2[-255.6528 - (-255.4859)] = 0.334,$$

which, with 2 degrees of freedom, gives $p = \text{Pr}(\chi^2(2) > 0.334) = 0.846$. The 2 degrees of freedom come from the constraints described earlier for adjacent-category logits 2 and 3. In general the degrees of freedom for this test are $[(K + 1) - 2] \times p$ where $K + 1$ is the number of categories and p is the number of covariates in each model. In work not shown we obtained the same result with the Wald test. Thus we cannot say that the adjacent-category model is different from the baseline model. Since the adjacent-category model summarizes the effect of smoking into a single odds ratio we might prefer to use this model. However, this discussion considered only one covariate and the final decision in any practical setting should consider all model covariates as well as an evaluation of model fit.

Next we consider the continuation-ratio model. As shown in equation (8.15) the coefficients for this model yield the log-odds for a birth in one of the weight categories relative to all lighter weight categories. The unconstrained model described in equation (8.15) can be fit via a set (three in this case) of binary logistic regressions. Each fit is based on a binary outcome, y_k^*, defined as follows:

$$y_k^* = \begin{cases} 1 & \text{if } y = k \\ 0 & \text{if } y < k \\ \text{Missing} & \text{if } y > k \end{cases}$$

Table 8.16   Estimated Coefficients, Standard Errors, z-Scores, and Two-Tailed p-Values for the Fitted Unconstrained Continuation-Ratio Model

Logit	Variable	Coeff.	Std. Err.	z	p	Log-Likelihood
1	SMOKE	0.623	0.4613	1.35	0.177	−62.8400
	Constant	−0.188	0.2511	−0.75	0.454	
2	SMOKE	0.508	0.3991	1.27	0.203	−77.7436
	Constant	−1.068	0.2471	−4.32	0.000	
3	SMOKE	0.704	0.3196	2.20	0.028	−114.9023
	Constant	−1.087	0.2147	−5.06	<0.001	
Total log-likelihood						−225.4859

for $k = 1, 2, 3$. The results of fitting the unconstrained continuation-ratio logit model containing SMOKE are shown in Table 8.16. The results of the three separate fits are summarized into one single table for purposes of emphasizing that we have fit a single multiple-category outcome. This model is, in terms of the number of parameters and log-likelihood, fully equivalent to the unconstrained baseline model. Note that, as shown at the bottom of Table 8.16, the sum of the values of the log-likelihoods from the three separate fits is equal to the log-likelihood from the unconstrained baseline model.

The three estimated coefficients in Table 8.16 are quite similar (all are approximately 0.6). The estimates indicate that the odds of a birth in the next lower weight category relative to higher weight categories among women who smoked during pregnancy is about $1.8 = \exp(0.6)$ times that of women who did not smoke.

To test for the equality of the three smoking coefficients, we make use of the fact that, as a result of the definition of the model, the three sets of parameter estimates are independent. Thus a simple test for equality is the 2 degrees of freedom chi-square statistic

$$W^2 = \frac{(0.623 - 0.508)^2}{[(0.4613)^2 + (0.3991)^2]} + \frac{(0.623 - 0.704)^2}{[(0.4613)^2 + (0.3196)^2]} = 0.056$$

which yields $p = \Pr[\chi^2(2) > 0.056] = 0.972$. Hence we cannot say, at the 0.05 level, that the three coefficients are different and we consider fitting the constrained continuation-ratio logit model in equation (8.16).

The results of fitting this model are shown in Table 8.17. The estimate of the odds ratio for smoking during pregnancy is $1.87 = \exp(0.627)$. The wording of the interpretation is the same as that given for the approximate value from the unconstrained model. This odds ratio is a bit larger than the estimate of 1.45 obtained under the adjacent-category model. The reason is that the reference group for the continuation-ratio model includes all heavier weight categories and not just the next highest, which is used in the adjacent-category model.

In general, the continuation-ratio model might be preferred over the baseline and adjacent-category model when the conditioning used in defining and fitting the model makes clinical sense. A common example is one where the number of

Table 8.17 Estimated Coefficients, Standard Errors, z-Scores, and Two-Tailed p-Values for the Fitted Constrained Continuation-Ratio Model

Variable	Coeff.	Std. Err.	z	p
SMOKE	0.627	0.2192	2.86	0.004
Constant1	−0.189	0.2204		
Constant2	−1.114	0.2129		
Constant3	−1.052	0.1862		

Log-likelihood = −255.5594

attempts to pass a test or attain some binary outcome is modeled. The first logit models the log-odds of passing the test the first time it is taken. The second logit models the log-odds of passing the test on the second attempt given that it was not passed on the first attempt. And this process continues until one is modeling the Kth attempt. Since this is not a common setting we do not consider the model in any more detail. Further elaboration and discussion can be found in the references cited earlier in this section.

The most frequently used ordinal logistic regression model in practice is the constrained cumulative logit model (called the *proportional odds model*) given in equation (8.17). Each of the previously discussed models for ordinal data compares a single outcome response to one or more reference responses (e.g., $Y = k$ versus $Y = k - 1$, or $Y = k$ versus $Y < k$). The proportional odds model describes a less than or equal versus more comparison. For example if the outcome is extent of disease the model gives the log-odds of no more severe outcome versus a more severe outcome. The constraint placed on the model is that the log-odds do not depend on the outcome category. Thus inferences from fitted proportional odds models lend themselves to a general discussion of direction of response and do not have to focus on specific outcome categories. The results are much simpler to describe than those from any of the unconstrained models but are of about the same order of complexity as results from the other constrained models.

This consistency of effect across response categories in the proportional odds model is similar to that described for the constrained adjacent-category and continuation-ratio models and, as such, should always be tested.

Ananth and Kleinbaum (1997) discuss modifications of the proportional odds model that allow one or more covariates to have category-specific effects. These "partial" proportional odds models have not, as yet, seen wide use in practice and we do not consider them further in this text.

One way of deriving the proportional odds model is via categorization of an underlying continuous response variable. This derivation is intuitively appealing in that it allows us to use some concepts from linear regression modeling. For example, the cutpoints used to obtain the four-category variable BWT4 are 2500, 3000 and 3500 grams. Because of the way packages handle the proportional odds model it turns out to be more convenient to code the ordinal outcome so it increases in the same direction as its underlying continuous response. Thus we define the outcome BWT4N as follows: 0 if BWT $\leq$ 2500, 1 if 2500 < BWT $\leq$ 3000, 2 if 3000 < BWT $\leq$ 3500, and 3 when BWT > 3500 and the specific cutpoints as $cp_1 = 2500$, $cp_2 = 3000$, and $cp_3 = 3500$.

We show in Figure 8.3 a hypothetical line or model, BWT $= \lambda_0 + \lambda_1 \times$ LWT, that describes mean birth weight as a function of mother's weight at the last menstrual period. The particular values used to obtain the line are $\lambda_0 = 100$ and $\lambda_1 = 20$ and are for demonstration purposes only. The actual linear regression of BWT on LWT could have been used; however, the resulting graph would not have had as large a range in the BWT axis or as steep a slope. It is the idea that is important not the actual numbers.

Suppose that instead of the usual normal errors linear regression model we have a model where the errors follow the logistic distribution. The statistical model for birth weight is then BWT $= \lambda_0 + \lambda_1 \times$ LWT $+ \sigma \times \varepsilon$, where σ is proportional to the variance and ε follows the standard logistic distribution with cumulative distribution function

$$\Pr(\varepsilon \leq z) = \frac{e^z}{1 + e^z}. \tag{8.19}$$

Evans et al. (2000) discuss this distribution.

The regression based on the continuous outcome models the mean of BWT as a function of LWT. In ordinal logistic regression we model the probability that BWT falls in the four intervals defined by the three cutpoints shown in Figure 8.3. For example, we show in Figure 8.4 the underlying logistic distribution for the regression model in Figure 8.3 at LWT = 125. The mean is 2600 grams. The probabilities for the four ordinal outcomes are the respective areas under this curve. The area below 2500 is the largest indicating that, among women who

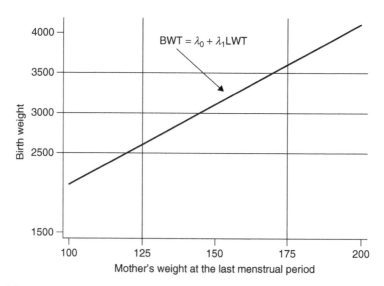

Figure 8.3   Plot of a hypothetical model describing mean birth weight as a function of mother's weight.

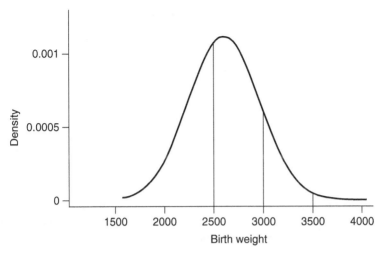

Figure 8.4 Plot of the hypothetical underlying distribution of birth weight among mothers with LWT = 125.

weigh 125 pounds, a birth weight less than or equal to 2500 grams (BWT4N = 0) is the most likely ordinal outcome. However, at 175 pounds the mean from the regression line is 3600 grams and the probability is largest for the BWT4N = 3 ordinal outcome and smallest for the BWT4N = 0 ordinal outcome. Under the proportional odds model we model the ratios of cumulative areas defined by the cutpoints.

Consider women who weigh 125 pounds. Under our coding of the four-category ordinal variable BWT4N we have

$$\Pr(\text{BWT4N} = 0 | \text{LWT} = 125) = \Pr(\text{BWT} \leq cp_1 | \text{LWT} = 125)$$

$$= \Pr[(\lambda_0 + 125 \times \lambda_1 + \sigma \times \varepsilon) \leq cp_1]$$

$$= \Pr\left[\varepsilon \leq \frac{cp_1 - (\lambda_0 + 125 \times \lambda_1)}{\sigma}\right]$$

$$= \Pr[\varepsilon \leq \tau_1 - 125 \times \beta] \tag{8.20}$$

where we let $\tau_1 = (cp_1 - \lambda_0)/\sigma$ and $\beta = \lambda_1/\sigma$. Under the assumption of errors with the distribution function in equation (8.19), the probability in equation (8.20) is

$$\Pr[\varepsilon \leq \tau_1 - 125 \times \beta] = \frac{e^{\tau_1 - 125 \times \beta}}{1 + e^{\tau_1 - 125 \times \beta}}. \tag{8.21}$$

It follows from equation (8.21) that

$$\Pr(\varepsilon > \tau_1 - 125 \times \beta) = 1 - \Pr(\varepsilon \leq \tau_1 - 125 \times \beta) = \frac{1}{1 + e^{\tau_1 - 125 \times \beta}}. \tag{8.22}$$

Hence the log-odds of a lighter weight baby at this cutpoint among 125 pound women is

$$\ln\left[\frac{\Pr(BWT4N \leq 0|LWT = 125)}{\Pr(BWT4N > 0|LWT = 125)}\right] = \ln\left[\frac{\Pr\left(\varepsilon \leq \tau_1 - 125 \times \beta\right)}{\Pr(\varepsilon > \tau_1 - 125 \times \beta)}\right]$$

$$= \ln\left[\frac{\frac{e^{\tau_1 - 125 \times \beta}}{1 + e^{\tau_1 - 125 \times \beta}}}{\frac{1}{1 + e^{\tau_1 - 125 \times \beta}}}\right] \qquad (8.23)$$

$$= \ln[e^{\tau_1 - 125 \times \beta}]$$

$$= \tau_1 - 125 \times \beta,$$

which is the proportional odds model in equation (8.17). If we follow the steps in equations (8.20)–(8.23) then we obtain identical expressions for the other outcome categories. For example, at the cutpoint cp_3 we have the log-odds

$$\ln\left[\frac{\Pr(BWT4N \leq 2|LWT = 125)}{\Pr(BWT4N > 2|LWT = 125)}\right] = \ln\left[\frac{\Pr\left(\varepsilon \leq \tau_3 - 125 \times \beta\right)}{\Pr(\varepsilon > \tau_3 - 125 \times \beta)}\right]$$

$$= \tau_3 - 125 \times \beta.$$

By similar calculations at $BWT4N = 1$ among 175 pound women the log-odds is

$$\ln\left[\frac{\Pr(BWT4N \leq 1|LWT = 175)}{\Pr(BWT4N > 1|LWT = 175)}\right] = \ln\left[\frac{\Pr\left(\varepsilon \leq \tau_2 - 175 \times \beta\right)}{\Pr(\varepsilon > \tau_2 - 175 \times \beta)}\right]$$

$$= \tau_2 - 175 \times \beta.$$

We can follow the same derivation for any covariate, x, and any number of categories for an ordinal outcome variable, Y, and we obtain as the log-odds for as small or smaller outcome the equation

$$\ln\left[\frac{\Pr(Y \leq k|x)}{\Pr(Y > k|x)}\right] = \ln\left[\frac{\Pr\left(\varepsilon \leq \tau_{k+1} - x \times \beta\right)}{\Pr(\varepsilon > \tau_{k+1} - x \times \beta)}\right] = \tau_{k+1} - x \times \beta, \qquad (8.24)$$

for $k = 0, 1, \ldots, K - 1$. It follows from equation (8.24) that the log of the odds ratio for $x = x_1$ versus $x = x_0$ is

$$\ln\left[\frac{\Pr(Y \leq k|x_1)}{\Pr(Y > k|x_1)}\right] - \ln\left[\frac{\Pr(Y \leq k|x_0)}{\Pr(Y > k|x_0)}\right] = (\tau_{k+1} - x_1 \times \beta) - (\tau_{k+1} - x_0 \times \beta)$$

$$= -\beta(x_1 - x_0). \qquad (8.25)$$

How we use the results from a package and equation (8.25) to estimate an odds ratio depends on the package used. For example, the results of fitting the proportional odds model in STATA with outcome BWT4N and covariate LWT are shown in Table 8.18. Note that the coefficient for LWT in Table 8.18 is positive reflecting the direction of the association seen in Figure 8.3. Hence increasing values of

Table 8.18   Results of Fitting the Proportional Odds Model to the Four Category Birth Weight Outcome, BWT4N, with Covariate LWT

Variable	Coeff.	Std. Err.	z	p	95% CI
LWT	0.013	0.0043	2.95	0.003	0.004, 0.021
Constant1	0.832	0.5686			
Constant2	1.707	0.5782			
Constant3	2.831	0.6027			

Log-likelihood $= -255.1477$

LWT are associated with increasing values of BWT4N. Thus the output is consistent with the underlying hypothetical continuous outcome model. The negative sign in equation (8.25) reflects the fact that, under a positive association, the covariate is protective (i.e., negatively associated with smaller values of the ordinal outcome). Hence the estimate of the effect of a 10 pound increase in LWT on the odds ratio for as light or lighter versus a heavier baby is

$$\widehat{OR} = \exp(-0.013 \times 10) = 0.88.$$

This estimate implies a 12% reduction in the odds for a lower weight baby per 10 pound increase in weight.

One feature of the proportional odds model that is identical to the binary logistic model is that we can reverse the direction of the model by simply changing the signs of the coefficients. For example, if we are interested in modeling heavier versus lighter weight babies then the estimate of the odds ratio for a 10 pound increase in weight is

$$\widehat{OR} = \exp(0.013 \times 10) = 1.14.$$

This estimate indicates that there is a 14% increase in the odds of a heavier baby per 10 pound increase in weight.

The output from SAS's PROC Logistic is identical to Table 8.18 except that the reported estimate of the coefficient for LWT is -0.013 as SAS uses a model that does not negate the coefficient, β, in equation (8.17).

As a second example we fit the model containing smoking status of the mother during pregnancy. Women who smoke during pregnancy tend to have lower weight births thus the association in the conceptual underlying continuous model is negative. The results of fitting this model in STATA are shown in Table 8.19 where the coefficient for SMOKE is negative.

Hence the estimate of the odds ratio for a lower versus a heavier weight baby is, from equation (8.25),

$$\widehat{OR} = \exp[-(-0.761)] = 2.14.$$

The interpretation is that women who smoke during pregnancy have 2.1 times the odds of a lower versus a heavier baby than women who do not smoke. Similar to

Table 8.19 Results of Fitting the Proportional Odds Model to the Four Category Birth Weight Outcome, BWT4N, with Covariate SMOKE

Variable	Coeff.	Std. Err.	z	p	95% CI
SMOKE	−0.761	0.2719	−2.80	0.005	−1.293, −0.228
Constant1	−1.116	0.1984			
Constant2	−0.248	0.1819			
Constant3	0.867	0.1937			

Log-likelihood = −255.6725

the discussion for LWT the estimate of the odds ratio for a heavier versus lighter weight baby is

$$\widehat{OR} = \exp(-0.761) = 0.47.$$

The interpretation of this estimate is that the odds of a heavier versus lighter weight baby are 53% less for women who smoke during pregnancy.

As with other constrained ordinal models, one should check to see whether the assumption of proportional odds is supported by the data. In addition, one should assess goodness of fit of the model. Several tests have been proposed for testing for the proportional odds assumption and each in some form compares the model in equation (8.17) to an augmented model in which the coefficients for the model covariates are allowed to be different namely

$$c_k(\mathbf{x}) = \ln\left[\frac{\Pr(Y \le k|\mathbf{x})}{\Pr(Y > k|\mathbf{x})}\right] = \tau_k - \mathbf{x}'\boldsymbol{\beta}_k, \tag{8.26}$$

where $\tau_k < \tau_{k+1}$ for $k = 1, \ldots, K$. Brant (1990) proposed a Wald test that compares estimates of the coefficients from a fit of the model in equation (8.26) to those from a fit of the model in equation (8.17). The test has degrees of freedom equal to $[(K + 1) - 2] \times p$. From a practical standpoint fitting the model in equation (8.26) is complex. Thus, Brant recommends obtaining estimates of the parameters by approximating the fit with separate binary logistic regression models using the outcomes

$$w_k = \begin{cases} 1, & y \le k \\ 0, & y > k \end{cases}, \quad k = 0, 2, \ldots, K - 1.$$

The fit is approximate, as it cannot be guaranteed that the constant terms and cumulative probabilities will be monotonic increasing. A command to compute the Brant test is available for STATA (to locate this command from within STATA run "findit Brant"). SAS compares the two models via a score test. An approximate likelihood ratio test is computed in STATA via the command "omodel."

As an example, to test the proportional odds assumption for the fitted model in Table 8.19 the value of Brant's Wald test is $W = 0.36$ with $p = 0.836$, the approximate likelihood ratio test from omodel in STATA is $G = 0.38$ with $p = 0.829$ and the score test from SAS yields $p = 0.644$, each with $(4 - 2) \times 1 = 2$ degrees of freedom. All three tests support the proportional odds assumption.

Fagerland and Hosmer (2012b) consider goodness of fit tests for the proportional odds model proposed by Lipsitz et al. (1996) and Pulkstenis and Robinson (2004), and propose a new test that is an extension of the Hosmer–Lemeshow test for the multinomial logistic regression model discussed in Section 8.1 [see Fagerland et al. (2008) and Fagerland and Hosmer (2012a)].

To obtain the new test assume that we have fit the proportional odds model in equation (8.17) containing, say, p covariates and use it to estimate the cumulative probabilities

$$\hat{\pi}_k(\mathbf{x}) = \frac{e^{\hat{c}_k(\mathbf{x})}}{1 + e^{\hat{c}_k(\mathbf{x})}}, \tag{8.27}$$

where $\hat{c}_k(\mathbf{x}) = \hat{\tau}_k - \hat{\boldsymbol{\beta}}'\mathbf{x}$. We use the cumulative probability estimates in equation (8.27) to estimate the individual outcome probabilities $\Pr(Y = k|\mathbf{x})$ as

$$\hat{\phi}_k(\mathbf{x}) = \begin{cases} \hat{\pi}_0(\mathbf{x}), k = 0 \\ \hat{\pi}_k(\mathbf{x}) - \hat{\pi}_{k-1}(\mathbf{x}), & k = 1, \ldots, K - 1. \\ 1 - \hat{\pi}_{K-1}(\mathbf{x}), k = K \end{cases} \tag{8.28}$$

We then use these estimated probabilities, as suggested by Lipsitz et al. (1996), to calculate an ordinal score for each subject

$$s_i = \sum_{k=0}^{K} k \times \hat{\phi}_k(\mathbf{x}_i). \tag{8.29}$$

Next we create a grouping variable by partitioning the ordinal score ranked subjects into g equal sized groups. We define g indicator variables for group membership for each subject as

$$I_{ij} = \begin{cases} 1 \text{ if } s_i \text{ is in group } j \\ 0 \text{ otherwise} \end{cases}.$$

Lipsitz et al. (1996) propose assessing goodness of fit by fitting the augmented model containing $g - 1$ indicator variables

$$c_k(\mathbf{x}_i, \mathbf{I}_i) = \tau_k - \mathbf{x}'\boldsymbol{\beta} + \sum_{j=1}^{g-1} \gamma_j I_{ij} \tag{8.30}$$

and performing the likelihood ratio test of the augmented model in equation (8.30) versus the model in equation (8.17). Under the hypothesis that $\gamma_j = 0, j = 1, \ldots, g - 1$ and a sufficiently large sample, the test follows a chi-square distribution with $g - 1$ degrees of freedom. In order to provide adequate numbers of subjects in each group and enough groups to provide power to detect departures from model assumptions, they recommend one choose $6 \le g \le n/5K$. One disadvantage of this Lipsitz test is that it is not based on a comparison of the observed frequencies to model estimated frequencies within outcome by score groups as is the case with the goodness of fit test described in Section 8.1. We say more on this point shortly.

Fagerland and Hosmer (2012b) propose an extension of the Hosmer-Lemeshow test for fit of the multinomial logistic regression model. The basis of the test is a $g \times (K + 1)$ table of observed and expected frequencies. The g rows are defined by the same g groups of ranked ordinal scores used in the Lipsitz test and the columns by the $K + 1$ values of the outcome variable. The basic layout is shown in Table 8.20.

If we denote the subjects in ordinal score group j by Ω_j with

$$O_{jk} = \sum_{i \in \Omega_k} z_{ik},$$

and

$$\hat{E}_{jk} = \sum_{i \in \Omega_k} \hat{\phi}_k(\mathbf{x}_i)$$

then the test statistic is

$$\widehat{C}_O = \sum_{l=1}^{g} \sum_{k=0}^{K} \frac{(O_{lk} - \hat{E}_{lk})^2}{\hat{E}_{lk}}. \tag{8.31}$$

The degrees of freedom for the multinomial goodness of fit test $\widehat{C}_M$ in equation (8.11) are $(K) \times (g - 2)$, as we have coded the outcome to have $K + 1$ values. The test in equation (8.31) has additional degrees of freedom because the individual column total estimated expected frequencies do not equal the observed total, $\sum_{l=1}^{g} \hat{E}_{lk} \neq \sum_{l=1}^{g} O_{lk}$ for $k = 0, 2, \ldots, K$. Since the overall totals are the same, namely

$$\sum_{l=1}^{g} \sum_{k=0}^{K} \hat{E}_{lj} = \sum_{l=1}^{g} \sum_{k=0}^{K} O_{lk} = n,$$

a degree of freedom is lost because of this summing constraint and another is lost because of the constraint that the estimated constant terms are monotonic increasing. Hence the distribution of $\widehat{C}_O$, under the null hypothesis that the fitted model is the correct model and assuming a large enough sample, is chi-square with $(K) \times (g - 2) + (K - 1)$ degrees of freedom. (Again, recall that the number of response levels is $K + 1$.) See Fagerland and Hosmer (2012b) for supporting simulation results. We defer illustrating the goodness of fit tests until after the multivariable example in Section 8.2.2.

Fagerland and Hosmer (2012a) use groups for the multinomial goodness of fit test $\widehat{C}_M$ based on the complement of $\Pr(Y = 0|\mathbf{x})$. Fagerland and Hosmer (2012b) show that frequencies based on forming groups based on the values of $1 - \hat{\phi}_0(\mathbf{x})$ are identical to those in Table 8.20 based on ordinal score groups. Lipsitz et al. (1996) suggest an alternative ordinal score that yields $s_i = \hat{\phi}(\mathbf{x}_i)$. Using this score also yields the same observed and expected frequencies as those in Table 8.20, although the rows are in reverse order.

Lipsitz et al. (1996) note that their test is based on $g - 1$ linear combinations of the $(O_{lj} - \hat{E}_{lj})$ thus the test has fewer degrees of freedom than $\widehat{C}_O$. In addition,

Table 8.20 Observed and Estimated Expected Frequencies by Ordinal Score Group and Outcome

Ordinal Score Group	$Y = 0$		$Y = 1$		$\cdots$	$Y = K$		Total
	Obs.	Exp.	Obs.	Exp.	$\cdots$	Obs.	Exp.	
1	O_{10}	$\hat{E}_{10}$	O_{12}	$\hat{E}_{12}$	$\cdots$	O_{1K}	$\hat{E}_{1K}$	n/g
2	O_{20}	$\hat{E}_{20}$	O_{22}	$\hat{E}_{22}$	$\cdots$	O_{2K}	$\hat{E}_{2K}$	n/g
$\vdots$	$\vdots$	$\vdots$	$\vdots$	$\vdots$	$\ddots$	$\vdots$	$\vdots$	$\vdots$
g	O_{g0}	$\hat{E}_{g0}$	O_{g2}	$\hat{E}_{g2}$	$\cdots$	O_{gK}	$\hat{E}_{gK}$	n/g

because there is no table analogous to that shown in Table 8.20 it is difficult to find regions where there are departures from model fit. Simulations in Fagerland and Hosmer (2012b) found that the Lipsitz test has better power to detect violations of the specification of the composition of the model, $\beta'\mathbf{x}$, than the $\hat{C}_O$ test, but $\hat{C}_O$ has higher power to detect a violation of the proportional odds assumption. Hence we recommend that both tests be used when evaluating a fitted proportional odds model.

In this section we considered three different models when the outcome is ordinal scaled: adjacent-category, continuation-ratio, and proportional odds. The choice of what model to ultimately use in any setting should consider which odds ratios are most informative for the problem as well as an assessment of model adequacy.

8.2.2 Model Building Strategies for Ordinal Logistic Regression Models

The steps in model building for an ordinal logistic regression model are essentially the same as described in Chapter 4 for the binary logistic regression model and in Section 8.1 for the multinomial logistic regression model. However, best subsets selection is not yet available for ordinal models. Following model building one should assess goodness of fit. For the proportional odds model one should use the Lipsitz and Fagerland–Hosmer test. For the adjacent-category and continuation-ratio one may assess fit via separate binary logistic regressions using, if possible, the coefficients from the ordinal model fit. Casewise diagnostics are, frankly, problematic as they have not yet been developed for ordinal models. What one must do is obtain them from separate binary regressions in the same way as illustrated in Section 8.1 for the multinomial logistic regression model.

To illustrate modeling and assessment of fit we could use any of the ordinal models but we chose to use the proportional-odds model as it is the one most frequently used in practice. The first example considers neuropsychiatric disturbance (NEURO) as the outcome variable from the Adolescent Placement data. Recall that it is coded: 0 = none, 1 = mild, 2 = moderate, and 3 = severe. The goal of the modeling is to explore what patient factors are associated with progressively severe disturbance. Using the method of purposeful selection we obtained a model containing the following variables: age, the square of age (using fractional polynomials), state custody (CUSTD), race (RACE), and emotional disturbance (EMOT). We choose to use age centered about its mean (AGE_c) and the square of age about its mean (AGE2_c) in order to control the magnitude of the three constant terms. The results of the fit are shown in Table 8.21.

Next we checked for the proportional odds assumption using both the Brant Wald and the approximate likelihood ratio test. The value of Brant's Wald test is $W = 14.71$ with $p = 0.258$; the approximate likelihood ratio test from omodel in STATA is $G = 21.64$ with $p = 0.042$. Each statistic is compared to a chi-square distribution with 12 degrees of freedom. The results are mixed with one p-value greater and the other slightly less than 0.05. The results of the Fagerland–Hosmer goodness of fit test are shown in Table 8.22. We used 10 groups as $508/(5 \times 4) = 25.4$.

Table 8.21   Results of Fitting the Proportional Odds Model to the Four-Category Outcome, NEURO, in the Adolescent Placement Data

Variable	Coeff.	Std. Err.	z	p	95% CI	
AGE_c	−2.059	0.8738	−2.36	0.018	−3.771,	−0.346
AGE2_c	0.071	0.0302	2.36	0.018	0.012,	0.130
CUSTD	−0.631	0.2087	−3.02	0.003	−1.040,	−0.222
RACE	0.593	0.2336	2.54	0.011	0.135,	1.051
EMOT	1.127	0.3282	3.43	0.001	0.484,	1.770
RxE	−0.849	0.4354	−1.95	0.051	−1.702,	0.004
Constant1	1.283	0.2081			0.875,	1.691
Constant2	2.253	0.2274			1.807,	2.699
Constant3	2.810	0.2452			2.329,	3.290

Log-likelihood = −461.7982

Table 8.22   Observed and Estimated Expected Frequencies within Each of the 10 Ordinal Score Groups and Level of Outcome

Group	NEURO = 0		NEURO = 1		NEURO = 2		NEURO = 3		Total
	Obs.	Exp.	Obs.	Exp.	Obs.	Exp.	Obs.	Exp.	
1	42	42.91	6	4.68	2	1.40	1	2.02	51
2	35	39.96	10	6.21	1	1.95	5	2.89	51
3	43	39.47	4	6.45	2	2.04	2	3.04	51
4	41	39.06	8	7.14	0	2.31	3	3.49	52
5	35	35.29	6	7.42	3	2.48	5	3.82	49
6	32	34.34	10	8.74	5	3.06	4	4.86	51
7	43	33.49	4	9.07	0	3.23	4	5.20	51
8	27	31.59	13	9.77	4	3.63	7	6.01	51
9	27	29.02	14	10.6	4	4.17	6	7.21	51
10	25	24.16	6	11.34	8	4.99	11	9.50	50

The value of the test statistic is $\widehat{C}_o = 29.782$, which, with $3(8) + 2 = 26$ degrees of freedom, results in $p = 0.277$. Among the 40 cells in Table 8.22 none of the estimated expected frequencies are less than 1 and 17 of them are less than 5, approximately 43% of the total. The significance level for the Lipsitz test is $p = 0.065$.

In aggregate, we feel that the various tests do support model fit and the assumption of proportional odds. We leave the computation of casewise diagnostic statistics from separate binary fits as an exercise. Ideally, one should compute these using the values of the parameter estimates in Table 8.21. See the discussion in Section 8.1 on this point.

The reader should have had considerable practice estimating odds ratios by this point in the text, so we leave estimation and interpretation of the odds ratios for the dichotomous covariates in the model as an exercise. The fitted model is quadratic in age, where age ranges from 11 to 19 with the minimum logit at 14.5 years. This is a setting where estimating the odds ratio for age versus the age at minimum log-odds at 14.5 is of clinical interest. As this is a bit more complicated we summarize the details of applying the four-step procedure discussed in Chapter 4 and then graph the estimator with 95% confidence intervals in Figure 8.5.

The first step is to write down the model at the "exposed" age, say a, and the referent age of 14.5. Since the model uses centered age these are centered as well yielding the following expression for the log-odds ratio

$$\ln[\widehat{\text{OR}}(a, 14.5)] = [\hat{\beta}_1(a - \bar{a}) + \hat{\beta}_2(a^2 - \bar{a}^2)] - [\hat{\beta}_1(14.5 - \bar{a}) + \hat{\beta}_2(14.5^2 - \bar{a}^2)]$$

$$= \hat{\beta}_1(a - 14.5) + \hat{\beta}_2(a^2 - 14.5^2)$$

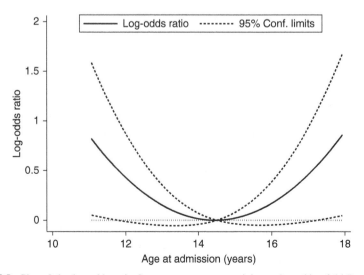

Figure 8.5 Plot of the log-odds ratio for age versus age at minimum log-odds of 14.5 with 95% confidence bands.

where the $\hat{\beta}$'s denote the estimated coefficients for AGE_c and AGE2_c and $\bar{a} = 14.2715$ is the mean age and $\bar{a}^2 = 206.53661$ is the mean of age squared. Simplifying the above expression yields

$$\ln[\widehat{OR}(a, 14.5)] = \hat{\beta}_1 \times f(a) + \hat{\beta}_2 \times g(a),$$

where $f(a) = (a - 14.5)$ and $g(a) = \hat{\beta}_2(a^2 - 14.5^2)$. It follows that estimator of the standard error of the log-odds ratio is

$$\widehat{SE}\{\ln[\widehat{OR}(a, 14.5)]\} = \left\{ \begin{array}{l} f(a)^2 \times \widehat{Var}(\hat{\beta}_1) + g(a)^2 \times \widehat{Var}(\hat{\beta}_2) \\ +2 \times f(a) \times g(a) \times \widehat{Cov}(\hat{\beta}_1, \hat{\beta}_2) \end{array} \right\},$$

and from output of the fit in Table 8.21 we obtain

$$\widehat{Var}(\hat{\beta}_1) = 0.76344139, \quad \widehat{Var}(\hat{\beta}_2) = 0.00091291 \text{ and } \widehat{Cov}(\hat{\beta}_1, \hat{\beta}_2) = -0.02634735.$$

These quantities are used in the usual manner to obtain the 95% confidence bands plotted in Figure 8.5.

The plot in Figure 8.5 shows that as age decreases and increases from 14.5 the log-odds ratio for increasingly severe neuropsychiatric disturbance increases. However the increase is only significant for ages younger than about 11.5 years and older than about 17 years as this is where the lower confidence limit line crosses the line equal to 0. The results in Figure 8.5 can be displayed on the odds ratio scale but the exponentiation increases the range on the y-axis to the point where it is difficult to plot. At this point one might, in practice, prepare a table containing estimated odds ratios for a few key ages to supplement the results in Figure 8.5.

In practice, the next step would be to obtain case-wise diagnostic statistics and, as noted earlier, these are not generally available from software packages for ordinal models. Thus, we would need to compute three sets of diagnostic statistics from separate binary fits where the binary outcomes are defined as

$$\tilde{y}_{ki} = \begin{cases} 1 & \text{if } y_i \le k \\ 0 & \text{if } y_i > k \end{cases}, \quad k = 0, 1, \ldots, K - 1. \tag{8.32}$$

The process is quite similar to obtaining the diagnostic statistics for a fitted multinomial model described in Section 8.1. As such, we leave this step as well as preparing a summary of the results in Table 8.21 as an exercise.

Fitting neuropsychiatric disturbance with a proportional odds model is an example where the fitted model supported the proportional odds assumption. As a second example, we consider as the outcome danger to others (DANGER) where we show that the proportional odds assumption is not supported by the data.

Using the method of purposeful selection we obtained the model shown in Table 8.23. The covariate violence (VIOL) was selected but ended up causing numerical problems. There is a zero frequency cell in the cross tabulation of it with DANGER. There are no subjects with a history of violence that were judged to be of little danger to others. It may be that this pair of values provides an example of what is called a *structural zero*, namely a cell with probability equal

Table 8.23 **Results of Fitting the Proportional Odds Model to the Four Category Outcome, DANGER, in the Adolescent Placement Data**

Variable	Coeff.	Std. Err.	z	p	95% CI
WEEKS	0.040	0.0202	1.97	0.049	0.0002, 0.080
BEHAV	0.614	0.0560	10.97	0.000	0.505, 0.724
GENDER	0.645	0.1815	3.55	0.000	0.289, 1.001
CUSTD	−0.492	0.1786	−2.76	0.006	−0.842, −0.142
Constant1	1.068	0.2958			0.488, 1.648
Constant2	2.893	0.3238			2.258, 3.527
Constant3	4.435	0.3540			3.741, 5.129

Log-likelihood = −546.8982

to 0 of occurring [see Agresti (2002)]. Trying to account for a structural 0 in the modeling introduces needless complexity when the point of this example is assessing the proportional odds assumption and what to do when it is not satisfied. So we decided not to include VIOL in the model. The preliminary final model is given in Table 8.23 where we used WEEKS = (LOS/7) to measure length of stay.

The results in Table 8.23 look reasonable and are clinically plausible with increasing length of stay, behavioral score, and being male associated with more danger to others while being in state custody is associated with decreasing danger to others. However, until we assess the model for adherence to model assumptions and fit it is not appropriate to consider the model in Table 8.23 as the final model.

The results of evaluating the proportional odds assumption using the four different tests yielded the following significance levels: Brant's test $p < 0.001$, approximate likelihood ratio test $p < 0.001$, Fagerland-Hosmer test $p = 0.001$, and Lipsitz test $p = 0.532$. Recall that the simulations in Fagerland and Hosmer (2012b) demonstrated that the Lipsitz test had the least power in detecting violations of the proportional odds assumption, doing best on linear predictor misspecification. Hence we conclude that the fitted model does not satisfy the proportional odds assumption.

There are several options available when the model does not satisfy the proportional odds assumption. The simplest approach, by far, is to fit a multinomial logistic regression model. The next simplest approach is to fit three binary logistic models using the outcomes defined in equation (8.32). The inferences are different in these two approaches. The multinomial model provides estimates of odds ratios of the referent outcome (e.g., DANGER = unlikely) versus each of the three higher levels of danger to others. The three separate binary fits provide estimates of odds ratios for less versus more danger at the three lowest levels. This latter analysis is a bit more complicated than the multinomial approach and may not be worth the effort unless it is vital to keep the outcome ordinal scaled. The most complicated approach is to fit the partial proportional odds model that modifies the model in equation (8.17) as follows

$$c_k(\mathbf{x}) = \ln\left[\frac{\Pr(Y \leq k|\mathbf{x},\mathbf{z})}{\Pr(Y > k|\mathbf{x},\mathbf{z})}\right] = \tau_k - \mathbf{x}'\boldsymbol{\beta} - \mathbf{z}'\boldsymbol{\theta}_k, \tag{8.33}$$

where the coefficients for the covariates in $\mathbf{x}$ are constant whereas those for the covariates in $\mathbf{z}$ are not constant over the K logit functions. Software to fit this model is not widely available and thus the model is not recommended at this time. A compromise model that is possible with current software is to fit the constrained multinomial logistic regression model

$$\ln \left[\frac{\Pr(Y = k|\mathbf{x})}{\Pr(Y = 0|\mathbf{x})} \right] = \alpha_k - \mathbf{x}'\beta - \mathbf{z}'\theta_k. \qquad (8.34)$$

Once one chooses which model to fit then model building and evaluation proceeds as usual, although admittedly not as simply as would be possible if the proportional odds assumptions held.

In summary, modeling an ordinal outcome with one of the ordinal logistic regression models described in this section follows the same methods described in Chapter 4 for binary outcomes and in Section 8.1 for multinomial outcomes. One should choose that ordinal model that yields estimates of the odds ratios that are clinically most useful within the context of the problem at hand. The multinomial logistic regression model is a good fall back when ordinal model assumptions do not seem to hold.

EXERCISES

1. The data for the low birth weight study are described in Section 1.6.2. These data are used in Section 8.2 to illustrate ordinal logistic regression models via the four-category outcome BWT4,

$$\text{BWT4} = \begin{cases} 0 \ \text{ if BWT} > 3500 \\ 1 \ \text{ if } 3000 < \text{BWT} \leq 3500 \\ 2 \ \text{ if } 2500 < \text{BWT} \leq 3000 \\ 3 \ \text{ if BWT} \leq 2500 \end{cases}.$$

However in this problem use the outcome variable *BWT4* and fit the multinomial or baseline logistic regression model with BWT4 = 0 as the referent outcome and consider as possible model covariates all other variables in Table 1.6, except birth weight.

The steps should include: (i) a complete univariate analysis, (ii) an appropriate selection of variables for a multivariate model (this should include scale identification for continuous covariates and assessment of the need for interactions), (iii) an assessment of fit of the multivariate model, (iv) preparation and presentation of a table containing the results of the final model (this table should contain point and interval estimates for all relevant odds ratios), and (v) conclusions from the analysis.

2. The following exercise is designed to enhance the idea expressed in Figure 8.3 and Figure 8.4 that one way to obtain the proportional odds model is via categorization of a continuous variable.

(a) Form the scatterplot of BWT versus LWT.

(b) Fit the linear regression of BWT on LWT and add the estimated regression line to the scatterplot in 2(a). Let $\hat{\lambda}_0$ denote the estimate of the intercept, $\hat{\lambda}_1$ the estimate of the slope and s the root mean squared error from the linear regression.

(c) It follows from results for the logistic distribution that the relationship between the root mean squared error in the normal errors linear regression and the scale parameter for logistic errors linear regression is approximately $\hat{\sigma} = s\sqrt{3}/\pi$. Use the results from the linear regression in 2(b) and obtain $\hat{\sigma}$.

(d) Use the results from 2(b) and 2(c) and show that the estimates presented in Table 8.18 are approximate, and

(e) By hand draw a facsimile of the density function shown in Figure 8.4 with the three vertical lines at the values 2500, 3000, and 3500. Using the results in equation (8.20), equation (8.21) and the estimates in Table 8.18 compute the value of the four areas under the hand-drawn curve. Using these specific areas demonstrate that the relationship shown in equation (8.23) holds at each cutpoint.

3. Obtain and evaluate the diagnostic statistics for the multinomial logistic regression model fit to the outcome PLACE3 in Table 8.10.

4. Obtain and evaluate the diagnostic statistics for the proportional odds model fit to the outcome NEURO shown in Table 8.21. This should use the separate binary regressions with outcome defined as in equation (8.32). If at all possible with the software package you are using calculate the diagnostics using the estimated coefficients in Table 8.21. If this is not possible use the diagnostics from the usual fit, but comment on any differences in these coefficients and those in Table 8.21.

5. Estimate and interpret the odds ratios for the dichotomous covariates in Table 8.21. Be sure to account for the interaction term.

6. Fit the multinomial logistic regression model using the DANGER as the outcome and covariates in Table 8.23. Compare the results of this fit to the one shown in Table 8.23.

CHAPTER 9

Logistic Regression Models for the Analysis of Correlated Data

9.1 INTRODUCTION

Up to this point in the text we have considered the use of the logistic regression model in settings where we observe a single dichotomous response for a sample of statistically independent subjects. However, there are settings where the assumption of independence of responses may not hold for a variety of reasons. For example, consider a study of asthma in children in which subjects are interviewed bi-monthly for 1 year. At each interview the date is recorded and the mother is asked whether, during the previous 2 months, her child had an asthma attack severe enough to require medical attention, whether the child had a chest cold, and how many smokers lived in the household. The child's age and race are recorded at the first interview. The primary outcome is the occurrence of an asthma attack. What differs here is the lack of independence in the observations due to the fact that we have six measurements on each child. In this example, each child represents a cluster of correlated observations of the outcome. The measurements of the presence or absence of a chest cold and the number of smokers residing in the household can change from observation to observation and thus are called *cluster-specific* or *time-varying covariates*. The date changes in a systematic way and is recorded to model possible seasonal effects. The child's age and race are constant for the duration of the study and are referred to as *cluster-level* or *time-invariant covariates*. The terms clusters, subjects, cluster-specific and cluster-level covariates are general enough to describe multiple measurements on a single subject or single measurements on different but related subjects. An example of the latter setting would be a study of all children in a household. Repeated measurements on the same subject or a subject clustered in some sort of unit (household, hospital, or physician) are the two most likely scenarios leading to correlated data.

Applied Logistic Regression, Third Edition.
David W. Hosmer, Jr., Stanley Lemeshow, and Rodney X. Sturdivant.
© 2013 John Wiley & Sons, Inc. Published 2013 by John Wiley & Sons, Inc.

The goals of the analysis in a correlated data setting are, for the most part, identical to those discussed in earlier chapters. Specifically, we are interested in estimating the effect of the covariates on the dichotomous outcome via odds ratios. However, the models and estimation methods are more complicated in the correlated data setting. Failure to appropriately handle correlations among the observations can lead to incorrect inferences on the effects of model covariates [Austin et al. (2003)].

Methods described earlier in this book were used to handle correlated data prior to development of new methodology and software tools. This approach has several potential pitfalls that are avoided by using in the models of this chapter. Returning to the example given earlier of measurements on each child, we could address this in a traditional logistic regression model using indicator variables to designate the visit number. This approach does account for the visit number in the model and may sometimes produce viable estimates of parameters. However, such a model does not account for the fact that, within each child, the data are not independent and this could lead to issues with estimation and inference accuracy. From a practical standpoint this approach quickly becomes infeasible in the presence of a large number of observations in each cluster (e.g., suppose the child is measured every week for a year).

Finally, it is likely that there will be some children with missing data in such a study design. It is also common for the intervals between observations to differ between children in such a study. Traditional logistic regression requires additional methodology, which we discuss in Chapter 10, to handle missing data so that important information in the data is not lost. The models in this chapter do not suffer from either issue [Gibbons et al. (2010)]. Thus, when the data are correlated, models designed to account for the correlation should be used rather than attempting to account for the effect using traditional modeling approaches.

There is a large and rapidly expanding literature on methods for the analysis of correlated binary data. The methods and models are referred to by a variety of terms such as: hierarchical models, multilevel models, mixed models, random coefficient models, variance components, and latent variable models. Most of the research in this area is at a mathematical level that is beyond this text. However, software to fit the more common and established models for correlated binary data is available in major packages such as SAS and STATA. Thus, the goal of this chapter is to introduce the models that can be fit with the major software packages and to discuss the strengths and limitations of these models as well as the interpretation of the resulting parameter estimates. Software packages designed specifically for correlated data modeling such as MLwiN [Rasbash et al. (2009)] and Mplus [Muthen and Muthen (2008)] may have additional options that are not covered in this chapter.

Several accessible review papers that discuss the models we consider are Neuhaus et al. (1991), Neuhaus (1992), Diez-Roux (2000), Guo and Zhao (2000), Goldstein et al. (2002), and Gibbons et al. (2010). Diggle et al. (2002) discuss methods for the analysis of longitudinal data and consider models for binary data. Ashby et al. (1992) provide a detailed annotated bibliography on methods for analyzing correlated categorical data. Collett's (2003) text discusses methods for analyzing correlated binary data at a level comparable to this text. A few texts that go into a bit more depth, useful for additional study, include Snijders and Bosker (1999), McCulloch and Searle (2001), Hedeker and Gibbons (2006), and Rabe-Hesketh and Skrondal (2008). Pendergast et al. (1996) also review methods for clustered binary data. Breslow and Clayton (1993) consider mixed models for generalized linear models. Agresti et al. (2000) present a summary of different methods for the analysis of correlated binary data via random effects models, one of which we discuss in this chapter. Their paper considers other models and different data settings where random effects models can be effectively used. Coull and Agresti (2000) consider extensions of a mixed model considered in this section. Rosner (1984) and Glynn and Rosner (1994) consider specialized models for the analysis of paired binary outcomes.

9.2 LOGISTIC REGRESSION MODELS FOR THE ANALYSIS OF CORRELATED DATA

Two approaches are commonly used to model correlated binary data: a random effects model and a population average model. The *random effects model* mimics the usual normal errors linear mixed effects model, where parameter estimates are conditional on the subject or cluster. Under the *population average model* estimates are, in a sense, averaged over the clusters. A third, more specialized, model is the *transitional model* that is, essentially, a random effects model using one or more of the previously observed values of the outcome as a covariate(s). Although we do not illustrate the transitional model here, a thorough discussion of the approach is available in references for longitudinal data analysis such as Molenberghs and Verbeke (2005). An example of the model is found in Azzalini (1994).

The random effects model is referred to in the literature as a "cluster-specific" or "conditional" model. Often the clusters are specific subjects, but we will use the cluster-specific terminology as this term is a bit more general than "subject-specific." It describes the case of multiple observations on a single subject and single observations on related subjects. The cluster-specific binary outcome model is formulated in the manner of the normal errors linear mixed effects model. Suppose we are in a setting with m clusters and n_i observations per cluster. We denote the dichotomous outcome variable as Y_{ij} and the collection of covariates as $\mathbf{x}'_{ij} = (x_{1ij}, x_{2ij}, \ldots, x_{pij})$ for the jth observation in the ith cluster. Under the logistic-normal cluster-specific model the correlation among individual responses within a cluster is accounted for by adding a random effect term, specific to the cluster, to the logit. The equation for the logit is

$$g(\mathbf{x}_{ij}, \alpha_i, \boldsymbol{\beta}_s) = \beta_0 + \alpha_i + \mathbf{x}'_{ij}\boldsymbol{\beta}_s, \qquad (9.1)$$

where the random effects, α_i, are assumed to follow a normal distribution with mean zero and constant variance, that is, $\alpha_i \sim N(0, \sigma_\alpha^2)$. In practice the random effect terms are unobserved and this leads to complications when we consider estimation of the regression coefficients, $\boldsymbol{\beta}_s$. The subscript s refers to the fact that the coefficients apply to a logistic regression model that is specific to subjects with random effect equal to α_i. Suppose that in our hypothetical asthma study the coefficient, β_s, for having had a chest cold in the previous 2 months is $\ln(2)$. The interpretation is that having a chest cold doubles the odds of having a severe asthma attack in the next 2 months, among children with the same value of the unobserved random effect. The interpretation applies either to a specific child or to an unobserved group of asthmatic children each with the same value of the random effect. As the covariate "chest cold" can change from month to month, the within-subject interpretation provides an easily understood estimate of the increase in the odds for a specific subject. On the other hand, suppose that race is a dichotomous covariate coded as either white or non-white and its coefficient is $\ln(2)$. The cluster-specific interpretation is that a nonwhite child with random effect α_i has odds of a severe asthma attack that is twice the odds of a white child with the same random effect. As both the race and random effect are constant within subject and cannot change, this odds ratio is not likely to be useful in practice. Thus, these two simple examples illustrate that the logistic-normal model is most likely to be useful for inferences about covariates whose values can change at the subject level. We will describe interpretation of the cluster-specific model in more detail using specific numeric examples in Section 9.4.

The effect of the term α_i in equation (9.1) is to increase the correlation among responses within a cluster relative to the correlation of the responses among clusters. The basic idea is that because the logistic model probabilities of the outcome within a cluster have a common value of α_i their outcomes will be more highly correlated than the outcomes from different clusters where the α_i's are different. The greater the heterogeneity in the values of the α_i's, the greater the difference in the within- and between-cluster correlations. The heterogeneity in the α_i's is controlled by the variance σ_α^2. Thus, as σ_α^2 increases the within-cluster correlation increases.

Another way to think of this model is in terms of "levels" or a hierarchy in the data (the terms *multilevel* or *hierarchical* models are commonly used to describe these models in some fields of inquiry). This is best seen by rewriting the model in equation (9.1) separating the (random) intercept from the vector of parameter estimates and defining the model as:

$$g(\mathbf{x}_{ij}, \beta_{0i}, \boldsymbol{\beta}_s) = \beta_{0i} + \mathbf{x}_{ij}'\boldsymbol{\beta}_s \quad \text{(level 1 model)} \tag{9.2}$$

and

$$\beta_{0i} = \beta_0 + \alpha_i \quad \text{(level 2 model).} \tag{9.3}$$

Here, expression 9.2 for the logit is level 1, the within-cluster level, but we see the subscript on the intercept term implies this is a random intercept with clusters having different values. The expression defining these random intercepts is the level 2 or the cluster level model given in equation (9.3) and shows that each cluster has intercept equal to the constant plus the cluster random effect. For example, level 1 might be patients and level 2 might be the hospitals. When we consider further extensions to the models (random slopes and more levels of clustering) this parameterization of the model is sometimes easier to understand.

An alternative to the cluster-specific model in equation (9.1) is the population average model or "marginal" model. Under this model we average probabilities of the outcome, in a sense, over the statistical distribution of the random effect and assume that this process yields the logit

$$g(\mathbf{x}_{ij}, \boldsymbol{\beta}_{PA}) = \beta_0 + \mathbf{x}_{ij}' \boldsymbol{\beta}_{PA}. \tag{9.4}$$

Probabilities based on the logit in equation (9.4) represent the proportion of subjects in the population with outcome present among subjects with covariates $\mathbf{x}_{ij}$. Note that we have not specified the statistical distribution of the random effects, only that the population proportions have logit function given by equation (9.4). As we show, the lack of any distributional assumptions presents problems when trying to estimate $\boldsymbol{\beta}_{PA}$. The interpretation of a coefficient equal to $\ln(2)$ for having had a cold during the previous 2 months is that the odds of a severe asthma attack among those who had a cold is twice the odds among those who did not have a cold. Thus the coefficient describes the effect of the covariate in broad groups of subjects rather than in individual subjects. If the coefficient for race is $\ln(2)$ then the log-odds of a severe asthma attack among non-whites is twice that of whites. We will give specific numeric examples in Section 9.4 of interpreting the population average model. Note that as specified so far, the logistic regression models covered earlier in the book that assume independence of the responses are no different from the population average model. In fact, the standard model may be thought of as a population average model. However, when we discuss the population average model we typically refer to models addressing correlation in the responses through the covariance structure, which will be discussed in the next section.

Both the cluster-specific and population average model may be fit to data containing subject-specific and cluster-level covariates. As a result, the choice of which model to use should be based on what types of inferences the fitted model is intended to provide. As described via the two covariates "having had a cold" and "race," the cluster-specific model is most useful when the goal is to provide inferences for covariates that can change within cluster, whereas the population average model is likely to be more useful for covariates that are constant within cluster. However, model choice is not always this straightforward. As an example, for clinical trials Lindsey and Lambert (1998) strongly oppose use of population average models as they may hide the true nature of an effect on each individual—in extreme cases leading to concluding a positive/negative effect overall when every individual observed has the opposite effect, negative/positive. By contrast, Diggle et al. (2002) support the use of a population average model for analyzing clinical trials data as the average effect of a treatment is the measure of interest. The cluster-specific models offer an advantage, as we see in later sections, in allowing the researcher to estimate a population average like effect as well as the cluster-specific effects. Clearly, both models have their place in practice. We return to this point via examples throughout this chapter.

9.3   ESTIMATION METHODS FOR CORRELATED DATA LOGISTIC REGRESSION MODELS

As we alluded to in the previous section, estimation in correlated data models is not as straightforward or easily described as in the uncorrelated data setting where a likelihood function can be derived from the binomial distribution. As it is the simpler model, we begin with the population average model.

In the population average model, estimation is based on generalized estimating equations (GEE). Liang and Zeger (1986) and Zeger et al. (1988) first used GEE with the binary data population average model. The GEE approach uses a set of equations that look like weighted versions of the likelihood equations shown in Chapters 1 and 2. The weights involve an approximation of the underlying covariance matrix of the correlated within-cluster observations, which requires an assumption about the structure of this correlation. The default assumption used by most packages is called exchangeable (or sometimes compound symmetry) correlation that assumes the correlation between pairs of responses within a cluster is constant, $Cor(Y_{ij}, Y_{il}) = \rho$ for $j \neq l$. Three other possible correlation structures that can be specified in most packages are independent, auto-regressive and unstructured. Under the independent model $Cor(Y_{ij}, Y_{il}) = 0$ for $j \neq l$ and the GEE equations simplify to the likelihood equations obtained from the binomial likelihood in Chapter 2. We do not consider this correlation structure further in this chapter. The auto-regressive structure is appropriate when there is a time or order component associated with the observations. The correlation among responses depends on the lag between the observations and is assumed to be constant for equally lagged observations. Settings where there is an explicit time component are a bit specialized and additional approaches to handling such data are covered in texts such as Diggle et al. (2002) or Hedeker and Gibbons (2006). In the unstructured correlation case one assumes that the correlation of the possible pairs of responses is different, $Cor(Y_{ij}, Y_{il}) = \rho_{jl}$ for $j \neq l$. At first glance this might seem to be the best choice. However, it requires estimating a large number of parameters that are, for the most part, of secondary importance. For example, if we have clusters with six observations per cluster we must estimate 15 correlations. In most applications we are only interested in estimating the regression coefficients and need to account for correlation in responses to obtain correct estimates of the standard errors of the estimated coefficients. For this reason Liang and Zeger (1986) refer to the choice of correlation structure to use in the GEE as the "working correlation." The idea is that one chooses a correlation structure for estimation that seems plausible for the setting and then this structure is used in adjusting the estimator of the variance. We discuss some methods of assessing the choice of correlation structure in later sections of the chapter. For data that does not have a clear choice of structure, a reasonable and parsimonious choice is the "exchangeable correlation" structure. One of the advantages of the GEE approach is the "robustness" of the estimates to choice of correlation structure [see for example Gardiner et al. (2009) or Goldstein et al. (2002)]. In other words, even if the correlation structure chosen is not the true structure the parameter estimates from GEE are often still valid. This property holds when the robust (or "sandwich") estimates discussed later are used. Thus we use the GEE method for population average models with exchangeable correlation as the working correlation unless the nature of the data clearly suggests another choice.

We need some additional notation to fully describe the application of GEE to the population average model. We denote the logistic probability obtained from the logit in equation (9.4) as

$$\pi_{PA}(\mathbf{x}_{ij}) = \frac{e^{g(\mathbf{x}, \boldsymbol{\beta}_{PA})}}{1 + e^{g(\mathbf{x}, \boldsymbol{\beta}_{PA})}},\tag{9.5}$$

where $g(\mathbf{x}, \boldsymbol{\beta}_{PA})$ is the usual linear expression of the logit consisting of the set of predictors and the corresponding parameters estimated under the population average model. We use two matrices to describe the within-cluster covariance of the correlated observations of the outcome variable. The first is an $n_i \times n_i$ (recall from the previous section that this is the number of observations in the cluster) diagonal matrix containing the variances under the model in equation (9.4) denoted

$$\mathbf{A}_i = \text{diag}[\pi_{PA}(\mathbf{x}_{ij}) \times (1 - \pi_{PA}(\mathbf{x}_{ij}))]\tag{9.6}$$

and the second is the $n_i \times n_i$ exchangeable correlation matrix denoted

$$\mathbf{R}_i(\rho) = \begin{bmatrix} 1 & \rho & \cdots & \rho \\ \rho & 1 & & \rho \\ \vdots & & \ddots & \vdots \\ \rho & \rho & \cdots & 1 \end{bmatrix}.\tag{9.7}$$

Using the fact that the correlation is defined as the covariance divided by the product of the standard deviations it follows that the covariance matrix in the ith cluster is

$$\mathbf{V}_i = \mathbf{A}_i^{0.5} \mathbf{R}_i(\rho) \mathbf{A}_i^{0.5},\tag{9.8}$$

where $\mathbf{A}_i^{0.5}$ is the diagonal matrix whose elements are the square roots of the elements in the matrix in equation (9.6). The contribution to the estimating equations for the ith cluster is $\mathbf{D}'_i \mathbf{V}_i^{-1} \mathbf{S}_i$ where $\mathbf{D}'_i = \mathbf{X}'_i \mathbf{A}_i$, $\mathbf{X}_i$ is the $n_i \times (p+1)$ matrix of covariate values and $\mathbf{S}_i$ is the vector with jth element the residual $s_{ij} = y_{ij} - \pi_{PA}(\mathbf{x}_{ij})$. The full set of estimating equations is

$$\sum_{i=1}^{m} \mathbf{D}'_i \mathbf{V}_i^{-1} \mathbf{S}_i = \mathbf{0}\tag{9.9}$$

and its solution is denoted as $\hat{\boldsymbol{\beta}}_{PA}$. Implicit in the solution of these equations is an estimator of the correlation parameter, ρ. Typically this is based on the average correlation among within-cluster empirical residuals and as such it is also adjusted with each iterative change in the solution for $\hat{\boldsymbol{\beta}}_{PA}$.

Liang and Zeger (1986) show that the estimator, $\hat{\boldsymbol{\beta}}_{PA}$, is asymptotically normally distributed with mean $\boldsymbol{\beta}_{PA}$. They derive, as an estimator of the covariance matrix, the estimator that is often referred to as the information sandwich estimator. The "bread" of the sandwich is based on the observed information matrix under the assumption of exchangeable correlation. The "bread" for the ith cluster is

$$\mathbf{B}_i = \mathbf{D}_i' \, \mathbf{V}_i^{-1} \mathbf{D}_i$$
$$= \mathbf{X}_i' \, \mathbf{A}_i (\mathbf{A}_i^{0.5} \mathbf{R}_i(\rho) \mathbf{A}_i^{0.5})^{-1} \mathbf{A}_i \mathbf{X}_i' \, .$$

The "meat" of the sandwich is an information matrix that uses empirical residuals to estimate the within-cluster covariance matrix. The "meat" for the ith cluster is

$$\mathbf{M}_i = \mathbf{D}_i' \, \mathbf{V}_i^{-1} \mathbf{C}_i \mathbf{V}_i^{-1} \mathbf{D}_i$$
$$= \mathbf{X}_i' \, \mathbf{A}_i (\mathbf{A}_i^{0.5} \mathbf{R}_i(\rho) \mathbf{A}_i^{0.5})^{-1} \mathbf{C}_i (\mathbf{A}_i^{0.5} \mathbf{R}_i(\rho) \mathbf{A}_i^{0.5})^{-1} \mathbf{A}_i \mathbf{X}_i' \, , \qquad (9.10)$$

where $\mathbf{C}_i$ is the outer product of the empirical residuals. Specifically, the jkth element of this $n_i \times n_i$ matrix is

$$c_{jk} = [y_{ij} - \pi_{PA}(\mathbf{x}_{ij})] \times [y_{ij} - \pi_{PA}(\mathbf{x}_{ij})].$$

The equation for the estimator is obtained by evaluating all expressions at the estimator $\hat{\boldsymbol{\beta}}_{PA}$ and the respective values of the covariates, namely

$$\widehat{\text{Cov}}(\hat{\boldsymbol{\beta}}_{PA}) = \left(\sum_{i=1}^{m} \hat{\mathbf{B}}_i \right)^{-1} \times \left(\sum_{i=1}^{m} \hat{\mathbf{M}}_i \right) \times \left(\sum_{i=1}^{m} \hat{\mathbf{B}}_i \right)^{-1}. \qquad (9.11)$$

We note that some packages may offer the user the choice of using the information sandwich estimator, also called the robust estimator, in equation (9.11) or one based only on the observed information matrix for the specified correlation structure, the "bread" $\mathbf{B}_i$. We recommend that unless there is strong evidence from other studies or clinical considerations that the working correlation structure is correct, one should use the estimator in equation (9.11).

One can use the estimated coefficients and estimated standard errors to estimate odds ratios and to perform tests for individual coefficients. Joint hypotheses must be tested using multivariable Wald tests because the GEE approach is not based on likelihood theory. This does make model building a bit more cumbersome, because in most packages it is more complicated to perform multivariable Wald tests than likelihood ratio tests. An alternative to Wald tests, available in some software packages, are Generalized Score statistics [Rotnitzky and Jewell (1990)]. Regardless, the fact that the method does not have a likelihood is a disadvantage of GEE. We will discuss other available tools for model building and comparison in later sections.

Unlike the population average model, it is possible to formulate a likelihood function for the cluster-specific model. If we assume that the random effects follow a normal distribution with mean 0 and constant variance, $\alpha_i \sim N(0, \sigma_\alpha^2)$, then the contribution of the ith cluster to the likelihood function as given in Section 1.2 is

$$f(\mathbf{y}_i|\mathbf{x}_i, \alpha_i) = \prod_{j=1}^{n_i} \frac{e^{y_{ij} \times (\alpha_i + \mathbf{x}_{ij}' \boldsymbol{\beta}_s)}}{1 + e^{\alpha_i + \mathbf{x}_{ij}' \boldsymbol{\beta}_s}}. \tag{9.12}$$

The difference is that now this expression is a function of not only the observed data but also the unobserved random effect. To obtain a likelihood that does not include this unknown, we "integrate out" the random effect as follows. First, the conditional likelihood in equation (9.12) is rewritten so that the conditioning is only on x by integrating over the distribution of α_i given by $g(\alpha)$:

$$f(y|x) = \int_\alpha f(y|x, \alpha)g(\alpha).$$

Substituting the expression from equation (9.12) and the assumed normal distribution for $g(\alpha)$ produces the cluster contribution to the likelihood

$$\Pr(\boldsymbol{\beta}_s)_i = \int_{-\infty}^{\infty} \left[\prod_{j=1}^{n_i} \frac{e^{y_{ij} \times (\alpha_i + \mathbf{x}_{ij}' \boldsymbol{\beta}_s)}}{1 + e^{\alpha_i + \mathbf{x}_{ij}' \boldsymbol{\beta}_s}} \right] \frac{1}{\sqrt{2\pi}} \frac{1}{\sigma_\alpha} \exp\left(-\frac{\alpha_i^2}{2\sigma_\alpha^2} \right) d\alpha_i. \tag{9.13}$$

The full log-likelihood is then the sum of the log of this likelihood over all clusters,

$$L(\boldsymbol{\beta}_s) = \sum_{i=1}^{m} \ln[\Pr(\boldsymbol{\beta}_s)_i]. \tag{9.14}$$

The problem is that complicated numerical methods are needed to evaluate the log-likelihood, obtain the likelihood equations, and then solve them. These methods are, in general, well beyond the mathematical level of this text. There are several approaches we do not discuss, including the use of the EM algorithm [Anderson and Aitken (1985)] and an empirical Bayesian approach [Wong and Mason (1985); Stiratelli et al. (1984)]. A fully Bayesian approach using Gibbs sampling (Markov Chain Monte Carlo, or MCMC, simulation) is discussed in Section 10.6 of this textbook as this approach has increased in popularity with the improvement in computing power.

Two classes of estimation method are most commonly used in standard software packages. The first is to avoid the difficulty of evaluating the integral in equation (9.13), which is a non-linear function of the parameters, by "linearizing" the model using a Taylor series approximation. These "linearized" models are then estimated using methods from linear mixed models. As the likelihood function is not actually used in the estimation, such procedures are referred to as "quasilikelihood" or "pseudolikelihood" estimation. The second approach is to evaluate the integral in the likelihood function using numerical integration techniques [Pinheiro and Bates (1995); Rabe-Hesketh et al. (2002)], namely quadrature (Gauss–Hermite quadrature). The basic idea of quadrature is to replace the integral over the random effects normal distribution in equation (9.13) with a sum. In other words, the continuous distribution is approximated by a discrete distribution. We will illustrate the choices and issues with both approaches using examples in Sections 9.4 and 9.5. The remainder of this section gives some additional details that may be skipped on the first read or that may be of interest only to more experienced users.

Software packages offer numerous options for the approximation and parameter estimation algorithms. We will provide recommendations later about selecting from these choices. For the quasi- and pseudolikelihood (PL) methods, marginal quasi-likelihood (MQL) [Goldstein (1991)] involves a Taylor series expansion around random effects of 0 (their theoretical mean value—or in essence expanding around the fixed effects or marginal model). The Taylor expansion may include a term for only the first derivative (first-order approximation) or, to improve accuracy, a second derivative term (second order). The choice of expansion is designated MQL-1 or MQL-2. Expansion around the current estimates of the random effects at each iteration is termed penalized quasilikelihood (PQL) estimation [Breslow and Clayton (1993); Goldstein and Rasbash (1996)] and again, may involve a first or second order approximation (designated PQL-1 or PQL-2). SAS uses a slight variation to these methods termed "pseudolikelihood" or PL [Wolfinger and O'Connell (1993)]. The approach includes two choices for the Taylor series expansion at each iteration. In the first, known as marginal pseudolikelihood (MPL), the expansion is around the expected values (corresponds to MQL). In the other, referred to as subject-specific pseudolikelihood (SPL), expansion is around the estimated random effects. An additional option with PL methods is to make use of the residuals at each optimization step, which reduces bias in the estimates. Estimation without using the adjustment is termed "maximum likelihood" and an "M" is added to the acronym (MMPL and MSPL). The corresponding methods using the residuals are RMPL and RSPL.

The primary option for adaptive quadrature estimation involves the choice of the number of discrete points (known as quadrature points) and their locations. They are chosen and given weights based upon the underlying normal distribution. With correlated data, issues with the method arise with large clusters or high intra-cluster correlation, which can lead to sharp peaks in the continuous distribution that may fall between the points chosen for the discrete approximation. Adaptive quadrature improves the approximation by scaling and shifting the locations chosen based upon the cluster data [Rabe-Hesketh et al. (2005)]. Increasing the number of points chosen improves the approximation.

The choice of estimation methods (and options—there are many not discussed here) is an issue in cluster-specific models as different methods will produce different results. Although the differences are often small there are examples in real data sets in which they can be quite striking [Lesaffre and Spiessens (2001); Masaoud and Stryhn (2010)]. We will discuss some strategies in the context of examples in later sections of this chapter. Our general preference is to use methods like adaptive quadrature or MCMC. These methods, in general, appear to suffer the least from bias in the estimates and offer the added advantage of an estimate of the likelihood function for use in model building and comparison such as the likelihood ratio tests used in earlier chapters [Zhang et al. (2011)]. The methods do have potential drawbacks however. Quadrature does not always produce the parameter estimates that truly maximize the likelihood [Lesaffre and Spiessens (2001)]; issues appear to be most likely in settings with high intra-cluster correlations. Adaptive quadrature suffers less from potential estimation bias. A more likely problem is the ability of the numerical methods to converge with a complicated model (i.e., those with more than two levels or multiple random effects). However, although one would prefer to use more quadrature points to improve approximations, increasing the number can lead to numerical convergence issues.

The quasi- or pseudolikelihood methods offer an advantage over numerical methods in their ability to converge and produce estimates for the parameters. However, there is substantial evidence [Rodriguez and Goldman (1995, 2001); Breslow (2003); Heo and Leon (2005); Masaoud and Stryhn (2010)] that they can suffer from bias in those estimates particularly in settings with small samples in the clusters or high intra-cluster correlation. PQL-2 seems to suffer less (RSPL for PL) but, like numerical methods, may not allow estimation computationally. Additionally, options to improve the methods using simulation [see Goldstein and Rasbash (1996), and Ng et al. (2006), for a review of some] techniques are proposed and may be available in some software packages.

9.4 INTERPRETATION OF COEFFICIENTS FROM LOGISTIC REGRESSION MODELS FOR THE ANALYSIS OF CORRELATED DATA

In this section we explore the similarities and differences in the estimates of effect from marginal (population average) and conditional (cluster-specific) models for correlated binary data. Specifically, we focus on the GEE model described in the previous section with exchangeable correlation structure and the corresponding random effects model using quasilikelihood and adaptive quadrature estimation methods. These models are available in most standard statistical software packages. The GEE model, for example, is fit using PROC GENMOD in SAS and XTGEE or XTLOGIT with the "PA" option in STATA. The random effects models in SAS are fit using PROC GLIMMIX and in STATA with XTLOGIT. Only quadrature estimation is available in STATA. In SAS the default method is PL estimation. SAS has the option to use quadrature, producing estimates very similar to STATA.

To provide an example we created another sampled data set from the GLOW data, as described in Section 1.6.3 called "GLOW_RAND" with 500 observations and the same covariates as described in Table 1.7. This data set is different from the GLOW500 data and was created in order to better illustrate features of correlated data models. In earlier chapters, the data set described in Section 1.6.3 was analyzed without accounting for two possible sources of correlation between observations on study subjects: the physician (PHYS_ID) and the study site (SITE_ID). As subjects are clustered by physician within sites it may be necessary to consider a three-level random effects model when analyzing the data. In this section, we begin by considering two-level models using only sites, SITE_ID, and a random intercept. The GLOW_RAND data has 6 sites with as few as 24 subjects in one site (site 4) and as many as 113 in one site (site 2). There are 124 physicians and the sizes of physician clusters vary from 1 to 13.

The outcome of interest is, again, whether a fracture occurred in the first year of follow-up (FRACTURE). In this section, we fit a model using the continuous covariate weight (kg) at enrollment divided by 5 (WEIGHT5), the dichotomous covariate arms needed to stand (ARMASSIST), and the three level categorical covariate self-reported risk of fracture (RATERISK). We divided weight by 5 in order for the coefficient to provide the change in log-odds for a 5 kg increase in weight (see Section 3.4).

We begin by fitting the standard logistic model that ignores the correlation among subjects within sites (i.e., SITE_ID). A summary of the results of this fit are shown in the second column of Table 9.1 under the heading labeled "Standard Model." Estimates from models that account for the correlation are presented in columns 3 and 5 and the percentage differences as compared to the standard model are calculated and presented in columns 4 and 6. Although not shown, all four variables are significant in all three models with p-values less than 0.02.

9.4.1   Population Average Model

The results shown from the fit of the population average model with exchangeable correlation are shown in the third column of Table 9.1. We used STATA's xtlogit

Table 9.1 **Estimated Coefficients and Standard Errors from the Standard Logistic Regression Model, the Population Average Model, and the Cluster-Specific Model**

Variable	Standard Model Coeff. (Std. Err.)	Population Average Model Coeff. (Std. Err.)	Population Average Model % Change	Cluster-Specific Model Coeff. (Std. Err.)	Cluster-Specific Model % Change
WEIGHT5	−0.121	−0.114	5.70	−0.116	4.13
	(0.040)	(0.025)	(−37.50)	(0.041)	(1.25)
RATERISK_2	0.721	0.678	−5.96	0.683	−5.27
	(0.293)	(0.128)	(−56.31)	(0.297)	(1.37)
RATERISK_3	0.771	0.734	−4.80	0.745	−3.37
	(0.309)	(0.248)	(−19.74)	(0.313)	(1.29)
ARMASSIST	0.901	0.903	0.22	0.923	2.33
	(0.223)	(0.189)	(−15.25)	(0.228)	(2.24)
Constant	−0.342	−0.466		−0.471	
	(0.613)	(0.309)		(0.642)	
/lnsig2u				−1.877	
				(0.927)	
Sigma_u				0.391	
				(0.181)	
Rho		0.022		0.044	
				(0.039)	

command with the "pa" option and the robust or "sandwich" estimates shown in equation (9.11) for the standard errors (option "vce(robust)"). The percentage change from the standard logistic model estimates is at most 6%. The small differences observed in estimated coefficients are often the case, in particular when the correlation between clusters is small as in this example where $\hat{\rho} = 0.022$. We discuss this estimate later. However, the estimated standard errors are considerably smaller, by 15–56%. Interestingly, in this case, by accounting for the correlation among subjects within sites we have more precision and thus tighter inferences and narrower confidence intervals. In the example, the overall conclusion about the significance of covariates is unchanged as the p-values are all less than 0.003.

One danger in ignoring correlation among responses is that the inferences could change and a covariate that is not significant appears to have statistical significance under the standard model, or an insignificant covariate could likewise appear significant. Rabe-Hesketh and Skrondal (2008) suggest that the type of covariate, cluster, or subject can determine how statistical inference is affected. For a cluster-level covariate the estimated standard error will be too small if the model ignores the correlation. The danger in this case is to conclude significance where none exists. The opposite is true for subject-level covariates. Austin et al. (2003) give an example of ignoring the correlation in a three-level model, patients clustered within physicians who are clustered within hospitals. In their example, failing to account for the correlation has the general effect of reducing the significance of physician level effects while increasing the significance of hospital level affects. These results agree with the opinion that higher (cluster) level covariates are ones likely to erroneously appear significant when correlation is ignored.

By using the exchangeable correlation structure we assume that the correlation between pairs of observations for a given subject is the same. Thus, the correlation matrix as given in equation (9.7) involves a single parameter ρ, which we have added to Table 9.1 as "Rho." In this case the estimated value $\hat{\rho} = 0.022$ is small suggesting the correlation within sites is not large. In the population average model, the working correlations are usually of little interest, and as a result tests of their significance are not typically conducted. We discuss the issue of determining whether the chosen correlation structure is best in the next two sections.

Estimators of the odds ratios from a fitted population average model are computed using the same steps described for the standard model in Chapter 3. Estimated odds ratios and their confidence intervals from the fitted models in Table 9.1 are shown in Table 9.2. For example the estimate of the odds ratio for ARMASSIST is:

$$e^{0.9034} = 2.468.$$

The end points of the 95% confidence interval are computed as in the standard model and are:

$$e^{0.9034 \pm 1.96(0.189)} = (1.704, 3.575).$$

The odds ratios from a population average model are based on proportions of subjects in the population at the different levels of the covariate of interest while holding all other covariates fixed. As a result, their interpretation is analogous to the

Table 9.2 Estimated Odds Ratios and Confidence Intervals from the Population Average Model in Table 9.1

Variable	Odds Ratio	95% CI
WEIGHT5	0.892	0.850, 0.937
RATERISK_2	1.970	1.534, 2.531
RATERISK_3	2.083	1.282, 3.385
ARMASSIST	2.468	1.704, 3.575

interpretation of odds ratios from the standard logistic regression model, discussed in Chapter 3. Hence, the population average model is likely to be the best model for correlated data when the objective of the study is to describe, in broad terms, the effects of the covariates. However, this broad interpretation comes at the cost of not using information available in repeated measurements of a covariate on study subjects.

In our example, the estimated population average odds ratio for ARMASSIST is 2.47. The interpretation is that the odds of a fracture in the first year computed from the proportion of subjects requiring arm assistance to stand is 2.47 times that based on the proportion of subjects not requiring arm assistance, holding self-reported risk of fracture and weight constant. The population average odds ratio for a 5 kg increase in weight is 0.89. The interpretation is that the odds of a fracture in the first year computed from the proportion of subjects weighing 5 kg more than some reference weight is about 11% lower than that based on the reference weight, holding self-reported risk and arm assistance constant. The fact that weight is linear in the logit implies this odds ratio holds for a 5 kg increase at any weight. The population average odds ratio for self-reported risk of fracture involves two comparisons to the reference group, RATERISK = 1, obtained via reference cell coding described in Section 3.3. As an example, we compare women who report that their risk of fracture is greater than other women the same age (RATERISK = 3) to women who report that their risk of fracture is less than women the same age (RATERISK = 1). Using the results from the fitted population average model in Table 9.2 the estimate of this odds ratio is 2.08. The interpretation is that the odds of fracture in the first year of follow-up computed from the proportion of subjects reporting higher risk than others in the same age group is 2.08 times the odds of fracture in the first year of follow-up based on the proportion of subjects who report lower risk than others in the same age, holding weight and arm assistance required constant.

9.4.2 Cluster-Specific Model

We next fit a cluster-specific model in STATA using adaptive quadrature with the same covariates. The results are shown in column 5 of Table 9.1. The estimated odds ratios and their 95% confidence intervals are shown in Table 9.3. We obtained

Table 9.3 Estimated Odds Ratios and Confidence Intervals from the Fitted Cluster-Specific Model Using Adaptive Quadrature Estimation in Table 9.1

Variable	Odds Ratio	95% CI
WEIGHT5	0.891	0.823, 0.964
RATERISK_2	1.980	1.106, 3.544
RATERISK_3	2.107	1.141, 3.890
ARMASSIST	2.516	1.609, 3.933

similar results using adaptive quadrature in SAS. In both packages all other options are at their default settings.

Table 9.1 contains additional output typically provided for cluster-specific models. The top panel of output contains results describing the estimates of the coefficients. The bottom panel contains results describing the estimate of the variance of the random effect due to site. For numerical stability reasons STATA chooses to estimate the log of the variance described in the row labeled "/lnsig2u" in Table 9.1. The resulting estimate of the standard deviation, displayed in the row labeled "sigma," is obtained as the square root of the exponentiated estimate of the log variance, for example, $0.391 = \sqrt{\exp(-1.88)}$. The result in the row labeled "rho" is an estimate of the intracluster correlation (ICC), a measure of the proportion of the total variance accounted for by the random effect. The proportion requires an estimate of the variance at level 1 and the most common practice is to use the value $\pi^2/3$, which is the assumed variance for an underlying "threshold" continuous model producing the binary responses [McCullagh and Nelder (1989)]. Based upon this assumption, the estimated proportion of the total variance explained is

$$0.044 = \frac{0.391^2}{\frac{\pi^2}{3} + 0.391^2}.$$

SAS provides similar or equivalent output for the fitted model. As we observed in the population average model, the ICC suggests little correlation between observations within sites.

The percentage differences between cluster-specific estimates and the standard model estimates are shown in the last column of Table 9.1. The cluster-specific estimates are similar in this example, differing by less than 6%. We note that the estimated coefficients from the cluster-specific model are all larger in absolute value than those from the population average model, a point we return to shortly. As both coefficient and standard error estimates are similar it is not surprising that the coefficients are statistically significant with p-values less than 0.03. This is not always the case with cluster-specific models for correlated data as we will demonstrate in the next section. Statistical significance for the random effects is not typically shown in this portion of the computer output. We also discuss tests for significance of random effects in the next section.

The interpretation of estimated odds ratios from a fitted cluster-specific model apply to subjects with a common but unobserved value of the underlying random effect, α_i. This could be a single subject or a group of subjects. For example the estimate of the cluster-specific odds ratio from Table 9.3 for use of arms in standing (ARMASSIST) is 2.52. The interpretation is that by needing to use arms to stand a woman has increased her odds of a fracture in the first year of follow-up by 2.52 times the odds if she did not require arm assistance, holding self-reported risk and weight constant. In this case the odds ratio makes sense because arm assistance is probably a modifiable risk factor at the subject level. However, an estimated odds ratio for a nonmodifiable factor such as race is more difficult to interpret. One would have to resort to comparisons of hypothetical groups of subjects with the same random effect who differ in their race holding other covariates constant. We leave the details as an exercise.

The cluster-specific odds ratio for a 5 kg increase in weight is 0.89. The interpretation is that the odds of having a fracture in the first year of follow up for a woman who gained 5 kg is 11% less than the odds at the current weight, holding self-reported risk and arm assistance constant. This odds ratio suggests, likely incorrectly, that by simply gaining weight a person can substantially reduce the risk of a fracture. What is needed in the model is a more objective measure of size of the woman such as body mass index. If the effect of weight gain is similar for both short and tall subjects then the odds ratio correctly estimates the effect of body size on fractures for subjects with the same random effect and holding all other covariates constant. The interpretation for the categorical self-reported risk odds ratios is similar to that of the dichotomous variable arm assist with each odds ratio comparing the odds to the reference group and is left as an exercise.

The covariates weight, arm assist and self-reported risk provide good examples of the strengths and weaknesses of population average and cluster-specific models. In a sense, the odds ratios for these covariates are easier to interpret from population average models as they describe effects in broad groups of subjects in the population. The clear weakness of the population average model is that it cannot address effects such as age. The cluster-specific model is best suited for such a covariate, as one does not have to argue that the inferences apply to some hypothetical and unobservable group of subjects with the same random effect. For example, an odds ratio of 2.0 for a 10 year increase in age in a population average model would be interpreted as the odds of fracture is twice as much for the population of subjects that is 10 years older than the odds for those in the 10 years younger population. Both models can be used to address important clinical questions and have their place in an analysis of clustered binary data.

There are two other estimates of effect that subject matter scientists find useful when interpreting results of cluster-specific models. These are the Median Odds Ratio (MOR) and the Interval Odds Ratio (IOR) described in Larsen et al. (2000) and Larsen and Merlo (2005). Currently, these measures are not calculated in software packages, but are both simple to compute and are being increasingly used when reporting results from cluster-specific models for binary outcomes.

The MOR is a measure of how much variability in the outcome exists between clusters. It compares the odds for randomly selected subjects from two different clusters holding all covariates in the model constant. Recall that the random effect for cluster i is α_i. Thus, the odds ratio for two such subjects is defined as $\exp(|\alpha_i - \alpha_j|)$. The absolute value is used to ensure that the difference between the random effects is positive; in other words, to compare the subject with higher odds to the one with lower odds. Hence, these odds ratios are always greater than or equal to 1. The MOR is the median value of the distribution of odds ratios for all such randomly chosen pairs. Thus, a value of the MOR near 1 suggests little difference between clusters as it implies that most of the differences, $|\alpha_i - \alpha_j|$, are small. A value much larger than 1 is indicative of variability in outcome between clusters. Using results from the standard normal distribution the estimate of the MOR is:

$$\widehat{\text{MOR}} = e^{z_{0.75}\sqrt{2\hat{\sigma}^2}}$$
$$= e^{0.6745\sqrt{2\hat{\sigma}^2}}, \quad (9.15)$$

where $z_{0.75}$ is the 75th percentile of the Standard Normal distribution function and $\hat{\sigma}^2$ is the estimator of the cluster variance. Using the results of the fitted cluster-specific model in Table 9.1 the estimate of the cluster variance is the estimated variance of the random intercept

$$\hat{\sigma}^2 = \exp(-1.877) = 0.152881,$$

which leads to an MOR estimate of

$$\widehat{\text{MOR}} = e^{0.6745\sqrt{2 \cdot 0.152881}} = 1.45.$$

The interpretation is that for two randomly chosen subjects from different sites (i.e., different clusters) with the same values of the covariates in the model (weight, arm assistance, and self-reported risk) the median odds for the higher risk subject of a fracture in the first year is 1.45 times that of the lower risk subject in all such pairs. In other words, for half of the possible pairs of randomly selected subjects from different sites the odds for the higher risk subject is more than 1.45 times that of the lower risk subject. The 50% increase in odds for half of the pairs suggests a difference in the risk of fracture between subjects at different sites. However, there is no formal test for how large the MOR needs to be to support this conclusion.

The interval odds ratio, IOR, is useful for examining the effect of cluster but not subject level covariates on risk of the outcome. It is defined as the interval covering the central 80% of odds ratios between two subjects from different clusters and with different cluster-level covariate values [note: we use 80% which is the value recommended by Larsen et al. (2000)]. Unlike the MOR, the distribution of the odds ratios used to form the IOR does not always involve comparing larger to smaller odds. Hence, the values used to compute the IOR can be less than 1 as well as greater than 1. The IOR has a different interpretation than the odds ratio computed from the coefficient of a cluster level covariate, namely the odds for a change in the covariate for a subject in a fixed cluster. The IOR considers the difference in the covariate, but for subjects from different clusters. Note that the IOR is not a confidence interval for an odds ratio, hence 80% is defined by the percentage of the population odds ratios one wishes to cover. For two hypothetical sets of covariate values, $\mathbf{x}_1$ and $\mathbf{x}_2$, the equations to estimate the IOR are:

$$\widehat{\text{IOR}}_{\text{lower}} = e^{\hat{\beta} \times (\mathbf{x}_1 - \mathbf{x}_2) - z_{0.9} \times \sqrt{2\hat{\sigma}^2}} \tag{9.16}$$

and

$$\widehat{\text{IOR}}_{\text{upper}} = e^{\hat{\beta} \times (\mathbf{x}_1 - \mathbf{x}_2) + z_{0.9} \times \sqrt{2\hat{\sigma}^2}}, \tag{9.17}$$

where $z_{0.9} = 1.28$ is the 90th percentile of the Standard Normal distribution.

In our example, we do not have any cluster level variables in the model. For purposes of illustrating the IOR, suppose that we had the dichotomous variable URBAN in the model where 1 represented an urban site and 0 a rural site and we wish to compare subjects from an urban to rural site holding other covariates constant. If the estimated coefficient for the URBAN variable were 0.8 the IOR estimate would be:

$$\widehat{\text{IOR}} = e^{0.8 \times (1-0) \pm 1.28 \times \sqrt{2(0.391)^2}}$$

$$= (1.097, 4.517).$$

There are two key insights the IOR can provide about the cluster covariate and cluster correlation. The first is based on the width of the interval. Wide intervals indicate that the variability between clusters (sites) is large relative to the effect of the (hypothetical in this case) cluster variable. A narrow interval suggests less variability between clusters. The second insight is based on whether or not the interval contains the value one. In this example, the interval does not contain one, which would suggest that the effect of the cluster-level variable is still significant even in the presence of the variability, σ_α^2, between clusters. Thus we would conclude the effect of URBAN is significant relative to the variability in the SITE. The interval is quite wide, however, suggesting there is additional variability due to SITE.

In cluster-specific models, unlike population average models, the cluster effects, α_i, may be of interest to the researcher. For example, we may wish to know which sites have larger or smaller probabilities of fracture 1 year after follow-up because there is some variability across sites as seen in the IOR. Regardless of estimation method, quadrature, or PL, software packages such as STATA and SAS can produce estimates and standard errors of the random effects in cluster-specific models. In most cases, the estimates are, in fact, predictions that are based on conditional distributions of the random effect for a cluster given the estimated values for the fixed and random parameters in the model. In Bayesian terminology (see Section 10.6), these are "posterior" distributions and the estimates for the random effect is usually the mode of that distribution. The predicted values are referred to as BLUPs (Best Linear Unbiased Predictions) or EBLUPs (Estimated Best Linear Unbiased Predictions). It is important to understand that due to the way they are calculated these predicted values are "shrunken" to the mean. In essence, they are shifted toward the overall population average from the observed value one might obtain using only the cluster average. The intuition is that the cluster estimate is based on a small sample and we would like to take advantage of information from the other clusters.

In STATA, we use xtmelogit to fit a model and produce the predicted values of the random effects. We used the xtlogit procedure to fit a model with a random intercept and covariates weight, self-reported risk, and arm assist with results shown in Table 9.1. The advantage of the xtlogit procedure is that it has an option to fit both the cluster-specific and population average models we used in this section. However, for more complicated random effects models the xtmelogit procedure must be used. The xtmelogit procedure provides the additional output options necessary to obtain the estimates of the predicted cluster random intercept values. In SAS, one adds the "solution" option to the random statement to estimate and report the predicted values within the GLIMMIX procedure. The estimates of the random effects and standard errors for the model fit in column 4 of Table 9.1 are shown in Table 9.4.

As we are fitting a model with a random intercept only, as shown in equation (9.3), the posterior predicted values are the estimates, $\hat{\alpha}_i$, for each cluster (site). When added to the model estimated intercept coefficient of -0.471 shown in Table 9.1, they provide a predicted value of the intercept for a given cluster (site). As an example, the predicted random effect for site 1 from Table 9.4 is -0.093. Thus the predicted intercept for site 1 is $-0.471 + (-0.093) = -0.564$. As the intercept acts to shift the fitted logistic function up or down, the random effects indicate whether the overall probability of a fracture in the first year is higher or lower than the average for the given cluster (site). For site 1, the probability is slightly lower as the effect estimate is negative. We see that in this example two sites (SITE_ID $= 5$ and 6) appear to differ in terms of predicted intercept from the other four in that they have higher (positive) predicted intercept values. The predicted intercept for site 5 adds 0.496 to the estimated fixed effect intercept which, in turn, raises the estimated probability of a fracture in the first year for subjects from that site. Likewise, for site 6 there is a positive random effect of 0.3. Among the other four, site 3 has a much larger negative value and shifts probabilities down.

A useful method of presenting the predicted random effects is the so-called caterpillar plot [Goldstein and Healy (1995)], which displays the posterior estimates of the random intercepts with 95% confidence interval error bars. Goldstein and Healy (1995) suggest a procedure to adjust the error bars so that the average Type 1

Table 9.4 Predicted SITE_ID Random Intercepts, $\hat{\alpha}_i$, Using Adaptive Quadrature Estimation

SITE_ID	Predicted $\hat{\alpha}_i$	Std. Err.	Predicted Intercept $\hat{\beta}_0 + \hat{\alpha}_i$
1	−0.093	0.202	−0.564
2	−0.036	0.197	−0.507
3	−0.460	0.254	−0.931
4	−0.164	0.311	−0.635
5	0.496	0.193	0.025
6	0.300	0.214	−0.171

error rate for comparing pairs of differences between estimates is 0.05. With only six clusters, the adjustment factor is fairly simple to compute but in cases with more clusters this becomes more difficult so the standard normal 95% confidence intervals (i.e., the estimate plus/minus 1.96 times its standard error) may be the only option. Alternatively, use of a specialized software program [e.g., MLWin, Rasbash et al. (2009)] that produces this plot with the scaling may be required. Hence we present in Figure 9.1 the simple 95% confidence interval estimates by adding and subtracting 1.96 times the standard error from the estimated predicted values for each random effect.

The plot displays the predicted posterior random intercepts ranked from smallest to largest for the six sites in the study with error bars to help visually identify sites that may differ. Although we cannot use these results for inference, it does appear that there is a significant difference between sites 5 and 3 where the confidence intervals clearly do not overlap. As the posterior estimates are shrunken toward the overall mean the conclusion is reasonably conservative.

The predicted random effects allow us to compute predicted probabilities of the outcome for each subject in the sample accounting for the effect of the cluster. Predicted probabilities for the first five subjects in the GLOW_RAND data set are shown in Table 9.5. To illustrate how these values are computed we use subject 3. As this subject does not use arm assistance and lists RATERISK of 2, the coefficients for ARMASSIST and RATERISK_3 are multiplied by the covariate value of 0. Using the values of WEIGHT5 and RATERISK_2 as well as the estimates for the intercept and the predicted random effect for site 3 in Tables 9.1 and 9.4 the estimated logit is computed:

$$\hat{g}(\mathbf{x}) = -0.471 - 0.116 \times 15.70 + 0.683 \times 1 + 0.745 \times 0 + 0.923 \times 0 - 0.46$$

$$= -2.0692$$

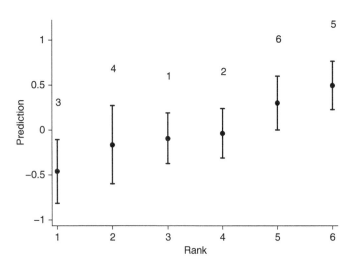

Figure 9.1 Plot of the ranked six predicted random intercepts, $\hat{\alpha}_i$, with 95% error bars for the six sites.

Table 9.5   Predicted Probabilities of FRACTURE for the First Five Subjects

SUBJECT_ID	SITE_ID	ARMASSIST	RATERISK	WEIGHT5	Predicted Probability
1	2	YES	3	14.52	0.373
2	3	YES	3	15.88	0.249
3	3	NO	2	15.70	0.112
4	4	YES	2	14.52	0.329
5	5	NO	3	9.70	0.412

and the probability estimate is

$$\hat{\pi} = \frac{e^{-2.0692}}{1 + e^{-2.0692}} = 0.112.$$

Most software packages will also include options to compute the predicted probabilities using only the fixed effects (in STATA the "fixedonly" option for predict). This produces predicted probabilities setting the random effects to their prior mean value of 0–in other words the probability for the subject visiting the "average" site (not the average probability over all sites). For our example with subject 3 using fixed effects only the logit is computed:

$$\hat{g}_F(\mathbf{x}) = -0.471 - 0.116 \times 15.70 + 0.683 \times 1 + 0.745 \times 0 + 0.923 \times 0 - 0$$

$$= -1.6092$$

and the probability estimate is

$$\hat{\pi}_F = \frac{e^{-1.6092}}{1 + e^{-1.6092}} = 0.167.$$

We see that this probability is higher as the subject was from site 3, which has a lower than average probability of a fracture in the first year (as indicated by the predicted value of the random intercept being negative).

9.4.3   Alternative Estimation Methods for the Cluster-Specific Model

As discussed in Section 9.3, there are several methods for estimating parameters in cluster-specific models. Some packages may not offer adaptive quadrature or there may be numerical issues that force the use of a different method. The most common alternatives are versions of quasi- or pseudolikelihood estimation. The results for the cluster-specific model using PL estimation from SAS are presented in Table 9.6. In this example, the results are fairly similar to those obtained using adaptive quadrature in Tables 9.1 and 9.3. SAS provides the variance estimate of 0.199, which corresponds to a standard deviation (Sigma) of 0.446; same order of magnitude as the value of 0.391 estimated in Table 9.3. One issue with PL estimation is that the random-effect estimate, $\hat{\sigma}_\alpha^2$, tends to be biased toward zero—we do

Table 9.6   Estimated Coefficients, Standard Errors, Odds Ratios, and Confidence Intervals for a Cluster-Specific Model Using Pseudo-Likelihood (PL) Estimation

Variable	Coeff.	Std. Err.	Odds Ratio	95% CI Odds Ratio
WEIGHT5	−0.115	0.040	0.892	0.824, 0.965
RATERISK_2	0.676	0.296	1.966	1.099, 3.519
RATERISK_3	0.738	0.312	2.092	1.133, 3.862
ARMASSIST	0.916	0.227	2.499	1.599, 3.906
Constant	−0.477	0.645		
Sigma_Squared	0.199	0.182		

not observe that in our example as the estimate is actually larger, $0.446 > 0.396$, using PL estimation. In general, the fixed effect estimates tend to be smaller in absolute value (coefficients closer to zero) for the PL fit. This is fairly common using the PL/PQL estimation methods—the fixed estimates can also be biased toward 0, although typically they are less so than the random effect estimates. As discussed in the previous section, the default method in SAS applies adjustments that reduce the bias. In our example, the ICC estimate is 0.044, which is small, and the number of subjects in each cluster is large, hence the estimated effects appear less impacted by the estimation method. The bias is generally most noted in cases with high ICC or small cluster sizes.

The adaptive quadrature and PL estimation methods for cluster-specific models presented here point out a difficulty one may encounter in practice. Software packages may give parameter estimates that can lead to different interpretation of the effects. The reason is that the solutions to the likelihood equations depend on the particular numerical method used. In addition, there are different rules used by the packages to stop the iteration process or control other parts of the optimization algorithms. For example, SAS's GLIMMIX procedure has numerous options and criteria that the user can specify. However, only expert users should even attempt to use anything but the default settings. STATA's xtlogit command uses the same basic method as SAS, under adaptive quadrature, but has far fewer optimization options. Again we think that modifying these options should be left to experienced users. Other packages such as R [R Development Core Team (2010)], MLwiN [Rasbash et al. (2009)], or SPSS [SPSS, Inc. (2012)] for such models may have an entirely different set of default settings and options.

9.4.4   Comparison of Population Average and Cluster-Specific Model

Neuhaus et al. (1991) and Neuhaus (1992) present results that compare the magnitude of the coefficients from the cluster-specific model and population average model. These authors show, for coefficients whose value is near 0, that

$$\beta_{PA} \approx \beta_s[1 - \rho(0)], \qquad (9.18)$$

where $\rho(0)$ is the intra-cluster correlation among the observations of the binary outcome. This result demonstrates that we expect the estimates from fitted population average models to be closer to the null value, 0, than estimates from the fitted cluster-specific model. The shrinkage to the null in equation (9.18) can also be obtained from results examining the effect of failing to include an important covariate in the model, see Neuhaus and Jewell (1993) and Chao et al. (1997).

We fit models to computer generated data to illustrate the effect of the intracluster correlation on the difference between the cluster-specific and population average coefficients. In each case, the fitted model contained a single continuous covariate distributed as normal with mean 0, standard deviation 3, and true cluster-specific coefficient $\beta_s = 1$. The random effects were generated from a normal distribution with mean 0 and standard deviation $\sigma_\alpha = 0, 0.5, 1.0, 1.5, \ldots, 10.0$. As we noted earlier in this section, the intracluster correlation increases with increasing σ_α. In these examples the resulting intracluster correlations, $\rho(0)$, range from 0 to about 0.84. For each set of parameter values we generated data for 200 clusters of size 4. Hence the equation of the logit is $g(x_{ij}, \beta_s) = \alpha_i + x_{ij}$ with $i = 1, 2, \ldots, 200$, $j = 1, 2, 3, 4$, $x_{ij} \sim N(0, 9)$ and $\alpha_i \sim N(0, \sigma_\alpha^2)$. We fit cluster-specific and population average models containing the covariate x. The values of the respective estimated coefficients are plotted versus the intracluster correlation in Figure 9.2. In addition, we plot an approximate population average coefficient obtained using equation (9.18), that is, $\tilde{\beta}_{PA} \approx \hat{\beta}_s[1 - \rho(0)]$.

The results shown in Figure 9.2 demonstrate that the attenuation to the null described in equation (9.18) holds in this example. We note that the estimate of the cluster-specific coefficient tends to fluctuate about the true value of 1.0 with increased variability for large values of the intracluster correlation. We observed

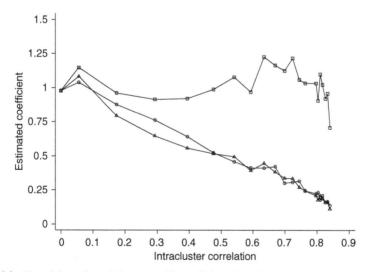

Figure 9.2 Plot of the estimated cluster-specific coefficient (□), estimated population average coefficient (○) and approximate estimated population average coefficient (△) versus the intracluster correlation obtained from fitting models with 200 clusters of size 4.

this same general pattern for varying numbers of clusters and observations per cluster.

Neuhaus (1992) shows that the variability in the estimates of the coefficients depends on the total sample size and intracluster correlation. In practice, the variability in the estimates of the population average coefficient depends to a greater extent on the number of clusters whereas that of the cluster-specific coefficient depends more on the total sample size and the intracluster correlation. The results in Neuhaus (1992) also show that the Wald statistics for population average coefficients under exchangeable correlation and the cluster-specific model should be approximately the same. This result also follows from the approximation shown in equation (9.18).

Some intuition behind the shrinkage to the null in the population average model can be gained by looking at an example using the cluster-specific model fit in this section. Using the estimates in Table 9.1 column 5, we plotted the probability of fracture in the first year for values of WEIGHT5 for subjects requiring arm assistance (ARMASSIST = 1) and the highest self-reported risk level (RATERISK_3 = 1). We produced curves for different possible random intercept values (dashed lines) in Figure 9.3. The random intercept values chosen are from 2 (highest curve) to −2 (lowest curve) by increments of 0.5. The average of these nine hypothetical clusters is shown with the solid line. We see that averaging across the clusters results in a curve that is not as steep as those for each cluster. This is due, mathematically, to the fact that the relationship between x and y is non-linear for a logistic regression model. More intuitively, we see that the more "extreme" clusters are "averaged out" by others with the opposite "extreme" (i.e., large positive and large negative random effects) so that the population average slope is closer to 0.

When the random effects are assumed to be normally distributed (typically the case in cluster-specific logistic regression) Zeger et al. (1988) develop a formula to equate coefficients between the cluster-specific and population average models that is easily computed from the basic model output and is given by

$$\tilde{\beta}_{PA} \approx \hat{\beta}_s \frac{1}{\sqrt{1 + \left(\frac{16}{15}\right)^2 \frac{3}{\pi^2} \hat{\sigma}^2}}. \tag{9.19}$$

In order to describe the effect of the intra-cluster correlation we calculate the approximate estimates from equation (9.18), using STATA's loneway to approximate the correlation, $\hat{\rho}(0)$, and those from equation (9.19). These approximations along with the coefficients from the population average model and cluster-specific (using adaptive quadrature) model are shown in Table 9.7.

The results show that the shrinkage to the null is well described by the approximation formulas in equations (9.18) and (9.19). The advantage of equation (9.19) is that one does not need to estimate $\rho(0)$. In this case the approximation in equation (9.19) is slightly better. We have seen instances where the reverse is the case, possibly due to violation of the normal assumption for the random effect. In general, one can be reasonably confident in the approximate population average effects

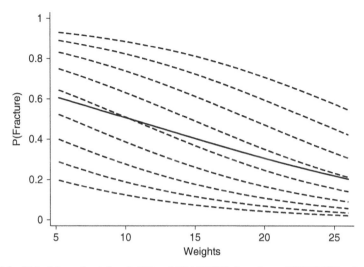

Figure 9.3 Plot of the estimated probability of FRACTURE for values of WEIGHT5 and values of the random intercept (dashed lines, 2, 1.5, 1, 0.5, 0, −0.5, −1, −1.5, −2) with the average of the clusters (solid line).

Table 9.7 Estimated Coefficients from the Cluster-Specific Model, Population Average Model and Two Approximations to the Population Average Model

Variable	Cluster-Specific Coeff., $\hat{\beta}_s$	Population Average Coeff., $\hat{\beta}_{PA}$	Approximate Pop. Averages Equation (9.18)	Equation (9.19)
WEIGHT5	−0.116	−0.114	−0.112	−0.113
RATERISK_2	0.683	0.678	0.658	0.665
RATERISK_3	0.745	0.734	0.717	0.726
ARMASSIST	0.922	0.903	0.887	0.899

computed from a cluster-specific model. If the primary goal of the analysis is population average inferences then one should fit the population average model. In the next section we discuss variable selection in the correlated binary data setting.

9.5   AN EXAMPLE OF LOGISTIC REGRESSION MODELING WITH CORRELATED DATA

Model building is as vital for correlated data as it is for uncorrelated data but has received relatively less attention in the statistical literature and practice than the uncorrelated case. Model complexity and lack of available tools for model checking and comparison have perhaps contributed to the problem. However, the modeling paradigm presented in detail in Chapter 4 may be applied to the models discussed in this chapter with only a few minor adjustments. Statistical variable selection methods such as stepwise and best subsets are not currently available for fitting correlated data models in software packages. Thus, one must use some form of purposeful selection using Wald or Score tests with the population average model and Wald or likelihood ratio tests (depending upon the estimation method) with the cluster-specific model. Checking the scale of continuous covariates is just as important with correlated as with non-correlated data models. One can always use the method of design variables because computer-intensive methods such as fractional polynomials have not yet been implemented for use with correlated data models. An alternative approach would be to assume the observations are not correlated and use spline functions or fractional polynomials to identify a potential nonlinear transformation. One would then try this transformation when fitting the appropriate correlated data model. Interactions should be specified and checked for inclusion in the same manner as described in Chapter 4. Diagnostic statistics, such as those described in Chapter 5, have not, as yet, all been extended for use in model checking with correlated data models. However, one could approximate the analysis by assuming the observations are not correlated and using the methods in Chapter 5. Although not specifically developed for this situation, this analysis is better than not doing any model checking. We focus on model building in this section and discuss ideas for model checking in Section 9.6.

We illustrate model building with correlated data using the polypharmacy data described in Section 1.6.8 and Table 1.12. The outcome of interest is whether the patient is taking drugs from three or more different classes (POLYPHARMACY) and researchers were interested in identifying factors associated with this outcome. Our purpose and approach to the data is from a model building perspective and, as such, we created a sample from the original data set useful in illustrating key points. Thus, the data set used here is a sample of 500 patients from among only those subjects with observations in each of the 7 years. Based on the suggestions of the principal investigator, we initially treated the covariates for number of inpatient and outpatient mental health visits (MHV) with categories described in Table 1.12. In addition we added a random number of months to the age, which was recorded only in terms of the year in the original data set. As our data set is a sample, the results in this section do not apply to the original study. Interested readers should refer to Fontanella et al. (2012) for results based on the full study.

9.5.1 Choice of Model for Correlated Data Analysis

An important component of analyzing correlated binary data is the choice of model to use. We tend to prefer cluster-specific models in the clinical trials setting, and generally feel the population average model is better suited for epidemiological studies. The key point, however, is that the appropriate model choice is not always obvious and one should carefully consider this selection prior to analyzing the data. When there is some doubt as to model choice, the type of inferences one can make from each model, as discussed in the previous section, may be the deciding factor. Finally, if the cluster effect is of interest itself (e.g., in this study we might be interested in comparing subjects) then a cluster-specific model must be used. If the goal is to merely account for the correlations that may result from the clusters, a population average model may be the better choice. In this example we would likely select the population average approach. For purposes of illustration, we demonstrate model building for both model types.

9.5.2 Population Average Model

For population average models fit using GEE, the first model building decision is choice of a correlation structure. We suggest using an exchangeable correlation initially, unless one has specific knowledge to suggest another choice. As an example, if the correlation is based upon repeated measures over time then an autoregressive correlation may be appropriate. Estimates from GEE are known to be robust to choice of correlation structure and the key, in preliminary model building, is to account for the correlations in some way. Using the "robust" or "sandwich" estimates for standard errors with the exchangeable correlation structure in model building is thus a good initial option in the absence of more knowledge about the correlation structure.

One measure for model comparison and selection that has been suggested for use with GEE models is the quasilikelihood information criteria (QIC) criteria [Pan (2001)]. This measure is a modification to the Akaike Information Criteria (AIC) discussed in Section 4.2 that was defined as

$$\text{AIC} = -2 \times L + 2 \times (p + 1),$$

where L is the log-likelihood of the fitted model and p is the number of regression coefficients estimated for nonconstant covariates. In GEE the likelihood is not estimated so the QIC is computed using the quasilikelihood function to replace the likelihood function and adjusts the "penalty" term, $2 \times (p + 1)$, based upon the use of a correlated model. The QIC is defined

$$\text{QIC} = -2 \times QL + 2\text{tr}(\widehat{\Omega_I} \widehat{V_R}), \tag{9.20}$$

where QL is the quasilikelihood function [McCullagh and Nelder (1989)] that, for binary data with dispersion parameter assumed to be 1, is the log-likelihood defined in equation (1.4) evaluated with the parameters estimated under the working correlation structure. $\hat{V}_R$ is the robust estimate of the covariance matrix of the parameters given in equation (9.11) in Section 9.3, and $\hat{\Omega}_I$ is the estimate of the inverse of the model-based covariance estimates (the "bread" of equation (9.11)) under the assumption of independence. The latter term is often referred to as the "model based" estimate of the covariance. If the covariance structure is correct the model based estimates and robust estimates are the same and the final term is the trace of the identity matrix of dimension $p + 1$ and the penalty term is the same used in QIC_u described in equation (9.21). As the expression in equation (9.20) involves the estimates of the covariance matrix, the QIC is potentially useful in variable selection as well as choice of working correlation structure. An approximation to QIC, referred to as QIC_u, uses the same penalty term as in AIC and is defined as follows:

$$QIC_u = -2 \times QL + 2 \times (p + 1). \tag{9.21}$$

QIC_u is only useful for variable selection and not correlation structure choice because the penalty term ignores the correlation. As with the AIC measure, smaller values are indicative of a "better" model. These measures are available in many software packages. SAS, for example, reports both.

For the polypharmacy data, we start modeling using an autoregressive correlation structure as the data are observed over time. We begin with the default lag of 1. (The assumption concerning correlation structure will be discussed later in the example.) We use robust estimates for the standard errors and purposeful variable selection (as described in Chapter 4) in building the model. The QIC statistic can be used to help assess the choice of a correlated data model. Using SAS, we fit the intercept-only model with the AR(1) correlation structure choice and then refit assuming exchangeable correlations. The QIC for the AR(1) is slightly higher at 3816.83 compared to 3815.92. We will discuss the choice further in the example but, at this point, with the values effectively the same, we opt for the AR(1) structure due to the repeated measurements that lead to the correlation in observations. The estimated working correlation in the exchangeable case is 0.45, suggesting there is a fairly strong correlation within subjects. As discussed in previous sections, we prefer modeling the correlation, even if the estimate is smaller and the independence model seems preferable statistically, when there is a clinical reason to believe correlation exists, as is the case in this example.

We begin purposeful model building with univariable analysis using GEE models with the AR(1) correlation structure at every step. Wald tests are used in determining whether a variable should be included in the model. Estimates for univariable analysis are presented in Table 9.8. In SAS the default multivariable test for polytomous covariates is a Score test; so use of the multivariable Wald test requires an option in the model statement. We present the results using both tests, for each of the five models, in Table 9.9. We have observed instances when the multivariable Score test appeared too conservative as it failed to reject although there were significant differences between levels of the covariates. We do not observe such an issue in this example as the two tests produce very similar results. We use the multivariate Wald option for subsequent model fitting. Note that the results in Tables 9.8 and 9.9 are based on SAS output because both Score and Wald tests are available. Wald test results in STATA are comparable although there are slight differences in estimates of the standard errors. None of the differences alters the resulting decisions to include or exclude a covariate from the first multivariable model.

Modeling proceeds as described in Chapter 4. In addition to checking statistical significance of covariates added and removed from the model using Wald tests, the delta beta hat percentage is also checked to insure that confounding is not an issue. We leave the details as an exercise. The univariable analysis results

Table 9.8 Estimates from Fitting the Univariable Analysis Population Average Logistic Regression Models to the Polypharmacy Data

Variable	Coeff.	Std. Err.	z	p
MHV4_1	0.161	0.131	1.22	0.221
MHV4_2	0.601	0.142	4.22	<0.001
MHV4_3	0.925	0.150	6.18	<0.001
INPTMHV3_1	0.447	0.227	1.97	0.049
INPTMHV3_2	0.403	0.340	1.18	0.236
GROUP_2	0.137	0.134	1.02	0.305
GROUP_3	0.331	0.226	1.46	0.143
URBAN_1	0.067	0.153	0.44	0.662
COMORBID_1	−0.171	0.094	−1.71	0.070
ANYPRIM_1	−0.007	0.071	−0.10	0.920
NUMPRIMRC_1	0.002	0.071	0.02	0.983
NUMPRIMRC_2	−0.396	0.211	−1.88	0.060
GENDER_1	0.525	0.201	2.61	0.009
RACE_1	−0.353	0.219	−1.62	0.106
RACE_2	−0.321	1.004	−0.32	0.750
ETHNIC_1	−0.982	0.647	−1.52	0.129
AGE	0.105	0.018	5.95	<0.001

Table 9.9 Wald and Score Tests for Polytomous Covariates from the Univariable Fits in Table 9.8

Variable	df	Wald Test		Score Test	
		W	p	S	p
MHV4	3	55.09	<0.001	46.46	<0.001
INPTMHV3	2	4.70	0.095	6.01	0.050
GROUP	2	2.65	0.266	2.69	0.260
NUMPRIMRC	2	3.82	0.148	3.30	0.192
RACE	2	2.69	0.261	3.01	0.222

in Table 9.8 suggest the possibility of collapsing categories for several covariates. One to five outpatient MHV was not statistically different ($p = 0.226$) from no outpatient MHV but we chose to maintain the four levels as there is clinical interest in comparing to no outpatient MHV. Inpatient MHV of 1 is not significantly different from more than 1 ($p = 0.91$) and there are very few observations in the data set of more than one visit so we created a dichotomous covariate (INPTMHV2) that is 0 for no inpatient MHV and 1 otherwise. Similarly, we combine BLACK and OTHER to create a dichotomous covariate, RACE2, that is 0 if WHITE and 1 otherwise. Finally, we combined the 0 and 1 categories of number of primary diagnoses. The preliminary main effects model includes the five covariates shown in Table 9.10: gender (GENDER), outpatient MHV (MHV4), age (AGE) and the dichotomous versions of inpatient MHV (INPTMHV2) and race (RACE2).

Table 9.10   Preliminary Main Effects Population Average Logistic Regression Model for the Polypharmacy Data

Variable	Coeff.	Std. Err.	z	p
GENDER_M	0.467	0.197	2.37	0.018
AGE	0.110	0.018	6.17	<0.001
MHV4_1	0.151	0.131	1.06	0.289
MHV4_2	0.601	0.153	3.93	<0.001
MHV4_3	0.917	0.163	5.62	<0.001
RACE2_1	−0.435	0.204	−2.14	0.033
INPTMHV2_1	0.368	0.193	1.91	0.056
Constant	−3.426	0.305	−11.23	<0.001

Rho = 0.571 ; QIC = 3517.75 ; QICu = 3504.15.

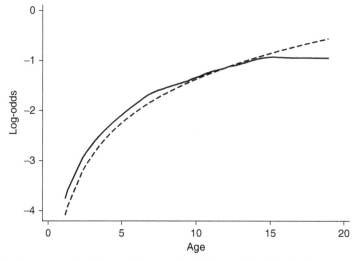

Figure 9.4   Lowess smooth of the log-odds for age (solid line) and fitted fractional polynomial ($m = 1$, natural log) for age (dashed line).

The multivariable Wald tests for the polytomous covariate outpatient MHV is significant with p-value less than 0.001.

The next step in model building is to check the scale of the continuous covariate, age, in the model. The Lowess smoothed plot can help identify potential issues with scale. The plot for age, shown in Figure 9.4, although reasonably linear, has enough curvature to suggest not treating the covariate as if it were linear in the logit. We see that the log-odds of polypharmacy increases with increased age, but eventually the increase in age has less impact. As discussed in Chapter 4, design variables can be used as another graphical check with other covariates included in the model. We leave this as an exercise.

Fractional polynomials can both confirm the graphical evidence and suggest possible transformations of the variables. In the population average model setting,

Table 9.11   Fractional Polynomial Results for Age Using the Standard Logistic Regression Model

AGE	df	Deviance	G	p	Powers
Not in model	0	3424.368	39.330	<0.001	
Linear	1	3387.273	2.235	0.525	1
$m = 1$	2	3385.345	0.307	0.858	0
$m = 2$	4	3385.838			−2 .5

however, the likelihood is not estimated making model comparisons more difficult. The shape of the plot in Figure 9.4 can help suggest a transformation of the covariate. For example, one might try a model using the square root or natural log of age. Additionally, one can fit the same model using standard logistic regression in order to produce fractional polynomial model comparisons to obtain ideas for an appropriate transformation. As the standard logistic model is, in essence, a population average model, the results from the fractional polynomial analysis will, generally, produce reasonable choices. This approach is not as useful in cases where the parameter estimate changes substantially between the two models. The results of using fractional polynomials in STATA for age with a standard logistic regression model are shown in Table 9.11.

Using the closed test method there is no significant improvement using a fractional polynomial transformation of age. The $m = 1$ transformation using the natural log improves the deviance by nearly 2 over the linear in the logit model but is not statistically significant with p-value $= 0.16$. Given the Lowess plot in Figure 9.4, we additionally test the proposed transformations suggested by the fractional polynomials by including them in the model fit with GEE estimation. Including the $m = 2$ (-2 .5) transformation in the model the inverse quadratic term is not statistically significant ($p < 0.257$). The best $m = 1$ transformation (0) does decrease both QIC and QIC_u values. Further, plotting the resulting fitted model with the Lowess smooth in Figure 9.4, adjusting the values so they have the same mean on the logit scale as the Lowess smooth, the transformation using the log of age appears to model the nonlinearity well.

Selection of interactions is performed as in Chapter 4. We first identify clinically plausible interactions for consideration. In practice this involves consulting subject matter experts. In this case no clinically meaningful interactions were significant at the 0.01 level. Hence our preliminary final model, shown in Table 9.12, has the five covariates inpatient MHV, outpatient MHV, race, gender and the natural log transformed age (AGEFP1).

We can perform one final check of the assumption about the underlying correlation structure. QIC_u is not appropriate for comparing correlation structures as it only involves fixed parameters so we focus on the QIC. For the final model of Table 9.12, using the exchangeable correlation assumption rather than AR(1), the QIC decreases from 3514.4 to 3504.1. This again suggests reviewing the choice of correlation structure and we explore this in Section 9.6. Note that the estimated

Table 9.12 Preliminary Final Population Average Logistic Regression Model for the Polypharmacy Data

Variable	Coeff.	Std. Err.	z	p
GENDER_M	0.464	0.197	2.35	0.019
AGEFP1	1.267	0.214	5.92	<0.001
MHV4_1	0.155	0.143	1.09	0.277
MHV4_2	0.608	0.153	3.97	<0.001
MHV4_3	0.927	0.163	5.68	<0.001
RACE2_1	−0.442	0.204	−2.17	0.030
INPTMHV2_1	0.366	0.192	1.90	0.057
Constant	−5.209	0.571	−9.12	<0.001

Rho = 0.570; QIC = 3514.43; QIC_u = 3500.43.

correlation with the exchangeable choice is 0.418, which is enough to support the need for modeling with the correlation.

This example illustrates the issues one encounters in working with population average models using GEE estimation. The primary difficulty is selecting a correlation structure. Our general approach is to use the correlation structure that seems most appropriate for the situation and proceed with model building using the methods of purposeful selection in Section 4.2. When a final model has been selected, we can perform a sensitivity analysis to the choice of correlation structure with QIC values. Finally, model checks described in Section 9.6 may suggest problems with the model that might lead to revisiting the correlation structure choice. If there are problems and a more complicated correlation structure is contemplated, then we recommend consulting a statistician experienced in analyzing correlated data using GEE. We reiterate that an advantage of the population average models is that parameter estimates and standard errors, particularly robust estimates, are often unchanged by choosing the incorrect correlation structure [Zeger and Liang (1986)] and the exchangeable structure, as demonstrated in this example, is often adequate for addressing the correlation.

9.5.3 Cluster-Specific Model

For cluster-specific models, we also use the purposeful method of covariate selection from Section 4.2. Here, we select a random-effects structure to account for the correlated data and then proceed with model building. Generally, the preliminary models are built assuming random intercept(s) only. After a preliminary main effects model is chosen we explore potentially more complicated correlation structures.

In the polypharmacy example, we have clustering at only one level, within subjects, and begin with a single random intercept and fit models using adaptive quadrature estimation. The first step is a univariable analysis of all covariates. During this step, we also fit an intercept only model with the random intercept included to examine the correlation within subjects. STATA output for this model

Table 9.13   Univariable Analyses of the Random Intercept of a Cluster-Specific Model Using Quadrature Estimation from Polypharmacy Data, $n = 3500$

Variable	Coeff.	Std. Err.	z	p	95% CI	
Constant	−2.400	0.162	−14.82	<0.001	−2.718,	−2.083
/lnsig2u	2.004	0.126			1.756,	2.252
Sigma_u	2.724	0.172			2.406,	3.083
Rho	0.693	0.027			0.638,	0.743

Likelihood ratio test of rho = 0 : chibar2(01) = 928.41 Prob >= chibar2 = 0.000

is shown in Table 9.13. In this case the estimate of the fixed intercept is below 0 reflecting that the proportion of observations of polypharmacy in the data set is less than 50%; the exact value is 23.4%. The estimate of the cluster standard deviation, $\hat{\sigma}_\alpha$, is 2.72 with a 95% confidence interval of (2.41, 3.08). STATA also reports the value of $\ln(\hat{\sigma}_\alpha^2)$ as "/lnsig2u". The corresponding estimate of the ICC (i.e., $\hat{\rho}$) is 0.69, and its confidence interval is (0.64, 0.74).

The confidence intervals for the ICC and standard deviation of the random effect do not include 0, which suggests that the ID random effect is significant. As we proceed in model building, we are interested in testing whether a random effect is significant. For models fit using numerical integration methods, a likelihood function is available and, thus, a likelihood ratio test is possible. However, there is a problem with the test for significance of random effects, as the null value, 0, is on the boundary of the parameter space. A solution proposed by Self and Liang (1987) is to use a "mixture" distribution placing 50% weight on 0 and 50% on an assumed normal distribution for positive values truncated at 0. However, if several random effects are tested simultaneously then the mixture distribution becomes increasingly complicated and packages such as STATA and SAS report an approximate p-value. STATA, for example, gives a "conservative" test result—an upper bound on the p-value meaning the effects are at least as significant as the reported value and may be more significant, and lets the user know that the results are not exact. At the bottom of Table 9.13 the likelihood ratio test is output in terms of "Rho" or the ICC and, in the case of a single random effect, this is equivalent to testing $\sigma_\alpha = 0$. The "chibar2(01)" term reflects the fact that the test is based on the mixture distribution. The reported p-value is less than 0.001 suggesting that the random intercept for the subject is significant. Note that this agrees with the 95% confidence intervals for both Rho and Sigma, neither of which contains 0. This is not always the case. When the results lead to different conclusions we prefer the likelihood ratio test. The significance implies $\sigma_\alpha > 0$ and thus we conclude that the probability of polypharmacy varies with the subject.

The univariable analysis for the potential predictors, each fit using a random intercept model, is shown in Table 9.14. In addition to the estimates of the coefficients, standard errors and the associated significance test, we have included the estimate of the random effect standard deviation from each fit in the last column. These estimates are all about 2.7. The amount of variability between subjects

Table 9.14   Estimates from Univariable Analysis Using a Cluster-Specific Logistic Regression Model Fit to the Polypharmacy Data

Variable	Coeff.	Std. Err.	z	p	$\hat{\sigma}_\alpha$
MHV4_1	0.403	0.278	1.45	0.147	2.37
MHV4_2	1.215	0.282	4.31	<0.001	
MHV4_3	1.757	0.286	6.15	<0.001	
INPTMHV3_1	1.140	0.280	4.07	<0.001	2.65
INPTMHV3_2	0.780	0.439	1.78	0.076	
GROUP_2	0.308	0.206	1.50	0.134	2.72
GROUP_3	0.753	0.418	1.80	0.071	
URBAN_1	0.081	0.264	0.31	0.760	2.72
COMORBID_1	−0.333	0.201	−1.66	0.098	2.68
ANYPRIM_1	0.059	0.127	0.47	0.641	2.73
NUMPRIMRC_1	0.076	0.128	0.60	0.549	2.72
NUMPRIMRC_2	−0.957	0.641	−1.49	0.135	
GENDER_1	0.882	0.346	2.55	0.011	2.70
RACE_1	−0.611	0.393	−1.55	0.120	2.71
RACE_2	−0.826	1.905	−0.43	0.664	
ETHNIC_1	−1.068	1.380	−0.77	0.439	2.72
AGE	0.219	0.027	8.15	<0.001	2.86

Table 9.15   Wald and Likelihood Ratio Tests for Polychotomous Covariates in Univariable Analysis in Table 9.14 for the Polypharmacy Data

Variable	df	Wald Test		Likelihood Ratio Test	
		W	p	G	p
MHV4	3	60.64	<0.001	59.48	<0.001
INPTMHV3	2	18.18	<0.001	18.48	<0.001
GROUP	2	4.58	0.101	4.44	0.108
NUMPRIMRC	2	2.86	0.239	3.14	0.208
RACE	2	2.56	0.278	2.44	0.295

appears to increase when the age is considered and we may consider a random effect, or random slope, for this covariate later in the model building. The increase could also reflect the issue of scale already observed in the population average modeling. The univariable parameter estimates for the covariates are similar but of greater magnitude than those produced using the population average model in Table 9.8, as discussed in Section 9.4. In the random effects model case we have the ability to use likelihood ratio tests as well as the Wald tests when deciding whether to include a covariate in the model. For the polychotomous covariates in Table 9.14 we conduct both tests and display the results in Table 9.15. The results were similar for all five polychotomous covariates. As discussed previously we prefer the likelihood ratio test and use it throughout the remainder of this example.

Once the univariable analyses are complete, we begin with a model including the random intercept and all covariates with $p < 0.25$ in Tables 9.14 and 9.15. In this

Table 9.16 Preliminary Main Effects Cluster-Specific Logistic Regression Model for Polypharmacy Data Fit Using Adaptive Quadrature

Variable	Coeff.	Std. Err.	Z	p	G	p
GENDER_M	0.736	0.329	2.24	0.025		
AGE	0.221	0.027	8.27	<0.001		
MHV4_1	0.326	0.285	1.15	0.252	56.73	<0.001
MHV4_2	1.190	0.289	4.11	<0.001		
MHV4_3	1.722	0.294	5.86	<0.001		
RACE2_1	−0.655	0.367	−1.78	0.074		
INPTMHV2_1	0.903	0.253	3.56	<0.001		
Constant	−6.450	0.518	−12.45	<0.001		
/lnsig2u	1.777	0.133				
Sigma_u	2.431	0.161				
Rho	0.642	0.030			662.07	<0.001

case these are the same variables selected in the population average model, with the exception of one variable, the ethnicity indicator. We collapsed categories of inpatient MHV, race and number of primary diagnoses as we did in the population average modeling. All models fit in this stage of variable selection include the random intercept as we want to build a model while accounting for the potential correlations between subjects. It is possible that the final model would have differed had we excluded a random intercept term even when it does not appear significant in an intermediate analysis. The fit of the preliminary main effects model is shown in Table 9.16. As the population average and cluster-specific models differ in how they model the expected value with the cluster-specific model including the subject, the two models will not always include the same covariates. In this case, the race is still moderately significant but less so and, as a result, could be removed from the model at the 0.05 level. We opt to retain the predictor in the model at this stage. The random intercept is statistically significant ($p < 0.001$) based on the likelihood ratio test.

We continue the model building process by checking the scale of the continuous covariates. The method of design variables described in Chapter 4 is an option for scale checks in random effects models. When using quadrature estimation the method of fractional polynomials is also an option because the likelihood function is estimated. As discussed for population average models, smoothed plots and splines can assist in determining the form of transformation. In cluster-specific models, one option when the number of clusters is not too large is to produce smoothed plots for each cluster. A single plot for all clusters is also of interest but averaging across all clusters could make the form of the transformation more difficult to assess. In our example, with many subjects and only seven observations in each cluster, smoothed plots for each subject are not revealing leaving the averaged Lowess plot of Figure 9.4 as our only option. The fractional polynomial analysis is presented in Table 9.17. Unlike the standard logistic model fractional polynomial

Table 9.17 Fractional Polynomial Results for Range to Target in the Cluster-Specific Model of Table 9.16

RANGE	df	Deviance	G	p	Powers	
Not in model	0	2799.578	85.655	0.000		
Linear	1	2725.199	11.276	0.010	1	
$m = 1$	2	2714.428	0.505	0.777	-1	
$m = 2$	4	2713.923	—	—	-2	0

Table 9.18 Preliminary Final Cluster-Specific Logistic Regression Model for the Polypharmacy Data

Variable	Coeff.	Std. Err.	z	p	G	p
GENDER_M	0.744	0.331	2.25	0.025		
AGEFP1[a]	0.259	0.030	8.56	<0.001		
MHV4_1	0.327	0.287	1.14	0.254	58.47	<0.001
MHV4_2	1.202	0.291	4.13	<0.001		
MHV4_3	1.741	0.295	5.90	<0.001		
RACE2_1	−0.672	0.370	−1.82	0.069		
INPTMHV2_1	0.887	0.254	3.49	<0.001		
Constant	−10.168	0.866	−11.75	<0.001		
/lnsig2u	1.796	0.133				
Sigma_u	2.454	0.163				
Rho	0.647	0.030			668.63	<0.001

[a] $AGEFP1 = \ln(AGE/10)$.

results shown in Table 9.11, the best m = 1 model is preferred using the closed test procedure with p-value of 0.001 when compared to the linear choice. The recommended transformation is the inverse of age (-1). Examining the possible m = 1 transformations, we find two other choices that produce statistically equivalent Deviance values, -0.5 and the natural log. Based on the shape of the Lowess smooth of age in Figure 9.4 and subject matter guidance we prefer to model age using the log transformation as we did for the population average model. The resulting model is shown in Table 9.18. Note that we divide age by 10 before applying the transformation and call this AGEFP1 to keep the coefficient on a similar scale to others in the model. This aids with numerical issues encountered in additional model building steps when examining random slopes.

The last step is to check for interactions between variables in the model. In random effects models we also check the possibility of additional random effects such as random slopes entering the model during this step. We may also do some sensitivity analyses of the choice of estimation method, in this case quadrature, in this final step. In the polypharmacy data, the random intercept is statistically significant. In cases where the intercept is not significant we must decide whether it should remain in the model. In addition to the likelihood ratio test, we recommend computing delta beta hat percentages of the estimated fixed effects parameters when removing the random intercept using the formula

$$\Delta\hat{\beta}\% = 100 \times \frac{\hat{\beta}_F - \hat{\beta}_R}{\hat{\beta}_R},$$

where $\hat{\beta}_R$ is the estimate with the random effect in the model and $\hat{\beta}_F$ is with no random effect. If any of the estimated parameters change substantially (say by more than 15–20%) we believe that a strong argument could be made for keeping the random intercept in the model even if it is not significant. Even if the estimates do not change dramatically we may retain the random intercept as the cluster effects themselves may be of interest. In general, as we began modeling with a random intercept to account for clustering in the data we tend toward leaving the random intercept in the model, regardless of its significance.

An additional modeling detail is to check for potential random slopes. As with interaction terms, we are interested in only those random slopes that are both statistically significant and clinically plausible. In Section 9.2, we describe the random intercept model using equations (9.2) and (9.3). Adding a single random slope these equations are rewritten as:

$$g(\mathbf{x}_{ij}, \beta_{0i}, \beta_{1i}, \boldsymbol{\beta}_s) = \beta_{0i} + \beta_{1i}x_1 + \mathbf{x}_{ij}'\boldsymbol{\beta}_s \text{ (level 1 model)}, \qquad (9.22)$$

$$\beta_{0i} = \beta_0 + \alpha_i \text{ (level 2 model)}, \qquad (9.23)$$

$$\beta_{1i} = \beta_1 + \tau_i \text{ (level 2 model)}. \qquad (9.24)$$

The level-2 portion of the model is now expressed using two equations [equations (9.23) and (9.24)] for the random intercept and random slope respectively. The assumption about the distribution of the random slope effect is similar to the random intercept, namely $\tau_i \sim N(0, \sigma_\tau^2)$ and we initially assume the two random effects, τ_i and α_i, are independent. In this model, the covariate has an overall slope coefficient, β_1, but there is variability in the slope, due to the clusters. Thus, the question of randomness in the slope is answered by considering whether the effect of the covariate on the response might differ depending upon the cluster.

In the preliminary final main effects model for the polypharmacy data in Table 9.18 there are five covariates to consider for random slopes. Using the continuous covariate of the natural log of age (AGEFP1) as an example, the estimated slope coefficient is 2.59. This estimate means that as age increases the probability of polypharmacy also increases. The question is whether the relationship differs by subject. In other words, would we expect different subjects to be more or less influenced by changes in age? If we decide that such variability is plausible, we test the random slope to determine if the amount of variability is statistically significant. Smooth plots by subject in cases with a small number of subjects and large cluster sizes can help determine if variability in slopes is present in the data. In this case, there are many small clusters making such graphical analysis impractical. Adding the random slope for transformed age to

Table 9.19 Tests of Random Slopes Added to Main Effects Cluster-Specific Logistic Regression Model for the Polypharmacy Data

Random Effect	$\hat{\sigma}_\tau$	Std. Err.	G	p
AGEFP1[a]	3.64	0.581	19.61	<0.001
GENDER	<0.0001	0.940	<0.0001	1
MHV4_1	0.787	0.539	0.60	0.437
MHV4_2	0.170	1.574	0.96	0.327
MHV4_3	0.294	0.795	0.04	0.851
RACE2	<0.0001	0.710	<0.0001	1
INPTMHV2	1.90	0.600	6.24	0.012

[a] $AGEFP1 = \ln(AGE/10)$.

the model results in an estimate for the standard deviation, $\hat{\sigma}_\tau$, of 3.64 and the standard error of this estimate is 0.581. We can test the significance of the estimate formally using a likelihood ratio test comparing the models with and without the random slope. The log-likelihoods for the two models differ by 9.805. Thus, the test statistic is $G = 19.61$ and $p < 0.001$ using the chi-square distribution with 1 degree of freedom. The results for the likelihood ratio test of each of the possible random slopes for all five covariates individually added to the model are shown in Table 9.19. Note that the categorical variable MHV4 involves three random slopes and as such is difficult to interpret.

We follow the same procedure for random slopes and interactions, testing each of those believed clinically plausible from the main effects in the model. In our example, the only statistically significant interactions are race with inpatient MHV ($p = 0.048$) and transformed age with outpatient mental health visits ($p = 0.041$). There is no particular clinical justification for considering either interaction, and neither is significant at the 0.01 level. Further, when added to models including the random slopes, both lose statistical significance. Thus, we choose not to include them in the final model. The inpatient MHV random slope is also significant, but it does not have an obvious clinical interpretation. This is a dichotomous covariate so the random slope is significant because, although higher inpatient MHV is on average indicative of higher probability of polypharmacy, some subjects do not exhibit this relationship. We are not interested in individual subjects here, and the parameter estimates all change by less than 5% if the random slope is added to the model, so we include only the random slope for age in the final model. As we added a random slope to the model we further test the assumption that the random slope and random intercept are independent by adding a covariance parameter between the two random effects and use the likelihood ratio test to determine significance. In this case, the covariance parameter is not significant ($p = 0.48$) so we do not include this in the model. Hence the final model, shown in Table 9.20, has the five covariates: inpatient MHV, outpatient MHV, race, gender, and transformed age with a random slope and the random intercept. As previously mentioned, we divided age by 10 prior to applying the fracpoly transformation so the coefficient is of similar magnitude to the other parameters in the model and to avoid numerical issues.

Table 9.20   Final Cluster-Specific Logistic Regression Model for the Polypharmacy Data

Variable	Coef.	Std. Err.	z	p	G	p
GENDER_M	0.742	0.364	2.04	0.041		
AGEFP1[a]	2.659	0.384	6.93	<0.001		
MHV4_1	0.378	0.311	1.21	0.225	52.48	<0.001
MHV4_2	1.270	0.319	3.98	<0.001		
MHV4_3	1.833	0.324	5.66	<0.001		
RACE2_1	−0.783	0.406	−1.93	0.054		
INPTMHV2_1	0.883	0.270	3.27	0.001		
Constant	−4.416	0.432	−10.21	<0.001		
Std. Dev. (AGEFP1)	3.643	0.581				
Std. Dev. (Cons)	2.575	0.185				

[a]$AGEFP1 = \ln(AGE/10)$.

9.5.4   Additional Points to Consider when Fitting Logistic Regression Models to Correlated Data

One must be careful when fitting cluster-specific models as the numerical methods are sensitive to the number of clusters and cluster size. Software improvements in recent years have made adaptive quadrature a more viable alternative, but the potential for numerical problems still exists. If the intracluster correlation is quite small then the software may fail to converge to a solution with an estimate of σ_α^2 that is effectively 0. For example, in these settings STATA typically stops and reports an estimate of the log variance of −14.0. In this case one should abandon the cluster-specific model in favor of the usual logistic regression model because the two models are equivalent when $\sigma_\alpha = 0$.

Convergence issues are usually noted in computer output and it is up to the user to be sure that the solution was reached. A statement in the output such as "convergence not achieved" implies the results should not be used. Even when the algorithms converge, checks of the sensitivity of the results to estimation methods are important. One tool, available in software packages, when models are fit using quadrature compares the effect of the number of discrete quadrature points (Q) chosen to approximate the integral in equation (9.13) to maximize the likelihood. Using between 5 and 10 points is, in most instances, adequate to achieve stable estimates. However, examples where even 20 points are insufficient can occur. leSaffre and Spiessens (2001) note that adaptive quadrature does not seem as sensitive, but we recommend always checking the sensitivity to the choice of Q before finalizing a cluster-specific model. In STATA, the default is 12 points using xtlogit. SAS GLIMMIX uses an algorithm to select the number of points to use if no number is specified. Both procedures offer the user an automated method of checking the sensitivity of the estimates to the choice of points: in SAS the "METHOD = QUAD(QCHECK)" option in the model statement and in STATA the "quadchk" statement after fitting the model. In models with random

Table 9.21   Partial Output from Quadrature Point Check for Model of Table 9.20

Quadrature points	−2 Log-Likelihood	Relative Difference to Converged
7	2685.437	
9	2685.320	−0.0000434
11	2685.298	−0.0000517
21	2685.310	−0.0000468
31	2685.311	−0.0000469

slopes, the quadrature check is not available in STATA so Table 9.21 shows partial output from SAS for our example model of Table 9.20. The procedure compares the model fit with $Q = 7$ to those with $Q = 9$, 11, 21 and 31. The impact of the choice of Q on the log-likelihood, estimates of the coefficients for all covariates in the model, and on the estimate of the random effect are provided in the output in STATA when available. In SAS, as in Table 9.21, only the deviance (−2 times the log-likelihood) is provided. The relative difference is the ratio of the change in the deviance to the deviance of the model fit with 7 quadrature points. (Seven is the default number of quadrature points in STATA for xtmelogit, the procedure we used to include a random slope in the model.) In this example, the relative difference is extremely small even when increasing the number of points to 31. If the computer program does not include changes to parameters in the output of quadrature checks, we recommend an additional check by refitting the model with increased points. If the differences are not small when comparing estimates for different Q, such as changes in parameter estimates of more than 5 or 10%, then one should consider using more points if computationally feasible. We refit the model of Table 9.20 using $Q = 11$ and all parameter estimates changed by less than 5%, and most by less than 1%, so we conclude the choice of seven points is adequate in this model. The check of quadrature can be performed at any point in the model building process. In situations where numerical issues occur, such as the algorithm failing to converge, one option is to reduce the number of quadrature points. In these instances the check is particularly important. At a minimum it should be used before presenting final model results.

In the presence of numerical problems with quadrature an option is to use pseudo- or quasilikelihood (PL or QL) estimation methods. Although these methods have the potential for bias, recent improvements in the algorithms implemented in software packages such as SAS have decreased that concern. When pseudo- or quasi-likelihood methods are used for estimation, the lack of a likelihood function reduces options for model comparisons. Packages may have tests based upon the PL function or offer other tests (Score test for example) that, although not as desirable as the likelihood ratio test, can give the user evidence about the significance of fixed as well as random effects. Sometimes one can use the PL/QL estimation to identify preliminary models that can be estimated with quadrature. In some software packages one can change the options for starting values of estimates and use PL/QL estimates to improve the ability of the numerical methods to converge.

Another option is the use of Markov Chain Monte Carlo (MCMC) estimation described in Chapter 10 under Bayesian methods.

Even when numerical problems do not impact model building there are still other issues worth noting. One is the type of tests used in variable selection. When possible, and if there are differences in the inferences from tests, the likelihood ratio test is preferred. As an example, STATA produces Wald tests of parameter estimates assuming the standard normal distribution for the test statistic. The default in SAS is a test statistic based on the t distribution. The two tests will usually coincide but the t-test may produce higher p-values and fail to reject when the z-test rejects. The difference is greater when the number of clusters is large when using the default degrees of freedom for the t-test in SAS. The degrees of freedom computation is complicated so we do not include it here but refer interested readers to the SAS user's manual. The exact calculation used is also complicated and we refer those interested in the details to the help files for the program. Essentially the formula reduces the degrees of freedom by the number of clusters even if only a single random effect is added to the model. The loss of degrees of freedom leads to a t distribution with more variation and is, therefore, less likely to reject. When adaptive quadrature estimation is used the degrees of freedom in this t-test are too conservative as only one parameter was actually estimated rather than a parameter for each cluster. We recommend using the "DDFM = none" option in SAS to produce, in essence, a Wald test. Again, the likelihood ratio test is preferred over other options. PL/QL methods do not allow the use of the likelihood ratio test so that inference using the Wald tests is the only option.

Population average models using GEE also have a few potential issues to note. Likelihood ratio tests are not available so one must use either Wald or Score tests. These tests are generally similar but we have found examples where they differ enough to change the model selected. We have observed examples where the multivariable Score test was too conservative and thus prefer the Wald tests. In such cases clinical knowledge assists in determining which model to choose. Additionally, the impact of the covariate on estimates of other parameters in the model can inform the decision to include or exclude a covariate.

Given the potential for numerical issues in the estimation methods for correlated data models care in the model building and interpretation is critical. Where possible we often use several methods of estimation as well as statistical inference in order to help identify problems if they exist. If methods do not agree then there may be issues that make these models inappropriate for drawing inference and caution is in order. Finally, we note that as models become more complicated so too do the interpretation and statistical issues. For example, random effects models may include more than two levels or several random effects. In such cases, model building proceeds as usual but will require care in checking for such effects in the interaction step. As with interactions, the interpretation of the results is impacted as clusters have different slope values. Presenting results by cluster using the posterior predicted slope values is appropriate when this occurs.

9.6   ASSESSMENT OF MODEL FIT

Diagnostic statistics, such as those described in Chapter 5, are not as readily available for use in model checking with correlated data models. Summary measures of
overall model fit, in particular, have not been developed or implemented in software
packages. Some case-wise diagnostic tools for individual subjects are available or
could be approximated by assuming the observations are not correlated and using
the methods in Chapter 5. Summary measures using this approach can also be used
but lack power in many correlated data settings [Sturdivant (2005)]. Although not
specifically developed for correlated data models, this analysis is generally regarded
as being better than not doing any model checking at all. In this section, we discuss
the available tools and offer recommendations for model checking with correlated
binary data.

9.6.1   Assessment of Population Average Model Fit

Although methods have not been implemented in many software packages, it is
possible to perform overall tests of fit for population average correlated data models.
Evans and Li (2005) examined the performance of the Hosmer–Lemeshow test and
extensions of the Pearson chi-square and other tests described in Section 5.2.2 to
the correlated data setting. Their results indicate that the usual Hosmer–Lemeshow
test may be used in some settings to assess fit of population average models.
In general, one must avoid using the test when there are many tied or nearly
tied values in the estimated probabilities. This is likely to occur under one or
more of the following conditions: the model contains many cluster-level covariates;
the intracluster correlation among the responses is large; the number of clusters
is small and there are many observations per cluster. In a particular setting if
none of these conditions hold then the test can be used. As an example, the fitted
population average model for the polypharmacy data in Table 9.12 does have a
relatively high intracluster correlation, $\hat{\rho} = 0.57$, but there are many clusters (500
subjects) with only seven observations in each cluster. The model contains the
cluster-level covariates gender and race, but the predicted probabilities have few
tied or nearly tied values due to the other covariates in the model. Thus, this
is a setting where the test might be used effectively. Most software packages
do not have the option for the test in population average models but one can
easily obtain the test statistic applying the methods described in Chapter 5. Use of
ten groups for the polypharmacy model of Table 9.12 produces the observed and
expected values for each decile of risk in Table 9.22. The corresponding value of the
Hosmer–Lemeshow test statistic is $\hat{C} = 40.571$ which, with 8 degrees of freedom,
results in $p < 0.001$ and calls into question model fit. There are differences in
observed and expected counts particularly in the highest risk deciles where the
model underestimates the risk.

   Horton et al. (1999) propose a statistic that is related to the Hosmer–Lemeshow
statistic. The test involves forming G groups based on deciles of risk and then creating $G - 1$ indicator variables to identify the group membership for each observation

Table 9.22 Observed (Obs) and Estimated Expected (Exp) Frequencies Within Each Decile of Risk Using the Fitted Population Average Model of Table 9.12

| | POLYPHARMACY = 1 | | POLYPHARMACY = 0 | | |
Decile	Obs	Exp	Obs	Exp	Total
1	18	28.28	332	321.72	350
2	40	43.08	311	307.92	351
3	55	52.60	295	297.40	350
4	40	60.98	309	288.02	349
5	68	69.29	282	280.71	350
6	80	78.28	272	273.72	352
7	95	87.08	254	261.92	349
8	110	99.79	243	253.21	353
9	130	113.50	216	232.50	346
10	183	141.12	167	208.88	350

in the data set. These indicator variables are added to the logistic regression model with all other predictors and a Score test, a chi-square test with $G - 1$ degrees of freedom, of the null hypothesis that the parameters for these indicator variables are all 0 performed. With ten groups, the resulting test statistic value is $\hat{C}_2 = 7.155$, which, with 9 degrees of freedom, produces $p = 0.62$ and supports model fit, in the sense that there is not a significant shift, up or down, in the estimated probabilities within each decile. The Hosmer–Lemeshow test does not support model fit. However the two tests address different aspects of model fit and are not numerically related.

Two residual based statistics for goodness of fit for models fit using GEE were proposed by Evans (1998), Pan (2002), and Evans and Hosmer (2004). Simulation results of Evans and Hosmer (2004) showed that the statistics were effective for assessing overall fit in many settings. The first statistic is an extension of the normal approximation to the Pearson chi-square test. The moments of the Pearson chi-square test statistic, defined in equation (5.2), computed using quantities defined in Section 9.3 for GEE estimation in equations (9.6)–(9.10), are

$$E(X^2 - N) = 0,$$
$$\widehat{\mathrm{Var}}(X^2 - N) = (1 - 2\hat{\pi})'\mathbf{A}^{-1}(\mathbf{I} - \mathbf{H_G})\mathbf{V}\mathbf{A}^{-1}(1 - 2\hat{\pi}), \qquad (9.25)$$

where $\mathbf{H_G}$ is a slightly modified version of an analog to the "hat" matrix proposed for GEE by Hall et al. (1994) and defined as $\mathbf{H_G} = \mathbf{D}(\mathbf{D}'\mathbf{V}^{-1}\mathbf{D})\mathbf{D}'\mathbf{V}^{-1}$ and $\hat{\pi}$ is the vector of predicted probabilities from the model. The test proceeds in similar fashion to the standard logistic model test described in Section 5.2. Specifically, the standardized statistic is computed using equation (9.25) as

$$z_{X^2} = \frac{X^2 - N}{\sqrt{\widehat{\mathrm{Var}}(X^2 - N)}}, \qquad (9.26)$$

with a two-tailed p-value computed using the standard normal distribution. The second statistic is based on the unweighted sum-of-squared residuals or

$$U(y_j, \hat{\pi}_j) = \sum_j (y_j - m_j \hat{\pi}_j).$$

The moments of the statistic are computed as

$$\widehat{E}(U) = \hat{\pi}(1 - \hat{\pi}),$$
$$\widehat{\text{Var}}(U) = (1 - 2\hat{\pi})'(\mathbf{I} - \mathbf{H_G})\mathbf{V}(\mathbf{I} - \mathbf{H_G})'(1 - 2\hat{\pi}), \qquad (9.27)$$

leading to the test statistic

$$z_U = \frac{U - \widehat{E}(U)}{\sqrt{\widehat{\text{Var}}(U)}} \qquad (9.28)$$

with a two-tailed p-value computed using the standard normal distribution. Pan (2002) proposes slight modifications to both statistics by using a different variance estimator. Evans and Li (2005) compare these, and other, goodness of fit statistics and suggest using more than one test in assessing model fit due to potential lack of power for any one measure. They also provide SAS code for computing the statistics.

In this example, the resulting Pearson residual test statistic value is $z_{\chi^2} = -1.9165$, which is marginally supportive of model fit ($p = 0.055$). The unweighted sum-of-squares residual test statistic value is $z_U = -0.4538$, which fails to reject model fit ($p = 0.65$). The versions of the statistics using Pan's modification produce similar values. In our example, one of the tests clearly suggests potential issues with model fit and a second marginal evidence of issues. This is worth noting as we continue to assess the model further.

The QIC criteria of Pan (2001) described in the previous section are the only readily available measures of fit useful for comparing choice of correlation structure in these models. Zeger and Liang (1986) point out, using empirical results, that the GEE method of fitting the models is robust to choice of the correlation structure. The implication is that even if the structure is misspecified the resulting parameter estimates may be unaffected. However, it is worth checking the sensitivity of the model to the choice of correlation structure, particularly in cases where it may not be clear what structure to select.

Vonesh et al. (1996) develop measures similar to R^2 for population average models as well as a chi-square test of the covariance structure choice using the PL function. However, the R^2 measure does not appear to perform well with binary data and the test is best when dealing with models involving an assumed normal distribution of the response. Although both statistics are not appropriate in logistic regression models, Vonesh et al. (1996) do describe useful strategies for checking the correlation structure without a test statistic. The first approach is to fit the model using an unstructured covariance and compare the results to those with the chosen correlation structure using their version of R^2. However, this is often not a viable option as the estimation may fail in settings where the data are unbalanced, with differences in cluster sizes, or for data with a large number of observations in each cluster. Further, an unstructured covariance implies some correspondence between observations in each cluster to those in other clusters. For example, this is the case when the observations are repeated measurements over time so that observation 1 in each cluster is the first-time measurement, observation 2 is the second-time measurement, and so forth. The second approach is to use the PL ratio test to compare the estimated covariance matrix of the parameter estimates from models with and without use of the robust or "sandwich" estimation.

As previously noted, the test statistics used by Vonesh et al. (1996) do not extend to binary data but one can apply the ideas of the tests. The clusters in our polypharmacy data set include seven observations (one each year) for each subject. The unstructured covariance matrix assumes a different correlation between each pair of years leading to the need to estimate 21 parameters. In data sets with more observations in each cluster the number of parameters may become too large to make these methods practical.

In approach 1, we fit the same model from Table 9.12 using an unstructured correlation yielding the correlation estimates shown in Table 9.23. We are interested in determining whether the estimated correlations suggest that the autoregressive correlation assumption is appropriate. In this case, we observe a pattern of decreasing correlations when the "lag" between years increases. Correlations for 1-year differences range from 0.45 to 0.624 and are, on average, higher than the correlations for 2-year differences that range from 0.331 to 0.528. The trend continues with only a few exceptions. The pattern supports an AR correlation structure. The AR(1) choice led to an estimated $\hat{\rho} = 0.57$ for lag 1 correlations. The lag 2 estimate is then $\hat{\rho}^2 = 0.57^2 = 0.3249$, which is lower than the observed correlation estimates in Table 9.23 using the unstructured model. The correlations continue to drop more quickly at higher lags than suggested by the unstructured model. The one statistical measure we have available to compare the models with different correlation structures is the QIC. In this case the QIC for the model with unstructured correlations is 3546.54, which is more than 30 higher than that of the AR(1) model of Table 9.12. The increase in QIC does not support adopting an unstructured correlation structure that would add a large number of additional parameters. Another option is to assume an exchangeable correlation. The QIC for this option is

Table 9.23 Example of Estimated Unstructured Correlation Matrix for Model of Table 9.12

	2002	2003	2004	2005	2006	2007	2008
2002	1.000						
2003	0.450	1.000					
2004	0.331	0.624	1.000				
2005	0.274	0.430	0.620	1.000			
2006	0.293	0.367	0.528	0.624	1.000		
2007	0.232	0.314	0.390	0.451	0.576	1.000	
2008	0.254	0.363	0.421	0.398	0.468	0.556	1.000

lower at 3504.1 by nearly 9 compared to the AR(1). The choice estimates a single correlation for all lags at 0.42. We feel the general trend to decrease correlation with time justifies an AR choice but note that the exchangeable option is defensible and that there are other more complicated structures possible that could address the issue with the AR(1) structure to decrease the estimated correlation too much with increasing lag. An example is the "banded" structure that estimates a separate correlation for each lag. Verbeke and Molenburghs (2009), as well as many of the references mentioned in Section 9.1, discuss possible structures.

Our example is the most common situation where this approach is likely to suggest a correlation structure choice other than exchangeable. The observations within a cluster become less "similar" from one to the next, in this case when measurements are taken over time. One disadvantage of this approach is that, even if feasible for the data set (which occurs only when clusters are small), it may not always be clear from the estimated unstructured correlation matrix what alternative is best. However, it is one method of at least checking the chosen structure.

The second approach is to compare the estimated covariance matrix of the parameter estimates with and without using the robust or "sandwich" estimates we recommended. The robust estimates "adjust" the standard errors based on the selected model correlation structure using the observed data. If the data do not support the choice of correlation structure the adjustments are larger. Thus, although the robust estimates allow for a degree of error in choosing a correlation structure, if the adjustment is large it suggests that the true structure has not been modeled well. Examining the complete covariance matrices for models with many covariates is daunting. We recommend, at a minimum, comparing the variances of the parameter estimates. For the polypharmacy data set modeled in Table 9.12 the covariance matrix is 8×8 and most of the estimated covariances are near 0 so we only display the results of the variance comparison in Table 9.24. If there are large changes, such as exceeding 15 or 20%, there could be reason to consider a more complicated correlation structure. Table 9.24 presents, for each parameter, the variance estimates using the robust "sandwich" estimators, the variance estimates when the robust option is not used, and the percentage change. The inpatient MHV (INPTMHV2) parameter estimate increases by a large amount, over 77%, when the robust estimation is used. Gender also changes by more than 20% but all other estimates change relatively little. A large change may be a concern if inference about the parameter estimate is affected. In this case we might consider a more complicated correlation structure. In this example, both the parameter for inpatient MHV and gender were selected for inclusion in the model using the robust standard errors and are even more significant with model based standard errors.

In the polypharmacy model, neither approach for checking the correlation structure is conclusive, and neither reveals enough of an issue to make us consider adopting a correlation structure with many additional parameters. As discussed, these checks are only an option in data with small cluster sizes. Regardless, we reiterate that the robust estimates are preferable. The impact of issues with the selected correlation structure concerns the precision of the standard errors of parameters. If robust standard errors are larger they are more conservative for inferences. In our

Table 9.24   Estimated Variances for Population Average Polypharmacy Model Using AR(1) Correlation Structure Using Robust Estimates and Model Based Estimates of Table 9.12

Parameter	Model Based Variance	Robust Variance	Percent Change
GENDER_M	0.0309	0.0389	25.89
AGEFP1	0.0530	0.0457	−13.77
MHV4_1	0.0220	0.0205	−6.82
MHV4_2	0.0244	0.0235	−3.69
MHV4_3	0.0261	0.0267	2.30
RACE2_1	0.0392	0.0416	6.12
INPTMHV2_1	0.0208	0.0369	77.40
Constant	0.3724	0.3259	−12.49

example, the largest changes, for gender and inpatient MHV, increase the standard errors using robust estimates. For gender, the increase does not modify significance. The increase in standard error does lead to inpatient MHV changing from significant ($p = 0.011$) to marginally significant ($p = 0.054$) with robust estimates. We retained the covariate in the model so, in this example, the final model is unchanged.

Vonesh et al. (1996) propose several measures for comparing the estimated covariance matrices explicitly using measures that compare how much two matrices differ. Using these measures, they compute the *concordance correlation*, which is interpreted much like R^2 in that it will be close to 0 if the matrices are not close and nearer to 1 if they are close. Finally, they form a PL ratio test using a discrepancy function between the two matrices. The measures require mathematical background beyond the scope of this text and are not currently available in standard software for models fit using GEE. SAS PROC GLIMMIX does produce the measures in population average models estimated with PL.

Selecting the appropriate correlation structure, given available tools, is the most difficult part of model fitting and assessment. In our example, we observed some evidence that the AR(1) structure may overestimate the reduction in correlation as lag between years increases but the unstructured choice is not preferable given the increased number of parameters. We recommend use of exchangeable correlation and robust estimates for standard errors for most situations, and the AR(1) structure for data such as the example in which correlations decrease with a variable such as time. If the analyst, by using the approaches described here, feels there are indicators that the choice is flawed, further research is required.

Individual subject-specific diagnostic statistics for population average models, similar to those discussed in Chapter 5, are useful in identifying possible covariate patterns that are poorly fit. Additional statistics for examining clusters have been developed [Preisser and Qaqish (1996)]. We recommend the same plots of individual covariate pattern diagnostic statistics discussed in Chapter 5 and similar plots of the cluster-level statistics. The actual diagnostic measures used will depend upon the software package. Regardless of the software package the standardized, or Pearson residual, is usually produced or easily computed using equation (5.1). As the likelihood is not estimated in models fit using GEE the deviance residual is not available.

The residuals for polypharmacy observations are positive and for those without polypharmacy are negative. The majority of the standardized residuals should fall between -2 and 2 and those larger than 3 in absolute value are usually considered outliers. Among the no polypharmacy observations, the largest Pearson residual is -1.02 and none appears as outlier. There is one extreme Pearson residual for polypharmacy, with a value of 6.41. The observation is for a female with no outpatient or inpatient MHV and race non-white; all indicators associated with reduced risk of polypharmacy. The outlier is the only observed polypharmacy for the subject and occurred when she was young, 5 years old. Although the value is somewhat suspicious with no observed polypharmacy in other years, we cannot exclude it from the data set.

Preisser and Qaqish (1996) propose a slightly different "hat" matrix than that of equation (9.25) for use in calculating the leverages. The equation, using the notation of Section 9.3, is given by

$$H = X(X'WX)^{-1}X'W, \qquad (9.29)$$

where W is the block diagonal matrix with block for subject i defined as

$$W_i = D_i^{-1}A_i^{-0.5}R_i^{-1}(\rho)A_i^{-0.5}D_i^{-1}.$$

The leverages are the diagonal elements of the "hat" matrix and are produced in standard software packages. A plot of leverages for our example is shown in Figure 9.5. None of the leverages falls well away from the rest of the values. The largest leverage, 0.0126, is a subject who is non-white, male, with more than 0 inpatient MHV and the highest category of outpatient MHV. Less than 1% of observations in the data set have such a covariate pattern and the observation belongs to the oldest, age 15, of these.

The influence statistics $\Delta\hat{\beta}_j$ and ΔX_j^2 discussed in Chapter 5 are not always produced in standard software for models estimated using GEE but can be computed using equations (5.15) and (5.16). The ΔD_j statistic is not available because a likelihood is not estimated. Plots of $\Delta\hat{\beta}_j$ and ΔX_j^2 are shown in Figures 9.6 and 9.7. As outlined in Chapter 5 we are interested in identifying subjects that appear to have influence on the overall model fit. There are large ΔX_j^2 values above the approximate cutoff value of 4 suggested in Chapter 5. There are ten observed values exceeding 10. One observation had a larger value than other subjects at 35.5 that we excluded from Figure 9.6, and a second at 15.4. The first is the same subject with the largest Pearson residual discussed earlier. The second is the second youngest subject with observed polypharmacy and the second lowest outpatient MHV category. The only younger observed polypharmacy corresponded to a subject with the highest category of outpatient MHV. In both large ΔX_j^2 cases the model based probability of polypharmacy is below 0.07 but the response is a 1. All of the values of the influence statistic $\Delta\hat{\beta}_j$ are small but three lie away from the

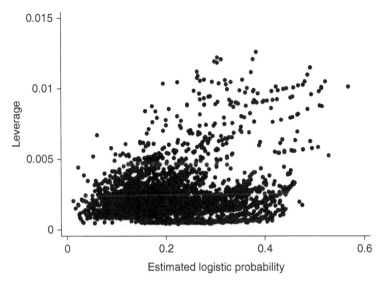

Figure 9.5 Plot of leverage verses the estimated logistic probability ($\hat{\pi}$) for the model of Table 9.12.

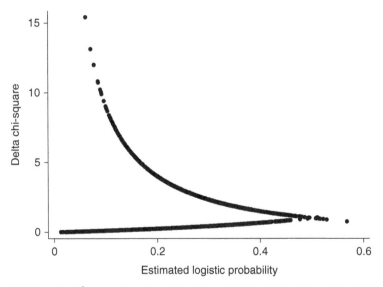

Figure 9.6 Plot of ΔX_j^2 verses the estimated logistic probability ($\hat{\pi}$) for the model of Table 9.12, excluding one large value.

rest of the values. The second largest, at 0.044, is the largest Pearson residual and ΔX_j^2 already discussed. The largest, 0.046, is the youngest subject with observed polypharmacy. The third point, at 0.043, is a case of observed polypharmacy in a relatively young subject who is a non-white female, categories associated with

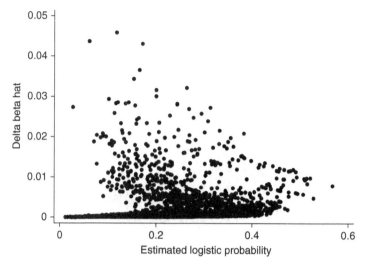

Figure 9.7   Plot of $\Delta\hat{\beta}_j$ verses the estimated logistic probability ($\hat{\pi}$) for the model of Table 9.12.

lower risk and also moderately high leverage as less than 4% of the observations are from such subjects.

As discussed in Chapter 5, we recommend removing any points that potentially indicate lack of fit or influence from the data set and examine their effect on parameter estimates and model fit. In analyses not shown, we did remove the four points discussed with the largest values of their Pearson residual, $\Delta\hat{\beta}_j$ or ΔX_j^2 and examined their effect on parameter estimates. On removing all four points, none of the parameter estimates changed by more than 15% except for the intercept. The largest change was the estimate of the parameter for race, which decreased by 14% from -0.442 to -0.504, an increase in effect. The covariate values are reasonable, and we conclude that these observations should remain in the data set.

The cluster level leverage defined by Preisser and Qaqish (1996) is the sum of the values on the diagonal of the "hat" matrix of equation (9.29) for a given cluster. For the polypharmacy model of Table 9.12 the cluster leverages are shown in Figure 9.8. As the sum of the leverages is the number of parameters in the model (8 in this example) the average cluster leverage is $8/500 = 0.016$. We see that most of the values are fairly close to the average value but there are a few subjects with high leverages relative to the others. The subjects with highest cluster leverages are those with nonzero inpatient MHV and non-white race categories (placing them in a subgroup comprising less than 1% of the subjects in the data set).

Preisser and Qaqish (1996) propose measures of cluster influence analogous to influence statistics for individual observations. The first, $DCLS_i$, measures the influence of removing cluster i on the overall model fit by approximating the influence of removing the cluster on the linear predictor and therefore the fitted values. The statistic is defined as:

$$DCLS_i = \frac{1}{p}\mathbf{E}_i'(\mathbf{W}_i^{-1} - \mathbf{Q}_i)^{-1}\mathbf{Q}_i(\mathbf{W}_i^{-1} - \mathbf{Q}_i)^{-1}\mathbf{E}_i \qquad (9.30)$$

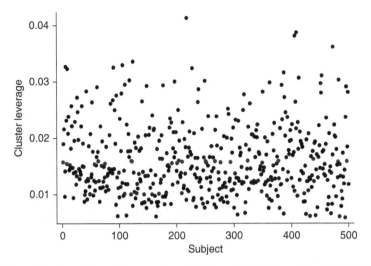

Figure 9.8 Plot of cluster leverages for each subject in the fitted model of Table 9.12.

where $\mathbf{Q}_i = \mathbf{X}_i(\mathbf{X'WX})^{-1}\mathbf{X}_i'$, $\mathbf{E}_i = \mathbf{D}_i(\mathbf{Y}_i - \hat{\boldsymbol{\pi}}_i)$, and p is the number of parameters in the model. A related measure is the "Studentized" version of $DCLS_i$, which scales the statistic based on the variance estimate of the parameters excluding the deleted cluster. This measure is a product of scaled residuals and cluster leverage and is defined as:

$$MCLS_i = \frac{1}{p}\mathbf{E}_i'(\mathbf{W}_i^{-1} - \mathbf{Q}_i)^{-1}\mathbf{H}_i\mathbf{E}_i. \qquad (9.31)$$

The $DCLS_i$ statistic is scaled using the variance estimate based on all clusters and, as a result, the statistic may decrease in magnitude and hide the influence to some extent. This makes the $MCLS_i$, in some instances, the preferable of the two [Welsch (1986)]. The $MCLS_i$, on the other hand, measures the influence of the cluster on the parameter estimates and their estimated variances simultaneously. These two statistics are available in SAS.

Plots of $DCLS_i$ and $MCLS_i$ in the polypharmacy example are identical with slight differences in scale. This is often the case in our experience. The $DCLS_i$ plot is shown in Figure 9.9. A possible cutoff for large values of the statistic is 1.0 [Kleinbaum et al. (1998)] so none of the subjects appears to have undue influence. A few subjects have large values relative to the others. Two of the three largest values are the same subjects with second- and third-highest leverages. The largest value is a relatively older non-white male subject with three observed polypharmacy events. We note nothing in the data for any of the three subjects that is suspicious, and removing all three from the data and refitting the model does not change the inferences or parameter estimates by more than 10% except for the estimated coefficient of race, which drops from -0.442 to -0.594, or 34%. This is not surprising as there are only 82 non-white subjects in the data set. The three

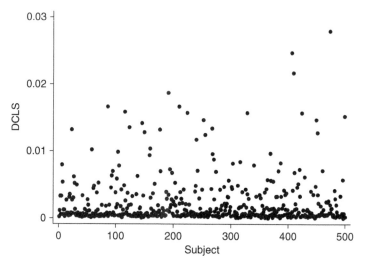

Figure 9.9   Plot of $DCLS_i$ for each subject in the fitted model of Table 9.12.

subjects have a polypharmacy percentage of 71% compared to 15.9% for the other subjects in that race category so removing them lowers the coefficient.

Preisser and Qaqish (1996) also propose a statistic to approximate the effect of removing a cluster on the parameter estimates, or $\hat{\boldsymbol{\beta}} - \hat{\boldsymbol{\beta}}_{(i)}$ where $\hat{\boldsymbol{\beta}}_{(i)}$ are the estimates with cluster i removed. The statistic is computed as:

$$DBETAC_i = (\mathbf{X}'\mathbf{W}\mathbf{X})^{-1}\mathbf{X}_i(\mathbf{W}_i^{-1} - \mathbf{Q}_i)^{-1}\mathbf{E}_i. \tag{9.32}$$

The plot of $DBETAC$ values for the subjects in the polypharmacy example is shown in Figure 9.10. There are three subjects with larger absolute values of $DBETAC$. They are all subjects that were young, between 4 and 10 years old, during the study yet with multiple years with observed polypharmacy. The two highest have observed polypharmacy all 7 years of the study. The highest corresponds to the subject with an observation producing the largest Pearson residual and ΔX^2_j discussed previously. The third largest was also identified in the diagnostics for individual observations with an observation with a high $\Delta\hat{\boldsymbol{\beta}}_j$. When these three subjects are removed only the parameter estimate of the transformed age covariate changes by more than 10%, increasing by 15.1%. We, again, conclude there is no reason to remove the subjects from the data set.

After analysis of all the diagnostic statistics we conclude that there are no overly influential subjects or observations, although a few are poorly fit. We discussed and illustrated how to compute odds ratios and their confidence intervals for population average models in Section 9.4. We present these values for the final model only for one covariate of interest, the outpatient MHV (Mental Health Visits), in Table 9.25. In our example, 0 outpatient MHV is the reference category. The results suggest that subjects are significantly more likely to have polypharmacy for more than 5 outpatient MHV. The odds of polypharmacy are 1.8 times as high for 6–14

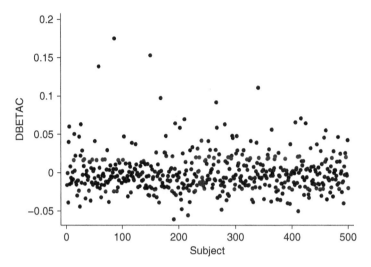

Figure 9.10 Plot of $DBETAC_i$ for each subject in the model of Table 9.12.

Table 9.25 Estimated Odds Ratios and Confidence Intervals for Outpatient MHV from the Population Average Model in Table 9.12

Outpatient MHV	Odds Ratio	95% CI
0	1	n/a
1–5	1.168	0.883, 1.546
6–14	1.836	1.360, 2.479
>14	2.528	1.836, 3.481

outpatient MHV and 2.5 times for more than 14 outpatient MHV than for no outpatient MHV. The odds for 1 to 5 visits is not significant. As we modified the data for this example all conclusions are hypothetical and do not apply to the original data. However, we note that the results are similar to the analysis with the original data. Interested readers are referred to Fontanella et al. (2012) for the conclusions of the study.

9.6.2 Assessment of Cluster-Specific Model Fit

Overall measures of fit for cluster-specific models are limited. The Hosmer–Lemeshow test may be used with the cluster-specific model using fitted values that include an estimate of the random effect term, as well as all the regression coefficients. The cluster-specific fitted values, as described in Section 9.4.2, are available from statistical software. Thus, one can calculate the test "by hand" using the results presented in Chapter 5. In STATA, the computation is available in the user created hl.ado program which can be found at the Website www.homepages.ucl.ac.uk/~ucakgam/stata.html. Specifically, equation (5.7) gives a formula for computing the test statistic and the discussion in that section provides guidance on forming the groups and computing the corresponding table as shown in Table 5.1. We calculated this test for the final cluster-specific model of polyphar-macy in Table 9.20, yielding $\hat{C} = 110.01$ which, with 8 degrees of freedom, produces $p < 0.0001$. Sturdivant (2005) conducted extensive simulations showing that the test rejects more than the nominal level when applied to fitted cluster-specific models. Thus, when interpreting the Hosmer–Lemeshow test in this setting a significant result does not necessarily indicate issues with the fitted model. The test statistic is particularly prone to issues when there are small cluster sizes and moderate to high correlation, which is exactly the case in our example. Thus, the test is not recommended in this example and is only presented for illustrative purposes.

Evans (1998) extended the normal approximation to the Pearson chi-square test for the cluster-specific model. This statistic is not available in software packages. With X^2 as defined in equation (5.2) and N observations in the data set, for cluster-specific models the moments are:

$$\widehat{E}(X^2 - N) = \mathbf{1}'\hat{\mathbf{W}}^{-1}\mathbf{g} - 2\boldsymbol{\pi}'\hat{\mathbf{W}}^{-1}\mathbf{g} + 2\mathbf{g}'\hat{\mathbf{W}}^{-1}\mathbf{g} - 2\,\text{trace}\,[\mathbf{M}'\hat{\mathbf{W}}^{-1}(\mathbf{I} - \mathbf{M})\mathbf{W}]$$
(9.33)

and

$$\widehat{\text{Var}}(X^2 - N) = (\mathbf{1} - 2\hat{\boldsymbol{\pi}})'\hat{\mathbf{W}}^{-1}(\mathbf{I} - \mathbf{M})\mathbf{W}(\mathbf{I} - \mathbf{M})'\hat{\mathbf{W}}^{-1}(\mathbf{1} - 2\hat{\boldsymbol{\pi}}),$$
(9.34)

where $\mathbf{1}$ is a vector of ones, $\hat{\mathbf{W}}$ a diagonal matrix with $\hat{\pi}_i(1 - \hat{\pi}_i)$ as diagonal elements, $\mathbf{M} = \mathbf{WQ}(\mathbf{Q}'\mathbf{WQ} + \mathbf{R})^{-1}\mathbf{Q}'$ and $\mathbf{g} = \mathbf{WQ}(\mathbf{Q}'\mathbf{WQ} + \mathbf{R})^{-1}\mathbf{R}\boldsymbol{\delta}$. In these expressions, $\mathbf{R}$ is a matrix with the inverse covariance matrix of the random effects in the lower right and zeros elsewhere, $\mathbf{Q}$ a matrix with the design matrix for the fixed effects augmented with the design matrix of the random effects and $\boldsymbol{\delta}$ a vector with fixed parameter estimates augmented with the estimates for the random effects. Using the estimates of the mean and variance the standardized statistic is then:

$$z_{X_c^2} = \frac{(X^2 - N) - \widehat{E}(X^2 - N)}{\sqrt{\widehat{\text{Var}}(X^2 - N)}},$$
(9.35)

which is compared to the standard normal distribution to obtain a p-value. In simulations by Evans (1998) involving large sample sizes and including a random intercept only, the proportion of times the null hypothesis was rejected using the statistic in equation (9.35) was close to the nominal level. However, in further simulation studies by Sturdivant (2005) of settings with more random effects and smaller sample sizes, the distribution of the statistic was both biased and skewed so that it rejected the null hypotheses sometimes more often and sometimes less often than the nominal level, casting doubt on its usefulness in assessing fit. Sturdivant and Hosmer (2007) proposed a smoothed version of the statistic with satisfactory performance in many simulated data settings. The performance of this statistic appears to hold under different methods of estimation [Sturdivant et al. (2007)]. Unfortunately, the test statistic is quite complicated to compute and is not currently implemented in software packages. Hence, we do not discuss it further. Cheng and Wu (1994) propose a test for choice of link function. As this test has not been implemented in software, and further study of its performance in binary correlated data is required, we do not discuss it here. Vonesh et al. (1996) propose use of their concordance correlation to assess model fit by computing the value with and without the random effect estimates. In essence this measures how much the random effects improve agreement between predicted and actual responses. However, currently the concordance correlation is only available in SAS GLIMMIX when fitting a population average model as discussed in the previous section. Further, the measure has not been adequately tested in cluster-specific models involving binary responses.

TenHave and Ratcliffe (2004) present an easily implemented approach to testing the assumption that the random effects are normally distributed. In Section 9.4.4 we discussed methods of approximating the population average coefficients from parameter estimates of a fitted cluster-specific model. They demonstrate that discrepancies between the approximate coefficients and the actual estimates from a fitted population average model may indicate two possible problems with the random effects model: (i) negative intra-cluster correlation and (ii) confounding between the cluster level random effects and the fixed effect covariates. We illustrate this by comparing the two estimates using the GLOW data presented in Table 9.7. The parameter estimates from the cluster-specific model are shown in column 2 and estimates from a corresponding population average model fit are displayed in column 3 of Table 9.7. The final two columns show the two approximate population average coefficients we compute from the cluster-specific model using equations (9.18) and (9.19). In this example, the approximations are both close to the estimates of the population average model so we do not have reason to suspect issues with the random effects model. In the examples of TenHave and Ratcliffe (2004) the differences were marked in cases with the two problems mentioned as discussed earlier. For example, they observed estimates in the population average model larger in absolute value than those of the cluster-specific model whereas the reverse is true when using the equations to convert from cluster-specific to population average estimates.

In population average models we were concerned with checking the choice for the covariance structure. The related check in cluster-specific models is the assumptions made about the distribution of the random effects in the model. Recall that for the basic model with a random intercept specified in equation (9.1), we assume the random intercept is normally distributed, or $\alpha_i \sim N(0, \sigma_\alpha^2)$. The assumption about the distribution of the random slope effect is similar to the random intercept, namely $\tau_i \sim N(0, \sigma_\tau^2)$ and we assume the two random effects, τ_i and α_i, are independent unless a covariance parameter between random effects is significant statistically.

The best method for assessing the normality assumption of a random effect is based on the predicted values of the random effects. One can then use standard tests and plots for normality such as the normal probability (PP) or normal quantile

(QQ) plots. The predicted random effects are discussed in Section 9.4.2. By appropriately standardizing, the estimates should have a standard normal distribution and it is the standardized values we use in the PP or QQ plots. There are several choices for estimating the standard error of the predicted random effects. The standard error produced in most software packages is the one Goldstein (2003) refers to as the "comparative" standard error. It is based on estimating the variance in prediction errors, $\hat{\alpha}_i - \alpha_i$, of the random effect in a given cluster. These standard errors are most useful in comparing random effects to see if there are differences between clusters [Skrondal and Rabe-Hesketh (2009)]. For diagnostic purposes, a better choice is the "diagnostic" standard error [Goldstein (2003)], which is an estimate of the variance of the predicted random effect, $\hat{\alpha}_i$. Unfortunately, the "diagnostic" standard error is not produced in SAS or STATA. A user developed routine in STATA, GLLAMM, which produces the estimates can be downloaded (www.gllamm.org). An additional concern in using the standardized predicted random effects is when the number of observations and variability differs in each cluster. Lange and Ryan (1989) offer a method of weighting the estimates to address this problem. Again, as with many of the methods for correlated binary data, the method is not implemented in current software.

We illustrate the use of these plots with the model in Table 9.20. In the examples to follow, we only consider the random slope. The random intercept should be similarly addressed and we leave this analysis as exercises. The PP plot using the "diagnostic" residuals is shown in Figure 9.11 and the plot using the "comparative" residuals in Figure 9.12. In this example, the plot using the comparative standard error appears less linear but both plots would cause us to question the assumption of normality for the random effect of subject. In our experience, using the standardized "comparative" residuals usually leads to similar conclusions about the normality assumption so that if the software package does not produce "diagnostic"

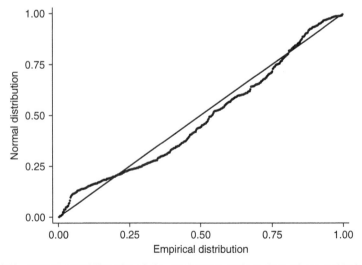

Figure 9.11 Normal probability plot of the standardized random slope of age residuals for the polypharmacy model using the diagnostic standard error estimate.

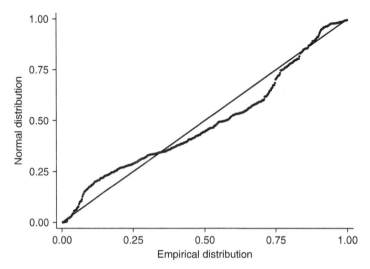

Figure 9.12 Normal probability plot of the standardized random slope of age residuals for polypharmacy model using the comparative standard error estimates.

standard errors, standardizing using the "comparative" standard errors can still lead to a useful diagnostic tool. This is not always true and issues with plots based on "comparative" errors do not necessarily mean the normality assumption is questionable. As we focus on the diagnostic standard errors, we observe that the curve in Figure 9.11 is reasonably linear but with clear departures from the line. We further test the normality using the Shapiro–Wilk test, which does reject the hypothesis of normality with $p < 0.001$. The test is fairly sensitive to departures from normality in large samples but the result should be noted and inferences about the random effects used cautiously. If only the "comparative" residuals were available the results would clearly suggest that care be exercised when making inferences that assume the normal distribution for the subjects or clusters in the study based on the model. If we are concerned with this aspect of the model a more complicated model for the random effects may be required and an experienced statistician consulted.

As was done in Chapter 5 for the standard logistic regression model, we should check for the effect of individual observations on model estimates and fit. We are interested in identifying subjects with high leverage, large residuals, or a large degree of influence on the model estimates. In the cluster-specific model we are also interested in detecting clusters that are poorly fit or exert leverage and influence on the model estimates. We follow the approach outlined in Langford and Lewis (1998) and begin with the highest level in the model.

Continuing with the polypharmacy model in Table 9.20 we have a two level model with the yearly observations (level 1) clustered by the subjects (level 2). We first look at the level 2 diagnostics for the individual subjects in the study. The posterior predicted values of the random effects can be considered the level 2 residuals and, as previously discussed, are more informative if standardized by one of the standard error estimates. Ideally, they are standardized by the "diagnostic" standard error, if available, but using the "comparative" standard error will still help identify poorly fit subjects.

Boxplots of the two types of standardized residuals for the random slopes for subjects in the polypharmacy data are shown in Figure 9.13. The advantage of using the diagnostic standardized residuals is that they may be compared with the standard normal distribution. Thus, we would expect roughly 95% of them to fall between the values of 2 and −2 as we observe in our example. The comparative standardization does not allow for this check because the standard error is smaller (it is based on the variance of the difference between the predicted and actual random effects). This generally leads to larger standardized residuals although not in this example. Both may be useful in looking for unusual observations that are potential outliers. In our example, the two produce different pictures and we focus on the diagnostic version. We see subjects with slightly higher values although, with 500 subjects, it is not unusual to have values as large as 3. The largest, in absolute value, is −2.97 for a white male with observed polypharmacy in the first 3 years, when he was youngest, and none thereafter. This pattern is unusual as polypharmacy is less likely for young subjects. This leads to the observed large negative random slope estimate to reverse the predicted probabilities for the subject so that they are higher when he was young. The large diagnostic random slope is thus well justified by the data.

Langford and Lewis (1998) proposed formulas to compute leverage and measures of influence but these have not been implemented in standard software packages. The previously referred to user written STATA program, GLLAMM,

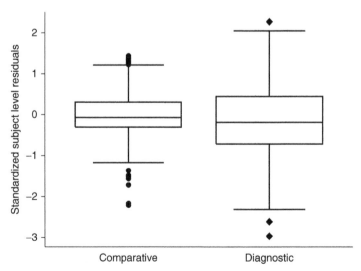

Figure 9.13 Boxplot of diagnostic random slope residuals for the fitted polypharmacy model in Table 9.20 using diagnostic and comparative standard errors.

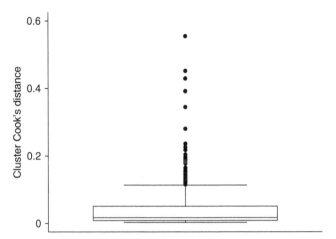

Figure 9.14 Boxplot of Langford–Lewis version of Cook's Distance of subjects for the fitted polyphar-macy model in Table 9.20.

does compute a measure of influence for the highest level cluster variable in the model, which is comparable to Cook's Distance in the standard logistic model. A boxplot of these values for the polypharmacy model in Table 9.20 is shown in Figure 9.14. We observe several subjects (clusters) with particularly high values relative to other subjects in the data set. The largest is the same subject with the largest standardized slope residual with a value of 0.55. The next largest value of 0.45 is a subject with a similar instance of polypharmacy in the 4 younger years and not in the 3 oldest years.

We identified potentially influential clusters and, in our example, identified a difference in these subjects that may be the reason for large cluster-level diagnostic values. The reason may not always be immediately apparent. In some instances the subject or cluster may differ in some way from others in the study. Alternatively, there may just be a few specific observations within the cluster that led to the diagnostic results observed. The third to fifth highest observed values in Figure 9.14 may fall into this category. In these subjects, polypharmacy is observed in the middle years of the study and those observations may lead to the potential influence. Thus, we also explore diagnostic measures for subject and year, or level 1, observations within the subjects. Neither SAS or STATA currently has options for producing measures of leverage or influence for the level 1 observations in cluster-specific models. Both packages do offer residuals similar to the Pearson and deviance residuals discussed in Section 5.2. In STATA the GLLAMM procedure is required. A plot of residuals for each individual observation grouped by cluster is a useful method for examining both the level one diagnostic statistic and the reasons clusters had high influential values. Such a plot of the Pearson residuals for each observation grouped by the subject is shown in Figure 9.15 for the subjects with the highest observed values in Figure 9.14. In data sets with fewer subjects such a plot can be produced for the entire data set. As expected, the two

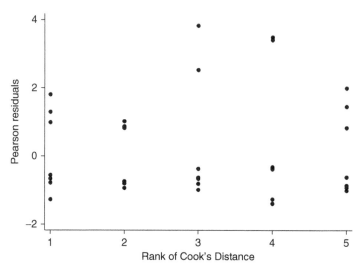

Figure 9.15 Scatter plot of level 1 Pearson residuals by subject for largest Cook's Distance of Figure 9.14.

subjects with the largest Cook's Distance do not have large residuals. The reason they are potentially influential is that they differ from other subjects in the study in their polypharmacy profile. The next two most influential subjects do have two large residuals each corresponding to the years they had observed polypharmacy. In both cases, the polypharmacy occurred in middle years of the study time frame making the points difficult to model using age and the random slope for age. The subject with the fifth largest Cook's Distance has a similar polypharmacy profile with two occurrences in the middle years of the study but slightly lower residuals due to an observed polypharmacy in the final year that is the other relatively large residual observed. In this example, we are able to readily identify the reason for the large Cook's Distance. As Cook's Distance measures influence (a function of the residuals and leverage) another reason for the large values may be leverage and not readily apparent. As mentioned, we have no measures of leverage but can explore each of the covariates in the model by cluster in such cases.

Once a cluster is identified as possibly influential, Langford and Lewis (1998) suggest two approaches to determining how it impacts model estimates. The first is to remove the entire cluster and refit the model. In settings with few clusters, with many observations in each cluster, this approach may delete too much data. This is not the case in the polypharmacy data. With 500 subjects in the study and only 7 observations per subject deleting a single subject removes only 0.2% of the data. We refit the model removing the two subjects with the largest values of Cook's Distance. The result was small changes in the estimates for the parameters with none greater than 15%. Thus we do not exclude the entire cluster. In general, the deletion approach works best for small clusters.

The second method is to include the potential outlying cluster in the fixed part of the model using an indicator variable to fit a separate intercept while excluding the cluster from the random portion of the model. If the results of analysis suggest the cluster is poorly fit using the random effects and that the model should be modified to fix the problem, this approach may be more desirable than deleting the entire cluster. In our example, the influential clusters do not impact the model to such an extent that we would consider this more complicated model.

In addition to looking at diagnostics in terms of clusters that might be outliers or influential we also recommend looking at the level 1 residuals for all observations using plots similar to those discussed in Section 5.3 for standard logistic regression diagnostics. An example is the plot of squared deviance residuals obtained from the GLLAMM procedure in STATA against the model predicted probabilities shown in Figure 9.16. A similar plot may be produced using the squared Pearson residuals.

We see two curves in Figure 9.16, starting small and rising for no polypharmacy ($y = 0$) and starting high and falling for polypharmacy ($y = 1$). We are looking for extreme values. For no polypharmacy there are three observations with values larger than 5. The interpretation is that the model based probability of polypharmacy was high, over 0.88, but the subjects did not have polypharmacy. All three are in the highest category of outpatient MHV with counts greater than 14 and relatively older males, factors associated with higher probability of polypharmacy. The subjects have increased risk based on either their white race or non-zero inpatient MHV and, in one case, both. The curve for polypharmacy observations in Figure 9.16 also has four values greater than 5.5 with two greater than 6. In these cases, the observation was polypharmacy when model based probabilities of this response were less than 8.8%. For all four, the observation is their only polypharmacy in the 7 years of the study, with indicators of lower risk. The largest is a relatively young female with no inpatient and only 1 outpatient MHV. The other three are

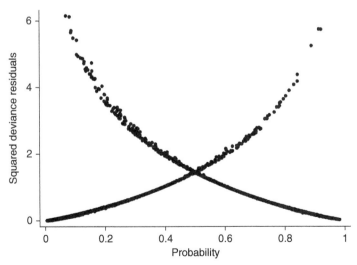

Figure 9.16 Scatter plot of level 1 squared deviance residuals by model predicted probabilities for the fitted polypharmacy model in Table 9.20.

Table 9.26   Estimated Odds Ratios and Confidence Intervals for
Outpatient MHV from the Cluster-Specific Model in Table 9.20

Outpatient MHV	Odds Ratio	95% CI
0	1	n/a
1–5	1.459	0.792, 2.685
6–14	3.560	1.906, 6.648
>14	6.252	3.314, 11.794

also relatively young with no inpatient MHV. One has no outpatient MHV and the
other two, one who is younger, a single outpatient MHV. None of the observed
large observations, for either response or non-response, is particularly suspicious
or alarming.

Analysis of potential outliers proceeds as described in Section 5.3. This typically
involves removing the observations, refitting the model and assessing the change in
model estimated parameters. We leave this as an exercise. One point worth noting
is that, in cluster-specific models, the removal of influential observations at level 1
may impact fit at higher levels in the model so the diagnostic measures for higher
levels should be reexamined if subjects are taken out of the data set.

Once diagnostics are complete we use the final model for estimation and interpretation of covariate effects. In the example, the odds ratios for one covariate
of interest comparing levels of higher outpatient MHV to no visits are shown in
Table 9.26. The subject-specific estimates of the effects, as discussed in Section
9.3, are larger than those of the population average model shown in Table 9.25.
The inferences in terms of the study questions are not changed using the subject-
specific interpretation. For a given subject, outpatient MHV categories above five
lead to significantly higher odds of polypharmacy. As in the population average
model, the odds of 1 to 5 outpatient MHV is not statistically different than none.
We remind the reader that our conclusions are provided as an example as they are
based on a sample and not the actual data set.

9.6.3   Conclusions

In most cases, the cluster-specific or population average models are appropriate
for modeling correlated binary data. The correlation must be due to recognizable
factors in the design of the study that allow one to explicitly identify clusters, or
sets of observations, that are correlated and those that are uncorrelated. The cluster-
specific model is likely to be most useful for describing the effect of covariates
that are repeatedly measured on the same subject. The population average model
is best suited to describe the effect of covariates that are constant within clusters.
However, both models may be fit with both types of covariates. One must pay
particular attention to signs of numerical problems when fitting both models. These
include failure of the program to converge to a solution and a "zero" estimate of
the variance of the random effect.

Logistic regression models for correlated binary data is an area of active statistical research with new developments appearing on a regular basis. As these developments are accepted by the statistical community as sound and worthwhile modeling tools, developers of software packages can be expected to add them to their routines.

EXERCISES

1. Suppose that a dichotomous covariate, D, for race comparing WHITE $(D = 1)$ to OTHER $(D = 0)$ is included in the GLOW models and the estimated coefficient is 2.

   (a) Interpret the odds ratio for race assuming that a population average model was fit.

   (b) Interpret the odds ratio assuming that a cluster-specific model was fit.

   (c) If interpretation of the race covariate is the primary study goal, which model do you think is more appropriate?

2. Show that if the correlation is 0 (i.e., an independent correlation structure is chosen) that the GEE of equation (9.9) reduces to the likelihood equations for a standard logistic regression model.

3. Interpret the odds ratios for self-reported risk (RATERISK) produced in the cluster-specific model of Table 9.3 of Section 9.4.

4. Interpret the odds ratios for a 2-year increase in age and the odds ratio for gender for the population average model of Table 9.12 and the cluster-specific model of Table 9.20 in Section 9.5. Are the differences in odds ratios from the two models what you expect? Explain.

5. Use equation (9.19) to approximate the population average coefficients using the parameter estimates for the final cluster-specific polypharmacy model of Table 9.20. Compare these approximations to the parameter estimates produced by fitting the corresponding population average model in Table 9.12. If there are large differences, what might this suggest about the assumptions for the model(s)?

6. Fit the population average model for the polypharmacy data of Table 9.12 using the independent correlation structure, in other words using a standard logistic regression model. Compare the two models. Does including the correlation due to subjects in the model seem necessary? Explain.

7. Using techniques described in this chapter, as well as design variables, examine the scale of the age covariate in the population average and cluster-specific models of Section 9.5. Do you agree with the transformations proposed?

8. Compute and interpret the MOR for the covariates in the final cluster-specific model for the polypharmacy data in Table 9.20.

9. Fit a univariable model for the polypharmacy data with the single cluster-level covariate, race dichotomized to white and other. Using the resulting model compute and interpret the IOR.

10. Develop a preliminary main effects model for the GLOW_RAND data using a population average model with exchangeable correlation structure.

11. Develop a preliminary main effects model for the GLOW_RAND data using a cluster-specific model with random intercept based on the SITE.

12. If you have a software package that can produce the QIC, examine the effect on the QIC statistics of adding two-way interactions for race by age and inpatient by outpatient MHV to the final polypharmacy population average model of Table 9.12. Are the changes in QIC consistent with other indicators of the significance of the interaction terms?

13. Fit the final polypharmacy cluster-specific model of Table 9.20 then produce the empirical Bayes predicted random intercept values. What do these values mean in the context of this model? Compare values for different subjects and comment on whether they make sense by examining the actual data for each subject. If possible produce these values using different software packages or procedures and compare.

14. Use the GLOW_RAND data from Section 9.4 and fit a cluster-specific model using adaptive quadrature for estimation. Use FRACTURE as the response and covariates: calculated fracture risk score (FRAC_SCORE), age (AGE), and self-perception of risk (RATERISK). Include a random intercept for physician id (PHY_ID).

    (a) Does the number of quadrature points appear to impact the model estimates?

    (b) What happens if you test each covariate for a random slope?

CHAPTER 10

Special Topics

10.1 INTRODUCTION

As is likely true in other textbooks there are important topics that should have been included, but do not seem to logically fit in the existing chapters. In Section 10.2 we provide an overview, with an example, of the use of propensity scores in logistic regression modeling, where the goal of the analysis is to estimate the effect of a treatment. Section 10.3 considers fitting a logistic regression model to sparse data where one cannot rely on large sample assumptions. This is often referred to as "exact" logistic regression. Throughout the text we have assumed any missing data would have no effect on the analysis. In Section 10.4 we consider methods for dealing with missing data. Section 10.5 considers choosing a sample size when the goal of the analysis is to estimate the effect of one covariate where the effect of others has been controlled using a logistic regression model. An introduction to the Bayesian approach to logistic regression modeling is presented in the Section 10.6. In Section 10.7 we consider regression modeling of a binary outcome using link functions other than the logit. The chapter concludes with sections on effect mediators and other modes of statistical interaction.

10.2 APPLICATION OF PROPENSITY SCORE METHODS IN LOGISTIC REGRESSION MODELING

In a typical observational study, subjects who received a particular treatment have likely not been randomly assigned to treatment. Thus, estimation of a treatment effect can be confounded by covariates whose distributions differ both with respect to the treatment groups (assumed to be two here) and the strength of the association between the covariates and the outcome. Model-based assessment of and adjustment for confounding is discussed in detail in Section 3.5. In Section 4.2 we explicitly

Applied Logistic Regression, Third Edition.
David W. Hosmer, Jr., Stanley Lemeshow, and Rodney X. Sturdivant.
© 2013 John Wiley & Sons, Inc. Published 2013 by John Wiley & Sons, Inc.

incorporated the ideas discussed in Section 3.5 into the Method of Purposeful Selection (of covariates). The strength of this model building approach is that by selecting covariates that are associated in a meaningful clinical or statistical manner with the outcome, and are believed to (or actually do) express statistical evidence of confounding of the treatment effect, adjusted estimates of the treatment effect that are assumed to be free of confounding may be obtained. However, the method does not explicitly balance covariate distributions within levels of the treatment covariate. Thus, there may be residual confounding and associated bias in the effect estimate. A method that is increasingly being used in observational studies that directly addresses the potentially confounding effects of covariate imbalance is to incorporate the propensity score, for treatment, into the analysis.

The propensity score is a function that models the probability of treatment assignment conditional on the covariates, namely

$$e(\mathbf{X}) = \Pr(Z = 1|\mathbf{X}), \tag{10.1}$$

where Z denotes the treatment indicator variable, assumed to be coded 0 or 1, and $\mathbf{X}$ denotes the collection of study covariates. Rosenbaum and Rubin (1983) developed many of the statistical properties of the propensity score and followed with a number of papers studying its application [e.g., Rosenbaum and Rubin (1984)]. There is quite an extensive literature now on the propensity score. A few papers the reader may find helpful that supplement the material presented here include: D'Agostino (1998), Austin and Mamdani (2006), Austin et al. (2007), Austin (2008), Hill (2008) and Williamson et al. (2011). Extensive citations of other relevant work may be found in these papers.

Before proceeding further with propensity score methods, we think it is helpful to review the model-based approach to assess the presence of confounding discussed in Section 3.5. In that section we considered a logistic regression model containing a dichotomous exposure/treatment variable, say Z, and a continuous potential confounder, say X, and assumed that the theoretically correct logit was linear in X, that is, $g(z, x) = \beta_0 + \beta_1 \times z + \beta_2 \times x$. Denote the logit for a model only containing Z as $g(z) = \theta_0 + \theta_1 \times z$. The statistic we proposed, and used in the *Method of Purposeful Selection*, to assess the amount of confounding due to X is

$$\Delta\hat{\beta}\% = 100 \times \frac{(\hat{\theta}_1 - \hat{\beta}_1)}{\hat{\beta}_1}, \tag{10.2}$$

where $\hat{\beta}_1$ and $\hat{\theta}_1$ are the estimators of the coefficients for Z in the two models, and the criterion we suggested using for evidence of confounding is $\Delta\hat{\beta}\% \geq 10 - 20\%$. We showed that, under these model assumptions, the difference between the crude and adjusted estimate of the effect of Z is

$$\hat{\theta}_1 - \hat{\beta}_1 \cong \hat{\beta}_2 \times (\bar{x}_1 - \bar{x}_0),$$

which is an expression that captures the essence of the two dimensions required for a covariate, X, to confound the effect of another covariate, Z: (i) The association between the treatment and confounder and (ii) the association between the confounder and the outcome. The term $(\overline{x}_1 - \overline{x}_0)$ is a measure of the difference in the distribution of X in the two groups defined by Z. If the estimators of the sample mean of X within the two groups are the same, then the covariate does not confound the effect of Z. Obviously, the potential confounder, X, must also be associated with the outcome, as measured by $\hat{\beta}_2$. If treatment is randomly assigned then, in theory, we expect that $(\overline{x}_1 - \overline{x}_0)$ should be small. In an observational study there is no such theoretical guarantee. In previous chapters we controlled for confounding by statistically adjusting for X (i.e., including it in the model). An alternative to modeling approaches, such as Purposeful Selection, is to create the propensity score, use it to form groups where the distribution of the covariates is balanced, $(\overline{x}_1 - \overline{x}_0) \cong 0$, and then estimate the effect of Z. The important thing to understand at this point is that the purpose of the propensity score is to explicitly balance the distribution of covariates, as opposed to handling imbalance via statistical adjustment (modeling).

The first step in propensity score adjustment is to estimate the probability of treatment by fitting a logistic regression model with the treatment covariate as the outcome. Austin et al. (2007) studied the properties of propensity scores formed from four different classes of covariates: (i) covariates associated with treatment assignment, basically the $(\overline{x}_1 - \overline{x}_0)$ part; (ii) covariates associated with the outcome, basically the $\hat{\beta}_2$ part; (iii) confounders of the effect of the treatment covariate, the whole of $\hat{\beta}_2 \times (\overline{x}_1 - \overline{x}_0)$; and (iv) all measured covariates.

Early users of propensity score methods tended to follow (iv). They included as many covariates, interactions and higher order terms as the data would support. The idea is that one should include any covariate that possibly is a confounder. Here overfitting can be a problem and one may be trying to balance over so many covariates that the sample finally used for analysis is unnecessarily reduced in size.

Austin et al. (2007) found, using simulations, that propensity scores formed from covariate classes (i) and (iii) had the best overall performance with respect to bias and mean squared error of the estimate of treatment effect. For now, assume that we have an estimate of the propensity score for each of n study subjects: $\hat{e}_i, i = 1, 2, \ldots, n$.

Before analyses are performed it is recommended, and we agree, that one should examine the distribution of $\hat{e}$ within the two treatment groups to determine the region of common support. There are two schools of thought on this. Some [e.g., Austin and Mamdani (2006)] suggest eliminating subjects on the control treatment, $z = 0$, with values of $\hat{e}$ less than the smallest value of $\hat{e}$ among those receiving the treatment, $z = 1$. Leuven and Sianesi (2003), in their STATA program psmatch2, eliminate subjects with $z = 1$ and a value of $\hat{e}$ that is larger than the largest value of $\hat{e}$ among those with $z = 0$. Our feeling is that one should drop both groups from the analysis; this is what we use to define the region of common support. After common support is determined, one should refit the propensity score model on the reduced data set before performing any of the analyses described next.

When the outcome of interest is binary and one uses a logistic regression model, there are essentially three different approaches to using the propensity score. The first, and simplest, is to fit the logistic regression model containing the indicator for treatment, z, and the estimated propensity score, $\hat{e}$. Since the propensity score is continuous one should carefully determine whether the logit is nonlinear and apply a transformation to it, if needed. For simplicity, assume that the logit is, indeed, linear in the estimated propensity score and the estimated logit is

$$\hat{g}(z, \hat{e}) = \hat{\beta}_0 + \hat{\beta}_1 z + \hat{\beta}_2 \hat{e}. \tag{10.3}$$

Based on this model, the propensity score adjusted estimate of the odds ratio for treatment is $\text{OR} = \exp(\hat{\beta}_1)$. The Wald-based confidence interval estimate uses the estimator of the standard error of $\hat{\beta}_1$ from the fit. This adjusted analysis assumes that two hypothetical subjects with the same value of the propensity score, who differ only in treatment, have no imbalances in the distribution of covariates used to obtain $\hat{e}$; that is, by including $\hat{e}$ in the model we control for confounding due to covariate imbalance.

One practical problem is that this analysis does not account for the fact that $\hat{e}$ is also a function of the data. Hence, the estimated standard errors from the fit of the model in equation (10.3) are likely to be too small. One approach is to use bootstrap methods. This process is a bit complex, in that, to do it properly requires that estimating the propensity score be part of the bootstrap process, not just multiple fits of the model in equation (10.3) with a bootstrap sample. This latter analysis is much easier to do than the former and it may be better than simply using the fit of equation (10.3).

The second approach is to fit separate models within each quintile of $\hat{e}$. Rosenbaum and Rubin (1983) show that if there is no imbalance in the covariates within the strata, then approximately 90% of the bias due to confounding is removed. Thus, it is vital to check that this assumption holds within each quintile before proceeding further with the stratified analysis. If there is imbalance, then practical solutions are to move the cutpoints defining the groups or use more than five groups. Assuming there is balance within the quintiles, then one fits stratum-specific models with estimated logit functions

$$\hat{g}_j(z) = \hat{\beta}_{0j} + \hat{\beta}_{1j} z, \, j = 1, 2, \ldots, 5. \tag{10.4}$$

The combined estimate of the log-odds ratio for treatment effect is

$$\ln(\widehat{\text{OR}}) = \frac{1}{5} \sum_{j=1}^{5} \widehat{\beta}_{1j}. \tag{10.5}$$

The five fits are independent of each other, thus the estimated standard error of the pooled log-odds ratio estimator is

$$\widehat{\text{SE}}[\ln(\widehat{\text{OR}})] = \left[\frac{1}{25} \sum_{j=1}^{5} \widehat{\text{Var}}\left(\hat{\beta}_{1j}\right) \right]^{0.5}, \tag{10.6}$$

which can be used in the usual manner to obtain the Wald-based confidence interval estimator of the odds ratio.

An alternative analysis using quintiles is to begin by fitting the model

$$g(z, \mathbf{s}) = \beta_0 + \sum_{k=2}^{5} \beta_{1k} \times s_k + \beta_2 \times z + \sum_{k=2}^{5} \beta_{3k} \times s_k \times z, \qquad (10.7)$$

where s_2, s_3, s_4, s_5 are the design variables for the quintiles using the first quintile as the reference group. Next we fit the model that excludes the four interaction terms

$$g(z, \mathbf{s}) = \beta_0 + \sum_{k=2}^{5} \beta_{1k} \times s_k + \beta_2 \times z. \qquad (10.8)$$

If the likelihood ratio test comparing the model in equation (10.7) to the model in equation (10.8) is significant, then estimates of effect are different for each stratum and we use methods for estimating odds ratios in the presence of interaction. One hopes that this test is not significant as it points to imbalance and residual confounding. If the two models are not significantly different, then we use the results from the fit of equation (10.8) to estimate treatment effect as $\widehat{OR} = \exp(\widehat{\beta}_2)$. We think that this model-based stratified analysis is the simpler analysis and may result in narrower confidence intervals than the group pooled estimator in equation (10.5).

The third approach is to create a matched sample. The matching is driven by the smaller of the two treatment groups. For discussion purposes, assume that the number of subjects with $z = 1$ is less than the number with $z = 0$. Using one of several possible metrics, one matches each subject with $z = 1$ to a subject from the group with $z = 0$. In the example, we use the STATA program psmatch2, see Leuven and Sianesi (2003), with caliper matching based on the logit($\widehat{e}$). The width of the caliper controls how many matches one is able to make among the controls. For each subject in the treatment group, all untreated subjects within caliper width of the treatment subject's score are identified, and one or more are selected at random. A problem is that, as one makes the matches, the pool of available controls shrinks, eventually reaching the point where there may be no controls whose score is within caliper width of the remaining unmatched treated subjects. One could solve the problem by using sampling with replacement. Alternatives when using sampling without replacement are to: (i) increase the caliper width or (ii) not match all treated subjects. The penalty for increasing the caliper width may be imbalance in covariates. Regardless of the method one should always check that there is no imbalance in the covariates over the matched subjects. For example, one can do this using a paired t-test for $1-1$ matched data and a continuous covariate.

Once the matched sample is chosen we believe that any analysis for treatment effect ought to take into account the correlation due to the matching. Two easily implemented approaches are: (i) fit the conditional logistic regression model stratifying on the covariate defining matches, as described in Chapter 7 or (ii) fit the GEE population average model discussed in Chapter 9, clustering on the covariate defining the matches. One problem with the conditional logistic regression approach is that matches where the outcome is constant do not contribute to the analysis. In the example, we illustrate both of these approaches. A third and less desirable option, in our opinion, is to use the usual logistic regression model with a robust estimator of the standard error of the estimated coefficients.

GLOW variables used to this point did not include bone medications. We now introduce an expanded GLOW data set, ALR3_GLOW_BONEMED, that includes, in addition to the variables in Table 1.7, information on whether or not a woman was taking any of 11 bone medications at enrollment, BONEMED ($0 = $ no, $1 = $ yes), and at follow-up, BONEMED_FU ($0 = $ no, $1 = $ yes). Since use is self-reported we have no information on compliance or dosage. We used these two covariates to create a new covariate that indicates whether a woman was taking bone medication at both enrollment and follow-up, BONETREAT ($0 = $ no, $1 = $ yes). Using this definition of treatment, 118 women among the 500 were taking bone medications. We leave propensity score analyses of other definitions of treatment as exercises.

The first step is to build the propensity score logistic regression model. To do this we focus on identifying covariates in class one, described above, namely factors associated with who received treatment. First we fit the logistic regression model with FRACTURE as the outcome and covariate BONETREAT. Denote the model coefficient for BONETREAT as $\hat{\theta}_1$. Next, we add a potential confounder to the model. Denote the coefficient for BONETREAT from this bivariable fit as $\hat{\beta}_1$. If the percent change in the coefficient (see eq. 10.2), for BONETREAT exceeds 10%, we conclude the added covariate is a confounder of the treatment effect. Following this process we identified as confounders the covariates: AGE, HEIGHT, BMI and PRIORFRAC (having had a prior fracture).

Next, we fit the logistic regression model with outcome BONETREAT and covariates AGE, HEIGHT, BMI and PRIORFRAC. Using the method of fractional polynomials, we found that the fractional polynomial $(3, 3)$ in age was significant. Several other transformations yielded a deviance that was trivially larger, including the quadratic model $(1, 2)$. Hence, for ease of interpretation, we used the quadratic model in the propensity score. The plot of the estimated logit versus age, done in a manner similar to that used in Chapter 4, showed that as age increases from age 55 there was an increase in the odds of receiving treatment until age 70 when the odds decreased. This is consistent with clinical practice. There was no evidence of a need to transform HEIGHT or BMI. No interactions were significant at the 5% level.

When we checked for common support we found that there were 43 subjects who did not take bone medications with an estimated propensity score less than the smallest value among those who did take bone medications. Three women who took bone medications had an estimated propensity score larger than the second largest* value among the women who did not take bone medications. Among the 454 women with estimated propensity scores within the region of common support, 115 were taking bone medications, BONETREAT $= 1$.

We refit the propensity score model and the results of the fit are shown in Table 10.1. Examining the fit using the decile of risk statistic we found that $\widehat{C} = 11.26$ with $p = 0.19$. The area under the ROC curve is 0.70. Thus, we conclude

---

*We choose the second largest value as the largest, 0.79, was the larger by 0.13 and the largest value of the 500.

Table 10.1   Fitted Propensity Score Model for Treatment Variable BONETREAT, $n = 454$

	Coeff.	Std. Err.	z	p	95% CI
AGE	0.602	0.2198	2.74	0.006	0.171, 1.033
AGE2	−0.004	0.0015	−2.68	0.007	−0.007, −0.001
HEIGHT	−0.060	0.0192	−3.15	0.002	−0.098, −0.023
BMI	−0.112	0.0260	−4.29	<0.001	−0.163, −0.061
PRIORFRAC	0.531	0.2581	2.06	0.039	0.026, 1.037
Constant	−10.238	8.1124	−1.26	0.207	−26.138, 5.662

that the model fits and has, at best, modest discrimination between those who did and those who did not receive bone medications. We feel that it is important to check for fit and, especially, the model's discrimination. A propensity score model that discriminates well may have a narrow range of common support, which would reduce the sample available for the analysis of the outcome.

The first, and simplest, propensity score analysis is to fit the model in equation (10.3). We checked, using fractional polynomials, and found no evidence of a need to transform the propensity score. Table 10.2 presents results of fitting the model containing only BONETREAT, and results when the propensity score (PSC) is included, the model in equation (10.3).

The estimated crude odds ratio for treatment is $\widehat{OR} = 1.63$ and is significant. The interpretation is, without considering other covariates, that women taking bone medications have an estimated odds of fracture that is 1.63 times larger than women not taking bone medications. This result seems counterintuitive, as one would expect that women on treatment should have lower, not higher, odds of fracture. Thus, there could be residual confounding of the treatment effect estimate.

At this point we feel it is important to remind the reader that, due to the sampling used to obtain the GLOW data used in this text, results in no way apply to the whole GLOW study or women, in this case, taking or not taking bone medications.

When we add the propensity score to the model the estimated odds ratio dropped to $\widehat{OR} = 1.48$ and, with $p = 0.108$, is no longer significant. Thus, while still indicating an increased odds of fracture for women on treatment the estimate does not achieve statistical significance. One problem with this analysis is that there

Table 10.2   Fitted Models to Assess the Treatment Effect of BONETREAT: Crude and Propensity Score Adjusted Model, $n = 454$

	Coeff.	Std. Err.	z	p	95% CI
BONETREAT	0.491	0.2346	2.09	0.036	0.032, 0.951
Constant	−1.159	0.1274	−9.10	<0.001	−1.408, −0.909
BONETREAT	0.395	0.2462	1.61	0.108	−0.087, 0.878
PSC	1.102	0.8480	1.30	0.194	−0.560, 2.764
Constant	−1.417	0.2396	−5.92	<0.001	−1.887, −0.948

may be residual confounding, because we have one large group and there can be imbalances in the distribution of the covariates between treatment groups. In fact, the two-sample tests of the four covariates over the two treatment groups are significant. This analysis is really not terribly different from the covariate-based modeling approach in previous chapters, since covariates could still remain unbalanced.

The next approach is to model within each quintile of the propensity score, after checking for balance in the covariates. That is, fitting the models in equation (10.4) and evaluating the estimator in equation (10.5). We did check for balance in the covariates and none of the two-sample tests were significant. The results of the fit of the within quintile models are shown in Table 10.3.

The estimate of the within quintile pooled estimator in equation (10.5) is $\widehat{OR} = 1.69$ with a 95% confidence interval $(1.01, 2.84)$. The estimate shows a 69% increase in the odds of fracture among women taking bone medications since 1 is not contained within the confidence interval, the increase is statistically significant.

An alternative to the pooled analysis is to use all 454 subjects in the region of common support and include the quintiles in the model using four design variables. We fit the interactions model in equation (10.7) and compared it to the main effects model in equation (10.8) via the likelihood ratio test, yielding $G = 3.01$ with $p = 0.57$. We conclude that no interaction exists, and proceed with the main effects model whose results are shown in Table 10.4.

The estimated odds ratio for bone medications from Table 10.4 is $\widehat{OR} = 1.49$ with a 95% confidence interval $(0.92, 2.42)$. The point estimate shows a 49% increase in the odds of fracture, but it is not significant as the confidence interval contains one and the Wald test has $p = 0.104$. The fact that the interactions between quintiles and treatment are not significant allows us to conclude that the variability in the estimates of the five coefficients for BONETREAT seen in Table 10.3 is not significant. We prefer the stratified analysis in Table 10.4 to the pooled analysis

Table 10.3   Fitted Models, within Quintiles of the Propensity Score, to Assess the Treatment Effect of BONETREAT, $n = 454$

Quintile		Coeff.	Std. Err.	z	p	95% CI
1	BONETREAT	0.872	0.7657	1.14	0.255	−0.628, 2.373
	Constant	−1.566	0.2939	−5.33	<0.001	−2.142, −0.990
2	BONETREAT	1.070	0.6619	1.62	0.106	−0.227, 2.368
	Constant	−1.253	0.2673	−4.69	<0.001	−1.777, −0.729
3	BONETREAT	0.548	0.5069	1.08	0.280	−0.446 1.541
	Constant	−1.059	0.2815	−3.76	<0.001	−1.610, −0.507
4	BONETREAT	−0.209	0.4978	−0.42	0.675	−1.185, 0.767
	Constant	−0.847	0.2817	−3.01	0.003	−1.399, −0.295
5	BONETREAT	0.353	0.4564	0.77	0.440	−0.542, 1.247
	Constant	−0.972	0.3138	−3.10	0.002	−1.587, −0.357

Table 10.4   Fitted Models to Assess the Treatment Effect of BONETREAT: Crude and Propensity Score Adjusted Model, $n = 454$

	Coeff.	Std. Err.	z	p	95% CI
BONETREAT	0.401	0.2461	1.63	0.104	−0.082, 0.883
Q_2	0.351	0.3618	0.97	0.332	−0.358, 1.060
Q_3	0.488	0.3592	1.36	0.174	−0.216, 1.192
Q_4	0.442	0.3618	1.22	0.222	−0.268, 1.151
Q_5	0.507	0.3638	1.39	0.163	−0.206, 1.220
Constant	−1.502	0.2713	−5.53	<0.001	−2.034, −0.970

in Table 10.3 since it uses the entire sample in the region of common support and allows testing for quintile differences in effect. Regardless of which analysis one chooses, it is critical that a test for covariate imbalance within quintiles is done.

One may add additional risk factors to any of the models shown in Tables 10.2 to Table 10.4. When we add history of fracture (MOMFRAC), need to use arms (ARMASSIST), and self-reported risk of fracture (RATERISK, using two design variables) to the model in Table 10.4, the estimate of the odds ratio for taking bone medications decreases from 1.47 to $\widehat{OR} = 1.26$ with 95% confidence interval (0.75, 2.10). The change suggests that the propensity score, as calculated in Table 10.1, may not account for all confounding of the treatment effect. However, to this point, all estimates of treatment effect that use the propensity score are not significant.

The final method we discuss most completely balances the distribution of the covariates used in the propensity score is a 1–1 matched analysis. To obtain the matched sample we used the STATA program psmatch2 [see Leuven and Sianesi (2003)] using the logit of the propensity score in Table 10.1 and caliper matching with width equal 0.2 times the standard deviation of the estimated logit. The program matched, using sampling without replacement, 108 of the 115 treated subjects in the common support region of the propensity score model. In order to match all 115 treated subjects the caliper had to be increased to 1.0 standard deviation of the logit. This increase seems unwarranted, as it could well result in an imbalance in the distributions of the covariates in the two treatment groups. Thus, we proceed with the analysis using a data set that consists of 108 matched pairs. We tested for balance in the distribution of the four covariates used to estimate the propensity score with paired-sample tests; no imbalances were found.

Austin (2008) notes that 73% of papers in the medical literature between 1996 and 2003 failed to account for the matching. He recommends using methods specifically designed for matched data. Hill (2008) is at odds with this recommendation, stating that there are many ways to account for the dependence induced by the pairs. To provide comparisons we analyzed the data using three different methods: conditional logistic regression, discussed in Chapter 7, stratifying on pairs; the GEE population average model, discussed in Chapter 9, clustering on pairs assuming an exchangeable correlation structure; and the standard logistic regression model using a robust estimator of the standard errors of estimated coefficients. Within each approach we fit two models: a "simple" model containing only BONETREAT and a "risk" model that added history of fracture (MOMFRAC), need to use arms (ARMASSIST) and self-reported risk of fracture (RATERISK, using two design variables). After adding the estimated propensity score to these models, its estimated coefficient was nearly infinite. This is expected, since the score is nearly constant within pairs, hence is collinear with treatment.

To simplify the discussion and to better focus on the primary question of estimating the odds ratio of fracture for BONETREAT, we depart from our preferred practice of reporting full fitted models and instead report final estimates of the odds ratio for BONETREAT from the six different fits. These are summarized in Table 10.5.

The results from the three different approaches are quite consistent. The three estimated odds ratios from the "simple" fits are about 1.3 each and from the "risk" fits are about 1.1–1.2 each. The widths of the three confidence intervals from the "simple" fits are about 1.6 each, while those from the "risk" fits vary from the most precise, 1.4 (GEE), to the least precise, 1.8 (conditional logistic regression). Based on these results the GEE model would be a good alternative to the conditional logistic model in settings, such as this example, where many pairs are deleted due to a constant outcome within pairs. Results here show that, regardless of method, when we control for confounding using propensity score matched pairs, the estimate of the odds ratio of treatment with bone medications is greater than one, but not significant. Again, we remind the reader that due to the sampling used to obtain these GLOW data, the inferences only apply to these data and do not generalize to the study as a whole or treatment with bone medications in the general population of women 55 and older. One modeling detail that we did not report on here is assessment of fit and the casewise diagnostics analysis. We leave this as an exercise.

In summary, propensity score methods provide an alternative to model-based adjustment for confounding of treatment in observational studies. Currently,

Table 10.5 Estimates, with 95% CI, of the Odds Ratio for BONETREAT from Six Different Fitted Logistic Regression Models to the Matched Pairs Data, $n = 218$

Method	Model	$\widehat{OR}$	95% CI	CI Width
Conditional logistic regression[a]	Simple[b]	1.300	0.726, 2.329	1.603
	Risk[c]	1.085	0.509, 2.311	1.802
GEE population average	Simple	1.306	0.723, 2.359	1.636
	Risk	1.151	0.614, 2.159	1.545
Ordinary logistic regression	Simple	1.306	0.726, 2.350	1.624
	Risk	1.158	0.628, 2.134	1.506

[a]Fit based on 46 pairs, outcome constant in 62 pairs.
[b]Simple: Contains only BONETREAT.
[c]Risk: Simple plus MOMFRAC, ARMASSIST and RATERISK.

propensity score adjustment can only be used with a dichotomous treatment covariate in most software packages. The main advantage of a propensity score approach is that it more directly balances the distributions of confounding covariates in the two treatment groups. Because the propensity score is a composite of many covariates, it is vital that the user test for balance in each covariate. To enhance the possibility of balance, analyses are typically restricted to a region of common support in the propensity score. A disadvantage is that when the propensity score has a large area under the ROC curve, that is, discriminates well, the range of common support may be quite narrow, and thus a large number of subjects could be eliminated from the analysis of treatment effect. A further point to emphasize is that the propensity score analysis is not assumption free. One must be attentive to selection of confounders and model building details at all stages of the analysis. Once one builds the propensity score model there are three different approaches to using it: (i) model-based adjustment via its inclusion as a covariate, (ii) a stratified analysis by quintiles of the score, and (iii) a 1–1, or other, matched analysis. The potential to balance the confounders increases as restriction on the analysis increases from (i) to (iii). However, one must keep in mind that the confounding controlled for is limited to the covariates in the model. Theoretical properties of a propensity score analysis usually assume that the score contains all confounders, basically an assumption one cannot test. Regardless of the approach, one should assess the fit of the final model, and use casewise diagnostics to assess adverse impact on the model of individual subjects before using the model for inferential purposes.

10.3 EXACT METHODS FOR LOGISTIC REGRESSION MODELS

The methods used for testing and inference up to this point in the text have required, in addition to mathematical assumptions, that the sample size is sufficiently large for parameter estimates to be normally distributed and for the likelihood ratio and Wald tests to follow chi-square and normal distributions, respectively. Of additional relevance is the fact that the maximum likelihood estimators can be quite biased for small samples. For a general discussion of bias in maximum likelihood see Cox and Hinkley (1974) and for specifics relative to logistic regression see McCullagh and Nelder (1989).

There may be occasions where one would like to fit a logistic regression model but the sample size is such that large sample assumptions are clearly not justified. Recent advances in computational methods now make it possible to fit models using alternative methods in such settings. We discuss two methods: an exact method and an approximate method based on a modification of the usual likelihood function. The "gold standard" is to use the exact method but, as we show, the computations required are so computer intensive that they may be impractical in some settings while those for the approximate method are of the same order as maximum likelihood.

The exact method for fitting a logistic regression model and then making inferences and tests about the parameters when the sample size is small is a complicated version of Fisher's exact test for a 2×2 contingency table. Cox and Snell (1989) note that the extension of the theory of Fisher's exact test to logistic regression models has been known since the 1970s. However, the computations required are extremely complex and were considered impractical until efficient algorithms were developed by Tritchler (1984), Hirji et al. (1987, 1988) and Hirji (1992). Mehta and Patel (1995) review the theory and provide a number of insightful examples. The exact methods have been incorporated into a number of statistical software packages, including SAS, STATA and the special purpose program LogXact 9 for Windows (2012). We used SAS and STATA to fit the models in this section.

The central idea behind the theory of exact methods for logistic regression is to construct a statistical distribution that can, with efficient algorithms, be completely enumerated. The starting point in this process is to construct a conditional likelihood similar to that used in Chapter 7 for matched studies. Assume we have n independent observations of a binary outcome and a vector of $p + 1$ covariates (i.e., $(y_i, \mathbf{x}_i)$, $i = 1, 2, \ldots, n$). We assume that the functional form of the logit is $g(\mathbf{x}, \boldsymbol{\beta}) = \sum_{j=0}^{p} x_j \beta_j$ with $x_0 = 1$. In settings where we are primarily interested in the slope coefficients we consider the intercept, β_0, as the nuisance parameter and condition on its sufficient statistic, $n_1 = \sum_{i=1}^{n} y_i$. As shown in Mehta and Patel (1995) the resulting conditional likelihood is

$$\Pr(Y_1 = y_1, Y_2 = y_2, \ldots, Y_n = y_n | n_1) = \frac{\exp\left(\sum_{i=1}^{n} y_i \times \sum_{j=1}^{p} x_{ij} \beta_j\right)}{\sum_{l \in R} \exp\left(\sum_{l=1}^{n} y_l \times \sum_{j=1}^{p} x_{lj} \beta_j\right)},$$

(10.9)

where R denotes the collection of

$$\binom{n}{n_1} = \frac{n!}{[n_1!] \times [(n - n_1)!]}$$

possible allocations of 0 and 1 to $(y_1, y_2, \ldots, y_n)$ such that $n_1 = \sum_{i=1}^{n} y_i$. The form of the likelihood in equation (10.9) suggests that the sufficient statistic for β_j is

$$t_j = \sum_{i=1}^{n} y_i x_{ij}.$$

(10.10)

Cox and Hinkley (1974) present a discussion of sufficient statistics and their role in conditional inference. Denote the vector of sufficient statistics for the slope coefficients as $\mathbf{t}' = (t_1, t_2, \ldots, t_p)$. The exact distribution of the collection of p sufficient statistics is given by the equation

$$\Pr(T_1 = t_1, T_2 = t_2, \ldots, T_p = t_p) = \frac{c(\mathbf{t}) \exp\left(\sum_{j=1}^{p} t_j \beta_j\right)}{\sum_{\mathbf{u} \in S} c(\mathbf{u}) \exp\left(\sum_{l=1}^{p} u_l \beta_l\right)}$$

(10.11)

where $c(\mathbf{t})$ denotes the number of possible allocations of 0 and 1 to $(y_1, y_2, \ldots, y_n)$ such that $t_j = \sum_{i=1}^{n} y_i x_{ij}$ and S denotes the set of allocations of 0 and 1 to

$(y_1, y_2, \ldots, y_n)$ such that $n_1 = \sum_{i=1}^{n} y_i$ and $u_j = \sum_{l=1}^{n} y_i x_{lj}$ denotes the resulting value of the jth sufficient statistic for the lth allocation. The distribution in equation (10.11) is used to obtain point and confidence interval estimates of the regression coefficients as well as tests of hypotheses that coefficients are equal to zero. The calculations required for the multivariable problem are quite complex. Thus, we present some of the details for the exact methods with a model containing a single dichotomous covariate.

As an example, suppose that we wish to model risk factors for having a low birth weight baby among women 30 years or older in the low birth weight study described in Section 1.6.2. There are 27 such women and four had a low birth weight baby. It is clear that, with only 27 observations and four LOW $= 1$ outcomes, we should not use methods requiring large sample sizes for their validity. Consider the covariate recording the number of previous pre-term deliveries dichotomized into none (0) or at least one (1) and denoted PTD. The cross-classification of LOW by PTD is shown in Table 10.6.

The results in Table 10.6 show that the observed value of the sufficient statistic for the intercept term is $t_0 = 4$ and for the coefficient for PTD it is $t_1 = 2$. The latter result follows from the fact that only two subjects had LOW $= 1$ and PTD $= 1$ (i.e., $2 = \sum_{i=1}^{27} \text{LOW}_i \times \text{PTD}_i$). It follows from equation (10.11) that the exact probability is

$$\Pr(T_1 = t_1) = \frac{c(t_1) \exp(t_1 \beta_1)}{\sum_{u \in S} c(u) \exp(u \beta_1)}. \tag{10.12}$$

The possible values of the sufficient statistic are $t_1 = 0, 1, 2, 3, 4$. Thus, the term $c(t_1)$ describes the number of possible allocations of 23 values of zero and four values of one to 27 subjects with the resulting value of $t_1 = \sum_{i=1}^{27} \text{LOW}_i \times \text{PTD}_i$. STATA has the option to save a data set with this exact distribution, which used to obtain the results in Table 10.7. We see that there are 5985 sequences of 23 zeros and four ones, where $0 = \sum_{i=1}^{27} \text{LOW}_i \times \text{PTD}_i$. The simplest exact inferential question is a test of the hypothesis that $\beta_1 = 0$. The values of equation (10.12) under the null hypothesis are given in the last column in Table 10.7.

Table 10.6 Cross-Classification of Low Birth Weight (LOW) by History of Pre-term Delivery (PTD) Among Women 30 Years of Age or Older

LOW	PTD 0	PTD 1	Total
0	19	4	23
1	2	2	4
Total	21	6	27

Table 10.7　Enumeration of the Exact Probability Distribution of the Sufficient Statistic for the Coefficient of PTD

t_1	Count: $c(t)$	Probability Under $H_0 : \beta_1 = 0$
0	5985	0.34103
1	7980	0.45469
2	3150	0.17949
3	420	0.02393
4	15	0.00086
Total	17550	1.0

These probabilities are calculated using the fact that $1 = \exp(t_1 \times 0)$ and S contains 17,550 sequences. Thus, the first probability is

$$\Pr(t_1 = 0) = \frac{5985}{17550} = 0.34103,$$

and the others are calculated in a similar manner. We calculate the two tailed p-value by summing the probabilities in Table 10.7 over values of the sufficient statistic that are as likely, or less likely, to have a smaller probability than the observed value of $t = 2$. Thus, we obtain

$$p = 0.17949 + 0.02393 + 0.00086 = 0.20428.$$

We note that the value is identical to the two-sided p-value for Fisher's exact test computed from Table 10.6. In this case we cannot conclude that having a history of pre-term delivery is a significant risk factor for having a low weight birth among women who are 30 years of age or older. STATA reports the p-value, we think incorrectly in this case, as twice this value or 0.408.

The exact conditional maximum likelihood point estimate of the coefficient is the value that maximizes the probability given in equation (10.12) which, given the counts in Table 10.7, is

$$\Pr(T_1 = 2) = \frac{c(2)\exp(2\beta_1)}{\sum_{u \in S} c(u)\exp(u\beta_1)}$$

$$= \frac{3150\exp(2\beta_1)}{5985\exp(0\beta_1) + 7980\exp(1\beta_1) + 3150\exp(2\beta_1)}{}.$$
$$+ 420\exp(3\beta_1) + 15\exp(4\beta_1)$$

Even in this rather simple example the required computations are lengthy. For comparative purposes we show the results from fitting the conditional exact maximum likelihood estimate (CMLE) as well as those from fitting the usual logistic regression model (MLE) in Table 10.8. In this example, as shown in Chapter 3,

Table 10.8 Results of Fitting the Usual Logistic Model (MLE), the Exact Conditional Model (CMLE), and the Firth Modified Likelihood to the Data in Table 10.6

	Method	Coeff.	Std.Err.	95% CI
PTD	MLE	1.558	1.1413	−0.679, 3.795
	CMLE	1.482	1.1059	−1.383, 4.370
	Firth	1.466	1.0949	−0.680, 3.612
Constant	MLE	−2.251	0.7434	−3.708, −0.794
	CMLE	[a]	[a]	[a]
	Firth	−2.054	0.6876	−3.402, −0.706

[a]Not computed using CMLE in this case.

the usual MLE is simply the log of the odds ratio computed from the frequencies in Table 10.6.

Both the point estimate of the coefficient for PTD and the estimate of the associated standard error are slightly smaller when the exact conditional model is used. The endpoints of the confidence internal for the MLE are obtained in the usual manner as $\hat{\beta}_1 \pm 1.96 \times \widehat{SE}(\hat{\beta}_1)$. The endpoints of the CMLE are obtained from the following procedure: Assume that the possible range of the sufficient statistic, given the observed value of t_0, is $t_{min} \le t_1 \le t_{max}$. In our example the range is $0 \le t_1 \le 4$. The lower endpoint of a $100(1-\alpha)\%$ confidence interval is the value of β_1 such that

$$\alpha/2 = \sum_{k=t_{1obs}}^{t_{max}} \Pr(T_1 = k) \tag{10.13}$$

where t_{1obs} denotes the observed value of t_1, 2 in our example, and $\Pr(T_1 = k)$ is given in equation (10.12). If $t_{1obs} = t_{min}$ then the lower limit is set to $-\infty$. The upper endpoint of a $100(1-\alpha)\%$ confidence interval is the value of β_1 such that

$$\alpha/2 = \sum_{k=t_{min}}^{t_{1obs}} \Pr(T_1 = k). \tag{10.14}$$

If $t_{1obs} = t_{max}$ then the upper limit is set to $+\infty$. The solutions to equations (10.13) and (10.14) for a 95% confidence interval in our example are shown in Table 10.8. We note that the CMLE interval is considerably wider than the MLE interval, reflecting the increased uncertainty in our estimate due to the small sample size.

Firth (1993) notes that there are two different approaches to correct the bias in the maximum likelihood estimators in logistic regression: (i) apply a correction to the usual maximum likelihood estimators of the coefficients or (ii) modify the likelihood function so that the resulting estimators are less biased. Schaefer (1983) provides a method for the first approach, which Firth notes is not as effective as using the second, a more direct approach to remove bias. Firth's (1993) modified likelihood function is of the form

$$l(\beta)^* = l(\beta) \times |\mathbf{I}(\beta)|^{0.5},$$

where $l(\boldsymbol{\beta})$ is the usual likelihood function in equation (1.3) and $|\mathbf{I}(\boldsymbol{\beta})|^{0.5}$ is the square root of the determinant of the information matrix with elements defined in equations (2.3) and (2.4). Heinze and Schemper (2002) show that the score equations that must be solved to obtain the Firth estimators are of the form

$$\frac{\partial L(\boldsymbol{\beta})^*}{\partial \beta_j} = \sum_{i=1}^{n}[y_i - \pi_i + h_i(0.5 - \pi_i)] \times x_{ij} = 0,$$

where $L(\boldsymbol{\beta})^*$ is the log modified likelihood function and h_i is the value of the leverage defined in equation (5.22). Furthermore they show that these score equations may be obtained from the usual log-likelihood function obtained when each observation is replaced by two observations: y_i with weight $1 + h_i/2$ and $(1 - y_i)$ with weight $h_i/2$. The attractive feature of this is that computations are no more complex than those described in Chapters 1 and 2. The Firth estimators are available in both SAS and STATA. Each package produces the same value for the estimator but there are slight differences in the estimators of the standard errors of the estimated coefficients. Results presented in this section are from SAS. The Firth estimate of the coefficient for PTD in Table 10.8 is slightly closer to the exact value than the MLE. The confidence interval for the Firth estimate is much narrower than that for the exact estimate. Bull et al. (2007) show that a profile confidence interval estimator of the type illustrated in Figure 1.3 has better coverage properties than the symmetric Wald-based confidence interval in Table 10.8. However, this confidence interval estimator is not currently available in software packages.

As a second example consider the cross classification of smoking status during pregnancy versus low birth weight among women 30 years of age or older shown in Table 10.9. We note that the table contains a cell with zero frequency. As shown in Chapter 4, Section 4 conventional logistic regression software cannot be used in this case. However, we are able to obtain a two-tailed p-value, point and confidence interval estimate using exact methods.

The exact probability distribution under the hypothesis of no effect due to smoking during pregnancy $\beta_1 = 0$, is shown in Table 10.10. The p-value in this case is 0.01197 since no other value had as small or smaller probability than the observed value of 4. Since the observed value of the sufficient statistic is $4 = t_{max}$ the upper limit of the 95% confidence interval is $+\infty$ and the solution to equation (10.13) is 0.308. In settings where $t_{1obs} = t_{min}$ or $t_{1obs} = t_{max}$ the CMLE does not have a

Table 10.9   Cross-Classification of Low Birth Weight (LOW) by Smoking Status of the Mother During Pregnancy (SMOKE) Among Women 30 Years of Age or Older

LOW	SMOKE 0	SMOKE 1	Total
0	17	6	23
1	0	4	4
Total	21	6	27

Table 10.10   Enumeration of the Exact Probability Distribution of the Sufficient Statistic for the Coefficient of SMOKE

t_1	Count: $c(t)$	Probability Under $H_o : \beta_1 = 0$
0	2380	0.13561
1	6800	0.38746
2	6120	0.34872
3	2040	0.11624
4	210	0.01197
Total	17550	1.0

finite solution and Hirji et al. (1989) suggest using the median unbiased estimator (MUE). This estimator is defined as the average of the endpoints of a 50% confidence interval estimator. In settings where $t_{1obs} = t_{\min}$ and the lower limit is $-\infty$ the MUE is set equal to the upper limit of the 50% interval. In settings where $t_{1obs} = t_{\max}$ and the upper limit is $+\infty$ the MUE is set equal to the lower limit of the 50% interval. In our example we have $t_{1obs} = t_{\max}$ and the lower limit of the 50% interval is $\hat{\beta}_{1MUE} = 2.510$. That is, the solution to equation (10.13) using $\alpha = 0.5$ is 2.510. Thus use of exact methods yields point and interval estimates as well as a test of significance when none are computable using the usual MLE. The Firth estimator of the coefficient for SMOKE is $\hat{\beta}_{Firth} = 3.1889$, which is 27% larger than the exact estimate. The 95% Firth confidence interval is (0.130, 6.245), which conveys considerably more precision than the exact method confidence interval.

We obtain point and interval estimators of odds ratios in the usual manner by exponentiating the respective estimators for the coefficient. The odds ratio for smoking during pregnancy obtained from the MUE is $\widehat{OR} = 12.3$ and the endpoints of the 95% confidence interval are $(1.36, +\infty)$. The interpretation is that the odds of a low birth weight baby among women 30 years or older who smoke during pregnancy is 12.3 times higher than the odds among women 30 years or older who do not smoke during pregnancy and it could be as little as 1.36 times with 95% confidence interval. Results based on the Firth estimate are obtained in the usual manner.

One can use exact methods as well as Firth's method to fit multivariable logistic regression models and perform tests of subsets of parameters. Thus, it is theoretically possible to use both methods with the modeling paradigm described in detail in Chapter 4. However, the required computations are extensive for the exact method and can be quite time consuming, even on a fast computer. Thus, we recommend that the use of exact analyses be restricted to those settings where the sample sizes are small enough to question the use of the large sample assumption. The exception to this recommendation might be a setting where one has a zero frequency cell in a clinically important dichotomous covariate or a polychotomous covariate, whose categories should not be combined to eliminate the zero frequency. As noted, Firth's method does not have these computational issues. The Firth estimates are closer to the exact than the MLE's and, in most settings, can provide a useful estimator, especially when the computations required for the exact method are too complex for the computer being used.

The exact methods as described in this section focus on exact CMLE of the slope coefficients. It is possible to extend the approach to estimation of the intercept, but in most settings the computations are much more time consuming than those required to just estimate the slope coefficients.

The basic idea is the same but one estimates each parameter conditioning on the sufficient statistic for all other parameters. The result is a fitted model similar to ones discussed in detail in Chapter 4. As an example we present, in Table 10.11, the results of fitting both the usual and exact logistic models using women 25 years or older in the low birth weight study. The covariates in the model are weight at the time of the last menstrual period (LWT), smoking status during pregnancy (SMOKE) and history of prior pre-term delivery (PTD). There are 69 women in this subgroup and 19 low birth weight babies.

The estimates of the slope coefficients from all three methods in Table 10.11 are similar and would result in effectively equivalent estimates of their respective odds ratios. However, the exact confidence intervals are the widest, reflecting the increased variability due to the small sample size. This variability is not accounted for in the Firth or MLE Wald confidence interval.

In addition to fitting all parameters, evaluating fit and computing diagnostic statistics is possible as described in Chapters 5 and 7. However, we do not recommend using the p-value for the Hosmer-Lemeshow test based on g groups using the chi-square distribution with $g - 2$ degrees of freedom, as it is based on the large sample assumption that one is trying to avoid by using exact methods. How many groups, g, one chooses should depend on the sample size and the distribution of the outcome. It is highly likely that 10 groups would be too many, yielding a table with many small frequency cells. For example, the model fit in Table 10.11 has $n = 69$ and $n_1 = 19$. We would likely use six groups. Regardless of the number of groups, we suggest that one should visually check the agreement between the observed

Table 10.11 Results of Fitting the Usual Logistic Model (MLE), the Exact Conditional Model (CMLE), and the Firth Modified Likelihood in the Low Birth Weight Study to Women 25 Years or Older

	Method	Coeff.	Std.Err.	95% CI	
LWT	MLE	−0.019	0.0117	−0.042,	0.004
	CMLE	−0.018	0.0113	−0.043,	0.002
	Firth	−0.017	0.0109	−0.038,	0.004
SMOKE	MLE	0.249	0.6087	−0.944,	1.442
	CMLE	0.256	0.5933	−1.111,	1.567
	Firth	0.273	0.5953	−0.893,	1.439
PTD	MLE	1.393	0.6687	0.082,	2.703
	CMLE	1.310	0.6440	−0.137,	2.798
	Firth	1.302	0.6616	0.005,	2.598
Constant	MLE	1.097	1.5599	−1.961,	4.154
	CMLE	*	*	*	
	Firth	0.808	1.4820	−2.096,	3.712

and expected frequencies in the $2 \times g$ table. One should examine the diagnostic statistics using the plots discussed in Chapter 5. Models can then be refit, deleting suspect cases. We leave assessing the adequacy of the model in Table 10.11 as an exercise.

In summary we feel that exact methods for logistic regression should be considered when one is fitting a model with a small sample size or unbalanced data that result in zero frequency cells. In settings where computations are an issue we recommend using the Firth modified likelihood approach.

10.4 MISSING DATA

We have used data sets in all our examples with no missing observations. In practice, missing data is likely and can impact the analysis. In this section, we aim to provide a brief introduction to methods of handling missing data that are readily available in standard software packages, such as SAS and STATA. We focus on missing values in covariates rather than the outcome or response variable. Missing data in the response is most prevalent in longitudinal studies, and references dealing with longitudinal data analysis [e.g., Molenberghs and Verbeke (2005)] discuss how to handle this problem. Here we illustrate the basic issues and assumptions using the methods available in SAS and STATA using a modified version of the GLOW data set described in Section 1.6.3. Specialized software packages are also available [e.g., see Horton and Lipsitz (2001)].

A great deal of work involving missing data, and in particular the method known as multiple imputation, has been done, for example, in Rubin (1976, 1987), Little and Rubin (2002), and Schafer (1997). Introductory presentations are available in Allison (2001), Schafer (1999), and Schafer and Graham (2002). References on the topic and an overview of methods found in software packages are available in Harle and Zhou (2007). The method of multiple imputation that we describe, as implemented in STATA, is discussed in more detail in Raghunathan et al. (2001) and Royston (2004, 2005a, 2005b, 2009). White et al. (2011) provide practical advice for using the method and may be a good place to start for those interested in learning more.

The framework for missing data established by Rubin (1976) is commonly used to describe methods for handling missing data and required assumptions. The strongest assumption about the missing data within this framework is that it is *Missing Completely at Random* (MCAR). Under the MCAR assumption, the probability of a missing value does not depend on the response or on any of the other observed data. Thus, the estimator for the probability that the value is missing is

$$\Pr(M = 1) = \frac{n_{\text{mis}}}{n},$$

where M is the variable denoting whether the observation is missing and is zero if the observation is not missing and one if it is missing and n_{mis} is the number of missing values out of the n possible values of the covariate.

MCAR is not a realistic assumption in most instances. A less stringent assumption is that the probability of a missing value depends on the observed values of the response and covariates. Data that satisfies this assumption is known as *Missing at Random* (MAR) and the probability of a missing value is determined through a model for

$$\Pr(M = 1|\mathbf{X}_{obs}, \mathbf{Y}_{obs}, \boldsymbol{\theta}),$$

where $\mathbf{X}_{obs}$ and $\mathbf{Y}_{obs}$ are the observed values of covariate and response respectively and $\boldsymbol{\theta}$ is a vector of parameters for the missing data model. Missing data is known as *ignorable* if it is MAR and the parameters for the missing data model and the model for the response are independent.

The method of multiple imputation described in this section assumes the data is MAR and treats the models for the missing data and response as ignorable. The MAR assumption is that missing values do not depend on unobserved values of the covariates. If this assumption does not hold the data is *Not Missing at Random* (NMAR). Thus, the model for the missing data is based upon both observed and unobserved missing values or

$$\Pr(M = 1|\mathbf{X}_{mis}, \mathbf{Y}_{mis}, \mathbf{X}_{obs}, \mathbf{Y}_{obs}, \boldsymbol{\theta}).$$

Under NMAR more information about the distribution of the missing values is required in order to use multiple imputation.

Multiple imputation involves three steps: (i) the imputation step, (ii) the analysis of the completed data sets, and (iii) pooling the results from the analysis of the multiple data sets. The imputation step requires specifying a model to predict values for the missing data (assuming MAR) to obtain a "complete" data set. The process is repeated m times. Each of the m complete data sets is analyzed using the data model, in our case a logistic regression model. Finally, the results of the m analyses are combined to produce summary estimates of model parameters and standard errors for inference. The strength of multiple imputation is that it improves efficiency in inference over using only complete cases while accounting for the uncertainty due to the imputed data.

If data are missing from just one covariate, both SAS and STATA support models for the missing data that depend on the scale of the covariate. For example, if the missing data are from a dichotomous covariate the model is a logistic regression model, while for continuous covariates the model is a linear regression. SAS and STATA perform the imputations in a slightly different way when data are missing from more than one covariate. In SAS, unless the missing data are monotone, which we discuss in the example, the only option is to assume a multivariate normal (MVN) distribution for the missing data [Schafer (1997)]. As a result, all covariates are treated as continuous. The MVN distribution is usually difficult to specify so the actual imputed values are the result of using a *Markov Chain Monte Carlo* (MCMC) simulation to sample from the MVN distribution under the MAR model. We discuss MCMC in more detail in Section 10.6 within the context of Bayesian logistic regression. The issues discussed in that section about burn-in, convergence, and length of the simulation hold in this setting and both SAS and

STATA include options to check and adjust the MCMC that correspond to those outlined in Section 10.6. Multiple imputation can be approached from the Bayesian perspective with the missing data modeled using the "posterior" distribution given the observed values, see Gelman et al. (2004) for details.

In STATA, multivariate missing data are handled using Imputation Chain equations (ICE) or imputation using fully conditional specifications (FCS) [see van Buuren et al. (2006)]. This is also referred to as sequential regression multivariate imputation (SRMI) [see Raghunathan et al. (2001)]. The idea of ICE is to iteratively produce the imputed values in a univariable model for each covariate, conditional on the others. The advantage of the approach is that each univariable model can then be of a form appropriate to the type of data for that covariate. This iterative algorithm compares to the Gibbs sampler discussed in Section 10.6. Unlike the Gibbs sampler, however, the univariable conditional distributions are not formed from a fully specified joint distribution. This is the disadvantage of ICE in that the selected conditional distributions may not be compatible with the joint distribution [see Arnold et al. (2001)]. Lee and Carlin (2010) compare the ICE method to using the MVN distribution.

Once the m complete data sets are created, each is analyzed using the logistic regression model and the final step is to then combine the results of the m fitted models. The rules proposed by Rubin (1987) are used by SAS and STATA to combine the results. If we denote the estimator for a particular logistic regression coefficient from the fit to the m data sets as $\hat{\beta}^i$, $i = 1, 2, \ldots, m$ and the estimator of its variance as $\hat{V}^i$, $i = 1, 2, \ldots, m$, then the combined multiple imputation estimate of the coefficient is

$$\overline{\beta} = \frac{1}{m}\sum_{i=1}^{m}\hat{\beta}^i \tag{10.15}$$

and the estimate of the variance of $\overline{\beta}$ is

$$\overline{T} = \overline{V} + \left(1 + \frac{1}{m}\right)B, \tag{10.16}$$

where

$$\overline{V} = \frac{1}{m}\sum_{i=1}^{m}\hat{V}^i$$

and

$$B = \frac{1}{m-1}\sum_{i=1}^{m}(\hat{\beta}^i - \overline{\beta})^2.$$

Inferences are based on a t distribution with degrees of freedom

$$\nu = (m-1) \times \left[1 + \frac{\overline{V}}{\left(1 + \frac{1}{m}\right)B}\right]^2.$$

Both SAS and STATA perform the calculations in equations (10.15) and (10.16) and display the results in the familiar tabular form used for logistic regression.

To illustrate multiple imputation we modified the GLOW500 data by randomly deleting 20% of the values for age, weight, height, mother had a hip fracture (MOMFRAC), self-reported risk of fracture (RATERISK), and history of prior fracture (PRIORFRAC). The replacement of observed with missing values was done separately for each covariate leading to a data set with only 128 complete cases designated as GLOW500_MISSING. We then performed five imputations of the missing data using the chained regression equation approach of STATA and MCMC in SAS. We discuss the choice of five imputations at the end of the section. The assumptions made in the multiple imputation process are more likely valid when as many covariates as possible are included in the missing data model (i.e., covariates with and without missing values as well as the response) so we used all available covariates as well as the response variable in the model producing the imputed values. We list the hypothetical newly observed missing data for three subjects in Table 10.12. The missing data are denoted by "•". The imputed values are shown from both software packages. We note that the imputed values for the continuous covariates age, weight and height differ between the two packages. Note that the goal of multiple imputation is not to best predict the true missing values but rather to produce values from their distribution to improve efficiency in performing inference when analyzing the data. Since the procedure in SAS assumes covariates are continuous, imputed values for the dichotomous variables MOMFRAC and PRIORFRAC lie between user specified values of a and b, usually set to $a = 0$ and $b = 1$ as in this example, while the values in STATA are exactly 0 or 1. Similarly, the categorical covariate RATERISK results in continuous values rather than ordinal. SAS does have the ability to fit binary and categorical data in multivariate data sets but only if the pattern of missing values is monotone. A missing data pattern in Table 10.12 would be monotone if a missing value of age implies weight is missing, and if weight is missing then height is as well, and if height is missing then mother fracture is missing, and when mother fracture is missing the rate risk is as well and finally, a missing rate risk means missing prior fracture. Since such a pattern does not exist in the example data regardless of the order the covariates are listed we do not have monotone missing data.

We next fit a logistic regression model to the imputed data sets produced by SAS and STATA with results shown in the bottom two panels of Table 10.13. The results from fitting a model to the original data set, $n = 500$, are shown in the top panel and from fitting the model to the complete cases, $n = 128$, in the second panel. In order to produce comparable models, in SAS we imputed a single continuous value of self-reported risk and then rounded the nearest possible category, for example, 1.32 rounds to 1 and 1.67 to 2. The rounded values were then used to create the two design variables. An alternative approach would be to create the design variables first and impute the missing values for each of them. The imputed values that are originally continuous are rounded to form dichotomous variables. In this case care should be taken to ensure both design variables are not set to one. Rounding of binary or categorical covariates in multiple imputation is

Table 10.12 Three Subjects with Missing Data (Obs) and the Five Imputations from SAS and STATA

Package		ID	Age	Weight	Height	Mother fracture	Rate risk	Prior fracture
	Obs	51	•	65.8	157	0	•	0
	1	51	63.04	65.8	157	0	2	0
	2	51	61.73	65.8	157	0	1	0
STATA	3	51	75.88	65.8	157	0	3	0
	4	51	69.68	65.8	157	0	2	0
	5	51	55.57	65.8	157	0	2	0
	1	51	56.51	65.8	157	0	1.95	0
	2	51	47.25	65.8	157	0	1.55	0
SAS	3	51	56.71	65.8	157	0	2.99	0
	4	51	59.04	65.8	157	0	1.65	0
	5	51	56.84	65.8	157	0	1.90	0
	Obs	109	70	110.7	168	•	•	•
	1	109	70	110.7	168	0	1	0
	2	109	70	110.7	168	0	1	0
STATA	3	109	70	110.7	168	0	3	1
	4	109	70	110.7	168	0	1	0
	5	109	70	110.7	168	0	2	1
	1	109	70	110.7	168	0.45	2.45	0.30
	2	109	70	110.7	168	0.06	2.42	0.62
SAS	3	109	70	110.7	168	0.32	1.61	0.60
	4	109	70	110.7	168	0.25	1.41	0.69
	5	109	70	110.7	168	0.17	2.31	0.74
	Obs	262	•	•	160	•	2	1
	1	262	72.40	70.10	160	0	2	1
	2	262	72.56	77.12	160	0	2	1
STATA	3	262	69.20	85.14	160	0	2	1
	4	262	89.52	25.26	160	1	2	1
	5	262	73.83	52.98	160	0	2	1
	1	262	70.08	69.31	160	0.23	2	1
	2	262	64.48	57.07	160	0.20	2	1
SAS	3	262	60.55	55.79	160	0.003	2	1
	4	262	81.18	79.98	160	0.40	2	1
	5	262	71.87	63.19	160	0.27	2	1

suggested by Schafer (1997) and Ake (2005). This presents no problem when the covariate is dichotomous but is so when the covariate has more than two levels and design variables are required. Horton et al. (2003) and Allison (2005) suggest that this could lead to biased results in some settings and recommend treating such covariates as continuous in analyzing the SAS imputed data.

The result of the model fit to the complete cases illustrates the loss of efficiency as indicated by its larger standard errors compared to the analysis of the imputed data sets. The statistical significance is less for all covariates and none are significant in the complete case analysis. The models fit to the imputed data sets from SAS and STATA produce similar results. However, the standard errors are reduced and age, history of prior fracture and self-reported risk are correctly determined to be statistically significant.

As the results of multiple imputations analysis may depend on the number of imputations we repeated the analysis in Table 10.13 using 10, 20, and 50 imputations. The results were similar to those reported for five imputations. Rubin (1987) reported that little additional efficiency is gained beyond five or ten imputations

Table 10.13 Results of Fitting the Logistic Regression Model to the Complete Data ($n = 500$), the Complete Cases in the Modified Data ($n = 128$), and the Imputed Data from SAS and STATA

		Coeff.	Std. Err.	z/t	p	95% CI	
COMPLETE	AGE	0.046	0.013	3.45	0.001	0.020,	0.072
DATA,	WEIGHT	0.011	0.007	1.51	0.131	−0.003,	0.026
$n = 500$	HEIGHT	−0.048	0.019	−2.50	0.012	−0.085,	−0.010
	MOMFRAC	0.639	0.307	2.08	0.038	0.036,	1.241
	PRIORFRAC	0.660	0.245	2.69	0.007	0.179,	1.140
	RATERISK = 2	0.454	0.278	1.63	0.103	−0.092,	0.999
	RATERISK = 3	0.832	0.292	2.84	0.004	0.258,	1.405
COMPLETE	AGE	0.045	0.028	1.63	0.104	−0.009,	0.100
CASE,	WEIGHT	0.020	0.014	1.38	0.168	−0.008,	0.048
$n = 128$	HEIGHT	−0.073	0.047	−1.55	0.120	−0.164,	0.019
	MOMFRAC	0.465	0.603	0.77	0.441	−0.716,	1.646
	PRIORFRAC	0.229	0.501	0.46	0.648	−0.753,	1.211
	RATERISK = 2	0.526	0.562	0.94	0.349	−0.575,	1.627
	RATERISK = 3	0.499	0.610	0.82	0.413	−0.696,	1.694
STATA MI	AGE	0.041	0.015	2.68	0.009	0.010,	0.072
DATA,	WEIGHT	0.010	0.008	1.25	0.214	−0.006,	0.026
$n = 500$	HEIGHT	−0.036	0.023	−1.52	0.138	−0.083,	0.012
	MOMFRAC	0.617	0.391	1.58	0.125	−0.183,	1.418
	PRIORFRAC	0.740	0.258	2.86	0.004	0.232,	1.248
	RATERISK = 2	0.458	0.308	1.49	0.139	−0.151,	1.068
	RATERISK = 3	0.668	0.307	2.18	0.030	0.065,	1.271
SAS MI DATA,	AGE	0.041	0.017	2.43	0.022	0.007,	0.076
$n = 500$	WEIGHT	0.012	0.008	1.50	0.135	−0.004,	0.027
	HEIGHT	−0.046	0.024	−1.94	0.061	−0.094,	0.002
	MOMFRAC	0.711	0.360	1.97	0.051	−0.002,	1.423
	PRIORFRAC	0.809	0.276	2.93	0.004	0.267,	1.351
	RATERISK = 2	0.407	0.289	1.40	0.160	−0.161,	0.974
	RATERISK = 3	0.768	0.329	2.33	0.022	0.115,	1.421

even in data with up to 50% missing cases. In our example, we had a much higher rate, 74.4%, of cases with missing data and still achieved reasonable results with only five imputations. However, Royston (2004) suggests an upper bound of 50% on the amount of missing data when using multiple imputation.

Aspects of model building also become more complex when using multiple imputation. Features of the model used to analyze the data, such as covariates and their interactions or transformations, should be included in the model used to create the imputed data sets or bias in estimates is possible. Unfortunately, some of these features, such as interactions and transformations, only become apparent during the model building process after including the imputed values. Imputing values after the model building process could lead to bias as well, as the modeling would then include only complete cases. Wood et al. (2008) discuss model building and offer practical suggestions. One possibility they describe is to perform variable selection using a data set combining all m imputed data sets and weighting observations based on the number of missing values for that covariate.

Other aspects of analysis discussed in earlier chapters are also applicable to the multiple imputation data, although sometimes there are additional considerations. Predictions, for example, are possible by averaging over the imputed data sets. One method of producing these predicted values would be to first obtain $\hat{\pi}_{ij}$ for observation i in imputed data set j and then average these values over the m imputed data sets. Alternatively, White et al. (2011) recommend producing an estimate of the linear predictor for each observation in the imputed data sets and averaging these values before applying the inverse logit to produce an estimated probability. Model checking is still important and the approaches described in Chapter 5 are applicable. White et al. (2011) recommend performing the assessment of fit on each of the m imputed data sets individually. Issues noted only in a few of the imputed data sets may indicate issues with the imputation model, while those observed across most of the m data sets suggest problems in the model selected to analyze the data. There are other options to assess fit, such as using the averaged values, making this an area requiring further research.

In conclusion, we have illustrated that application of methods for multiple imputation of missing data in covariates can produce more efficient estimates of model parameters. We recommend using multiple imputation when a moderate amount of data are missing and assumptions about the randomness of the missing values are met. As always, one should pay close attention to issues in model building and, in the imputation setting, those corresponding to the combination of imputation and model building.

10.5 SAMPLE SIZE ISSUES WHEN FITTING LOGISTIC REGRESSION MODELS

In our experience there are two sample size questions, prospective and retrospective. The prospective question is: How many subjects do I need to observe to have specified power to detect that the new treatment is significantly better than the old or a placebo treatment? The retrospective question is: Do I have enough data to fit this model? There has been surprisingly little work on sample size for logistic regression. The available methods to address sample size selection have been implemented in just a few specialty software packages. The key element in determining whether one has adequate data to fit a particular model involves the number of events per covariate. Research by Peduzzi et al. (1996) and Vittinghof and McCulloch (2006) provides some guidance. In this section we consider methods for choosing a sample size first and then discuss the issue of events per covariate.

The basic sample size question is as follows: What sample size does one need to test the null hypothesis that a particular slope coefficient is equal to zero (without loss of generality we assume it is the first of p covariates in the model) versus the alternative that it is equal to some specified value, that is, $H_o : \beta_1 = 0$ versus $H_a : \beta_1 = \beta_1^*$. If the logistic regression model is to contain only this single dichotomous covariate, then one may use conventional sample size methods to test for the equality of two proportions [see Agresti (2002) or Fleiss et al. (2003)]. Alternatively one may use results in Whitemore (1981) and refinements in Hsieh (1989), Hsieh et al. (1998), Sheih (2001), and Demidenko (2007) for a logistic regression model containing a single dichotomous covariate. The difference in the two approaches is that the former is based on the sampling distribution of the difference in two proportions and the latter on the sampling distribution of the log of the odds ratio.

We illustrate the two approaches using the data from the GLOW study described in Section 1.6.3. Suppose that we consider these data as being either pilot data or data from an earlier study to help determine what sample size would be needed in a new study to test for a 50% increase in the odds of fracture among women whose mothers have had a fracture. In terms of the logistic regression model the null and alternative hypotheses are $H_o : \beta_1 = \ln(1) = 0$ versus $H_a : \beta_1 = \ln(1.5)$. To determine the sample size with either approach we need an estimate of the probability of fracture among women with no family history, $P_0 = \Pr(Y = 1 \mid x = 0)$. Cross-classifying the outcome variable (FRACTURE) by mother's history of fracture (MOMFRAC) shows that 23.2% of women whose mother did not have fracture had one during follow up. We round this to 20% for ease of calculation and use this as our response probability. The fracture probability yielding an odds ratio of 1.5 is

$$P_1 = \Pr(Y = 1 \mid x = 1) = \frac{1.5 \times 0.20}{(1 - 0.20) + 1.5 \times 0.20} = 0.2727.$$

Thus, stated in terms of proportions, the null and alternative hypotheses are $H_o : P_0 = P_1 = 0.20$ and $H_a : P_0 = 0.2, \; P_1 = 0.2727$.

Suppose that we plan to use an equal number of women in the two MOMFRAC groups. The sample size needed in each group for a one-sided test at the α level of significance of $H_o : P_0 = P_1$ and power $1 - \theta$ for the alternative $H_a : P_0 < P_1$ is given by the equation

$$n = \frac{\left(z_{1-\alpha}\sqrt{2\overline{P}\left(1 - \overline{P}\right)} + z_{1-\theta}\sqrt{P_0(1 - P_0) + P_1(1 - P_1)} \right)^2}{(P_1 - P_0)^2}, \tag{10.17}$$

where $\overline{P} = (P_0 + P_1)/2$ and $z_{1-\alpha}$ and $z_{1-\theta}$ denote the upper α and $\theta\%$ points respectively of the standard normal distribution. We use a one-sided test here for better comparability with the results in Whitemore (1981). For a two-sided test one would replace $z_{1-\alpha}$ with $z_{1-\alpha/2}$ in equation (10.17).

Thus, the number we would need in our two treatment groups for a 5% level test to have power 80% is

$$n = \frac{\left(1.645\sqrt{2 \times 0.2364 \times 0.7636} + 0.842\sqrt{0.20 \times 0.80 + 0.2728 \times 0.7272}\right)^2}{(0.2728 - 0.20)^2}$$

$$= 420.3,$$

or 421 women in each group for a total sample size of approximately 842 women.

Whitemore (1981) approaches the sample size problem via the sampling distribution of the Wald statistic for the estimate of the logistic regression coefficient. For a univariable logistic regression model containing a single dichotomous covariate, x, coded 0 or 1 the total sample size needed to test $H_o : \beta_1 = 0$ versus $H_a : \beta_1 = \beta_1^*$ is

$$n = (1 + 2P_0) \times \frac{\left(z_{1-\alpha}\sqrt{\dfrac{1}{1-\pi} + \dfrac{1}{\pi}} + z_{1-\theta}\sqrt{\dfrac{1}{1-\pi} + \dfrac{1}{\pi e^{\beta_1^*}}}\right)^2}{P_0\beta_1^{*2}}, \qquad (10.18)$$

where $\pi = P(X = 0)$ denotes the fraction of subjects in the study expected to have $x = 0$. In our example we want the sample size for an odds ratio of 1.5 or $\beta_1^* = \ln(1.5)$ and we plan to use equal numbers of women in the two groups. Thus, the value of equation (10.18) with $\pi = 0.5$ is

$$n = (1 + 2 \times 0.20) \times \frac{\left(1.645\sqrt{\dfrac{1}{0.5} + \dfrac{1}{0.5}} + 0.842\sqrt{\dfrac{1}{0.5} + \dfrac{1}{0.5e^{[\ln(1.5)]}}}\right)^2}{0.20 \times [\ln(1.5)]^2}$$

$$= 1.4 \times \frac{(1.645 \times 2 + 0.842\sqrt{2 + 2 \times 0.6667})^2}{0.20 \times 0.1644}$$

$$= 992.2.$$

This suggests that, rounding up to be divisible by 2, we would need approximately 994 subjects or 497 in each group, which is 76 more subjects per group than the sample size given by equation (10.17). The difference in the two sample sizes stems from a number of assumptions made by Whitemore to obtain equation (10.18). This equation is derived under the assumption that the logistic probabilities are small. The lead term in equation (10.18) is proposed as a way to adjust the sample size when this is not the case. To our knowledge no research has been published that compares the results from equations (10.17) and (10.18) in a systematic manner. Our recommendation for univariable models is that one should use equation (10.17) as it relies on fewer assumptions than equation (10.18).

Suppose that instead of an equal number of women in the two mothers' history groups we decided to use numbers that better reflect the proportions observed in the pilot study of 13% with mothers who had a fracture and 87% who did not. Suppose that we round to 15% and 85%, respectively. The ratio of the two sample sizes would be $r = (0.85/0.15) = 5.667$. Fleiss et al. (2003) show that the number in the exposed or women whose mothers did have a fracture is

$$n_1 = \frac{\left(z_{1-\alpha}\sqrt{(r+1)\,\overline{P}(1-\overline{P})} + z_{1-\theta}\sqrt{r \times P_0(1-P_0) + P_1(1-P_1)}\right)^2}{r \times (P_1 - P_0)^2} \qquad (10.19)$$

and the number in the unexposed group (or women whose mothers did not have a fracture) is $n_0 = r \times n_1$. Under the same null and alternative hypotheses we find, using equation (10.19), that $n_1 = 241$ and $n_0 = 1365$ for a total sample size of 1606. This is almost twice the sample size needed for equal numbers in the two groups. One reason to choose the latter allocation is a setting where the investigators know that they are not going to be able to obtain the additional 180 exposed women needed for an equal allocation. Hsieh et al. (1998) show, in their Appendix I, a modification of equation (10.18) that handles an unequal allocation of subjects to two groups.

If the single covariate we plan to include in the model is continuous and modeled as linear in the logit, then we use results for this setting derived by Whitemore (1981) and refined by Hsieh (1989) and Hsieh et al. (1998). These results are based on the assumption that the covariate is standardized to have mean 0 and standard deviation 1.0. Thus, the logistic regression coefficient is the change in the log-odds of a one standard deviation increment in the unstandardized covariate. The sample size needed for a one-sided test, at the α level of significance and power $1 - \theta$, of $H_o : \beta_1 = 0$ versus $H_a : \beta_1 = \beta_1^*$ is given by the equation

$$n = (1 + 2P_0\delta) \times \frac{(z_{1-\alpha} + z_{1-\theta}e^{-0.25\beta_1^{*2}})^2}{P_0\beta_1^{*2}}, \qquad (10.20)$$

where

$$\delta = \frac{1 + (1 + \beta_1^{*2})e^{1.25\beta_1^{*2}}}{1 + e^{-0.25\beta_1^{*2}}} \qquad (10.21)$$

and P_0 is the value of the logistic probability evaluated at the mean of the standardized covariates, that is,

$$P_0 = \frac{e^{\beta_0}}{1 + e^{\beta_0}}. \qquad (10.22)$$

Again, one replaces $z_{1-\alpha}$ with $z_{1-\alpha/2}$ in equation (10.20) if one is going to use a two-sided test.

As an example, suppose that we consider the covariate age in the GLOW study and ignore all of the other covariates. In these data the mean age of the subjects is approximately 68.5 years with a standard deviation of 9 years. We would like to determine the sample size we would need in order to be able to detect that the effect of a one standard deviation increase in age is a 50% increase in the odds of fracture (i.e., $\beta_1^* = \ln(1.5)$). To obtain an estimate of P_0 in equation (10.22) we fit a univariable logistic regression model containing the standardized covariate $AGES = (AGE - 68.5)/9$. The estimate of the intercept term is $\hat{\beta}_0 = -1.1561$ (results not shown) and equation (10.22) becomes

$$P_0 = \frac{e^{-1.1561}}{1 + e^{-1.1561}} = 0.239,$$

which, for ease of calculations, we round to 0.24.

The value of equation (10.21) in this example is

$$\delta = \frac{1 + (1 + [\ln(1.5)]^2)e^{1.25[\ln(1.5)]^2}}{1 + e^{-0.25[\ln(1.5)]^2}} = 1.24$$

and the sample size from equation (10.20)

$$n = (1 + 2 \times 0.24 \times 1.24) \times \frac{(1.645 + 0.842e^{-0.25[\ln(1.5)]^2})^2}{0.24[\ln(1.5)]^2}$$

$$= 243.3.$$

This result suggests that, if the true effect of age is to increase the odds of fracture for every nine year increase in age by 50%, then we need a total 244 subjects in our study. This same result may also be obtained from Table II in Hsieh (1989) or from the PASS 11.0 (2012) software package.

However, it is rare in practice to have final inferences based on a univariable logistic regression model. Hsieh (1989) and Hsieh et al. (1998) show that a simple and useful multivariable model adaptation of equation (10.20) simply inflates the univariable sample size by the inverse of the squared multiple correlation, ρ^2, of the covariate of interest, x_1, with the remaining $p - 1$ covariates in the model, yielding

$$n = \frac{(1 + 2P_0\delta)}{(1 - \rho^2)} \times \frac{(z_{1-\alpha} + z_{1-\theta}e^{-0.25\beta_1^{*2}})^2}{P_0\beta_1^{*2}}. \quad (10.23)$$

This is the equation used by the PASS 11.0 package.

As a first multivariable example we consider the sample size needed to test for an age effect of $\ln(1.5)$ per 9-year increase in age, where we include the other covariates in the fitted model shown in Table 4.9: HEIGHT, PRIORFRAC, MOMFRAC, ARMASSIST, and RATERISK3. In this example we consider treatment to be just another potential confounder of the age effect. The results of fitting a logistic regression model to the GLOW data with age standardized as, $AGES = (AGE - 68.5)/9$ and height standardized as $HEIGHTS = (HEIGHT - 161.4)/6.36$ are shown in Table 10.14.

Based on the results in Table 10.14 the estimated probability of fracture with all covariates equal to zero is

$$P_0 = \frac{e^{-1.795}}{1 + e^{-1.795}} = 0.1425.$$

Table 10.14   Results of Fitting a Logistic Regression Model to the GLOW Data

Variable	Coeff.	Std. Err.	z	p
AGES	0.299	0.1165	2.56	0.010
HEIGHTS	−0.295	0.1153	−2.55	0.011
PRIORFRAC	0.664	0.2452	2.71	0.007
MOMFRAC	0.664	0.3056	2.17	0.030
ARMASSIST	0.473	0.2313	2.04	0.041
RATERISK3	0.458	0.2381	1.92	0.054
Constant	−1.795	0.1800	−9.98	0.000

In this case, a woman with all covariates equal to zero corresponds to one who is 68.5 years old, is 161.4 cm tall, has not had a prior fracture, has a mother who did not have a fracture, does not need arm assistance when rising from a chair, and does not consider herself to be of much greater risk of fracture than other women of her age.

Suppose that we perform our test at the $\alpha = 0.05$ level and would like power $1 - \theta = 0.8$. Using a multiple linear regression package with AGES as the dependent variable and the remaining variables as covariates yields $R^2 = 0.1664$. The value of equation (10.21) is the same as that determined for the univariable model, $\delta = 1.24$, and the sample size from equation (10.23) is

$$n = \frac{(1 + 2 \times 0.1425 \times 1.24)}{(1 - 0.1664)} \times \frac{(1.645 + 0.842 \times e^{-0.25[\ln(1.5)]^2})^2}{0.1425 \times [\ln(1.5)]^2} = 417.04.$$

Thus, the application of the modification of the Whitemore formula suggests that only about 418 subjects are needed to have 80% power to test for the stated effect of age. We note that if the average fitted logistic probability is approximately equal to $P_0 = 0.1425$ then we would expect to have only 60 "events" or subjects who have a fracture during follow up. We comment on the importance of this number shortly.

As a second multivariable example we consider sample size for a study where mother having had a fracture is the main covariate of interest. What sample size is necessary to have 80% power to detect a treatment coefficient $\ln(1.5)$ when we adjust for the other covariates shown in Table 10.14? Application of Hsieh's correction factor for multiple covariates to equation (10.18) yields sample size

$$n = \frac{(1 + 2P_0)}{1 - \rho^2} \times \frac{\left(z_{1-\alpha}\sqrt{\frac{1}{1-\pi} + \frac{1}{\pi}} + z_{1-\theta}\sqrt{\frac{1}{1-\pi} + \frac{1}{\pi e^{\beta_1^*}}}\right)^2}{P_0 \beta_1^{*2}}. \tag{10.24}$$

In this example, since the covariate of interest is dichotomous, we suggest using one of the R^2 measures discussed in Chapter 5. One possibility is the squared correlation between the values of the dichotomous covariate and fitted values from a logistic regression of this covariate on all other variables in the model (i.e., the value of equation (5.12). In our example this yields $\rho^2 = (0.1370)^2 = 0.0188$. Thus, the multivariable adjusted sample size from equation (10.24) is

$$n = \frac{(1 + 2 \times 0.1425)}{(1 - 0.0188)} \times \frac{\left(1.645\sqrt{\frac{1}{0.5} + \frac{1}{0.5}} + 0.842\sqrt{\frac{1}{0.5} + \frac{1}{0.5e^{[\ln(1.5)]}}}\right)^2}{0.1426 \times [\ln(1.5)]^2}$$

$$= 1.31 \times \frac{(1.645 \times 2 + 0.842\sqrt{2 + 2 \times 0.6667})^2}{0.1425 \times 0.1644}$$

$$= 1303.05.$$

This suggests that, rounding up to be divisible by 2, a total sample size of about 1304, or 652 per treatment group would be required.

There are a number of potential problems with the sample size formula in equation (10.24). One is the ad-hoc use of the Hsieh's correction factor to account for multiple covariates. A second problem involves the earlier noted discrepancy in sample sizes suggested by equations (10.17) and (10.18). We think that the sample size suggested by equation (10.24) may be unnecessarily large but could be the starting point for a more in-depth sample size analysis using pilot data to do some model fitting. For example, one way to assess the precision obtained from modeling with a sample of 1304 subjects is to construct a pseudo-study as follows: expand the original 500 subjects by threefold to obtain 1500 subjects and then take an 87% random sample. We would then fit the proposed multivariable logistic regression model and examine the estimated coefficient for mother's fracture, its estimated standard error, Wald statistic and p-value. These results can be used to provide guidance as to how significant the results might be in the new, larger study. Ideally we would repeat the sampling portion of this process a number of times to obtain approximate sampling distributions of the estimated quantities. If, in the end, we think the estimated standard error is unnecessarily small with confidence intervals that are too narrow then we would repeat the process using a smaller sample size. This could be repeated until we had empirical evidence that the sample size provides about the desired precision in the multivariable model.

A second consideration, and one relevant to any model being fit, is the issue of events per covariate. Peduzzi et al. (1996) examine the issue of how many events per covariate are needed to obtain reliable estimates of regression coefficients when fitting a logistic regression model. Peduzzi et al. consider single term main effects models. In order to extend their ideas to more complex models that may have multiple terms for a number of covariates, we prefer to use the terminology *events per parameter*. In general the relevant quantity is the frequency of the least frequent outcome, $m = \min(n_1, n_0)$. In our experience this is usually the number of subjects with the event present, $y = 1$, but it could just as well be the number with the event absent, $y = 0$. Peduzzi et al. show that a minimum of 10 events per parameter are needed to avoid problems of over estimated and under estimated variances and thus poor coverage of Wald-based confidence intervals and Wald tests of coefficients. Thus, the simplest answer to the "do I have enough data" question is to suggest that the model contain no more than $p + 1 \leq \min(n_1, n_0)/10$ parameters. Vittinghof and McCulloch (2006) examined the question with more extensive simulations than those used by Peduzzit et al. and conclude that in many applications the aforementioned "rule of 10" may be too conservative. Vittinghof and McCulloch's simulations showed that with 5–9 events per parameter the coverage of confidence intervals was, in general, acceptable and that bias only contributed about 10% to mean squared error. They caution that with as few as 5–9 events per parameter one must be careful when interpreting the results from fitted models.

For example, in the GLOW study we have $125 = \min(125, 375)$ events. The rule of 10 suggests that models should contain no more than 12–13 parameters. The model fit in Table 10.14 using the GLOW data contains 6 parameters. Note that with the sample size of 167 when the goal is to test the coefficient for age we expect about 24 events. In this case the rule of 10 suggests that models should contain no more than 2–3 parameters. Using a more liberal rule of five events would suggest that a model with 4–5 parameters might be able to be fit.

As is the case with any overly simple solution to a complex problem, the rule of 10 (or 5–9) should only be used as a guideline and a final determination must consider the context of the total problem. This includes the actual number of events, the total sample size and most importantly the mix of discrete, continuous and interaction terms in the model. Peduzzi et al. considered only discrete covariates and provide no information about the bivariate distributions of outcome by continuous covariates. However, Vittinghof and McCulloch (2006) consider multivariable models containing both dichotomous and continuous covariates. We think that the ten events per parameter rule may be a good conservative working strategy for models with continuous covariates and discrete covariates with a balanced distribution over its categories. However, we are less certain about its applicability in settings where the distribution of discrete covariates is weighted heavily to one value, as often is the case in practice. Here one may require that the minimum observed frequency be, say, 10 in the contingency table of outcome by covariate.

In summary, having an adequate sample size is just as important when fitting logistic regression models as any other regression model. However, the performance of model-based estimates may be determined more by the number of events rather than the total sample size.

10.6 BAYESIAN METHODS FOR LOGISTIC REGRESSION

Bayesian methods are increasingly used for statistical analysis including logistic regression. Improvements in computational methods and capabilities have made these methods viable in practice, and allow estimation of model parameters in settings where other approaches fail, such as some of the more complicated random effects models described in Chapter 9. As we show in this section, the Bayesian method is easily adapted to the hierarchical type cluster-specific models for correlated data but this is not its only appeal. Gelman et al. (2004), Greenland (2007) and Congdon (2010) among others articulate the advantages of Bayesian approaches and we highlight a few here. Bayesian models take advantage of the knowledge gained from observations that are related in some way such as those belonging to the same group. The framework also allows comparison of models that are not nested, leading to the possibility of improvements in model selection. The interpretation of the parameters in Bayesian models is often viewed as more natural. Further, the methods provide an estimated density for the parameters so that there is no need to assume a distribution in order to perform inference or produce interval estimates. Finally, and perhaps the primary feature that distinguishes Bayesian methods from standard approaches, is that they allow the analyst to incorporate additional knowledge, not explicitly contained in the data set, into the model. This last feature has tremendous appeal in many situations, such as cases where sample size is small, but it also sparks debate due to the potential for subjective choices that could impact conclusions. We discuss the issue in more detail in the example to follow.

Use of Bayesian methods typically requires specialized software or that the user write their own program to perform the estimation. SAS recently added the ability to fit these models for logistic regression using PROC GENMOD or PROC MCMC. In this section we primarily utilized the software package BUGS, or Bayesian inference Using Gibbs Sampling [Gilks et al. (1994)], a product available for download in its most current version as OpenBUGS [Lunn et al. (2009)]. BUGS can be run from R and user contributed packages such as BRugs [Thomas (2004)] can be installed to provide an interface between the programs. Another package, similar to BUGS, is JAGS, or Just Another Gibbs Sampler [Plummer (2003)], designed to interface with R through the package rjags [Plummer (2012)] that has advantages of portability to more computing platforms.

The goal of this section is to introduce the Bayesian logistic regression model using a simple example. We cover some of the most salient features so that basic models can be fit and utilized. The material in the section provides a foundation for further study for those interested in more advanced topics involving Bayesian logistic regression. Many textbooks on Bayesian data analysis cover regression models and a few include logistic regression examples. Congdon (2003, 2006, 2010) and Gelman et al. (2004) offer an applied approach. The most comprehensive coverage of binary data is provided in Congdon (2005). Kruschke (2011) presents material at a level accessible to those new to Bayesian analysis and includes computer code for fitting models using BUGS and R. Ntzoufras (2009) is another text focused on methods using BUGS. Gelman and Hill (2007) and Albert (2009) are more advanced texts, but include code and examples. A review article by Agresti and Hitchcock (2005) includes a section on logistic regression with references for further reading. Kass et al. (1998) provides practical advice on many issues associated with use of the Markov Chain Monte Carlo (MCMC) methods discussed in the section.

The remainder of the section is organized into three parts. In Section 10.6.1 we describe the basic model and introduce the notion of a prior distribution. Section 10.6.2 is devoted to the most popular computational method used with Bayesian models known as *Markov Chain Monte Carlo* (MCMC) simulations. In addition to an overview of the basic algorithm we discuss some of the issues one must consider when using MCMC to ensure the simulation has run properly. This section may be skimmed on a first read. In the final Section 10.6.3 we present example results from a Bayesian logistic regression model using MCMC simulations. We discuss the difference in interpreting the results of such a model highlighting some of the advantages the Bayesian methods provide in this area. We also briefly discuss a few of the tools available for comparing models and performing diagnostics.

10.6.1 The Bayesian Logistic Regression Model

The basic Bayesian model differs from standard logistic regression by assuming the model parameters are random variables. As an example, we write the logit for the standard logistic regression model with a single predictor as

$$g(\mathbf{x}_i, \boldsymbol{\beta}) = \beta_0 + \beta_1 \mathbf{x}_i. \tag{10.25}$$

The Bayesian version of the model would assume a distribution for the two model parameters. A common choice [Gelman et al. (2004)] is the normal distribution in which case one might assume

$$\beta_0 \sim N(\mu_0, \sigma^2{}_0) \tag{10.26}$$

and

$$\beta_1 \sim N(\mu_1, \sigma^2{}_1). \tag{10.27}$$

The distribution chosen for the parameters is called the *"prior" distribution* and we discuss it in detail shortly. The word "prior" reflects the fact that distribution is formulated before analyzing the data observed in the study. Prior distributions are typically defined using the "tolerance" or "precision" parameters τ_0 and τ_1 instead of the variance. The reason for this specification is that tolerance is inversely related to the variance, as $\tau_i = 1/\sigma_i^2$, $i = 0, 1$. Thus, if the prior variance is large the tolerance is small. The interpretation is that the prior distribution in such a case is not "precise" in terms of specifying possible values of the parameter before the data are analyzed. Conversely, small variances lead to large tolerances and are highly precise in prior estimates for parameter values.

We would like to determine the distribution of the parameters based on the study data or the conditional distribution of the parameters given the binary observations denoted

$$f(\beta_0, \beta_1 | \mathbf{y}). \tag{10.28}$$

In equation (10.28) the vertical line denotes a conditional distribution and the statement is read the distribution of Beta0 and Beta1 as in (10.28) "given" the observed binary data. Recall that we can write an expression for the likelihood of the data given the parameters as

$$f(\mathbf{y} | \beta_0, \beta_1) = \prod_{i=1}^{n} \pi(x_i)^{y_i} [1 - \pi(x_i)]^{1-y_i}. \tag{10.29}$$

Note that the conditioning in the expressions of equations (10.28) and (10.29) are reversed. Bayes' Theorem allows us to relate such conditional distribution expressions. In particular, the distribution of the parameters given the data is known as the "posterior" distribution, as it is computed after the observed data are considered and is given by

$$f(\beta_0, \beta_1 | \mathbf{y}) = \frac{f(\beta_0, \beta_1) f(\mathbf{y} | \beta_0, \beta_1)}{f(\mathbf{y})}. \qquad (10.30)$$

The numerator in this expression is the joint density of the data and parameters. The denominator in this expression is the distribution of the observed data and is computed by integrating the joint density over all possible parameter values, in essence summing all the probability for the data using the expression

$$f(\mathbf{y}) = \iint f(\beta_0, \beta_1) f(\mathbf{y} | \beta_0, \beta_1) d\beta_0 d\beta_1.$$

In essence, the "posterior" distribution represents an "updating" of beliefs about the distribution of the parameters used to form the "prior" distribution based on the observed data. Unfortunately the expression in equation (10.30), and particularly the integral in the denominator, is computationally difficult to evaluate. Several approaches have been proposed and utilized. One is to use numerical methods and approximate the integral involved with a sum. This method becomes infeasible for large data sets. A second approach is to use an asymptotic approximation for the posterior distribution, such as the normal distribution. Methodology and computational power have made simulation methods possible to essentially sample from the posterior distribution rather than find the exact distribution with results closer to the true distribution than the asymptotic approximation. This approach is called *Markov Chain Monte Carlo (MCMC)* and we focus on these methods for the remainder of the section.

10.6.2 MCMC Simulation

MCMC methods select a sequence of values from the posterior distribution such that each depends only on the previous value. The dependence on only the previous value gives rise to a Markov Chain [Ross (1995)], a "random walk" around the posterior distribution of the parameters. Since the result is a sample over possible parameter values, the denominator of equation (10.30) is ignored as it merely acts as a normalizing constant to ensure the posterior probability totals one. The most general form of MCMC used in practice is the Metropolis Algorithm [first described in Metropolis and Ulam (1949) and Metropolis et al. (1953)]. This algorithm is described in the following steps:

1. Pick starting values for the parameters and set them as the current values, $\beta_{current}$.
2. Use the current parameter values to compute the unstandardized posterior density $f(\beta_{current} | \mathbf{y})$ using the numerator of equation (10.30).

3. Use a "proposal distribution" based on the current parameter values to generate new proposed parameter values β_{proposed}. As an example, the proposal distribution might be a normal distribution centered on the current parameter values.

4. Use the proposed parameter values to compute the unstandardized posterior density $f(\beta_{\text{proposed}}|\mathbf{y})$ using the numerator of equation (10.30).

5. Compute the "probability of moving" as $p_{\text{move}} = \min\left[\frac{f(\beta_{\text{proposed}}|\mathbf{y})}{f(\beta_{\text{current}}|\mathbf{y})}, \ 1\right]$.

6. Generate a random value between 0 and 1, $u = U(0, 1)$.

7. "Move" to the proposed parameter values if $u < p_{\text{move}}$, otherwise maintain the current values. In other words the next simulated values are the proposed value if we "move". If we do not move, the next simulated parameter values are the same as the previous iteration.

8. Repeat steps 2–7.

As a simple example of an iteration of the algorithm, suppose that the unstandardized posterior density for the current parameters is 2 and for the proposed parameters it is 4. This means that the posterior probability is higher for the proposed parameters. The probability of moving in step 5 is then $p_{\text{move}} = \min(4/2, 1) = \min(2, 1) = 1$. Thus, we replace the current values with the proposed values in step 7 since the probability of moving is 1 and any random value between 0 and 1 is less than this probability. Alternatively, suppose that the posterior density value for the current parameters is 4 and for the proposed parameters it is only 2. In this case, the probability of moving is $p_{\text{move}} = \min(2/4, 1) = \min(0.5, 1) = 0.5$. In this case we are equally likely to move to the new parameters or just remain at the current values. The reason we may move even though the current values have higher probability is that we want to explore the entire distribution of possible values of the parameters and not just a few. The algorithm would become "stuck" in certain higher probability portions of the distribution if the probability of moving in a situation like the second example were zero.

We discuss some of the issues with using MCMC algorithms in an example, but note here that there are some important considerations in examining the simulation output to ensure the algorithm runs with reasonable efficiency. The starting values should be selected so that there is non-zero posterior probability or it may take a large number of iterations just to reach parameter values that are part of the distribution. The choice of the "proposal distribution" is also important. A common choice is the multivariate normal distribution centered on current parameter values. If the variance or spread of the proposal distribution is large it may take a long time to move as the proposed values may be far from the current values and therefore extreme, or low probability, values of the posterior distribution. Alternatively if the proposal distribution is narrow relative to the posterior distribution it may take a long time to "explore" the entire posterior distribution as new parameter values are close to the current values. Fortunately, methods to choose appropriate proposal distributions have been developed and are automated in software packages [Gilks et al. (1995)].

Variations of the Metropolis algorithm are implemented in MCMC software packages. In the basic algorithm, the proposal distribution is symmetric so that it is equally likely to move 1 unit left or right from a current value. The implication of this is that the probability of returning to the previous value is the same as it was to move to the current value. The Metroplis–Hastings (M–H) algorithm [Hastings (1970)] uses a proposal distribution that is not symmetric. This may improve efficiency in the number of simulation iterations required by allowing the proposal distribution to more closely reflect the target posterior distribution [Gelman et al. (2004)] but requires a modification to the probability of moving:

$$p_{\text{move,M-H}} = \min \left[\frac{f(\boldsymbol{\beta}_{\text{proposed}} \mid \mathbf{y})}{f(\boldsymbol{\beta}_{\text{current}} \mid \mathbf{y})} \frac{f(\boldsymbol{\beta}_{\text{current}} \mid \boldsymbol{\beta}_{\text{proposed}})}{f(\boldsymbol{\beta}_{\text{proposed}} \mid \boldsymbol{\beta}_{\text{current}})}, 1 \right].$$

The additional term in this expression is the odds of moving to or from the proposed value added to incorporate the lack of symmetry of the proposal distribution. For more details about the M–H algorithm see Chib and Greenberg (1995).

The Gibbs Sampler [Geman and Geman (1984)] is a special case of the general Metropolis algorithm that is often more efficient and avoids the need to "tune" the proposal distribution. Rather, the proposal distribution is simply chosen as the conditional distribution of one, or a group, of parameter values given the current values of the other parameters. Once a sample is taken from the conditional proposal distribution of the parameter(s) they are updated to the new values and the next parameter or group of parameters is sampled in a similar fashion. When all parameters in the model are updated a single step of the algorithm is complete. As an example, in a model with an intercept and one slope parameter, the algorithm would first select a new intercept value from the conditional distribution of the intercept given the current slope parameter. Then, the new slope value would be chosen from the conditional distribution of the slope given the intercept. Note that this algorithm always uses the proposed values, or always moves. The Gibbs Sampler requires computation of the conditional distributions of parameters, which may not always be computationally efficient. However, often these conditional distributions are simpler to compute than the conditional distribution for all parameters. There is also the potential for the algorithm to take a great deal of time if the parameters are highly correlated. Gelfand et al. (1990) and Gelfand and Smith (1990) first extended the method for use in Bayesian data analysis settings. For a more general discussion of the method see Casella and George (1992).

Software packages such as BUGS, JAGS and SAS include variations and modifications of the basic methods described here to improve efficiency of the algorithms. One example is adaptive rejection sampling [Gilks and Wild (1992)]. Details and additional references are found in the more advanced texts such as Gelman et al. (2004). For the Bayesian logistic regression model when computational complexity leads to issues with MCMC, Albert and Chib (1993) describe an approach using "augmenting" variables in order to approximate the logistic regression model using a normal or t distribution, which may make computation feasible.

MCMC methods may be useful for models other than those arising from Bayesian approaches. As mentioned in Chapter 9, complicated random effects models for correlated data are often estimated using MCMC algorithms. The random effects models closely resemble the Bayesian model with prior distributions for the parameters. In a fully Bayesian implementation, the parameters of the random effects would themselves have a prior distribution (with "hyperparameters"). We do not demonstrate this more complicated model in this section. Gelman and Hill (2007) consider models from this perspective.

We illustrate aspects of Bayesian logistic regression models using the GLOWBAYES data set used in Chapter 4 and described in Table 1.7. Initially we include a single predictor, the continuous covariate weight (kg) at enrollment, in order to focus on the key issues with Bayesian models. Thus, the model fit is described in equation (10.25) and we use the normal prior distributions for the parameters as defined in equations (10.26) and (10.27). Initially we use a prior mean of zero and set the precision parameters to small values so that $\tau_0 = \tau_1 = 0.00001$. Assuming a prior mean of zero suggests that we do not have any knowledge about the relationship between the weight and probability of a fracture. Recall that the precision is inversely related to the variance so the small values mean we are assuming a prior distribution with a large variance, $\sigma^2 = 100{,}000$. This means we are quite uncertain about the true values of the parameters and the prior distribution reflects this and is said to be "diffuse" and "non-informative".

The first important aspect of fitting the model using MCMC methods involves checks of performance of the algorithm itself. The MCMC method randomly samples from the posterior distribution of the parameters. There are, however, three primary concerns with the resulting sequence of values. All of the concerns play a role in answering the basic question of how many iterations of the simulation should be run. The first concern is that if the algorithm does not start with values in the posterior distribution then early simulations may produce values not representative of the true parameter values. The second concern is that the samples in consecutive iterations are related so that the algorithm may result in many values taken from one region of the posterior distribution thus producing results that do not reflect the true probabilities of different values. The third concern is that the algorithm converges to the posterior distribution and, if so, when convergence is achieved how many values should be produced after that. We address each of the concerns in turn.

The first concern about the early values not representing the true posterior distribution is reduced if the starting values are reasonable. One approach is to first fit the model using standard logistic regression and use the parameter estimates as the initial values. Software packages often do this automatically. An additional strategy is to include a "burn in" period of iterations that are discarded. Gelman et al. (2004) conservatively recommend discarding half of the iterations. The actual number of total iterations depends upon tests of convergence that are discussed shortly. Since the computation time increases with the number of runs, Gelman et al. (2004) recommend beginning with a small number of runs such as 200 and then increasing as needed. SAS, JAGS, and BUGS all include options to declare the number of burn-in iterations for exclusion. The trace plot is a simple graphical tool that can help with several of the MCMC concerns. The trace plot shows the sampled

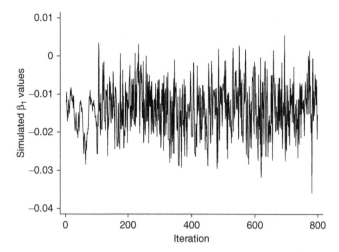

Figure 10.1   Trace plot of 800 MCMC iterations of the slope parameter for WEIGHT.

values for a given parameter by iteration. An example for the slope parameter in our single parameter model is shown in Figure 10.1. In this example, there were 800 iterations run with the first 400 iterations discarded as the burn-in. The plot shows all 800 simulated values. Using a burn-in of 400 values appears adequate as the simulated values appear to reach the posterior distribution before iteration 200 after which the samples fluctuate randomly within a band of values roughly between 0 and −0.03. Notice that for the first 100 to 150 iterations the graph does not have the tendency to fluctuate randomly, a sign that the early values are not representative of the posterior distribution.

The second concern involves the relationship between consecutive iterations leading to the MCMC algorithm spending too much time in small regions of the posterior distribution. This is known as *clumping*, a condition caused by high auto-correlation between sampled values, and is sometimes observable in the trace plot. In Figure 10.1 we have little evidence of this issue, but do see a few places where the amount of change in sample values is less over consecutive iterations. The plot should demonstrate a random fluctuation within the region of sampled values. When the trace plot does not clearly confirm or dismiss the concern that autocorrelation is a problem, another plot that may be useful is the autocorrelation function (ACF). The ACF for the slope parameter in our model is shown in Figure 10.2. Correlations are plotted by their "lag". "Lag 0" is the correlation of sampled parameter values to themselves and is therefore always equal to one. As an example, "Lag 20" is the correlation of all sampled values that are 20 iterations apart. A non-zero lag correlation equal to one means that the sampled parameter values at the given lag are identical. The ideal ACF quickly drops to low values near zero. In our example the correlation does drop and is below 0.1 for all lags except one and two. The autocorrelation is a particular concern if it drops slowly as lag increases

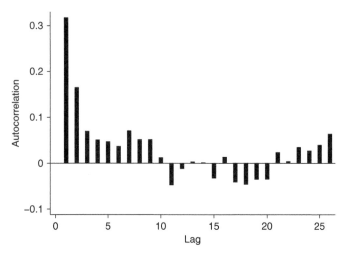

Figure 10.2   Plot of the autocorrelation function (ACF) for the slope parameter for WEIGHT.

[Albert (2009)]. Note that even with high ACF the MCMC sample could represent the posterior distribution but likely requires a much longer sequence to achieve convergence. When high autocorrelation is present, an option is "thinning" the simulated values. Thinning uses only 1 in every k simulated values to ensure a sample that is reasonably independent. As an example, if the ACF function did not drop below 0.1 until after lag twenty we might thin by keeping one in every twenty values. Note that this would mean that we would need 8000 samples after burn-in to produce a sample of 400 values. The higher the correlation at higher lags the more thinning is required. In our example, the autocorrelation does not appear to be an issue so we do not thin the samples.

The third concern is that the MCMC simulation has not completely converged to the posterior distribution, or that the samples are drawn too often or too little from specific areas of the distribution. The trace plot, again, is a useful tool for initially checking the convergence. If we see a trend in the sampled values, such as a steady increase in the values, the simulation has not converged. In our example, the values appear to center on about the same value but we noted some possible "clumping" that may indicate the simulation has not effectively converged or sampled from the entire posterior distribution. Burn-in and thinning may mitigate convergence issues. An additional tool is to produce multiple chains starting at different initial values of simulated samples. Kass et al. (1998) recommend choosing starting values using the mean and standard deviation of the prior distribution. For three chains, they suggest the mean of the prior distribution and then 1 standard deviation above and below that mean. Software packages allow the user to input initial values themselves or use default settings that attempt to choose reasonably different values while ensuring the chains start within the posterior distribution. Trace plots of all the chains can then indicate if convergence to the posterior distribution occurred as the simulated values should merge or "mix". Each chain should center on the same

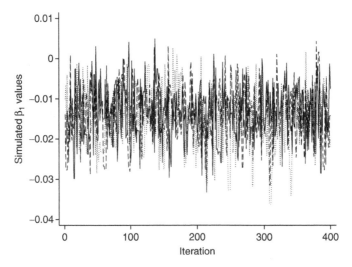

Figure 10.3 Plot of the three chains for the slope parameter for WEIGHT.

value with similar random fluctuations around that value. A plot of three chains for our example, with starting values randomly selected by the BUGS software, is shown in Figure 10.3. Since the three chains produce similar trace plots we have some evidence that the chains have converged.

In addition to graphical checks a number of diagnostic statistics have been developed to help assess convergence of MCMC chains. Many are included in software packages such as SAS and in BUGS or JAGS with R using the "CODA" package written by Plummer et al. (2006). One statistic is the Brooks–Gelman–Rubin (BGR) statistic [Brooks and Gelman (1998); Gelman and Rubin (1992)]. The BGR statistic is based on the ratio of two sources of variability when multiple chains are run. One source is variability of the observations within each chain, and the other is the variability between the chains. If the chains converged on the posterior distribution, then the variability between the chains should be small relative to the variation within each chain. Suppose that we run $j = 1, \ldots, m$ chains, each with $i = 1, \ldots, n$ sampled values denoted θ_{ij}. The variance of the parameter values in a single chain j is given by

$$s_j^2 = \frac{1}{n-1} \sum_{i=1}^{n} (\theta_{ij} - \overline{\theta}_{\cdot j})^2$$

where $\overline{\theta}_{\cdot j}$ is the average of the parameter values in chain j. The within chain variability, W, is defined as the average of the variances for the chains run or

$$W = \frac{1}{m} \sum_{j=1}^{m} s_j^2. \tag{10.31}$$

The between chain variability, B, is defined as

$$B = \frac{1}{m-1} \sum_{i=1}^{m} n(\bar{\theta}_{\cdot j} - \bar{\theta}_{\cdot\cdot})^2, \tag{10.32}$$

where $\bar{\theta}_{\cdot\cdot}$ is the average of all sampled values from all chains. The quantity in equation (10.32) then compares the average from each chain to the overall average parameter value. The estimated marginal posterior variance of the parameter is a weighted average of these two variances defined as

$$\hat{V}_\theta = \frac{n-1}{n} W + \frac{1}{n} B \tag{10.33}$$

and the BGR statistic is then given by

$$\hat{R} = \sqrt{\frac{\hat{V}_\theta}{W}}. \tag{10.34}$$

If the chains converge to the same posterior distribution, the between variability in equation (10.33) is small relative to the within variability and $\hat{R}$ in equation (10.34) should be close to one. If the chains have not "mixed", the between variability is larger and $\hat{R}$ is greater than one. A rule of thumb [Gelman et al. (2004)] is that $\hat{R}$ values above 1.1 are evidence that the chains have not converged. For the three chains from the example shown in Figure 10.3 the BGR statistic is below 1.10 by the ninth iteration confirming the graphical evidence that the chains have "mixed".

Other diagnostic measures are available in some software packages. Spiegelhalter et al. (2002) propose the "effective" sample size computed as

$$n_{eff} = nm \frac{\hat{V}_\theta}{B}. \tag{10.35}$$

For poorly mixed chains, the between chain variability is higher than the estimated posterior variability and the quantity in equation (10.35) is smaller than the total number of samples obtained from the MCMC simulation. Gelman and Hill (2007) propose a conservative effective sample size of 100 as the minimum to conclude that sufficient MCMC samples have been obtained. In our example using three chains the effective sample size is 714.8. The number of samples is sufficient although we did effectively lose nearly 500 due to the correlation at lags 1 and 2.

The Monte Carlo Standard Error (MCSE) is also reported in software packages. The MCSE is, in essence, the standard error of the mean of the posterior sampled values adjusted for the correlation in the Markov chain sampled values. The MCSE is computed by multiplying the variance of the sampled values by the inverse of the effective sample size to account for the correlation. A rule of thumb is that the MCSE should be less than 5% of the standard deviation of the estimated parameter. We demonstrate this statistic in the example to follow.

Geweke (1992) proposed statistics for checking convergence of each chain. If the chain has converged on the posterior distribution, the mean of the first runs after burn-in should be similar to the mean of the final runs. The Geweke test then compares the means of the first a runs to the final b runs with a typical choice of the number of runs being the first 10% and final 50%. If convergence is achieved, the Geweke statistic computed using the averages and variances of the two sets of runs,

$$Z_G = \frac{\overline{\theta}_a - \overline{\theta}_b}{\sqrt{V_a + V_b}}, \tag{10.36}$$

follows a standard normal distribution. A two-tailed hypothesis test at the 5% significance level rejects the null hypothesis of convergence for values of the statistic larger than 1.96 in absolute value. In our example the Geweke statistics from equation (10.36) for the three chains are -1.048, 0.435 and -0.792. All three statistics are below the 1.96 threshold so we fail to reject the hypothesis that the chains failed to converge.

Additional diagnostic statistics are proposed and may be available in software packages. Examples include the Heidelberger–Welch [Heidelberger and Welch (1981), (1983)] stationarity test of the sampled values and Raftery–Lewis [Raftery and Lewis (1992), (1996)] tests of the precision of posterior percentiles. In addition to thinning and burn-in, standardizing the explanatory variables is a common practice when fitting Bayesian models with MCMC methods that may improve efficiency and result in convergence with fewer simulations. An additional consideration is the precision of the prior distribution. Choosing a low precision, non-informative, prior as we did leads to less efficient MCMC simulation. We discuss the choice of prior distributions later in the section.

After examining convergence diagnostics and plots we conclude the MCMC samples appear to converge on the posterior distribution using a burn-in of 400 samples and 400 additional samples. We did note moderate correlation at lags 1 and 2 and a corresponding loss of effective samples and so choose to thin by selecting one of every three sampled values. Running this new MCMC with three chains reduces the ACF at all lags to below 0.1. The output is not shown and left as an exercise. We next turn our attention to an example of performing a Bayesian analysis.

10.6.3   An Example of a Bayesian Analysis and Its Interpretation

In the standard logistic model, we obtain estimates of the parameters in the model, their standard errors and form confidence intervals and test the null hypothesis that the true parameter is equal to zero. In the model for GLOWBAYES data using only WEIGHT the standard model output is displayed in Table 10.15.

The Bayesian analysis using MCMC is a sample from the posterior distribution of the parameters given the observed data and choice of prior. Using the three chains with 400 observations each after burn-in described in the previous section we thus have 1200 observations from the distribution of each parameter. A plot of the distribution for the slope parameter based on the 1200 observations is shown in Figure 10.4. The distribution looks normal, as was our assumed prior distribution.

Table 10.15 Output from Fit of the Standard Logistic Regression Model with WEIGHT as Predictor

	Coeff.	Std. Err.	z	p	95% CI
WEIGHT	−0.0136	0.0069	−1.957	0.0503	−0.0272, 0.0000
Constant	−0.1377	0.4961	−0.277	0.7814	−1.1100, 40.8346

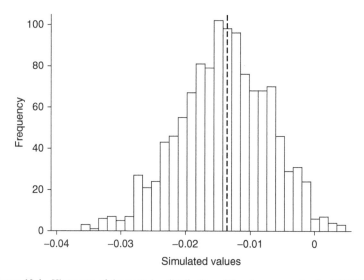

Figure 10.4 Histogram of the posterior distribution of the slope parameter for WEIGHT.

We see that most of the values from the simulation were less than zero, and the most common values were close to the value of −0.0136, shown as a dashed line in the figure, obtained from the standard logistic model.

We can also compute the summary statistics for the sampled values from the posterior distribution. A set of such statistics that are often of interest is shown in Table 10.16 for both the slope and intercept parameters. Focusing on the parameter values for the WEIGHT predictor, we see that the mean and median are close to the value of the parameter estimate in the standard logistic regression model. Further, the standard deviation from the posterior distribution sample is similar to the standard error for the standard logistic parameter estimate. The reason for the similarity is that we used a non-informative prior. The posterior distribution essentially takes a weighted average of the prior and likelihood. With little precision for the prior distribution, greater weight is given to the likelihood. If the MCMC converges and enough samples are obtained the summary statistics from the posterior distribution should be similar to the maximum likelihood estimates from standard logistic regression when using such a prior distribution. We discuss the role of the prior choice in more detail later. Additionally, note that while the summary statistics are similar there are differences in interpretation of the Bayesian results that we discuss shortly.

Table 10.16   Summary Statistics from Posterior Distributions of Intercept and Slope from 1200 MCMC Samples

	Mean	Std. Dev.	MCSE	2.5%	Median	97.5%
WEIGHT	−0.0141	0.0070	0.0003	−0.0276	−0.0140	−0.0013
Intercept	−0.1125	0.4964	0.0210	−1.0440	−0.1222	0.8951

Additional information presented in Table 10.16 includes the MCSE discussed earlier. The estimated standard deviation of the slope parameter based on the simulated posterior distribution, shown in Table 10.16 is 0.0070 and the estimated MCSE is 0.0003. The ratio of the two is $0.0003/0.007 = 0.043$, or 4.3%, which is less than the 5% rule of thumb suggesting the error due to simulation is not large enough to warrant concern. The 2.5 and 97.5 percentiles are also shown meaning that 95% of the sampled values fall in the interval between the resulting values, an interval known as an equal-tailed credible interval. In the case of the slope parameter, 95% of the sampled values are between −0.0276 and −0.0013. This interval is similar to a confidence interval from standard logistic regression models but has a slightly different and perhaps more intuitive interpretation. In the standard logistic regression case the 95% confidence interval for the WEIGHT parameter is from −0.0272 to 0. The interpretation is that if we repeated the data collection numerous times we would expect the interval we construct to contain the true parameter value 95% of the time. Thus, we say, we believe the true parameter falls in the interval with 95% confidence. The Bayesian credible interval is more directly interpreted as the probability of the values in the interval, given the observed data, totaling 95%. An additional advantage of the credible interval is that we have the sample from the posterior distribution for the parameter so the interval need not be constructed so that it is symmetric around the parameter estimate. An alternative to the equal tailed credible interval often used is the Highest Density Interval (HDI) sometimes referred to as the Highest Posterior Density (HPD) interval. To form the HDI we select the 95% of parameter values with the highest posterior probability. Computer software produces the interval automatically. In our example, the HDI is −0.0276 and −0.0013. This is similar to the equal-tailed credible interval but shifted slightly to the left to account for the skew in the posterior distribution. The posterior distribution shown in Figure 10.4 is close to normal but with a slightly higher probability for lower values than higher in the tails. The histogram of the posterior distribution in Figure 10.5 illustrates the slight shift of the HDI to the left due to higher probability of smaller values. The HDI is depicted in the figure with a heavy bold line.

The HDI and credible intervals are useful in assessing the significance of the predictor in the same manner as a confidence interval. Since both intervals include only negative values the probability that the parameter for WEIGHT is positive is less than 5% and the results suggest that the increase in weight decreases the probability of a fracture. In standard models we also perform a test of the null hypothesis that the true parameter value is zero. A small p-value rejects the null

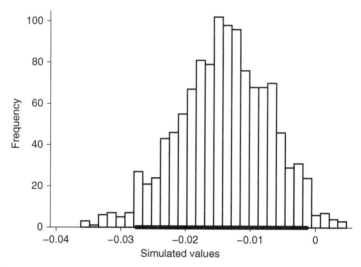

Figure 10.5 Histogram of the posterior distribution of the slope parameter for WEIGHT showing the HDI interval in bold on the axis.

hypothesis meaning the probability of observing the estimated slope parameter if the true slope was zero is small. In a Bayesian analysis, we use the posterior distribution to directly compute probabilities of parameter values. For example, we can compute the probability that the parameter is not negative. Using 3 chains of 400 sampled values we have 1200 observations from the posterior distribution of the parameter. Of these, 17 values are not negative. Thus, the probability is:

$$\Pr(\beta_1 \geq 0|\mathbf{y}) = \frac{17}{1200} = 0.0142.$$

Note that in the traditional hypothesis test we typically use the alternative hypothesis that the parameter is not equal to zero. In the Bayesian approach we compute a posterior probability that is more like a one-sided test since we do not formulate the problem in terms of the alternative hypothesis.

An advantage of the Bayesian approach is that it allows us to compute probabilities for outcomes of clinical interest directly from the posterior distribution. As an example, suppose that a clinician considers decreases of 5% or more in the odds of fracture relevant. The probability of such a decrease in odds for a 5-kg gain in weight would be of interest. The exponentiated coefficient represents the odds ratio for a 1-kg increase in weight. We are interested then in the probability statement:

$$\Pr(e^{5\beta_1} < 0.95).$$

To answer this question we compute $\exp(5\beta_1)$ for each of the 1200 sampled parameter values and count the number of times the resulting value is less than 0.95. Of our 1200 sampled values 837, or 69.8%, produce odds ratios below 0.95 for a 5-kg increase in weight. Thus, the probability that the odds of a fracture in the first year decrease by more than 5% for a 5-kg increase in weight is 0.698.

We next turn our attention to the choice of prior distribution. In our example, we chose a non-informative or "improper" normal prior distribution for the parameters. The tolerance was set to a small value so that the variance of the prior distribution was large. The large variance led to what is known as a "diffuse" prior distribution placing essentially equal and small probability on all possible values of the parameters. Such a choice would be appropriate if we had no knowledge about the parameter prior to the modeling effort. As mentioned previously, increasing the precision of the prior distribution may help improve convergence of the MCMC simulations. Further, the prior distribution provides an opportunity to utilize existing knowledge and potentially improve the quality of the model. In situations where a small sample is obtained this advantage is particularly attractive as the prior distribution acts as a mechanism to "add data" from other studies and effectively increase the sample size.

Recall that we used a mean of zero and tolerance of $\tau_0 = \tau_1 = 0.00001$ for the prior distribution in our example. Recognizing that weight is protective of fractures, we prefer a prior distribution in which the possibility of positive slope parameters is removed. To do so we first need to select a mean that is less than zero. The small tolerance we used corresponds to a variance of slightly more than 100,000 and a standard deviation of 316.2. The slope parameter represents the change in log-odds for a 1-kg change in weight. Thus, a coefficient of negative 10 would correspond to an odds ratio for a 1-kg decrease in weight of $\exp(10) = 22,026.5$, a completely unrealistic value. The slope parameter value is likely to be smaller in absolute value. A prior distribution with probabilities only between 0 and negative two would thus appear more realistic. A normal distribution with mean -1 and standard deviation 0.5 places approximately 95% of the probability in that range. The standard deviation of 0.5 corresponds to a tolerance given by

$$\tau_1 = \frac{1}{0.5^2} = 4.$$

The tolerance is the key to how much weight the prior information is given relative to the observed data. To illustrate the point, we refit the model using a prior mean of negative one and changing the tolerance used for the slope parameter prior distribution from 0.0001 to 4 and then to 10,000. The results are shown in Table 10.17. In the first row, when the tolerance is 0.0001, the summary statistics are identical to those from the MCMC simulation using a prior mean of zero shown in Table 10.16. The small tolerance or precision gives no weight to the prior mean and the result is based completely on the observed data. The second row results from using a prior standard deviation of 0.5 meaning a variance of 0.25 and tolerance of 4. We see that there is essentially no impact of decreasing the variance of the prior distribution to 0.25. The mean and median of the posterior distribution are closer to the prior mean of negative one but only by a small amount. We can safely use a prior with more precision than in the original example and not impart any undue knowledge while potentially improving the efficiency of the

Table 10.17 Summary Statistics from Posterior Distributions of the Slope Parameter for MCMC Samples with Prior Mean Negative One and Different Prior Tolerances

Prior Tolerance	Mean	Std. Dev.	MCSE	2.5%	Median	97.5%
$\tau_1 = 0.00001$	-0.0141	0.0070	0.0003	-0.0276	-0.0140	-0.0013
$\tau_1 = 4$	-0.0143	0.0070	0.0003	-0.0279	-0.0142	-0.0015
$\tau_1 = 10,000$	-0.8147	0.0086	0.0004	-0.8297	-0.8156	-0.7967

MCMC algorithm. The final row results from a run with prior standard deviation of 0.01. The mean, median, and percentiles are all now closer to the prior mean of negative one so the prior is weighted more heavily than the observed data.

In changing the prior distributions to create Table 10.17 we were interested in choosing a more precise prior without placing too much weight on the prior mean over the data at hand, as the prior mean was chosen arbitrarily. There may be instances where we wish to take advantage of knowledge about a predictor, perhaps from previous studies, and essentially include that previous knowledge with current study data. As an example, suppose that a previous study found weight to be a strong predictor of fracture with an estimated coefficient of -0.02 for weight and standard deviation of the parameter of 0.01. We wish to include the information from the previous study in our results. We incorporate the parameter estimate from the previous study as the mean of the prior distribution, assuming $\beta_1 \sim N(-0.02, \tau_1)$. The choice of the tolerance parameter could be based on the standard deviation of the parameter estimate from the previous study of 0.01, which corresponds to a variance of 0.0001 and tolerance of 10,000. For comparison and discussion to follow, we also used tolerance values of 1,000 and 100 and display the summaries of the posterior distribution in Table 10.18. The impact of choice of prior tolerance is clear in Table 10.18. With higher precision the mean and standard deviation of the posterior distribution are closer to the prior distribution.

The dependence on the prior choice as shown Tables 10.17 and 10.18 is one criticism of Bayesian methods. Simply put, changing the prior distribution led to substantial changes in results of the analysis. The posterior distribution is essentially a weighted average of the likelihood based on the current data and the prior distribution. In our example, using only the information from the current data set, or only the likelihood, the mean of the posterior distribution of the slope parameter

Table 10.18 Summary Statistics from Posterior Distributions of the Slope Parameter for MCMC Samples from Three Different Prior Distributions Based on Prior Study Results

Prior	Mean	Std. Dev.	MCSE	2.5%	Median	97.5%
$\tau_1 \sim N(-0.02, 10,000)$	-0.0158	0.0057	0.0002	-0.0271	-0.0158	-0.0053
$\tau_1 \sim N(-0.02, 1,000)$	-0.0142	0.0069	0.0002	-0.0276	-0.0142	-0.0019
$\tau_1 \sim N(-0.02, 100)$	-0.0141	0.0070	0.0003	-0.0276	-0.0140	-0.0014

is −0.014 and the estimate from the previous study used in the prior is −0.02. When we placed high precision with tolerance 10,000 on the prior distribution, the posterior mean is shifted closer to the prior mean at −0.0158. Low precision, or tolerance of 100, led to a posterior mean nearer to the likelihood-based estimate at −0.014. The posterior mean is essentially a weighted average of the prior mean and the likelihood estimate. The tolerance determines how much weight to give the prior distribution mean relative to the observed data. The weighting is related to the sample sizes, as the standard error of a mean is a function of the sample size. Increasing the sample size reduces the standard error or increases precision. Thus, when considering how much weight to place on the prior one consideration is the size of the sample both for the current study and for previous studies upon which the prior is based. If the current sample is small and the previous study large, we might weight the prior information more by using more precision in the prior distribution. Congdon (2003) suggests moderately increasing the standard error from previous studies to produce the prior tolerance in keeping with the notion of Browne and Draper (2000) who refer to this approach as "gently data determined". Kruschke (2011) similarly argues for a "mildly informative" prior distribution. The choice of prior distribution should be clearly articulated and defended when results are published. Further, performing sensitivity analysis to determine the impact of the choice of prior tolerance is important. If the inferences do not change for a range of prior tolerance choices it lends credibility to the analysis. When changing the prior distribution impacts study conclusions reporting the sensitivity analysis allows readers to see how. Further, the analyst can then provide support for the prior distribution choice in the context of the sensitivity analysis.

Including data from previous studies through the prior distribution, when appropriate, also illustrates an advantage of the Bayesian approach. In effect, the sample size of the study increases, which can lead to improved precision of the results. In our example from Table 10.18 the standard deviation of the sampled values of the slope parameter is smaller when the precision of the prior increased. The reduction in standard deviation occurs even when precision increases from 100 to 1,000 and the mean and median of the posterior distribution do not change much. In situations where a small sample is collected adequate previous research to warrant a precise prior distribution on one or more of the parameters may improve the analysis. In particular, one may use such priors on variables that are not of primary interest allowing a model with more predictors than otherwise possible [Kruschke (2011)].

Modeling within the Bayesian framework proceeds in similar fashion to the standard logistic setting described in Chapter 4. However, the time to run MCMC simulations and assessing the model output makes the process more difficult and time consuming than the standard analysis. There are methods proposed to compare Bayesian logistic regression models, including models that are not nested, useful for model building and variable selection. Suppose that we have two competing models, $M1$ and $M2$. The posterior probability of the two models given the data, or $\Pr(M1|\mathbf{y})$ and $\Pr(M2|\mathbf{y})$ are used to compare the two choices. From equation

(10.30) the posterior distribution for a given model M is given by:

$$Pr(M|\mathbf{y}) = \frac{Pr(M)\,Pr(\mathbf{y}|M)}{Pr(\mathbf{y})}.$$ (10.37)

Since the denominator in equation (10.37) is not a function of the model, but only the data that are the same for both models, we form a ratio of posterior distributions for the two models as

$$\frac{Pr(M_2|\mathbf{y})}{Pr(M_1|\mathbf{y})} = \frac{Pr(M_2)\,Pr(\mathbf{y}|M_2)}{Pr(M_1)\,Pr(\mathbf{y}|M_1)} = \frac{Pr(M_2)}{Pr(M_1)} \times \frac{Pr(\mathbf{y}|M_2)}{Pr(\mathbf{y}|M_1)}.$$ (10.38)

The final term in equation (10.38) is known as the Bayes factor (BF):

$$BF_{21} = \frac{Pr(\mathbf{y}|M_2)}{Pr(\mathbf{y}|M_1)}.$$ (10.39)

The BF is a ratio of conditional likelihoods often used in comparing Bayesian models and, if the models are nested, is equivalent to the likelihood ratio test used in standard logistic regression model comparison. Note that solving for the BF in equation (10.38) yields

$$BF_{21} = \frac{Pr(\mathbf{y}|M_2)}{Pr(\mathbf{y}|M_1)} = \frac{Pr(M_2|\mathbf{y})}{Pr(M_1|\mathbf{y})} \times \frac{Pr(M_1)}{Pr(M_2)}.$$ (10.40)

The second ratio in equation (10.40) is the prior probability for each of the two models being compared. If the two are equally likely *a priori*, the BF is computed as the ratio of the posterior probabilities of the two models. In logistic regression, however, this is rarely the case as typical models differ in terms of number and types of predictors. A rule of thumb for the BF is that if the $\log_{10}(BF_{21})$ is greater than 2 there is "decisive support" for M_2 compared to M_1. Values of $\log_{10}(BF_{21})$ between 0.5 and 2 suggest some support for M_2 and values below 0.5 are deemed inconclusive [Kass and Raftery (1995)].

Computing the BF is not simple in practice but a variety of approaches to approximate the value from the output of MCMC methods have been proposed. George and McCulloch (1993) describe Stochastic Search Variable Selection (SSVS), Green (1995) the reversible jump method and Dellaportas et al. (2000, 2002) the Gibbs Variable Selection (GVS) method. Carlin and Chib (1995), Chib (1995), Lewis and Raftery (1997) and Kuo and Mallick (1998) also propose methods. Reviews of some of the methods are available in Ntzoufras (2002), which includes computer code for BUGS, and in Han and Carlin (2001). All methods require some computer programming and many are either more complicated than the level of this book or require the user to carefully consider assumptions such as choice of "pseudo-priors" or "tuning parameters". Thus, we present the simplest method of Kuo and Mallick (1998) here as an example. The KM approach is not always the most efficient but is easy to implement using BUGS.

The KM approach is to add indicator variables γ_j, that are either 0 or 1 depending upon whether the covariate is included in the model. As an example, suppose that we are interested in whether to add HEIGHT to our model with WEIGHT. We could include two indicator variables in the model, one for each predictor, producing an expression for the logit

$$g(\mathbf{x}_i, \boldsymbol{\beta}, \boldsymbol{\gamma}) = \beta_0 + \beta_1 \gamma_1 \mathbf{x}_{1i} + \beta_2 \gamma_2 \mathbf{x}_{2i}. \tag{10.41}$$

In this example, if an indicator variable is a 0 then the covariate is not included in the model and if it is a 1 the covariate remains in the model. There are four possible models. The first is when neither predictor is included and both indicator variables are set to 0. The second includes both predictors with indicator variables both equal to 1. The remaining two models include one or the other of the two predictors with one indicator 0 and the other 1. The indicator variables are given Bernoulli prior distributions with parameter p representing the probability the indicator is 1. In our example setting $p = 0.5$ would mean the prior probability of the four models was equally likely and the BF would then be computed using only the posterior probability of the models using equation (10.40). The posterior distribution for a given model involves determining the proportion of MCMC samples when the indicator variables correspond to a given model. The KM method tends to be inefficient meaning many MCMC runs are often required to ensure the simulation has ample opportunity to "visit" the proposed models. An approach to ensure a less likely model is sampled from is to set the prior probability of that model higher than the others and use equation (10.40) to compute the BF. Additionally, Kuo and Mallick (1998) recommend standardizing the covariates in the model by subtracting the mean value and dividing by the standard deviation for each. They also recommend prior variances between 0.25 and 16 for the coefficients of the standardized predictors.

In data with many possible predictors one might not wish to consider all possible model combinations. Subsets of all possible models are selected by using functions of the indicator variables. For example, we consider three of the four possible models involving HEIGHT and WEIGHT. M_1 is the model with only WEIGHT, M_2 the model with only HEIGHT, and M_3 the model including both predictors. We set the probability, p_1, of first indicator variable, for WEIGHT, to a function of the second given by

$$p_1 = (1 - \gamma_2) + 0.5\gamma_2.$$

If HEIGHT is not in the model $\gamma_2 = 0$ and $p_1 = (1 - 0) + 0.5 \cdot 0 = 1$ so that WEIGHT is included in the model corresponding to model M_1. If HEIGHT is included in the model $\gamma_2 = 1$ and $p_1 = (1 - 1) + 0.5 \times 1 = 0.5$ so that there is equal probability of models M_2 or M_3 depending upon whether the indicator for WEIGHT is one. By setting the prior probability of the second indicator variable to 2/3, the three models are equally likely *a priori*. We standardized both covariates, and chose normal prior distributions for the three coefficients in the model with mean 0 and variance 16 as recommended by Kuo and Mallick (1998). The results for 100,000 MCMC samples using BUGS with 500 burn-in runs are shown in Table 10.19. The model with both covariates included was observed the least of the three models and we used it as the base model for computing the BFs shown in

Table 10.19   Results of Kuo and Mallick Model Selection Method Using 100,000 MCMC Runs

Model	Prior probability	Observed runs	BF
M_1: WEIGHT	1/3	50,340	13.717
M_2: HEIGHT	1/3	45,990	12.531
M_3: WEIGHT5 + HEIGHT	1/3	3,670	1.000

the final column of the table. An example of the computation of the BF comparing M_1 to M_3 using equation (10.40) is

$$BF_{13} = \frac{\Pr(\mathbf{y}|M_1)}{\Pr(\mathbf{y}|M_3)} = \frac{\Pr(M_1|\mathbf{y})}{\Pr(M_3|\mathbf{y})}\frac{\Pr(M_3)}{\Pr(M_1)} = \frac{0.50340}{0.03670}\frac{1/3}{1/3} = 13.717.$$

To apply the rule of thumb we compute $\log_{10}(13.717) = 1.137$ meaning we have modest support for the model with WEIGHT only compared to the model including both predictors. In a standard logistic regression, the p-value for HEIGHT added to a model containing WEIGHT is 0.16 so in both approaches we prefer the one variable model.

Spiegelhalter et al. (2002) proposed the Deviance Information Criteria (DIC) for Bayesian model comparisons. The DIC is produced by software packages such as BUGS and SAS. The deviance is a function of the likelihood as in the BF defined:

$$D(\mathbf{y}, M) = -2\log[p(\mathbf{y}|M)]. \tag{10.42}$$

Note that a lower deviance implies a higher likelihood. Using equation (10.42) and defining $\boldsymbol{\theta}_i$ as the values of the parameters at a given run of the MCMC runs, the average deviance for all n MCMC simulation runs is

$$\overline{D} = \frac{1}{n}\sum_{i=1}^{n} D(\mathbf{y}, \boldsymbol{\theta}_i). \tag{10.43}$$

The deviance for the average parameter values from the runs is then

$$\hat{D} = D(\mathbf{y}, \overline{\boldsymbol{\theta}}_i). \tag{10.44}$$

The DIC is the average deviance in equation (10.43) but penalized for the number of parameters in the model, as adding parameters always decreases the deviance. The DIC uses an estimate of the "effective number of parameters" defined as

$$p_D = \overline{D} - \hat{D} \tag{10.45}$$

leading to the expression:

$$DIC = \overline{D} + p_D. \tag{10.46}$$

Table 10.20   DIC Results for Models of Table 10.19

Model	$\overline{D}$	$\hat{D}$	p_D	DIC
M_1: WEIGHT	560.3	558.3	1.975	562.3
M_2: HEIGHT	560.4	558.4	1.943	562.3
M_3: WEIGHT5 + HEIGHT	559.3	556.4	2.916	562.2

A smaller DIC indicates a better model and a rule of thumb given by Spiegelhalter et al. (2002) is that changes in DIC greater than 4 offer significant support for the model with a smaller value.

The DIC and associated values for the three models of Table 10.19 considered in the BF example are shown in Table 10.20. The conclusions from the DIC values agree with those obtained from the BF. We see modest differences between models with the WEIGHT model similar to the model with only HEIGHT. Adding HEIGHT to the model with WEIGHT does not improve the DIC, suggesting the single variable model is preferable. Notice that the effective sample size for the model with only WEIGHT is close to 2, corresponding to the two parameters actually in the model. For the model adding height, the value is 2.92 so that the effective number of parameters in the model is not as close to the actual number of parameters supporting the contention that adding HEIGHT to the model is not preferred.

Model comparison and variable selection has received a great deal of attention in Bayesian data analysis literature. More advanced users may wish to explore additional approaches. One idea is to use a single prior distribution for a set of coefficients. As an example, one might assume all predictors in the model have parameters from the same normal prior distribution with mean zero [Kruschke (2011) discusses this approach]. As most of the distribution is near zero the result is that insignificant parameters have posterior sampled values that are small in absolute value. A more conservative choice to avoid excluding potentially significant variables from the model is to use a t distribution, as it has more probability in the tails of the distribution. A second approach is model averaging [Hoeting et al. (1999)] in which the BF values are weights used to average over the proposed models.

Assessing the fit when using Bayesian techniques is just as important as it was with standard logistic models. In addition to the sensitivity to choice of prior distribution already discussed we are concerned with how well the final model fits the observed data. Gelman et al. (2004) proposed "posterior predictive checking" as a method of assessing fit. The posterior predicted values are simulated values of the response using draws from the posterior distribution of the parameters for given values of the predictors. As an example, we return to the model using only WEIGHT and the MCMC simulation results shown in Table 10.16. We obtained 1200 simulated observations from the posterior distribution of the model intercept and slope. For each of the 500 observed values in the data set we can simulate 1200 values of the binary response for the given value of WEIGHT. To illustrate, the first subject in the data set had a weight equal to 74.4. The first posterior sample intercept is -0.1223 and the slope is -0.0138. For these values, the posterior probability of a fracture is computed by first obtaining the estimated logit:

$$g(74.4) = -0.1223 - 0.0138 \times 74.4 = -1.149$$

and then the probability

$$\pi(74.4) = \frac{e^{-1.149}}{1 + e^{-1.149}} = 0.240.$$

The probability of 0.24 is then the parameter for a random Bernoulli distribution used to generate a binary simulated value of whether a fracture occurred.

Once the posterior simulated values are obtained, they are compared to the observed data. For example, for the first observation in the data set 287 of the 1200, or 23.9%, of simulated values using the posterior sample were fractures. The observed value was not a fracture. We perform the computation for all 500 observations in the data set and plot the difference between the observed value of the response and the proportion of simulated responses in Figure 10.6. In the figure, the upper line of positive values is for responses of one and the other line is for those without a fracture. A few observations differ from the simulated values obtained from the model by more than the rest. The largest observed difference of 0.842 is a subject with observed fracture with WEIGHT of 108.9 kg. The 1200 simulated values from the posterior distribution produced only 190 fractures, or 15.8%, but the subject did have a fracture in the first year. The result is not surprising as the model suggests subjects who weigh more are less prone to fracture. This subject is the third heaviest in the data set of those who did have a fracture. The simulated values for the two heavier women with fractures are the next highest predicted differences at 0.8367 and 0.829. The largest predicted difference for those without a fracture is a subject weighing 46.7 kg, the sixth lightest in the data set. In this case, simulations from the posterior distribution predict a fracture is more likely than for other women in the data set but the subject did not have a fracture.

Posterior predictive checks can be used not just for individual observations but also for groups. An example using categories of weight is shown in Table 10.21. We form 10 groups from the subjects weighing the least to the most and compute the observed proportion in each group with fractures compared to the simulated posterior predicted values. While the general trend in the observed data is decreasing fractures as weight increases for many deciles the proportion actually increases. Thus, the model predictions are not as accurate as we would prefer in many deciles. The results may indicate that other predictors need to be included in the model.

Bayesian residuals are closely related to posterior predictive checks. Chaloner and Brant (1988) and Chaloner (1991) define residuals in Bayesian linear regression and they are extended to binary models by Albert and Chib (1995) who describe two versions of Bayesian residuals. One version is based upon a latent variable formulation of the model and uses results of Gibbs sampling with augmenting variables as outlined in Albert and Chib (1993). We focus on the second version

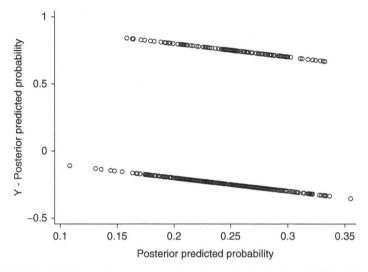

Figure 10.6 Plot of differences between observed and posterior simulated probabilities of response.

Table 10.21 Posterior Simulated and Observed Proportion of Fractures by Decile of Weight

Decile	Subjects	$Y = 1$	Observed Proportion	Simulated Proportion
WEIGHT5 < 54	47	14	0.298	0.311
54 ≤ WEIGHT < 58.1	57	15	0.263	0.288
58.1 ≤ WEIGHT < 61.2	34	11	0.324	0.275
61.2 ≤ WEIGHT < 65.8	59	19	0.322	0.269
65.8 ≤ WEIGHT < 69.4	49	10	0.204	0.258
69.4 ≤ WEIGHT < 72.6	56	15	0.268	0.247
72.6 ≤ WEIGHT < 77.1	53	13	0.245	0.234
77.1 ≤ WEIGHT < 83.18	45	8	0.178	0.225
83.18 ≤ WEIGHT < 91.65	50	9	0.180	0.204
91.65 ≤ WEIGHT	50	11	0.220	0.178

as it is readily computed using output of the basic MCMC runs we have used in this section and is similar to residuals from standard logistic regression discussed in Chapter 5. The residual is defined in terms of the probability of the response computed as in the standard logistic setting. As an example, for a single predictor the probability is

$$\pi_i = \frac{e^{\beta_0 + \beta_1 x_i}}{1 + e^{\beta_0 + \beta_1 x_i}}. \tag{10.47}$$

The residual is then defined as

$$r_i = y_i - \pi_i. \tag{10.48}$$

The residual is a function of the parameters and therefore has a distribution based upon the posterior distributions of the parameters. Given a sample from the posterior distributions we can produce a sample of the posterior distribution of the residual for each observation in the data set by computing equation (10.48) for all simulated values of the parameters. Key quantities of the posterior distribution, such as percentiles including the median, can be computed and may help identify outliers or unusual observations. Albert and Chib (1995) discuss several methods of identifying poorly fit subjects using the posterior residual distribution. We demonstrate two of these for the example model using WEIGHT from Table 10.16.

Using the MCMC simulated values for the intercept and slope we produce 1200 residuals for each of the 500 subjects in the data set using equations (10.47) and (10.48). We first graphically display the sampled posterior distributions of the residuals for each subject using boxplots in Figure 10.7. The boxplots fall into two lines depending upon the response value with the upper set corresponding to subjects with fractures and the lower to those without fractures. For subjects without an observed fracture, the largest residuals occur when the model predicted probability of response is largest and poorly fit subjects are those with large portions of the distribution near negative one. In this case, none of these distributions lie near negative one, but there is one subject with a boxplot further from zero that is a possible outlier. The subject has a model-based probability of a fracture equal to 0.34. The relatively higher probability is due to the subject being the lightest in the data set among those without a fracture at 40.8 kg. As increasing weight decreases the probability that a fracture occurs, this subject is not well modeled when weight is the only predictor. The distributions of Bayesian residuals are further from zero for subjects with fractures. There are three times as many subjects in the data set without a fracture and with only a single predictor in the model none of the subjects have average probabilities of fracture above 0.5. The subject with the largest posterior residuals is the heaviest among subjects with a fracture at 113.4 kg.

Plots of the posterior distributions of residuals such as Figure 10.7 can help identify outliers but the ability to differentiate between subjects even in modest sized data may be difficult. One option is to look at percentiles, such as the median or the 90th percentile, of the distributions for each subject. Albert and Chib (1995) recommend an additional approach that takes full advantage of having a sample from the entire distribution of the Bayesian residuals. When the response is one, poorly fit subjects are those with low model-based probabilities leading to residual values near one. Alternatively for response values of zero the poorly fit subjects are those with high probabilities and corresponding residual values near negative one. Thus, poor fit is reflected in a large portion of the posterior residual distribution near one in absolute value. Identification of subjects with poor fit is accomplished by computing the posterior probability of residuals exceeding a large absolute value. Albert and Chib (1995) suggest 0.75 as a possible choice. Using this cutoff, we compute the posterior probability of residuals exceeding this value for each subject by determining the proportion of the 1200 Bayesian residuals larger than 0.75 in absolute value. The ten subjects with the highest probability of a Bayesian residual above 0.75 are shown in Table 10.22. The heaviest subjects with fractures have

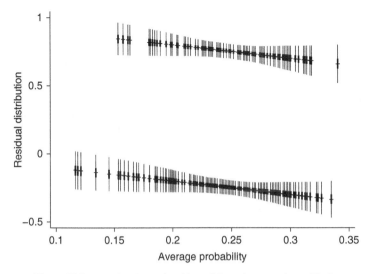

Figure 10.7 Boxplots for each subject of Bayesian posterior residuals.

Table 10.22 Observations with Highest Posterior Probability of Bayesian Residuals Greater than 0.75 in Absolute Value

WEIGHT	FRACTURE	Average Probability of Fracture	Probability Residual > 0.75
113.4	1	0.154	0.978
111.1	1	0.158	0.978
108.9	1	0.162	0.978
108.0	1	0.164	0.977
99.8	1	0.180	0.965
99.3	1	0.181	0.964
98.4	1	0.183	0.963
97.5	1	0.185	0.962
96.6	1	0.187	0.960
95.3	1	0.190	0.953

the highest probability of large residuals. The average probability of a fracture for these subjects in the model is low, as higher weight is less likely to lead to the response. The results are not surprising based upon the boxplots in Figure 10.7.

We have presented a simple example to illustrate the Bayesian approach and discussed some of the issues surrounding such an analysis. The section serves as an introduction designed to allow readers to fit basic models in a Bayesian framework and provides a foundation for further study. The references throughout the section offer a wealth of additional information on the subject. Bayesian regression modeling is an area of active research with advances both in methods and software implementation likely in the future.

10.7   OTHER LINK FUNCTIONS FOR BINARY REGRESSION MODELS

Up to this point in the text we have used the logit link/logistic regression function to model binary, multinomial, and ordinal outcomes. In this section we only consider a binary outcome as alternative link functions for multinomial and ordinal scaled outcomes are not as well developed. We motivated the choice of the logit link model in Chapter 1[†] where we noted that any model for a binary outcome must have a mean that lies between zero and one. In addition, for ease of estimation, there should be no constraints on the regression coefficients in the model. Put another way, this means that all possible values for the regression coefficients yield a model mean between zero and one. There are several other link functions that satisfy these two properties and two others that do not but have been used in practice in some settings. The goals of this section are to introduce each of these alternative link functions, illustrate their application to real data, compare their fit to that of the logit link, and suggest settings where these alternative links might provide a clinically useful analysis.

For ease of notation and to provide a setting where it is easy to compare the different models graphically we begin by describing and fitting a model containing a single continuous covariate. In general, let $\pi(\mathbf{x})$ denote the probability of the binary outcome being present. Under the logistic regression model

$$\pi(\mathbf{x}) = \frac{e^{\beta_0 + \beta_1 x}}{1 + e^{\beta_0 + \beta_1 x}} \qquad (10.49)$$

and its linearizing transformation is the logit function

$$g(x) = \ln\left(\frac{\pi(x)}{1 - \pi(x)}\right) = \beta_0 + \beta_1 x. \qquad (10.50)$$

Three of the five alternative link functions we consider are discussed in McCullagh and Nelder (1989, Section 4.3.1) and to a lesser extent in Cox and Snell (1989, Section 1.5) and Collett (2003, Section 3.5). These are the Probit, complementary log–log and log–log models. Each of these models has a mean that is constrained to be between zero and one and have no restrictions on their parameter values.

The Probit or integrated normal uses the standard normal distribution to model the probability as

$$\pi(x) = \Phi(\beta_{P0} + \beta_{P1} x), \qquad (10.51)$$

where the subscript "P" stands for "Probit" and Φ denotes the standard normal distribution function. In this case the linearizing transformation is

$$g_P(x) = \Phi^{-1}[\pi(x)] = \beta_{P0} + \beta_{P1} x, \qquad (10.52)$$

[†]We encourage readers to review the material Section 1.1 again to refresh their memory on the rationale for using the logistic regression model.

where Φ^{-1} is the inverse normal distribution. Unlike the logit transformation in equation (10.50) it is not a closed form expression of the coefficients. This has implications for the usefulness of the coefficients for estimating effects of covariates. The Probit model has a long history and predates the logistic regression model's use for binary data. Ashton (1972, Chapter 1) provides some of the background, while the earliest work on the Probit can be found in Bliss (1934).

The expression for the probability or mean for the complementary log–log model is

$$\pi_{CL}(\mathbf{x}) = 1 - \exp[-\exp(\beta_{CL0} + \beta_{CL1}x)] \qquad (10.53)$$

and its linearizing transformation is

$$g_{CL}(x) = \ln[-\ln(1 - \pi_{CL}(\mathbf{x}))] = \beta_{CL0} + \beta_{CL1}x, \qquad (10.54)$$

where we use the subscript CL to denote this model. The respective equations for the log–log model are

$$\pi_{LL}(\mathbf{x}) = \exp\{-\exp[-(\beta_{LL0} + \beta_{LL1}x)]\} \qquad (10.55)$$

and

$$g_{LL}(x) = -\ln[-\ln(\pi_{LL}(\mathbf{x}))] = \beta_{LL0} + \beta_{LL1}x, \qquad (10.56)$$

where we use subscript LL to indicate the model. The additional minus sign in the inner exponentiation in equation (10.55) is required in order to have the coefficients for the two log–log models to have the same signs.

Epidemiologists favor the log link function as its coefficients may be used to provide a direct estimate of relative risk. The equations for this link function are

$$\pi_L(\mathbf{x}) = \exp(\beta_{L0} + \beta_{L1}x) \qquad (10.57)$$

and

$$g_L(x) = \ln(\pi_L(\mathbf{x})) = \beta_{L0} + \beta_{L1}x, \qquad (10.58)$$

where the subscript L is used to denote the log link model. The problem with this model is that the mean can exceed one and there can be problems attaining convergence with maximum likelihood estimation. Blizzard and Hosmer (2006) studied the use of this link function with extensive simulations and note estimation problems occur when the probability in equation (10.57) approaches one. Their simulations show that using the estimated probabilities from a fit of a logistic regression model as the initial guess for the iterative solution of likelihood equations can improve convergence. They also show that the decile of risk goodness of fit statistic discussed in Section 5.2 may be used to assess fit.

The final link function considered in this section is the linear or identity function whose equation is

$$\pi_I(\mathbf{x}) = \beta_{I0} + \beta_{I1}x, \qquad (10.59)$$

where the subscript I is used to denote this model. This model can yield probabilities less than zero and greater than 1. It has not been studied in as serious a statistical manner as the other link functions. Its use in applications has been mostly by epidemiologists to provide an additive measure of effect, the risk difference, as an alternative to the multiplicative measures of effect from the logistic regression model discussed in detail in Section 3.5. This point is explored further in Section 10.9.

Given a sample of data we recommend using maximum likelihood to estimate the parameters for each of the five link functions. The form of the likelihood, $l(\beta)$, and log-likelihood, $L(\beta)$, functions are given in equations (1.3) and (1.4), respectively. The likelihood equations for the logistic regression model are given in equations (1.5) and (1.6). The likelihood equations for the alternative link functions are obtained by differentiating the log-likelihood with respect to the unknown parameters, replacing the logistic probability in equation (10.49) with the relevant expression for the alternative link function. The calculus is straightforward and so we do not present the equations. Estimators of the variances and covariances of the parameters come from the respective matrices of second order partial derivatives. We note that these equations are considerably more complex than those given for the logistic regression model in equations (2.3) and (2.4) and are thus not presented. The good news for users is that these models may be fit, for the most part, quite easily in many statistical packages.

Before proceeding to our example, we give our view of the role of the various alternative link functions in a regression analysis of a binary outcome. If the goal of the analysis is to obtain estimates of the probability of the outcome and estimates of effect for individual model covariates are, at best, of secondary importance, then we recommend that one consider the Probit, complementary log–log or log–log link models. One of these models may provide better probability estimates when the logistic regression model seems to have problems. Some guidance on what alternative model to choose can be obtained from an enhancement to Stukel's test discussed in Section 5.2. We discuss and illustrate this in the example to follow. If the goal of the analysis is to provide an alternative to the odds ratio as a measure of the effects of model covariates then we recommend using either the log link or identity link. We illustrate in the example that the estimated coefficients from the fit of the log link model can be used to estimate relative risk while those from the identity link can be used to estimate risk difference, where risk is defined as the probability that the binary outcome takes the value of interest.

As we noted above, one may encounter computational issues when fitting the log and identity link models. This is particularly true when the model contains continuous covariates measured over a broad enough range that model probabilities begin to approach one and/or zero (for the identity model). Unfortunately there is not much that one can do, short of using approximate estimation procedures, which we describe but do not recommend. For the log link Zou (2004) shows how one may use a Poisson regression routine to obtain parameter estimates. Blizzard and Hosmer (2006) studied this estimator and showed that while convergence is assured, obtaining probability estimates that are less than one is not. For the identity link one may obtain estimates from a linear regression program, but unless one uses iteratively adjusted weights equal to $[\pi_I(x) \times (1 - \pi_I(x))]^{-1}$ one will not obtain the same estimated coefficients as obtained from maximum likelihood. In any case a robust-sandwich type variance estimator should be used.

We use the Burn Study data to provide an example for fitting the Probit, complementary log–log and log–log link functions. For each of these link functions there are no computational issues. We show, in Table 10.23, the results of fitting the logistic regression models and the three other link functions containing the covariate total burn surface area (TBSA). We plot the fitted models versus TBSA in Figure 10.8.

Table 10.23   Results of Fitting the Logit, Probit, Complementary Log–Log, and Log–Log Link Function Models Containing the Covariate Total Burn Surface Area (TBSA) from the Burn Study, $n = 1000$

Link	DEATH	Coeff.	Std. Err.	z	p	95% CI
Logit	TBSA	0.085	0.0070	12.27	<0.001	0.072, 0.099
	Constant	−3.345	0.1757	−19.04	<0.001	−3.689, −3.001
Probit	TBSA	0.046	0.0032	14.21	<0.001	0.040, 0.052
	Constant	−1.884	0.0832	−22.64	<0.001	−2.048, −1.721
Comp. Log–log	TBSA	0.050	0.0029	17.5	<0.001	0.044, 0.056
	Constant	−2.880	0.1305	−22.06	<0.001	−3.135, −2.624
Log–log	TBSA	0.049	0.0039	12.57	<0.001	0.042, 0.057
	Constant	−1.432	0.0677	−21.14	<0.001	−1.564, −1.299

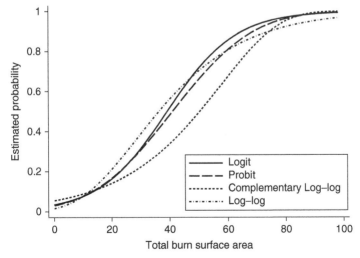

Figure 10.8   Plot of the estimated probabilities from fitted logit, Probit, complementary log–log and log–log link models containing total burn surface area.

The results in Table 10.23 show widely different values for the estimated coefficients. This is not unexpected as the link functions have different nonlinear transformations to the probability scale. We can see in Figure 10.8 that the fits from logit and Probit links are similar to each other (this is well known and, thus, expected). Each is symmetric about 0.5 with the Probit having shorter tails than the logit. The two log–log models are asymmetric with the complementary log–log model having a long left and short right tail. The log–log model has the reverse shape. In order to compare the fit of the four models we computed the decile of risk statistic using 10 groups based on the ranked probabilities from the logit fit. We do not evaluate the significance of the statistics, as the distributional properties of the decile of risk test have not been studied for the four alternative link functions. Regardless, the statistic does provide a comparable relative measure of fit. The values of the statistic from the four models (in the order listed in Table 10.23) are 14.2, 13.5, 34.8, and 8.7. The results support what we see in Figure 10.8, in that the logit and Probit models are similar and the complementary log–log model is different from the other three. What is perhaps surprising is the apparent better fit of the log–log model, 8.7, versus the logit model, 14.2. Comparing the two fits, logit versus log–log, in Figure 10.8 we might conclude that the logit model underestimates the probability of death between 18% and 50% burn area and over estimates it for burn area exceeding 50%.

The Stukel test discussed in Section 5.2 is based on adding two additional covariates to the model that measure the tail weight relative to the logit model. As described in Section 5.2, one uses a score test of the null hypothesis that the coefficients for the two additional variables are equal to zero. If one rejects this test then there is evidence that one might obtain a better fit with an alternative link function. If one is serious about considering an alternative link function then we suggest that one fits the logistic regression model adding the two covariates z_1 and z_2, defined in Section 5.2, as

$$z_1 = 0.5 \times [\hat{g}(x)^2] \times I[\hat{\pi}(x) \geq 0.5]$$

and

$$z_2 = -0.5 \times [\hat{g}(x)^2] \times I[\hat{\pi}(x) < 0.5],$$

to the model and use their estimated coefficients to guide the choice of an alternative link function. Stukel (1988) shows that if the two coefficients are about 0.165 then one might choose the lighter tailed and symmetric Probit model. The analysis supports choosing the log–log model if the coefficients are $(-0.037, 0.620)$ and the complementary log–log model if they are $(0.620, -0.037)$. Obviously, in any analysis there is variability in the estimates so one should examine their confidence interval estimates as well. When we add z_1 and z_2 to the logit model containing TBSA their estimated coefficients are $(-0.13, 0.38)$ and their confidence interval estimates contain -0.037 and 0.62, respectively, suggesting the log–log link function. The results of including z_1 and z_2 in the logit model should be viewed as just adding one more piece of information to the final decision process, which must include consideration of the clinical plausibility of any alternative link function as well as balancing the potential need for estimates of the effects of model covariates.

Next we consider the log and identity link models. In order to successfully fit these two models on the same set of data we had to restrict total burn surface area to $5 \leq TBSA \leq 60$. The results of these two fits as well as the logit model to the restricted range are shown in Table 10.24 and the fits are plotted in Figure 10.9.

Each of the estimated coefficients for total burn surface area in Table 10.24 expresses the effect on a different scale of the probability of death (respectively, the log-odds, log and the probability itself). We return to this point after we compare the shape of the three models.

The shapes of the three models shown in Figure 10.9 are distinctly different from each other. The logit is, as expected, "S-shaped", the log is exponential shaped and

Table 10.24 Results of Fitting the Logit, Log, and Identity Link Function Models Containing the Covariate Total Burn Surface Area ($5 \leq TBSA \leq 60$) from the Burn Study, $n = 542$

Link	DEATH	Coeff.	Std. Err.	z	p	95% CI
Logit	TBSA	0.096	0.0104	9.28	<0.001	0.076, 0.117
	Constant	−3.412	0.2573	−13.26	<0.001	−3.916, −2.908
Log	TBSA	0.041	0.0030	13.61	<0.001	0.035, 0.047
	Constant	−2.623	0.1546	−16.96	<0.001	−2.926, −2.320
Identity	TBSA	0.014	0.0011	12.55	<0.001	0.012, 0.017
	Constant	−0.054	0.0135	−4.00	<0.001	−0.080, −0.028

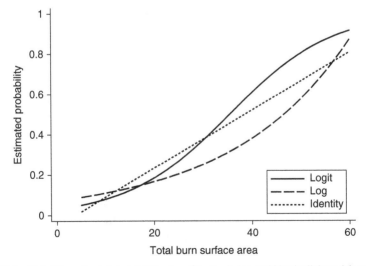

Figure 10.9 Plot of the estimated probabilities from fitted logit, log, and identity link models containing total burn surface area, $5 \leq TBSA \leq 60$.

the identity is a straight line. When we evaluate the decile of risk statistic over 10 groups, formed from the ranked estimated logit probabilities computed from the model in Table 10.24, we obtain values, in the order of the models in Table 10.24, of 13.2, 29.1, and 14.9. It is clear that the log model fits the least well and the logit and linear model provide similar fit, at least as measured by the decile of risk statistic.

The estimate of the odds ratio for a 5% increase in total burn surface area is, using the estimated coefficient for TBSA for the logit model in Table 10.24,

$$\widehat{OR} = \exp(5 \times 0.096) = 1.62.$$

The interpretation is that, for every 5% increase in TBSA, the odds of dying increases by 62%. It is easy to show, using the four-step procedure, that the estimate of effect for the log link model is the relative risk that, for a 5% increase in burn surface area, is

$$\widehat{RR} = \frac{\hat{\pi}_L(x+5)}{\hat{\pi}_L(x)} = \exp(5 \times 0.041) = 1.2.$$

Here the interpretation is that, for every 5% increase in TBSA, the risk of dying increases by 20%. This demonstrates that the odds ratio overestimates the relative risk when the outcome is not "rare", which is why some subject matter scientists (e.g., epidemiologists) would prefer to use the log link, when it does not run into estimation problems. We leave as an exercise fitting the logit and log link models showing that the two estimates become closer when death becomes a progressively rarer outcome.

The estimate of effect for the identity link model is the risk difference and, for a 5% increase in burn surface area, is

$$\widehat{RD} = \hat{\pi}_I(x+5) - \hat{\pi}_I(x) = 5 \times 0.014 = 0.07.$$

The interpretation is that, for every 5% increase in TBSA, the risk of dying increases by 7%.

Confidence interval estimates for both the relative risk and risk difference are easy to obtain from standard output from the model fits. For relative risk one simply multiplies the end points of the confidence interval for the coefficient by the clinically relevant change and then exponentiates the two new values. From Table 10.24 the confidence interval for a 5% increase is

$$\exp(5 \times 0.035) \leq RR \leq \exp(5 \times 0.047)$$

or $0.0175 \leq RR \leq 0.235$. For the identity link model one multiplies the endpoints by the change to obtain $(5 \times 0.012) \leq RD \leq (5 \times 0.017)$ or $0.06 \leq RD \leq 0.085$. For more complicated models containing interactions or other nonlinear terms we recommend following the 4-step procedure.

We demonstrated the fit and estimation of effects of the alternative links in Table 10.24 with the continuous covariate total burn surface area, as it yielded fitted models that clearly illustrate the difference in the shape of the probability as a function of the covariate. We leave as exercises fitting and estimation of effects for models containing dichotomous covariates and multivariable models.

In summary, we have considered five alternative link functions for regression models for a binary outcome that may be fit in most software packages. We suggest that the three link functions, Probit, complementary log–log and log–log, be considered as an alternative to the logit model when the primary focus of the analysis is modeling the probability of the outcome and the logit model does not seem to fit the data well. Estimates of effect from these models are not simple, easily interpreted functions of model parameters. On the other hand, when estimates of covariate effect are the primary focus, one can consider the log link model as an alternative to the logit link when it can be fit.[‡] Likewise, one can use the identity link model to obtain an additive effect estimate. For the log link, Blizzard and Hosmer (2006) derive casewise diagnostic statistics for evaluating fit and show that the decile of risk goodness if fit test may be used to assess model fit. Equivalent work for the other link functions has yet to be done. Model building steps are the same for the alternative links as for the logit link described in Chapter 4. Additional detail about interactions in the logit and identity link models is presented in Section 10.9.

10.8 MEDIATION[‡]

10.8.1 Distinguishing Mediators from Confounders

In Section 3.5 the motivation for using multivariable models to statistically adjust the effect of each variable for differences in the distributions of and associations among the other independent variables was discussed. We suggested that this statistical adjustment is necessary when two variables, each with an effect on the outcome, are associated with each other. As an example, we used hypothetical data on the difference in weight between two groups of boys, who differed in their age distribution. Because age influences weight, the unadjusted weight difference between the two groups of boys would reflect not only the effect of group membership, but also the effect of age. To isolate the effect of group membership, we need to compare boys in the different groups who are of the same age as we described in that section.[¶]

In interpreting the meaning of these adjusted effects, however, it is important to distinguish two different types of covariates—confounders and mediators. Both confounders and mediators are covariates that have an effect on the outcome and are associated with another independent variable; both produce a change in the coefficient of the independent variable when entered into a regression model. What

---

[‡]The log link model is appropriate only for prospectively collected data. It is not useful for binary outcome regression in case–control studies.

[§]Sharon Schwartz from the Department of Epidemiology and Melanie Wall from the Departments of Psychiatry and Biostatistics at Columbia University are the primary authors of this section.

[¶]Much of the discussion in this section requires familiarity with the material in Section 3.5. As such, we recommend that readers review that section before proceeding.

distinguishes them is the process that gives rise to the association between them and the independent variables.

It is easiest to describe this distinction if we focus on a particular independent variable of interest. Confounders are variables that *cause* the independent variable of interest or share a common cause with it. Mediators in contrast are consequences of the independent variable of interest. These relationships are depicted in three diagrams in Figure 10.10 where arrows between variables indicate causal relationships.

From the vantage point of explaining the relationship between the independent variable, X, and the outcome, Y, Z, is a confounder in diagrams A and B (where U represents other unmeasured variables) and Z is a mediator in Diagram C. The dashed arrow between X and Y may or may not be present. A covariate, labeled "Z" may be associated with an independent variable of interest because Z causes the independent variable (diagram A), because Z and the independent variable share a common cause, U, (diagram B) or because the independent variable of interest causes Z (diagram C). In each of these scenarios there may, but need not, be an arrow leading directly from the independent variable X to the outcome (indicated by a dashed arrow).

For example, suppose that we are interested in the effect of physical inactivity on experiencing a myocardial infarction. There are many other variables that have

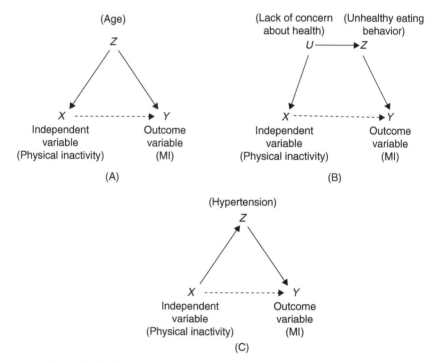

Figure 10.10 Distinction between the role of Z as a confounder or a mediator.

an effect on myocardial infarction that may be associated with physical inactivity, such as age, unhealthy eating habits and hypertension. To assess whether these covariates are confounders or mediators, we need to consider why they are associated with physical inactivity. The relationship between physical inactivity and age is best represented by diagram A. Physical inactivity and age are associated because as people age they are more likely to become less physically active, older age causes physical inactivity. The relationship between physical inactivity and unhealthy eating habits is best represented by diagram B; these two variables are associated because they share common causes, for example, lack of concern about health. Physical inactivity and hypertension are likely to be associated because physical inactivity has an effect on blood pressure as shown in diagram C where the independent variable, physical inactivity, is a cause of hypertension. So while age, unhealthy eating habits, and hypertension are all causes of myocardial infarction that are associated with physical inactivity, age and unhealthy eating habits are confounders whereas hypertension is a mediator. We emphasize that this distinction between confounder versus mediator is not made based on data analysis, but instead is based on subject matter knowledge.

10.8.2 Implications for the Interpretation of an Adjusted Logistic Regression Coefficient

When a covariate Z is included with another independent variable of interest, X, in a multivariable model the logit is given by the equation

$$g(x, z) = \beta_0 + \beta_1 x + \beta_2 z.$$

Assuming the goal is to assess the causal effect of X on the outcome, the *interpretation* of the logistic regression coefficient, β_1, will be very different if the covariate, Z, is a confounder versus a mediator. If Z is a confounder then we interpret β_1 as the *effect* of X on the outcome, assuming there are no other confounding variables. By including the confounder in the model, the estimated β_1 is expected to be closer to the true causal effect than if the confounder were not included. Specifically, β_1 represents the change in the logit associated with a one unit change in X, among subjects with a common value of Z.

If Z is a mediator, however, β_1 does not represent the effect of a one unit change in X on the outcome. Rather it represents only part of the effect of X on the outcome, the part that does not work through the mediator, Z. In the literature on mediation, this effect is referred to as the *direct effect* of X on the outcome. The effect of X on the outcome is then this direct effect, measured by β_1, plus the *indirect effect*, the effect of X that works through the mediator. The term *total effect* is often used in the context of mediational analysis to distinguish the effect of X on the outcome through all causal pathways from the direct and indirect effects that comprise this total effect. Outside the context of mediational analyses, the term "effect" implies total effect. We elaborate on the reasons for the differences in these interpretations next.

A confounder is a variable that leads to an association between the independent variable of interest and the outcome but is not part of the causal effect of the independent variable of interest on the outcome. Therefore, if we want to estimate the effect of the independent variable on the outcome, we need to isolate it from the effects of the confounders. That is, we want the coefficient to reflect only the effect of the independent variable and not the effect of differences in the distribution of the covariate with which it is associated. If the independent variable, X, is dichotomous, we would like the coefficient for x, β_1, in the logit, to be distinct from the effects z. Using the paradigm discussed in Section 3.5 and illustrated via $\Delta\hat{\beta}\%$ in equation (3.9), the effects of z amount to $\beta_2(\bar{z}_2 - \bar{z}_1)$ in the current context. In this scenario the coefficient for the independent variable of interest adjusted for the confounder provides our best estimate of the total effect of the independent variable. When Z is a confounder, if β_1 in the multivariable model, $g(x, z)$, is closer to zero than the coefficient, β_1^*, in the unadjusted model, $g(x) = \beta_0^* + \beta_1^* x$, this would indicate that part of β_1^* reflects the mixing of the effect of the confounder, Z, with X; part of the unadjusted coefficient, β_1^*, includes $\beta_2(\bar{z}_2 - \bar{z}_1)$. If the adjusted coefficient, β_1, is still appreciably greater than zero, this would indicate that the independent variable, X, does have an effect on the outcome, albeit an effect that is different than the crude (unadjusted) association, β_1^*. This scenario is consistent with the presence of the dashed arrow indicated in diagrams A, B, and C in Figure 10.10. If, however, the adjusted coefficient is not appreciably greater than the null (i.e., $\beta_1 = 0$) we would conclude that there is no effect of the independent variable on the outcome; there is no dashed arrow going from X to the outcome. The association between X and the outcome in the unadjusted model was simply a reflection of the different distribution of the confounder Z between those with and without X.

A mediator, in contrast, is a consequence of the independent variable and therefore represents a mechanism through which the independent variable influences the outcome. If Z is a mediator in the multivariable model, $g(x, z)$, β_1 represents the effect of X on the outcome net of the effect that works through the mediator. The coefficient, β_1, is the direct effect of X on the outcome. If the coefficient β_1, for x, in the adjusted model is close to 0, this indicates that the effect of X on the outcome works entirely through the effect of X on the mediator, Z. If β_1 in the adjusted model is different from 0 but smaller than the β_1^* in the unadjusted model, this would indicate that part, but not all, of the effect of X works through Z; there is an arrow leading directly from X to the outcome in Figure 10.10, diagram C.

Therefore, the interpretation of $\beta_1 = 0$ in model $g(x, z)$ is quite different when Z is a confounder and when it is a mediator. When Z is a confounder, if $\beta_1 = 0$ we say that X has no effect on the outcome; when Z is a mediator if $\beta_1 = 0$ we say that X has an effect on the outcome and we know the mechanism through which it works, Z.

10.8.3 Why Adjust for a Mediator?

If the coefficient without adjustment for the mediator provides the better estimate of the total effect of the independent variable on the outcome, why would we ever want to adjust for a mediator? The purpose would be to test hypotheses about how the independent variable causes the outcome, that is, to identify some of the causal pathways that make up the total effect [Hafeman and Schwartz (2009)]. For example, a researcher may want to know why individuals with strong social support networks are less likely to develop depression than those without such support. One hypothesis is that social networks encourage adherence to healthy lifestyles that are likely to be protective for the development of depression; there is an indirect effect of social networks on developing depression that works through the mediator of healthy lifestyles. An alternative hypothesis is that there is a direct effect of social networks on depression. By direct, we mean that social support works through some (unnamed) general mechanism other than encouraging healthy lifestyles. One could then use logistic regression to test these hypotheses. If the direct effect of social networks fully explains the association with depression such that there is no indirect effect through healthy lifestyles, the coefficient adjusted for a measure of healthy lifestyles, β_1, would be appreciably greater than 0 and negligibly different from the unadjusted effect, β_1^*. To the extent that the effect of social networks on depression works through the indirect effect of healthy behaviors, the coefficient adjusted for healthy behaviors, β_1, should be appreciably smaller than the unadjusted effect $(\beta_1 < \beta_1^*)$ and the adjusted coefficient should be close to 0. Of course it is possible that there is both an indirect effect through healthy behaviors and a direct effect of social networks through other mechanisms (as indicated by the inclusion of the dashed arrow in diagram C in Figure 10.10). In this instance, the adjusted estimate would be smaller than the unadjusted $(\beta_1 < \beta_1^*)$, but the adjusted would still be appreciably greater than 0.

10.8.4 Using Logistic Regression to Assess Mediation: Assumptions

The basic method for assessing mediation and controlling for confounding are essentially the same and are as described in Section 3.5. The main difference between estimating effects controlling for confounders and assessing mediation lies in the interpretation of the controlled coefficients and in the meaning of the difference between the unadjusted and adjusted coefficients as described above. A variation of the "*delta-beta-hat-percent*" useful in this context is

$$\Delta\hat{\beta}\% = \frac{100 \times (\hat{\beta}_1^* - \hat{\beta}_1)}{\hat{\beta}_1^*},$$

which can be interpreted as the indirect effect of the exposure—the proportion of the total effect of the independent variable of interest that works through the measured mediator.

To illustrate how to use logistic regression to test for mediation, we use the example of the effect of height on the development of a new fracture in the GLOW data introduced in Section 1.6.3. A reasonable hypothesis about how height influences the development of a new fracture is through the effect of height on the history of prior fractures—experiencing a fracture in the past may lead to bone

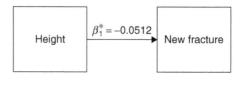

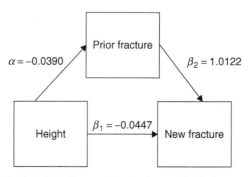

Figure 10.11 The total effect of height on new fracture is presented in the upper diagram. The indirect and direct effect of height on new fracture is presented in the lower diagram where the indirect effect is through prior fracture. All estimates are the on the logit scale.

weakening that leaves the individual more vulnerable to a fracture in the future. Figure 10.11 presents the assumed causal diagrams.

If the mediational hypothesis is correct then the following should hold:

1. Height should be significantly associated with new fracture in the unadjusted model,

$$\text{Pr(new fracture)} = \frac{e^{\hat{\beta}_0 + \hat{\beta}_1^* \times \text{height}}}{1 + e^{\hat{\beta}_0 + \hat{\beta}_1^* \times \text{height}}}.$$

2. Height should be significantly associated with prior fractures in the model,

$$\text{Pr(prior fracture)} = \frac{e^{\hat{\alpha}_0 + \hat{\alpha}_1 \times \text{height}}}{1 + e^{\hat{\alpha}_0 + \hat{\alpha}_1 \times \text{height}}}.$$

3. Prior fractures should be significantly associated with new fractures while controlling for height in the model,

$$\text{Pr(new fracture)} = \frac{e^{\hat{\beta}_0 + \hat{\beta}_1 \times \text{height} + \hat{\beta}_2 \times \text{prior fracture}}}{1 + e^{\hat{\beta}_0 + \hat{\beta}_1 \times \text{height} + \hat{\beta}_2 \times \text{prior fracture}}}$$

and

4. The association between height and new fractures in a model that includes prior fractures $\hat{\beta}_1$, should be smaller than the association between height and new fractures in the model that does not include prior fractures, $\hat{\beta}_1^*$ [Baron and Kenny (1986)].

Note that in Step 3 it is not sufficient just to correlate the mediator with the outcome; the prior fracture and future fracture may be correlated because they are both caused by the independent variable, height. Thus, height may play the role of a confounder in the association between prior fracture and new fracture and therefore must be controlled in establishing the effect of prior fracture on new fracture. The steps to test this hypothesis are outlined in Table 10.25.

Table 10.25a shows that height is associated with new fractures. Assuming the causal diagrams in Figure 10.11 are correct, this means there is a significant effect of height on new fracture. The coefficient -0.0512 says that each centimeter of height decreases the log-odds of developing a new fracture by 0.0512. Height is also associated with prior fracture (Table 10.25b)—each centimeter of additional height decreases the log-odds of a prior fracture by 0.039. Prior fractures are associated with new fractures while controlling for height, $\hat{\beta}_2 = 1.0122$ (Table 10.25c). Finally, in this model with both prior fracture and height, the direct effect of height on new fractures is -0.0447. This is a 12.7% decrease from the effect of height in the model without prior fractures: $(0.0512 - 0.0447)/0.0512 = 12.7\%$. This suggests that approximately 13% of the total effect of height is an indirect effect due to the mediational pathway of prior fractures.

We have summarized above a commonly used method for assessing mediation. However, there are several fairly stringent assumptions necessary for this simple method to validly assess mediation. First, there must be no uncontrolled confounding of the relationship between the independent variable and the outcome. Any confounding must be controlled before mediation is assessed. Second, there must be no uncontrolled confounding of the relationship between the mediator and the outcome [Robins and Greenland (1992); Judd and Kenny (1981)]. Third, there must be no effect measure modification, or interaction, between the independent variable of interest and the mediator on the log-odds scale [Robins and Greenland (1992); Hafeman (2009)]. Dealing with these complexities goes beyond the scope of this textbook. For a fuller discussion of these issues in the context of dichotomous outcomes

Table 10.25   Logistic Regression Results for Assessment of Mediation for the Causal Model in Figure 10.11

Variable	Coeff.	Std. Err.	z	p
a: Height as a Predictor of New Fracture				
HEIGHT	−0.0512	0.0171	2.99	0.003
Constant	7.1350	2.7441	2.60	0.009
b: Height as a Predictor of Prior Fracture				
HEIGHT	−0.0390	0.0168	2.32	0.020
Constant	5.1842	2.6981	1.92	0.055
c: Height and Prior Fracture as Predictors of New Fracture				
HEIGHT	−0.0447	0.0174	2.57	0.010
PRIORFRAC	1.0122	0.2254	4.49	<0.001
Constant	5.7851	2.7980	2.07	0.039

and logistic regression we refer the reader to VanderWeele and Vansteelandt (2010), Hafeman (2009), Cole and Hernan (2002) and Chapter 11 of Mackinnon (2008).

10.9   MORE ABOUT STATISTICAL INTERACTION[||]

In Section 3.5 *statistical interaction* or *effect modification* was introduced and defined to mean that the effect of one predictor variable on the outcome is not constant over the levels of another predictor variable. In the present section we will elaborate on the fact that the determination of whether there is effect modification or not depends upon the measure used to assess an effect. We will introduce the use of risk differences as an alternative to the odds ratio as a measure of effect and show how to assess for interaction directly on the probability scale (risk difference scale) as compared with the log-odds scale (as was done in Section 3.5). There is a literature, predominately in epidemiologic methods, that has focused on the distinctions between these types of interaction assessments [Rothman et al. (2008); VanderWeele (2009); Darroch (1997); Greenland (1983), (1993); Schwartz (2006); Elandt-Johnson (1984)]. The assessment of interaction on the probability scale is often referred to as "additive" or "biological" interaction while the assessment on the log-odds scale is called "*multiplicative*" or "*statistical*" or "*public health*" *interaction*. This is because when we use a probability (risk) scale, we assume that, absent interaction, risks add in their effects. In contrast, when we use logistic regression, a log-odds scale, we assume that, absent interaction, odds multiply in their effects. So interaction (effect modification) is defined to be deviation from what is expected under no interaction, which is scale dependent.

We will demonstrate that it is possible (even common) to come to different conclusions regarding whether there is effect modification depending on which scale is used to assess an effect.

10.9.1   Additive versus Multiplicative Scale – Risk Difference versus Odds Ratios

Throughout this text, odds ratios (or equivalently differences on the log-odds scale) are used to estimate effects. In the left hand panel of Figure 10.12 (similar to Figure 3.2) we show the log-odds of coronary heart disease (CHD; yes/no) by age for females and males. When comparing the lines for females (F) and for males (M) we see that there is a constant log-odds difference between these two lines across all ages (i.e., the lines are parallel on the log-odds scale). We can conclude that the odds ratio of CHD associated with a one unit increase of age is the same for females as it is for males; or, equivalently, the increased odds of CHD in men as compared with women is the same at every age. In other words, in terms of odds ratios, there is no effect modification by gender on the way age is associated

---

[||]Melanie Wall from the Departments of Psychiatry and Biostatistics and Sharon Schwartz from the Department of Epidemiology at Columbia University are the primary authors of this section.

with CHD, nor is there effect modification by age on the way gender is related to CHD. For example, the odds ratio comparing a 70-year-old with a 35-year-old is $5.7 = \exp(1.75)$ (where 1.75 is the difference in log-odds of CHD between a 70 and 35 year old) and this odds ratio is the same whether we are comparing two men or two women. The equation for the logit of CHD is

$$g(\mathbf{x}) = \beta_0 + \beta_1 \text{age} + \beta_2 \text{male} + \beta_3 \text{age} \times \text{male},$$

and the cross-product term would have coefficient $\beta_3 = 0$. Indeed the formula used to plot the lines on the left panel of Figure 10.12 is

$$g(\mathbf{x}) = \beta_0 + \beta_1 \text{age} + \beta_2 \text{male} = -5 + 0.05 \text{age} + 1.25 \text{male},$$

with no cross-product. But we can also express the relationship among age, gender and CHD using risk, $\Pr(\text{CHD} = 1 | \text{age}, \text{male})$, rather than log-odds by back-transforming the log-odds on the y-axis to the risk, probability, scale using the inverse logit (i.e., $\pi(\mathbf{x}) = e^{g(\mathbf{x})}/1 + e^{g(\mathbf{x})}$). When we present the results on the risk scale (see the right hand panel of Figure 10.12), we find that the lines are no longer straight and are not parallel. Now when we consider the risk difference between a 70-year-old female and a 35-year-old female we find the difference to be $18.2\% - 3.7\% = 14.5\%$, and the risk difference between a 70-year-old male and a 35-year-old male is $43.8\% - 11.9\% = 31.9\%$. Thus, the effect of increasing age in men leads to a larger increase in percentage points of CHD risk (31.9%) than the effect of increasing age in women that only leads to a 14.5% increase in

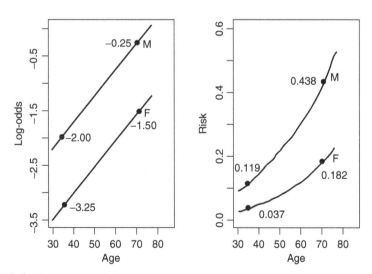

Figure 10.12 Demonstration that parallel lines on the log-odds scale (left) will lead to non-parallel lines when transformed to the risk scale (right). There is no effect modification (interaction) on the odds ratio scale (left) but there is effect modification on the risk difference scale (right).

percentage points of CHD risk. If we consider modeling the risks using the linear link function, discussed in Section 10.7, rather than the logit link,

$$\pi(\text{age, male}) = \beta_0 + \beta_1\text{age} + \beta_2\text{male} + \beta_3\text{age} \times \text{male} \qquad (10.60)$$

where $\pi(\text{age, male}) = \text{Pr}(\text{CHD} = 1|\text{age, male})$, we would find that the best fitting linear link model would have β_3 not equal to zero. That is, the risk of CHD is not just a sum of the effects of age and gender separately but also depends on the specific age by gender combination, such that being male has a stronger effect (in terms of risk differences) at higher ages.

This simple example illustrates that when there is no effect modification on the log-odds scale there will be effect modification on the risk difference scale and the opposite is true as well. This example is one where there was "super-additivity" meaning that the risk of CHD was larger than the sum of the risks of age and gender alone, that is, there was additional risk due to the combination of being male with increasing age. But, it is also an example of "perfect multiplicity (on the odds scale)" since the odds of CHD associated with increasing age and being male is simply the product of the odds for increasing age and the odds for being male.

Figure 10.13 provides a comparison of the different ways that two variables A and B can interact to affect an outcome on the additive (risk difference) versus the multiplicative (odds ratio or risk ratio) scale. Consider that the effect on the additive scale is 5 for A and 5 for B. Perfect additivity would mean that the increment in the risk due to the presence of both A and B would be $5 + 5 = 10$. By contrast on the multiplicative scale the increment in the risk due to the presence of both A and B, if there was no multiplicative interaction and hence perfect multiplicity, would be $5 \times 5 = 25$. The line plot on the bottom of Figure 10.13 represents the increment in the risk when both A and B are present and the labels indicate what conclusion would be drawn on the additive or the multiplicative scale. First

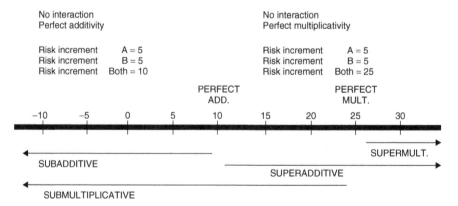

Figure 10.13 Comparison of interaction findings for additive and multiplicative scales. Reprinted with permission from Figure E-2, Appendix E, p315, of Schwartz (2006), by the National Academy of Sciences. Courtesy of the National Academies Press, Washington, D.C.

we note that if the increment in the risk when both A and B are present is <10 or >25 then we would find interaction on both the additive and multiplicative scale, albeit negative interaction (i.e., subadditivity and submultiplicativity) on the low end and positive interaction (i.e., superadditivity and supermultiplicativity) on the high end. But when the increments in the risk are between 10 and 25 we find that the answers to whether there is interaction or not and which direction it is can differ depending on the scale. When there is no multiplicative interaction (i.e., effect $= 25$) there is superadditivity, the scenario described in the example with age and gender above. When there is no additive interaction (i.e., effect $= 10$), there will be a submultiplicative interaction on the log-odds multiplicative scale. Moreover, for effects between 10 and 25, opposite conclusions about the direction of the interaction would be made with the additive scale finding positive interaction and the multiplicative scale finding negative interaction. This demonstration highlights the importance of choosing which effect measure (risk differences or odds ratios) is used.

10.9.2 Estimating and Testing Additive Interaction

Given two predictors of a dichotomous outcome, the most common method for statistically testing for effect modification is to include a cross-product term of the two predictors in a logistic regression model and test for the statistical significance of the coefficient of the cross-product term. As described above, this test of the cross-product coefficients in logistic regression examines whether there is *multiplicative interaction* between the variables in terms of how they affect the odds of the outcome. If, however, we want to test whether there is an *additive interaction*, that is, whether there is an effect modification on the additive risk scale between the predictors, we need to use the linear link model in equation (10.59).

The linear link binomial regression model can be fit using maximum likelihood in most statistical software [Spiegelman and Hertzmark (2005)]. For example, using STATA's glm command provides results similar to ordinary least squares regression in that the estimates of the regression coefficients, $\beta_0, \beta_1, \beta_2$, and β_3 are the same as in ordinary least squares but differ in the estimates of the standard errors. As shown in Section 10.7 the linear link binomial model fit using maximum likelihood takes into account the fact that the outcome is Bernoulli distributed rather than treating the residual errors as if they are normally distributed. A test for *additive interaction* is then performed by testing the null hypothesis that $\beta_3 = 0$, using a Wald or likelihood ratio test.

Given the simplicity of the linear link binomial model, it might be tempting to ask why this model rather than the logit link logistic regression model has not been used throughout this text. The answer is that if the linear link model is used there is a potential problem, as it can lead to predicted probabilities, $\hat{\pi}$, that are less than zero or greater than one. As noted in Section 10.7, it is common to have numerical convergence problems using maximum likelihood estimation for the linear link binomial model particularly with continuous predictors and data with risks of outcomes that are near zero or one. Thus, in some sense, application in practice may not be possible.

Nevertheless, in the simple case of two dichotomous predictors and their cross-product, the linear link binomial model can be straightforward to fit. We consider an example of this simple, yet common, scenario in detail using data from the study of Myopia in children described in Section 1.6.6. The outcome variable is an indicator of whether the child became myopic (MYOPIC) in the first 5 years of follow up. The two dichotomous predictors examined for interaction are whether the father of the child was himself myopic (DADMY) and whether the baseline spherical equivalent refraction was less than or greater than 0.50 (SPHEQ.50 coded so that $\leq$ $0.05 = 1$ and $> 0.50 = 0$). Previously, baseline spherical equivalent refraction has been used as a continuous predictor but here we have dichotomized it for simplicity of presentation of the method for testing for additive interaction. The value of 0.50 used for dichotomization corresponds to the 25th percentile of the distribution of baseline spherical equivalent refraction in the sample such that approximately 25% of the sample has values lower than 0.50 at baseline. For this study, myopia is defined as having any follow-up measurement of spherical equivalent refraction less than -0.75. None of the children were myopic at baseline. Table 10.26 presents the $2 \times 2 \times 2$ table of these data and Figure 10.14 plots the associated risks.

Table 10.26   Relating Myopic Outcome in Children with Father's Myopic Status and Baseline Spherical Equivalent Refraction (Higher or Lower than 0.50)

DADMY	SPHEQ.50	Child Becomes Myopic During Follow-up		Risk of myopia	Label
		No	Yes		
Dad is not myopic	High SPHEQ	225	7	3.0%	R_{00}
Dad is not myopic	Low SPHEQ	60	18	23.1%	R_{01}
Dad is myopic	High SPHEQ	196	14	6.7%	R_{10}
Dad is myopic	Low SPHEQ	56	42	42.9%	R_{11}
Total		537	81	13.1%	

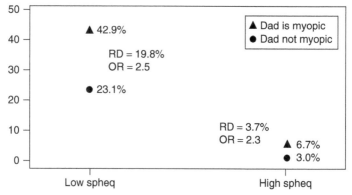

Figure 10.14   Plot of risk of myopia by categories of father's myopic status and whether baseline SPHEQ is low or high.

The question of interest is whether there is an interaction effect between father's myopic status and baseline SPHEQ.50 on risk for myopia in the child. Modern epidemiologic textbooks [e.g., Rothman et al. (2008)] define what is called the *interaction contrast* by taking the difference in risk differences and comparing it to zero in order to determine if there is an additive interaction. Specifically, in the case of two dichotomous predictors, using the risk label notation from Table 10.26, the interaction contrast (IC) is

$$IC = (R_{11} - R_{01}) - (R_{10} - R_{00})$$
$$= (R_{11} - R_{10}) - (R_{01} - R_{00}).$$

In our myopic example, the interaction contrast is estimated as

$$IC = (42.9 - 23.1) - (6.7 - 3.0)$$
$$= 19.8 - 3.7$$
$$= 16.1.$$

The interaction contrast can be interpreted in the following equivalent ways:

- the effect of having a father who is myopic is 16.1% greater when the child also has low SPHEQ.50 at baseline,
- the effect of having low SPHEQ.50 at baseline is 16.1% greater when the child has a father who is also myopic,
- the effect of having both a father who is myopic and a low SPHEQ.50 at baseline is 16.1% greater than the sum of the independent effects of a myopic father or low SPHEQ.50 at baseline alone.

If we fit the linear link binomial model,

$$\pi(DADMY, SPHEQ.50) = \beta_0 + \beta_1 DADMY + \beta_2 SPHEQ.50$$
$$+ \beta_3 DADMY \times SPHEQ.50$$

to this data using STATA's glm command we obtain the results shown in Table 10.27.

Table 10.27 Fit of the Linear Link Model Containing DDMY, SPHEQ.50 and Their Interaction

Variable	Coeff.	Std. Err.	z	p	95% CI	
DADMY	0.036	0.0206	1.78	0.076	−0.004,	0.077
SPHEQ.50	0.201	0.0490	4.09	<0.001	0.105,	0.297
DADMYxSPHEQ.50	0.161	0.0721	2.24	0.025	0.020,	0.303
Constant	0.030	0.0112	2.69	0.007	0.008,	0.052

The relationships between the estimates of the coefficients from the fit of the model in Table 10.27 and the risk estimates in Table 10.26 are (up to round off error) as follows:

$$R_{00} = \hat{\beta}_0 = 0.030,$$

$$R_{01} = \hat{\beta}_0 + \hat{\beta}_2 = 0.030 + 0.201 = 0.231,$$

$$R_{10} = \hat{\beta}_0 + \hat{\beta}_1 = 0.030 + 0.036 = 0.066,$$

and

$$R_{11} = \hat{\beta}_0 + \hat{\beta}_1 + \hat{\beta}_2 + \hat{\beta}_3 = 0.030 + 0.036 + 0.201 + 0.161 = 0.428.$$

We see that the estimated interaction coefficient is $\hat{\beta}_3 = 0.161$ (with standard error equal to 0.0721, Wald 95% confidence interval $(0.020, 0.303)$ and $p = 0.025$) indicating that the coefficient for the interaction is significantly different from zero and, thus, there is a statistically significant additive interaction. Note that the estimate for β_3 is equivalent (i.e., 0.161=16.1%) to the estimate of IC obtained by forming the difference in risk differences.

By comparison, when we consider odds ratios from the fit of the logit link model shown in Table 10.28, we find that the odds ratio of the father being myopic is similar for both levels of the child's SPHEQ.50. Specifically,

$$\widehat{OR}(DADMY, SPHEQ.50 = 0) = e^{(0.831)} = 2.3$$

versus

$$\widehat{OR}(DADMY, SPHEQ.50 = 1) = e^{(0.831+0.085)} = 2.5.$$

The same results can be obtained from Table 10.26. The odds ratio (OR) for father's myopic status being related to the child's myopic status given the child had low SPHEQ.50 at baseline is

$$\widehat{OR}(DADMY, SPHEQ.50 = 1) = \frac{R_{11}/(1 - R_{11})}{R_{01}/(1 - R_{01})} = 2.5,$$

and the OR when the child had high SPHEQ.50 at baseline is

$$\widehat{OR}(DADMY, SPHEQ.50=0) = \frac{R_{10}/(1 - R_{10})}{R_{00}/(1 - R_{00})} = 2.3.$$

Table 10.28 Fit of the Logit Link Model Containing DDMY, SPHEQ.5 and Their Interaction

Variable	Coeff.	Std. Err.	z	p	95% CI	
DADMY	0.831	0.4731	1.76	0.079	−0.096,	1.758
SPHEQ.50	2.266	0.4685	4.84	0.000	1.348,	3.185
DADMYxSPHEQ.50	0.085	0.5811	0.15	0.883	−1.054,	1.224
Constant	−3.470	0.3838	−9.04	0.000	−4.222, −2.718	

From the logit fit in Table 10.28, the estimate for the interaction coefficient is $\hat{\beta}_3 = 0.085$, with standard error of 0.5811 and $p = 0.883$. This evidence is not consistent with multiplicative interaction.

The previous example is one where there was a statistically significant additive interaction that was "superadditive" (i.e., the increased risk due to low SPHEQ.50 was made even stronger by the existence of another risk factor, DADMY), but there was no evidence of a significant multiplicative interaction. Next, we continue the example initially presented in Table 3.12 where there was a statistically significant multiplicative interaction that was "submultiplicative" (i.e., the increased risk of future fracture due to age was lessened among those who had already had the risk factor of having a prior fracture) and we will show that it does not have a significant additive interaction. If we fit the linear link binomial model

$$\pi(\text{AGE, PRIORFRAC}) = \beta_0 + \beta_1 \text{AGE} + \beta_2 \text{PRIORFRAC}$$

$$+ \beta_2 \text{AGE} \times \text{PRIORFRAC}$$

to the same data fit in Table 3.12 using STATA's glm command, we obtain the results shown in Table 10.29.

In Table 10.29 we see that the additive interaction term, $\hat{\beta}_3 = -0.008$, with a p-value of 0.109 indicates that there is not enough statistical evidence to support effect modification on the additive scale. This is in contrast to the finding in Table 3.12 where the interaction on the logit scale was -0.057 with a p-value of 0.022 indicating statistically significant effect modification on the multiplicative odds scale.

The method for estimating and testing additive interaction from the fit of the linear link model described above relies on direct estimation of the risk differences and their standard errors. Other methods for exploring additive interaction have been considered in the literature including most popularly the Relative Excess Risk due to Interaction or *RERI* [Rothman et al. (2008); Hosmer and Lemeshow (1992)]. The *RERI* is defined by taking the *IC* and dividing it by the overall baseline risk when neither risk factor is present, that is,

$$RERI = \frac{IC}{R_{00}} = \frac{R_{11}}{R_{00}} - \frac{R_{01}}{R_{00}} - \frac{R_{10}}{R_{00}} + 1$$

$$= RR_{11} - RR_{01} - RR_{10} + 1,$$

Table 10.29 Fit of the Linear Link Model Containing AGE, PRIORFRAC and Their Interaction (Compared to Table 3.12)

Variable	Coeff.	Std. Err.	z	p	95% CI	
PRIORFRAC	0.778	0.3805	2.04	0.041	0.323,	1.524
AGE	0.010	0.0024	4.10	0.000	0.005,	0.014
PRIORFRAC $\times$ AGE	-0.008	0.0053	-1.60	0.109	-0.019,	0.002
Constant	-0.455	0.1533	-2.97	0.003	-0.756,	-0.155

where RR_{XZ} indicates the risk ratio of the outcome given the status of X and Z compared with neither X nor Z being present. Here we test if $RERI = 0$, similar to the test that $IC = 0$ for the existence of additive interaction. Standard errors for testing the $RERI = 0$ have been developed using bootstrapping methods [Assmann et al. (1996)] as well as with approximations using the delta method [Hosmer and Lemeshow (1992); Lundberg et al. (1996)]. Implementation of the $RERI$ in the literature has typically involved substituting the odds ratio, OR_{XZ}, in place of the risk ratio in the formula [Hosmer and Lemeshow (1992); Richardson and Kaufman (2009); Knol et al. (2007)]. This approach can lead to misleading results in cases where the odds ratio is not a good approximation for the risk ratio [Kalilani and Atashili (2006)].

When statistically exploring effect modification we have demonstrated that scale matters (i.e., using a logit link can lead to different results than using a linear link). Although not discussed here, the reader should be aware that the exploration of interaction also can be influenced by the inclusion (or not) of confounding variables. The way in which the confounding variables change results can also depend on whether the logit or linear link is used. For further reading about additive versus multiplicative interaction in the presence of confounding, the reader is referred to Rothman et al. (2008), VanderWeele (2009), Darroch (1997), and Skrondal (2003).

EXERCISES

1. In the development of a propensity score for treatment in the GLOW study we defined treatment as being under treatment on enrollment and during follow up. Repeat the analysis using treatment on follow up.

2. Perform a full model assessment of the propensity score model in Table 10.1.

3. Perform a full model assessment of the propensity score model in Table 10.2.

4. Use the GLOW500_MISSING data and repeat the analysis of Section 10.4 by producing five imputed data sets using multiple imputations. How do your results compare to those presented in Section 10.4? If there is a large difference, why is this case and what does it suggest?

5. Produce diagnostic plots as in Chapter 5 for each of the five logistic regression models fit to the imputed data sets from Problem 4. Is there evidence of issues with the imputation models? Is there evidence of issues with the logistic regression model used to analyze the data?

6. Consider the low birth weight study. What sample size would be needed in a new study to be able to detect that the odds of a low birth weight baby among women who smoke during pregnancy is 2.5 times that of women who do not smoke, using a 5% type I error probability and 80% power?

7. Consider the low birth weight study. What sample size would be needed in a new study to be able to detect that the odds of a low birth weight baby decreases at a rate of 10% per 10 pound increase in weight at the last menstrual period, using a 5% type I error probability and 80% power?

8. Repeat Problem 6 assuming that you plan to use a model that contains age, weight of the mother at the last menstrual period and race.

9. Repeat Problem 7 assuming that you plan to use a model that contains age, smoking status during pregnancy and race.

10. Use MCMC simulation for the GLOW_RAND data set with WEIGHT5 as the only predictor. Use three chains, a burn-in of 400 and thin every three steps and check the convergence diagnostics for both intercept and slope. In particular, consider trace plots, the ACF, the BGR statistic, MCSE and the Geweke diagnostic statistic to confirm that the samples represent the posterior distribution.

11. For the MCMC simulation of Problem 10, change the thinning and look at the impact on the ACF. Explain the results.

12. Perform model building using MCMC and at least two additional predictors from the GLOW_RAND data set along with WEIGHT and HEIGHT. For the final model, perform diagnostic checks to ensure you have a viable MCMC sample and then interpret your results in a Bayesian framework including a credible interval for the odds ratios.

13. For the model of the Problem 12, use Bayesian residuals and/or posterior simulated values to examine the model fit.

14. Explore using an alternative link function to predict the probability of death using the same covariates as in the logit model in Table 4.27. As part of this process see what model is suggested when you add Stukel's two additional covariates. Did prediction improve?

15. Explore using the log link model and the identity link model with the covariates in Table 4.27. Is it possible to fit the model on the full data set? If not what restrictions are required to be able to fit the models?

References

Agresti, A. (2002). *Categorical Data Analysis, Second Edition*, Wiley Inc., New York.

Agresti, A. (2010). *Analysis of Ordinal Categorical Data, Second Edition*, Wiley Inc., New York.

Agresti, A., Booth, J. G., Hobert, J. P., and Caffo, B. (2000). Random effects modeling of categorical response data. *Sociological Methodology*, **30**, 27–80.

Agresti, A., and Hitchcock, D. (2005). Bayesian inference for categorical data analysis. *Statistical Methods & Applications*, **14**, 297–330.

Akaike, H. (1974). A new look at the statistical model identification. *IEEE Transactions on Automatic Control*, **19**, 716–723.

Ake, C. (2001). *Rounding after Multiple Imputation with Non-Binary Categorical Covariates*, Paper presented at the annual meeting of the SAS Users Group International, Philadelphia, PA.

Ake, C. (2005). Rounding after multiple imputation with non-binary categorical covariates. Paper presented at the annual meeting of the SAS Users Group International, Philadelphia, PA.

Albert, A., and Anderson, J. A. (1984). On the existence of maximum likelihood estimates in logistic models. *Biometrika*, **71**, 1–10.

Albert, J. (2009). *Bayesian Computation with R, Second Edition*, Springer, Dordrecht.

Albert, J., and Chib, S. (1993). Bayesian analysis of binary and polychotomous response data. *Journal of the American Statistical Association*, **88**, 669–679.

Albert, J., and Chib, S. (1995). Bayesian residual analysis for binary response regression models. *Biometrika*, **82**, 747–769.

Allison, P. (2001). *Missing Data*, Sage Publications, Thousand Oaks, CA.

Allison, P. (2005). *Imputation of Categorical Variables with PROC MI*, Paper presented at the annual meeting of the SAS Users Group International, Philadelphia, PA.

Ambler, G., and Royston, P. (2001). Fractional polynomial model selection procedures: Investigation of type I error rate. *Journal of Statistical Computation and Simulation*, **69**, 89–108.

Ananth, C. V., and Kleinbaum, D. G. (1997). Regression models for ordinal data: A review of methods and application. *International Journal of Epidemiology*, **26**, 1323–1333.

Anderson, D., and Aitken, M. (1985). Variance component models with binary response: interviewer variability. *Journal of the Royal Statistical Society, Series B*, **47**, 203–210.

Anderson, T. W. (1984). *An Introduction to Multivariate Statistical Analysis, Second Edition*, Wiley Inc., New York.

Arbogast, P. G., and Lin, D. Y. (2005). Model-checking techniques for stratified case-control studies. *Statistics in Medicine*, **24**, 229–247.

Archer, K. (2001). Goodness of fit tests for logistic regression models developed using data from complex sample surveys. Ph.D. Thesis, The Ohio State University.

Archer, K. J., and Lemeshow, S. (2006). Goodness of fit test for the logistic regression model fitted using sample survey data. *Stata Journal*, **6**, 97–105.

Archer, K. J., Lemeshow, S., and Hosmer, D. W. (2007). Goodness-of-fit tests for logistic regression models when data are collected using a complex sampling design. *Computational Statistics and Data Analysis*, **51**, 4450–4464.

Arnold, B., Castillo, E., and Sarabia, J. (2001). Conditionally specified distributions: An introduction. *Statistical Science*, **16**, 249–274.

Aschengrau, A., and Seage III,, G. R. (2008). *Essentials of Epidemiology in Public Health, Second Edition*, Jones and Bartlett Publishers, Sudbury, MA.

Ashby, M., Neuhaus, J. M., Hauck, W. W., Bacchetti, P., Heilbron, D. C., Jewell, N. P., Segal, M. R., and Fusaro, R. E. (1992). An annotated bibliography of methods for analyzing corrrelated categorical data. *Statistics in Medicine*, **11**, 67–99.

Ashton, W.D. (1972). *The Logit Transformation with Special Reference to its use in Bioassay*. Grifftn's Statistical Monographs & Courses, Number 32, Hafner, New York.

Assmann, S. F., Hosmer, D. W., Lemeshow, S., and Mundt, K. A. (1996). Confidence intervals for measures of interaction. *Epidemiology*, **7**, 286–290.

Austin, P. C. (2008). A critical appraisal of propensity-score matching in the medical literature between 1996 and 2003. *Statistics in Medicine*, **27**, 2037–2049.

Austin, P. C., Grootendorsi, P., and Anderson, G. M. (2007). A comparison of the ability of different propensity score models to balance measured variables between treated and untreated subjects: A Monte Carlo study. *Statistics in Medicine*, **26**, 734–753.

Austin, P. C., and Mamdani, M. M. (2006). A comparison of propensity score methods: A case-study estimating the effectiveness of post-AMI statin use. *Statistics in Medicine*, **25**, 2084–2106.

Austin, P. C., Tu, J. V., and Alter, D. A. (2003). Comparing hierarchical modeling with traditional logistic regression analysis among patients hospitalized with acute myocardial infarction: Should we be analyzing cardiovascular outcomes data differently? *American Heart Journal*, **145**, 27–35.

Azzalini, A. (1994). Logistic regression for autocorrelated data with application to repeated measures. *Biometrika*, **81**, 767–775.

Baron, R. M., and Kenny, D. A. (1986). The moderator-mediator variable distinction in social psychological research: Conceptual, strategic and statistical considerations. *Journal of Personality and Social Psychology*, **51**, 1173–1182.

Begg, C. B., and Gray, R. (1984). Calculation of polychotomous logistic regression parameters using individualized regressions. *Biometrika*, **71**, 11–18.

Belsley, D. A., Kuh, E., and Welsch, R. E. (1980). *Regression Diagnostics: Identifying Influential Data and Sources of Collinearity*, Wiley Inc., New York.

Bendel, R. B., and Afifi, A. A. (1977). Comparison of stopping rules in forward regression. *Journal of the American Statistical Association*, **72**, 46–53.

Bliss, C. I. (1934). The method of probits—a correction. *Science*, **79**, 38–39.

Bliss, C.I.(1937). The method of probits—a correction. *Science*, **79**, 409–410

Blizzard, L. and Hosmer, D.W. (2006) Parameter estimation and goodness of fit it in log binomial regression, *Biometrical Journal*, **48**, 5–22.

Brant, R. (1990). Assessing proportionality in the proportional odds model for ordinal logistic regression. *Biometrics*, **46**, 1171–1178.

Breslow, N. E. (1996). Statistics in epidemiology: The case-control study. *Journal of the American Statistical Association*, **91**, 14–28.

Breslow, N. (2003). *Whither PQL?* University of Washington Biostatistics Working Paper Series, 192, www.bepress.com/uwbiostat/paper192.

Breslow, N. E., and Cain, K. C. (1988). Logistic regression for two-stage case-control data. *Biometrika*, **75**, 11–20.

Breslow, N. E., and Clayton, D. G. (1993). Approximate inference in generalized linear mixed models. *Journal of the American Statistical Association*, **88**, 9–25.

Breslow, N. E., and Day, N. E. (1980). *Statistical Methods in Cancer Research. Vol. 1: The Analysis of Case-Control Studies*. International Agency on Cancer, Lyon, France.

Breslow, N. E., and Zhao, L. P. (1988). Logistic regression for stratified case–control studies. *Biometrics*, **44**, 891–899.

Brooks, S., and Gelman, A. (1998). General methods for monitoring convergence of iterative simulations. *Journal of Computational and Graphical Statistics*, **7**, 434–455.

Browne, W., and Draper, D. (2000). Implementation and performance issues in the Bayesian fitting of multilevel models. *Computational Statistics*, **15**, 391–420.

Bryson, M. C., and Johnson, M. E. (1981). The incidence of monotone likelihood in the Cox model. *Technometrics*, **23**, 381–384.

Bull, S. B., Lewinger, J. P., and Lee, S. S. F. (2007). Confidence intervals for multinomial logistic regression in sparse data. *Statistics in Medicine*, **26**, 903–918.

Bursac, Z., Gauss, H. C., Williams, D. K., and Hosmer, D. W. (2008). Purposeful selection of variables in logistic regression. *Source Code for Biology and Medicine*, **16**, 3–17.

Canary, J. (2013). A comparison of three goodness of fit tests for the logistic regression model. Unpublished Doctoral Dissertation, University of Tasmania, Hobart Tasmania Australia.

Carlin, B., and Chib, S. (1995). Bayesian model choice via Markov Chain Monte Carlo methods. *Journal of the Royal Statistical Society, Series B*, **57**, 473–484.

Casella, G., and George, E. (1992). Explaining the Gibbs sampler. *The American Statistician*, **46**, 167–174.

Chaloner, K. (1991). Bayesian residual analysis in the presence of censoring. *Biometrika*, **78**, 637–644.

Chaloner, K., and Brant, R. (1988). A Bayesian approach to outlier detection and residual analysis. *Biometrika*, **75**, 651–659.

Chambless, L. E., and Boyle, K. E. (1985). Maximum likelihood methods for complex sample data: Logistic regression and discrete proportional hazards models. *Communications in Statistics: Theory and Methods*, **14**, 1377–1392.

Chao, W-H., Palta, M., and Young, T. (1997). Effect of omitted confounders in the analysis of correlated binary data. *Biometrics*, **53**, 678–689.

Cheng, K., and Wu, J. (1994). Testing goodness of fit for a parametric family of link functions. *Journal of the American Statistical Association*, **89**, 657–664.

Chib, S. (1995). Marginal likelihood from the Gibbs output. *Journal of the American Statistical Association*, **90**, 1313–1321.

Chib, S., and Greenberg, E. (1995). Understanding the Metropolis-Hastings algorithm. *American Statistician*, **49**, 327–335.

Cole, S. R., and Hernan, M. A. (2002). Fallibility in estimating direct effects. *International Journal of Epidemiology*, **31**, 163–165.

Collett, D. (2003). *Modelling Binary Data, Second Edition*, Chapman & Hall/CRC, London.

Congdon, P. (2003). *Applied Bayesian Modelling*, Wiley, Chichester.

Congdon, P. (2005). *Bayesian Models for Categorical Data*, Wiley, Chichester.

Congdon, P. (2006). *Bayesian Statistical Modelling, Second Edition*, Wiley, Chichester.

Congdon, P. (2010). *Applied Bayesian Hierarchical Methods*, CRC Press/Chapman and Hall, Boca Raton.

Cook, R. D. (1977). Detection of influential observations in linear regression. *Technometrics*, **19**, 15–18.

Cook, R. D. (1979). Influential observations in linear regression. *Journal of the American Statistical Association*, **74**, 169–174.

Cook, R. D., and Weisberg, S. (1982). *Residuals and Influence in Regression*. Chapman & Hall, New York.

Copas, J. B. (1983). Plotting p against x. *Applied Statistics*, **32**, 25–31.

Cornfield, J. (1951). A method of estimating comparative rates from clinical data: Applications to cancer of the lung, breast and cervix. *Journal of the National Cancer Institute*, **11**, 1269–1275.

Cornfield, J. (1962). Joint dependence of the risk of coronary heart disease on serum cholesterol and systolic blood pressure: A discriminant function analysis. *Federation Proceedings*, **21**, 58–61.

Costanza, M. C., and Afifi, A. A. (1979). Comparison of stopping rules in forward stepwise discriminant analysis. *Journal of the American Statistical Association*, **74**, 777–785.

Coull, B. A., and Agresti, A. (2000). Random effects modeling of multiple binomial responses using the multivariate binomial logit-normal distribution. *Biometrics*, **56**, 73–80.

Cox, D. R. (1958). Two further applications of a model for binary regression. *Biometrika*, **45**, 562–565.

Cox, D. R. (1970). *The Analysis of Binary Data*, Methuen, London.

Cox, D. R., and Hinkley, D. V. (1974). *Theoretical Statistics*, Chapman & Hall, London.

Cox, D. R., and Snell, E. J. (1989). *Analysis of Binary Data, Second Edition*, Chapman & Hall, London.

D'Agostino, Jr.,, R. B. (1998). Tutorial in Biostatistics: Propensity score methods for bias reduction in the comparison of a treatment to a non-randomized control group. *Statistics in Medicine*, **17**, 2265–2281.

Darroch, J. N. (1997). Biologic Synergism and Parallelism. *American Journal of Epidemiology*, **145**, 661–668.

Day, N. E., and Byar, D. P. (1979). Testing hypotheses in case-control studies – equivalence of Mantel-Haenszel statistics and logit score tests. *Biometrics*, **35**, 623–630.

Dellaportas, P., Forster, J., and Ntzoufras, I. (2000). Bayesian variable selection using the Gibbs sampler. In *Generalized Linear Models: A Bayesian Perspective*, edited by D. Dey, S. Ghosh, and B. Mallick, Marcel Dekker, New York.

Dellaportas, P., Forster, J., and Ntzoufras, I. (2002). On Bayesian model and variable selection using MCMC. *Statistics and Computing*, **12**, 27–36.

Demidenko, E. (2007). Sample size for logistic regression revisited. *Statistics in Medicine*, **26**, 3385–3397.

Diez-Roux, P. (2000). Multilevel analysis in public health research. *Annual Reviews of Public Health*, **21**, 171–192.

Diggle, P. J., Heagerty, P. K., Liang, K. Y., and Zeger, S. L. (2002). *Analysis of Longitudinal Data, Second Edition*, Oxford University Press, New York, NY.

Dobson, A. (2002). *An Introduction to Generalized Linear Models: Second Edition*, Chapman & Hall, London.

Efron, B. (1975). The efficiency of logistic regression compared to normal discriminant function analysis. *Journal of the American Statistical Association*, **70**, 892–898.

Elandt-Johnson, R. (1984). *Statistical Interaction Revisited, Research Report*. Dept of Biostatistics University of Chapel Hill, Chapel Hill, N.C, http://www.stat.ncsu.edu /information/library/mimeo.archive/ISMS_1984_1457.pdf.

Evans, M., Hastings, N., and Peacock, B. (2000). *Statistical Distributions: Third Edition*, Wiley Inc., New York.

Evans, S. R. (1998). Goodness-of-fit in two models for clustered binary data. Unpublished doctoral dissertation. University of Massachusetts, Amherst, MA.

Evans, S., and Hosmer, D. (2004). Goodness of fit tests for the logistic GEE models: simulation results. *Communications in Statistics Simulation and Computation*, **33**, 247–258.

Evans, S., and Li, L. (2005). A comparison of goodness of fit tests for the logistic GEE model. *Statistics in Medicine*, **24**, 1245–1261.

Fagerland, M. W. (2009). *Performance of Significance Tests, with Emphasis on Three Statistical Problems in Medical Research*. Series of Dissertations Submitted to the Faculty of Medicine, No. 853, University of Oslo.

Fagerland, M. W., and Hosmer, D. W. (2012a). A generalized Hosmer-Lemeshow goodness of fit test for multinomial logistic regression. *Stata Journal*, **12**(3), 447–453.

Fagerland, M. W., and Hosmer, D. W. (2012b). A goodness of fit test for the proportional odds regression model. *Statistics in Medicine*, Epub ahead of print, doi:10.1002/ sim5645.

Fagerland, M. W., Hosmer, D. W., and Bofin, A. M. (2008). Multinomial goodness-of-fit tests for logistic regression models. *Statistics in Medicine*, **27**, 4238–4253.

Farewell, V. T. (1979). Some results on the estimation of logistic models based on retrospective data. *Biometrika*, **66**, 27–32.

Farrington, C. P. (1996). On assessing goodness of fit of generalized linear models to sparse data. *Journal of the Royal Statistical Society, Series B*, **58**, 344–366.

Fears, T. R., and Brown, C. C. (1986). Logistic regression methods for retrospective case-control studies using complex sampling procedures. *Biometrics*, **42**, 955–960.

Firth, D. (1993). Bias reduction of maximum likelihood estimates. *Biometrika*, **80**, 27–38.

Flack, V. F., and Chang, P. C. (1987). Frequency of selecting noise variables in subset regression analysis: A simulation study. *American Statistician*, **41**, 84–86.

Fleiss, J. (1979). Confidence intervals for the odds ratio in case-control studies: State of the art. *Journal of Chronic Diseases*, **32**, 69–77.

Fleiss, J., Levin, B., and Paik, M. C. (2003). *Statistical Methods for Rates and Proportions*, *Third Edition*, Wiley Inc., New York.

Fontanella, C. A., Early, T., and Phillips, G. (2008). Need or availability? Modeling aftercare decisions for psychiatrically hospitalized youth. *Children and Youth Services Review*, **30**, 758–773.

Fowlkes, E. B. (1987). Some diagnostics for binary regression via smoothing. *Biometrika*, **74**, 503–515.

Freedman, D. A. (1983). A note on screening regression equations. *American Statistician*, **37**, 152–155.

Furnival, G. M., and Wilson, R. W. (1974). Regression by leaps and bounds. *Technometrics*, **16**, 499–511.

Gardiner, J. C., Luo, Z. H., and Roman, L. A. (2009). Fixed effects, random effects and GEE: What are the differences? *Statistics in Medicine*, **28**, 221–239.

Gart, J. J., and Thomas, D. G. (1972). Numerical results on approximate confidence limits for the odds ratio. *Journal of the Royal Statistical Society, Series B*, **34**, 441–447.

Gelfand, A., Hills, S., Racine-Poon, A., and Smith, A. (1990). Illustration of Bayesian inference in normal data models using Gibbs sampling. *Journal of the American Statistical Association*, **85**, 972–985.

Gelfand, A., and Smith, A. (1990). Sampling-based approaches to calculating marginal densities. *Journal of the American Statistical Association*, **85**, 398–409.

Gelman, A., Carlin, J., Stern, H., and Rubin, D. (2004). *Bayesian Data Analysis*, *Second Edition*, CRC Press/Chapman and Hall, Boca Raton.

Gelman, A., and Hill, J. (2007). *Data Analysis Using Regression and Multilevel/Hierarchical Models*, Cambridge University Press, Cambridge.

Gelman, A., and Rubin, D. (1992). Inference from iterative simulation using multiple sequences (with discussion). *Statistical Science*, **7**, 457–511.

Geman, S., and Geman, D. (1984). Stochastic relaxation Gibbs distributions, and the Bayesian restoration of images. *IEEE Transactions on Pattern Analysis and Machine Intelligence*, **6**, 721–741.

George, E., and McCulloch, R. (1993). Variable selection via Gibbs sampling. *Journal of the American Statistical Association*, **88**, 881–889.

Geweke, J. (1992). Evaluating the accuracy of sampling-based approaches to calculating posterior moments. In *Bayesian Statistics 4*, Edited by J. Bernardo, J. Berger, A. David, and A. Smith, Clarendon Press, Oxford.

Gibbons, R., Hedeker, D., and DuToit, S. (2010). Advances in analysis of longitudinal data. *Annual Review of Clinical Psychology*, **6**, 79–107.

Gilks, W., Best, N., and Tan, K. (1995). Adaptive rejection Metropolis sampling. *Applied Statistics*, **44**, 455–472.

Gilks, W., Thomas, A., and Spiegelhalter, D. (1994). A language and program for complex Bayesian modelling. *The Statistician*, **43**, 169–177.

Gilks, W., and Wild, D. (1992). Adaptive rejection sampling for Gibbs sampling. *Applied Statistics*, **41**, 337–348.

Glynn, R. J., and Rosner, B. (1994). Comparison of alternative regression models for paired binary data. *Statistics in Medicine*, **13**, 1023–1036.

Goeman, J. J., and le Cessie, S. (2006). A goodness-of-fit test for multinomial logistic regression. *Biometrics*, **62**, 980–985.

Goldstein, H. (1991). Nonlinear multilevel models, with an application to discrete response data. *Biometrika*, **78**, 45–51.

Goldstein, H., Browne, W., and Rasbash, J. (2002). Multilevel modelling of medical data. *Statistics in Medicine*, **21**, 3291–3315.

Goldstein, H. (2003). *Multilevel Statistical Models*, 3rd Edition, London, Arnold.

Goldstein, H., and Healy, M. (1995). The graphical presentation of a collection of means. *Journal of the Royal Statistical Society, Series A*, **158**, 175–177.

Goldstein, H., and Rasbash, J. (1996). Improved approximations for multilevel models with binary responses. *Journal of the Royal Statistical Society, Series A*, **159**, 505–513.

Green, P. (1995). Reversible jump Markov Chain Monte Carlo computation and Bayesian model determination. *Biometrika*, **82**, 711–732.

Greenland, S. (1983). Tests for interaction in epidemiologic studies: a review and a study of power. *Statistics in Medicine*, **2**, 243–251.

Greenland, S. (1989). Modelling variable selection in epidemiologic analysis. *American Journal of Public Health*, **79**, 340–349.

Greenland, S. (1993). Additive risk versus additive relative risk models. *Epidemiology*, **4**, 32–36.

Greenland, S. (1994). Alternative models for ordinal logistic regression. *Statistics in Medicine*, **13**, 1665–1677.

Greenland, S. (2007). Bayesian perspectives for epidemiological research II. Regression analysis. *International Journal of Epidemiology*, **36**, 195–202.

Griffiths, W. E., and Pope, P. J. (1987). Small sample properties of probit models. *Journal of the American Statistical Association*, **82**, 929–937.

Grizzle, J., Starmer, F., and Koch, G. (1969). Analysis of categorical data by linear models. *Biometrics*, **25**, 489–504.

Groeger, J. S., Lemeshow, S., Price, K., Nierman, D. M., White, P., Klar, J., Granovsky, S., Horak, D., and Kish, S. (1998). Multicenter Outcome Study of Cancer Patients Admitted to the Intensive Care Unit: A Probability of Mortality Model. *Journal of Clinical Oncology*, **16**, 761–770.

Guo, G., and Zhao, H. (2000). Multilevel modeling for binary data. *Annual Review of Sociology*, **26**, 441–462.

Hafeman, D. M. (2009). Proportion explained: A causal interpretation for standard measures of indirect effects. *American Journal of Epidemiology*, **170**, 1443–1448.

Hafeman, D. M., and Schwartz, S. (2009). Opening the Black Box: a motivation for the assessment of mediation. *International Journal of Epidemiology*, **38**, 838–845.

Hall, C., Zeger, S., and Bandeen-Roche, K. (1994). *Added Variable Plots for Regression with Dependent Data, Technical Report*. Department of Biostatistics, John Hopkins School of Hygiene and Public Health, Baltimore, MD.

Halpern, M., Blackwelder, W. C., and Verter, J. I. (1971). Estimation of the multivariate logistic risk function: A comparison of the discriminant function and maximum likelihood approaches. *Journal of Chronic Disease*, **24**, 125–158.

Han, C., and Carlin, B. (2001). Markov Chain Monte Carlo methods for computing Bayes Factors: A comparative review. *Journal of the American Statistical Association*, **96**, 1122–1132.

Harle, O., and Zhou, X-H. (2007). Multiple imputation: Review of theory, implementation and software. *Statistics in Medicine*, **26**, 3057–3077.

Harrell, F. E. (2001). *Regression Modeling Strategies with Applications to Linear Models, Logistic Regression and Survival Analysis*, Springer, New York.

Harrell, F. E., Lee, K. L., and Mark, D. B. (1996). Tutorial in biostatistics: Multivariable prognostic models: Issues in developing models, evaluating assumptions and measuring and reducing errors. *Statistics in Medicine*, **15**, 361–387.

Haseman, J. K., and Hogan, M. D. (1975). Selection of the experimental unit in teratology studies. *Teratology*, **12**, 165–172.

Haseman, J. J., and Kupper, L. L. (1979). Analysis of dichotomous response data from certain toxicological experiments. *Biometrics*, **35**, 281–293.

Hastings, W. (1970). Monte Carlo sampling methods using Markov chains and their applications. *Biometrika*, **57**, 97–109.

Hauck, W. W., and Donner, A. (1977). Wald's test as applied to hypotheses in logit analysis. *Journal of the American Statistical Association*, **72**, 851–853.

Hedeker, D., and Gibbons, R. (2006). *Longitudinal Data Analysis*, Wiley Inc., Hoboken, NJ.

Heidelberger, P., and Welch, P. (1981). A spectral method for confidence interval generation and run length control in simulations. *Communications of the ACM*, **24**, 233–245.

Heidelberger, P., and Welch, P. (1983). Simulation run length control in the presence of an initial transient. *Operations Research*, **31**, 1109–1144.

Heinze, G. (2006). A comparative investigation of methods for logistic regression with separated or nearly separated data. *Statistics in Medicine*, **25**, 4216–4226.

Heinze, G., and Schemper, M. (2002). A solution to the problem of separation in logistic regression. *Statistics in Medicine*, **21**, 2409–2419.

Heo, M., and Leon, A. (2005). Comparison of statistical methods for the analysis of binary observations. *Statistics in Medicine*, **24**, 911–923.

Hill, J. (2008). Discussion of research using propensity score matching: Comments on "A critical appraisal of propensity score matching in the medical literature between 1996 and 2003". *Statistics in Medicine*, **27**, 2055–2061.

Hirji, K. F. (1992). Exact distributions for polytomous data. *Journal of the American Statistical Association*, **87**, 487–492.

Hirji, K. F., Mehta, C. R., and Patel, N. R. (1987). Computing distributions for exact logistic regression. *Journal of the American Statistical Association*, **82**, 1110–1117.

Hirji, K. F., Mehta, C. R., and Patel, N. R. (1988). Exact inference for matched case-control studies. *Biometrics*, **44**, 803–814.

Hirji, K. F., Tsiatis, A. A., and Mehta, C. R. (1989). Median unbiased estimation for binary data. *The American Statistician*, **43**, 7–11.

Hjort, N. L. (1988). *Estimating the Logistic Regression Equation when the Model is Incorrect. Technical Report*. Norwegian Computing Center, Oslo, Norway.

Hjort, N. L. (1999). Estimation in moderately misspecified models. Statistical Research Report, Department of Mathematics, University of Oslo, Oslo.

Hoeting, J., Madigan, D., Raftery, A., and Volinsky, C. (1999). Bayesian Model Averaging (with discussion). *Statistical Science*, **14**, 382–417.

Horton, N., Bebchuk, J., Jones, C., Lipsitz, S., Catalano, P., Zahner, G., and Fitzmaurice, G. (1999). Goodness-of-fit for GEE: an example with mental health service utilization. *Statistics in Medicine*, **18**, 213–222.

Horton, N., and Lipsitz, S. (2001). Multiple imputation in practice: Comparison of software packages for regression models with missing values. *The American Statistician*, **55**, 244–254.

Horton, N., Lipsitz, S., and Parzen, M. (2003). A potential for bias when rounding in multiple imputation. *The American Statistician*, **57**, 229–232.

Hosmer, T., Hosmer, D. W., and Fisher, L. L. (1983). A comparison of the maximum likelihood and discriminant function estimators of the coefficients of the logistic regression model for mixed continuous and discrete variables. *Communications in Statistics*, **B12**, 577–593.

Hosmer, D. W., Hosmer, T., Le Cessie, S., and Lemeshow, S. (1997). A comparison of goodness-of-fit tests for the logistic regression model. *Statistics in Medicine*, **16**, 965–980.

Hosmer, D. W., Jovanovic, B., and Lemeshow, S. (1989). Best subsets logistic regression. *Biometrics*, **45**, 1265–1270.

Hosmer, D. W., and Lemeshow, S. (1980). A goodness-of-fit test for the multiple logistic regression model. *Communications in Statistics*, **A10**, 1043–1069.

Hosmer, D. W., and Lemeshow, S. (1992). Confidence interval estimation of interaction. *Epidemiology*, **3**, 452–456.

Hosmer, D. W., and Lemeshow, S. (2000). *Applied Logistic Regression Analysis, Second Edition*, John Wiley and Sons Inc., New York.

Hosmer, D. W., Lemeshow, S., and Klar, J. (1988). Goodness-of-fit testing for multiple logistic regression analysis when the estimated probabilities are small. *Biometrical Journal*, **30**, 911–924.

Hosmer, D. W., Lemeshow, S., and May, S. (2008). *Applied Survival Analysis: Regression Modeling of Time to Event Data, Second Edition*, John Wiley and Sons Inc., New York.

Hsieh, F. Y. (1989). Sample size tables for logistic regression. *Statistics in Medicne*, **8**, 795–802.

Hsieh, F. Y., Bloch, D. A., and Larsen, M. (1998). A simple method of sample size calculation for linear and logistic regression. *Statistics in Medicine*, **17**, 1623–1634.

Jennings, D. E. (1986). Outliers and residual distributions in logistic regression. *Journal of the American Statistical Association*, **81**, 987–990.

Judd, C. M., and Kenny, D. A. (1981). Process analysis: estimating mediation in treatment evaluations. *Evaluation Review*, **5**, 602–619.

Kalilani, L., and Atashili, J. (2006). Measuring additive interaction using odds ratios. *Epidemiologic Perspectives & Innovations*, **3**, 5.

Kass, R., Carlin, B., Gelman, A., and Neal, R. (1998). Markov Chain Monte Carlo in practice: a roundtable discussion. *The American Statistician*, **52**, 93–100.

Kass, R., and Raftery, A. (1995). Bayes Factors. *Journal of the American Statistical Association*, **90**, 773–795.

Kay, R., and Little, S. (1986). Assessing the fit of the logistic model: A case study of children with haemalytic uraemic syndrome. *Applied Statistics*, **35**, 16–30.

Kelsey, J. L., Thompson, W. D., and Evans, A. S. (1986). *Methods in Observational Epidemiology*, Oxford University Press, New York.

Kleinbaum, D. G., Kupper, L. L., and Morgenstern, H. (1982). *Epidemiologic Research: Principles and Quantitative Methods*, Nostrand Reinhold, New York.

Kleinbaum, D. G., Kupper, L. L., Muller, K. E., and Nizam, A. (1998). *Applied Regression Analysis and Other Multivariable Methods*, *Third Edition*, Duxbury, Belmont, CA.

Knol, M. J., van der Tweel, I., Grobbee, D. E., Numans, M. E., and Geerlings, M. I. (2007). Estimating interaction on an additive scale between continuous determinants in a logistic regression model. *International Journal of Epidemiology*, **36**, 1111–1118.

Korn, E. L., and Graubard, B. I. (1990). Simultaneous testing of regression coefficients with complex survey data: Use of Bonferroni t statistics. *American Statistician*, **44**, 270–276.

Kruschke, J. (2011). *Doing Bayesian Data Analysis: A Tutorial with R and BUGS*, Academic Press/Elsevier, Amsterdam.

Kuo, K., and Mallick, B. (1998). Variable selection for regression models. *Sankhya: The Indian Journal of Statistics, Series B*, **60**, 65–81.

Kuss, O. (2002). Global goodness of fit testing in logistic regression with sparse data. *Statistics in Medicine*, **21**, 3789–3801.

Lachenbruch, P. A. (1975). *Discriminant Analysis*, Hafner, New York.

Landwehr, J. M., Pregibon, D., and Shoemaker, A. C. (1984). Graphical methods for assessing logistic regression models. *Journal of the American Statistical Association*, **79**, 61–71.

Lange, N., and Ryan, L. (1989). Assessing normality in random effects models. *The Annals of Statistics*, **17**, 624–642.

Langford, I., and Lewis, T. (1998). Outliers in multilevel data. *Journal of the Royal Statistical Society, Series A*, **161**, 121–160.

Larsen, K., and Merlo, J. (2005). Appropriate assessment of neighborhood effects on individual health: integrating random and fixed effects in multilevel logistic regression. *American Journal of Epidemiology*, **161**, 81–88.

Larsen, K., Petersen, J., Budtz-Jorgensen, E., and Endahl, L. (2000). Interpreting parameters in the logistic regression model with random effects. *Biometrics*, **56**, 909–914.

Lawless, J. F., and Singhal, K. (1978). Efficient screening of non-normal regression models. *Biometrics*, **34**, 318–327.

Lawless, J. F., and Singhal, K. (1987a). ISMOD: An all subsets regression program for generalized linear models I. Statistical and computational background. *Computer Methods and Programs in Biomedicine*, **24**, 117–124.

Lawless, J. F., and Singhal, K. (1987b). ISMOD: An all subsets regression program for generalized linear models II. Program guide and examples. *Computer Methods and Programs in Biomedicine*, **24**, 125–134.

Le Cessie, S., and van Houwelingen, J. C. (1991). A goodness-of-fit test for binary data based on smoothing residuals. *Biometrics*, **47**, 1267–1282.

Le Cessie, S., and van Houwelingen, J. C. (1995). Testing the fit of a regression model via score tests in random effects models. *Biometrics*, **51**, 600–614.

Lee, K., and Carlin, J. (2010). Multiple imputation for missing data: Fully conditional specification versus multivariate normal imputation. *American Journal of Epidemiology*, **171**, 624–632.

Lee, K., and Koval, J. J. (1997). Determination of the best significance level in forward stepwise logistic regression. *Communication in Statistics B*, **26**, 559–575.

Legler, J. M., and Ryan, L. M. (1997). Latent variable models for teratogenesis using multiple binary outcomes. *Journal of the American Statistical Association*, **92**, 13–20.

Lemeshow, S., and Hosmer, D. W. (1982). The use of goodness-of-fit statistics in the development of logistic regression models. *American Journal of Epidemiology*, **115**, 92–106.

Lemeshow, S., and Le Gall, J. (1994). Modeling the severity of illness of ICU patients: A system update. *Journal of the American Medical Association*, **272**, 1049–1055.

Lemeshow, S., Teres, D., Avrunin, J. S., and Pastides, H. (1988). Predicting the outcome of intensive care unit patients. *Journal of the American Statistical Association*, **83**, 348–356.

Lemeshow, S., Teres, D., Klar, J., Avrunin, J. S., Gelbach, S. H., and Rapoport, J. (1993). Mortality probability models (MPM II) based on an international cohort of intensive care unit patients. *Journal of the American Medical Association*, **270**, 2478–2486.

Lesaffre, E. (1986). Logistic discriminant analysis with applications in electrocardiography. Unpublished D.Sc. Thesis, University of Leuven, Belgium.

Lesaffre, E., and Albert, A. (1989). Multiple-group logistic regression diagnostics. *Applied Statistics*, **38**, 425–440.

Lesaffre, E., and Spiessens, B. (2001). On the effect of the number of quadrature points in a logistic random effects model; an example. *Applied Statistics*, **50**, 325–335.

Leuven, E., and Sianesi, B. (2003). PSMATCH2: Stats module to perform full Mahalanobis and propensity score matching, common support graphing and covariate imbalance testing. http://ideas.repec.org/c/boc/bocode/s432001.html, version 4.0.5 18apr2012.

Lewis, S., and Raftery, A. (1997). Estimating Bayes Factors via posterior simulation with the Laplace-Metropolis estimator. *Journal of the American Statistical Association*, **92**, 648–655.

Liang, K. Y., and Zeger, S. L. (1986). Longitudinal data analysis using generalized linear models. *Biometika*, **73**, 13–22.

Lilienfeld, D. E., and Stolley, P. D. (1994). *Foundations of Epidemiology, Third Edition*, Oxford University Press, New York.

Lin, D. Y., Pstay, B. M., and Kronmal, R. A. (1998). Assessing the sensitivity of regression results to unmeasured confounders in observational studies. *Biometrics*, **54**, 948–963.

Lindsey, C., and Sheather, S. (2010). Variable selection in linear regression. *The Stata Journal*, **10**, 650–669.

Lindsey, J., and Lambert, P. (1998). On the appropriateness of marginal models for repeated measurements in clinical trials. *Statistics in Medicine*, **17**, 447–469.

Lipsitz, S. R., Fitzmaurice, G. M., and Molenberghs, G. (1996). Goodness-of-fit tests for ordinal response regression models. *Applied Statistics*, **45**, 175–190.

Little, R., and Rubin, D. (2002). *Statistical Analysis with Missing Data, Second Edition*, Wiley, New York.

LogXact 9 for Windows. (2012). *Logistic Regression Software Featuring Exact Methods*, Cytel Software, Cambridge, MA.

Lundberg, M., Fredlund, P., Hallqvist, J., and Diderichsen, F. (1996). A SAS program calculating three measures of interaction with confidence intervals. *Epidemiology*, **7**, 655–656.

Lunn, D., Spiegelhalter, D., Thomas, A., and Best, N. (2009). The BUGS project: evolution, critique and future directions (with discussion). *Statistics in Medicine*, **28**, 3049–3067.

Lyles, L. H., Guo, Y., and Hill, A. N. (2009). A fresh look at the discriminant function approach for estimating crude or adjusted odds ratios. *American Statistician*, **63**, 320–327.

Lynn, H. S., and McCulloch, C. E. (1992). When does it pay to break the matches for an analysis of a matched-pairs design. *Biometrics*, **48**, 397–409.

MacKinnon, D. P. (2008). *Mediation in Categorical Data Analysis. In Introduction to Statistical Mediation Analysis*, Taylor and Francis, New York.

Maldonado, G., and Greenland, S. (1993). Interpreting model coefficients when the true model form is unknown. *Epidemiology*, **4**, 310–318.

Mallows, C. L. (1973). Some comments on Cp. *Technometrics*, **15**, 661–676.

Martin, N., and Pardo, L. (2009). On the asymptotic distribution of Cook's distance in logistic regression models. *Journal of Applied Statistics*, **36**, 1119–1146.

Masaoud, E., and Stryhn, H. (2010). A simulation study to assess statistical methods for binary repeated measures data. *Preventive Veterinary Medicine*, **93**, 81–97.

Mathematical Equation Editor. (2008). Math Type 6.0, Design Sciences, Inc., Long Beach, CA.

McCullagh, P. (1985a). On the asymptotic distribution of Pearson's statistics in linear exponential family models. *International Statistical Review*, **53**, 61–67.

McCullagh, P. (1985b). Sparse data and conditional tests. *Proceedings of the 45th Session of the ISI* (Amsterdam), Invited Paper 28, **3**, 1–10.

McCullagh, P. (1986). The conditional distribution of goodness-of-fit statistics for discrete data. *Journal of the American Statistical Association*, **81**, 104–107.

McCullagh, P., and Nelder, J. A. (1989). *Generalized Linear Models, Second Edition*, Chapman & Hall, London.

McCulloch, C., and Searle, S. (2001). *Generalized, Linear, and Mixed Models*, Wiley Inc, New York.

McFadden, D. (1974). Conditional logit analysis of qualitative choice behavior. In *Frontiers in Econometrics*, edited by P. Zarembka, Academic Press, New York.

Mehta, C. R., and Patel, N. R. (1995). Exact logistic regression: Theory and examples. *Statistics in Medicine*, **14**, 2143–2160.

Metropolis, N. and Ulam, S. (1949). The Monte Carlo method. *Journal of the American Statistical Association*, **44**, 335–341.

Metropolis, N., Rosenbluth, A., Rosenbluth, M., Teller, A., and Teller, E. (1953). Equation of state calculations by fast computing machines. *Journal of Chemical Physics*, **21**, 1087–1092.

Mickey, J., and Greenland, S. (1989). A study of the impact of confounder-selection criteria on effect estimation. *American Journal of Epidemiology*, **129**, 125–137.

Microsoft Corporation. (1998). *Microsoft® Word 98, Word Processing Program for the Apple® Macintosh™*, Microsoft Corporation, Bellevue.

Miettinen, O. S. (1976). Stratification by multivariate confounder score. *American Journal of Epidemiology*, **104**, 609–620.

Miller, M. E., Hui, S. L., and Tierney, W. M. (1991). Validation Techniques for logistic regression models. *Statistics in Medicine*, **10**, 1213–1226.

Mittlböck, M., and Schemper, M. (1996). Explained variation for logistic regression. *Statistics in Medicine*, **15**, 1987–1997.

Mittlböck, M., and Schemper, M. (2002). Explained variation for logistic regression – Small sample adjustments, confidence intervals and predictive precision. *Biometrical Journal*, **44**, 263–272.

Molenberghs, G., and Verbeke, G. (2005). *Models for Discrete Longitudinal Data*, Springer, New York.

Moolgavkar, S., Lustbader, E., and Venzon, D. J. (1985). Assessing the adequacy of the logistic regression model for matched case-control studies. *Statistics in Medicine*, **4**, 425–435.

Moore, D. S. (1971). A chi-square test with random cell boundaries. *Annals of Mathematical Statistics*, **42**, 147–156.

Moore, D. S., and Spruill, M. C. (1975). Unified large-sample theory of general chi-square statistics for tests of fit. *Annals of Statistics*, **3**, 599–616.

Muthen, B., and Muthen, L. (2008). *Mplus User's Guide*, Muthen and Muthen, Los Angeles.

Nagelkerke, N., Smits, J., le Cessie, S., and van Houlwelingen, H. (2005). Testing goodness of fit of the logistic regression model in case-control studies using sample reweighting. *Statistics in Medicine*, **24**, 121–130.

Neuhaus, J. M. (1992). Statistical methods for longitudinal and clustered designs with binary data. *Statistical Methods in Medical Research*, **1**, 249–273.

Neuhaus, J. M., Kalbfleisch, J. D., and Hauck, W. W. (1991). A comparison of cluster-specific and population-average approaches for analyzing correlated binary data. *International Statistical Review*, **59**, 25–35.

Neuhaus, J. M., and Jewell, N. P. (1993). A geometric approach to assess bias due to omitted covariates in generalized linear models. *Biometrika*, **80**, 807–815.

Neuhaus, J. M., and Segal, M. R. (1993). Design effects for binary regression models fitted to dependent data. *Statistics in Medicine*, **12**, 1259–1268.

Ng, E., Carpenter, J., Goldstein, H., and Rasbash, J. (2006). Estimation in generalized linear mixed models with binary outcomes by simulated maximum likelihood. *Statistical Modeling*, **6**, 23–42.

NHANES III Reference Manuals and Reports. (2012). Centers for Disease Control and Prevention (CDC). National Center for Health Statistics (NCHS). National Health and Nutrition Examination Survey Data. U.S. Department of Health and Human Services, Centers for Disease Control and Prevention, Hyattsville, MD, http://www.cdc.gov/nchs/nhanes/nhanes2011-2012/nhanes11_12.htm.

Ntzoufras, I. (2002). Gibbs variable selection using BUGS. *Journal of Statistical Software*, **7**, 1–19.

Ntzoufras, I. (2009). *Baysian Modeling using WinBUGS*, Wiley, Hoboken.

Oleckno, W. A. (2008). *Epidemiology: Concepts and Methods*, Waveland Press Inc., Long Grove, Illinois.

Osius, G., and Rojek, D. (1992). Normal goodness-of-fit tests for multinomial models with large degrees-of-freedom. *Journal of the American Statistical Association*, **87**, 1145–1152.

Osler, T., Glance, L. G., and Hosmer, D. W. (2010). Simplified estimates of the probability of death after burn injuries: extending and updating the baux score. *The Journal of Trauma*, **68**, 690–697.

Pan, W. (2001). Akaike's information criterion in generalized estimating equations. *Biometrics*, **57**, 120–125.

Pan, W. (2002). Goodness of fit tests for GEE with correlated binary data. *Scandinavian Journal of Statistics*, **29**, 101–110.

PASS Users Guide. (2012). PASS 11.0: Power and Sample Size for Windows. Number Cruncher Statistical Software, Kaysville, UT.

Paul, P., Pennell, M. L., and Lemeshow, S. (2013) Standardizing the power of the Hosmer-Lemeshow goodness of fit test in large data sets. *Stat Med.* **32**(1), 67–80.

Peduzzi, P. N., Concato, J., Kemper, E., Holford, T. R., and Feinstein, A. (1996). A simulation study of the number of events per variable in logistic regression analysis. *Journal of Clinical Epidemiology*, **99**, 1373–1379.

Pendergast, J. F., Gange, S. J., Newton, M. A., Lindstrom, M. J., Palta, M., and Fisher, M. R. (1996). A survey of methods for analyzing clustered binary response data. *International Statistical Review*, **64**, 89–118.

Pigeon, J. G., and Heyse, J. F. (1999a). An improved goodness of fit test for probability predication models. *Biometrical Journal*, **41**, 71–82.

Pigeon, J. G., and Heyse, J. F. (1999b). A cautionary note on assessing fit of logistic regression models. *Journal of Applied Statistics*, **26**, 847–853.

Pinheiro, J., and Bates, D. (1995). Approximations to the log-likelihood function in the non-linear mixed-effects model. *Journal of Computational and Graphical Statistics*, **4**, 12–35.

Plummer, M. (2003). JAGS: A program for analysis of Bayesian graphical models using Gibbs sampling. Available at http://mcmc-jags.sourceforge.net/.

Plummer, M. (2012). Package 'rjags'. Available from http://cran.r-project.org/web/packages/rjags/rjags.pdf.

Plummer, M., Best, N., Cowles, K., and Vines, K. (2006). CODA: Convergence Diagnosis and Output Analysis for MCMC. *R News*, **6**, 7–11.

Poirier, D. J. (1973). Piecewise regression using cubic splines. *Journal of the American Statistical Association*, **68**, 515–524.

Pregibon, D. (1981). Logistic regression diagnostics. *Annals of Statistics*, **9**, 705–724.

Pregibon, D. (1984). Data analytic methods for matched case-control studies. *Biometrics*, **40**, 639–651.

Preisser, J., and Qaqish, B. (1996). Deletion diagnostics for Generalized Estimating Equations. *Biometrika*, **83**, 551–562.

Prentice, R. L. (1986). A case-cohort design for epidemiologic cohort studies and disease prevention trials. *Biometrika*, **73**, 1–11.

Prentice, R. L., and Pyke, R. (1979). Logistic disease incidence models and case-control studies. *Biometrika*, **66**, 403–411.

Pulkstenis, E., and Robinson, T. J. (2002). Two goodness-of-fit tests for logistic regression models with continuous covariates. *Statistics in Medicine* **21**, 79–93.

Pulkstenis, E., and Robinson, T. J. (2004). Goodness-of-fit test for ordinal response regression models. *Statistics in Medicine*, **23**, 999–1014.

R Development Core Team. (2010). *R: A Language and Environment for Statistical Computing*. R Foundation for Statistical Computing, Vienna, Austria.

Rabe-Hesketh, S., and Skrondal, A. (2008). *Multilevel and Longitudinal Modeling Using Stata, Second Edition*, StataCorp LP, College Station, Texas.

Rabe-Hesketh, S., Skrondal, A., and Pickles, A. (2002). Reliable estimation of generalized linear mixed models using adaptive quadrature. *The Stata Journal*, **2**, 1–21.

Rabe-Hesketh, S., Skrondal, A., and Pickles, A. (2005). Maximum likelihood estimation of limited and discrete dependent variable models with nested random effects. *Journal of Econometrics*, **128**, 301–323.

Raftery, A., and Lewis, S. (1992). One long run with diagnostics: implementation strategies for Markov Chain Monte Carlo. *Statistical Science*, **7**, 493–497.

Raftery, A., and Lewis, S. (1996). The number of iterations, convergence diagnostics and generic Metropolis algorithms. In *Markov Chain Monte Carlo in Practice*, edited by W. Gilks, D. Spiegelhalter, and S. Richardson, Chapman and Hall, London.

Raghunathan, T., Lepkowski, J., Van Hoewyk, J., and Solenberger, P. (2001). A multivariate technique for multiply imputing missing values using a sequence of regression models. *Survey Methodology*, **27**, 85–95.

Rao, C. R. (1973). *Linear Statistical Inference and its Application*, Second Edition, Wiley Inc., New York.

Rasbash, J., Charlton, C., Browne, W., Healy, M., and Cameron, B. (2009). MLwiN Version 2.1. Centre for Multilevel Modelling, University of Bristol.

Richardson, D. B., and Kaufman, J. S. (2009). Estimation of the relative excess risk due to interaction and associated confidence bounds. *American Journal of Epidemiology*, **169**, 756–760.

Roberts, G., Rao, J. N. K., and Kumar, S. (1987). Logistic regression analysis of sample survey data. *Biometrika*, **74**, 1–12.

Robertson, C., Boyle, P., Hsieh, C. C., Macfarlane, G. J., and Maisonneuve, P. (1994). Some statistical considerations in the analysis of case-control studies when the exposure variables are continuous measurements. *Epidemiology*, **5**, 164–170.

Robins, J. M., and Greenland, S. (1992). Identifiability and exchangeability for direct and indirect effects. *Epidemiology*, **3**, 143–155.

Rodriguez, G., and Goldman, N. (1995). An assessment of estimation procedures for multilevel models with binary responses. *Journal of the Royal Statistical Society, Series A*, **158**, 73–90.

Rodriguez, G., and Goldman, N. (2001). Improved estimation procedures for multilevel models with binary responses. *Journal of the Royal Statistical Society, Series A*, **164**, 339–355.

Rosenbaum, P. R., and Rubin, D. B. (1983). The central role of the propensity score in observational studies. *Biometrika*, **70**, 41–55.

Rosenbaum, P. R., and Rubin, D. B. (1984). Reducing bias in observational studies using subclassification on the propensity score. *Journal of the American Statistical Association*, **79**, 516–524.

Rosner, B. (1984). Multivariate methods in ophthalmology with application to other paired-data situations. *Biometrics*, **40**, 1025–1035.

Ross, S. (1995). *Stochastic Processes*, Wiley, Hoboken.

Rothman, K. J., Greenland, S., and Lash, T.L. (2008). *Modern Epidemiology*, *Third Edition*, Lippincott-Raven, Philadelphia.

Rotnitzky, A., and Jewell, N. (1990). Hypothesis testing of regression parameters in semiparametric generalized linear models for cluster correlated data. *Biometrika*, **77**, 485–497.

Royston, P. (2004). Multiple imputation of missing values. *The Stata Journal*, **4**, 227–241.

Royston, P. (2005a). Multiple imputation of missing values: Update. *The Stata Journal*, **5**, 188–201.

Royston, P. (2005b). Multiple imputation of missing values: Update of ice. *The Stata Journal*, **5**, 527–536.

Royston, P. (2007). Profile likelihood estimation and confidence intervals. *The Stata Journal*, **7**, 376–387.

Royston, P. (2009). Multiple imputation of missing values: Further update of ice with an emphasis on categorical variables. *The Stata Journal*, **9**, 466–477.

Royston, P., and Altman, D. G. (1994). Regression using fractional polynomials of continuous covariates: Parsimonious parametric modelling (with discussion). *Applied Statistics*, **43**, 429–467.

Royston, P., and Altman, D. G. (2010). Visualizing and assessing discrimination in the logistic regression model. *Statistics in Medicine*, **29**, 2508–2520.

Royston, P., Altman, D. G., and Sauerbrei, W. (2006). Dichotomizing continuous predictors in multiple regression: A bad idea. *Statistics in Medicine*, **25**, 127–141.

Royston, P., and Ambler, G. (1998). Multivariable fractional polynomials. *Stata Technical Bulletin*, **STB–43**, 24–32.

Royston, P., and Ambler, G. (1999). Multivariable fractional polynomials: update. *Stata Technical Bulletin*, **STB–49**, 17–22.

Royston, P., Ambler, G., and Sauerbrei, W. (1999). The use of fractional polynomials to model continuous risk variables in epidemiology. *International Journal of Epidemiology*, **28**, 964–974.

Royston, P., and Sauerbrei, W. (2008). *Multivariable Model Building: A Pragmatic Approach to Regression Analysis Based on Fractional Polynomials for Modelling Continuous Variables*, John Wiley & Sons Ltd., Chichester.

Rubin, D. (1976). Inference and missing data. *Biometrika*, **63**, 581–592.

Rubin, D. (1987). *Multiple Imputation for Nonresponse in Surveys*, John Wiley & Sons Inc., New York.

Ryan, L. M. (1992). Quantitative risk assessment for developmental toxicity. *Biometrics*, **48**, 163–174.

Ryan, T. (1997). *Modern Regression Methods*, Wiley Inc., New York.

Santner, T. J., and Duffy, D. E. (1986). A note on A. Albert's and J. A. Anderson's conditions for the existence of maximum likelihood estimates in logistic regression models. *Biometrika*, **73**, 755–758.

SAS Institute Inc. (2009). *SAS Guide for Personal Computers, Version 9.2*, SAS Institute Inc., Cary, NC.

Sauerbrei, W. (1999). The use of resampling methods to simplify regression models in medical statistics. *Applied Statistics*, **48**, 313–329.

Sauerbrei, W., Meier-Hirmer, A., Benner, C., and Royston, P. (2006). Multivariable regression model building by using fractional polynomials: Description of SAS, STATA and R programs. *Computational Statistics and Data Analysis*, **50**, 3464–3485.

Sauerbrei, W., and Royston, P. (1999). Building multivariable prognostic and diagnostic models: Transformations of the predictors using fractional polynomials. *Journal of the Royal Statistical Society, Series A*, **162**, 71–94.

Schaefer, R. L. (1983). Bias correction in maximum likelihood regression. *Statistics in Medicine*, **2**, 71–78.

Schaefer, R. L. (1986). Alternative estimators in logistic regression when the data are collinear. *Journal of Statistical Computation and Simulation*, 25, 75–91.

Schafer, J. (1997). *Analysis of Incomplete Multivariate Data*. Chapman and Hall, New York.

Schafer, J. (1999). Multiple imputation: A primer. *Statistical Methods in Medical Research*, 8, 3–15.

Schafer, J., and Graham, J. (2002). Missing data: Our view of the state of the art. *Psychological Methods*, 7, 147–177.

Schlesselman, J. J. (1985). *Case-Control Studies: Design, Conduct, Analysis*, Oxford University Press, New York.

Schoenberg, I. J. (1946). Contribution to the problem of approximation of equidistant data by analytic functions. Part A – On the problem of smoothing or graduation. A first class of approximation formulae. *Quarterly Journal of Applied Mathematics*, 4, 45–99.

Schwartz, S. (2006). *Committee on Assessing Interactions Among Social, Behavioral, and Genetic Factors in Health. "Appendix E Modern Epidemiologic Approaches to Interaction: Applications to the Study of Genetic Interactions." Genes, Behavior, and the Social Environment: Moving Beyond the Nature/Nurture Debate*, The National Academies Press, Washington, D.C.

Scott, A. J., and Wild, C. J. (1991). Fitting models under case-control or choice based sampling. *Journal of the Royal Statistical Association, Series B*, 48, 170–182.

Self, S., and Liang, K. (1987). Asymptotic properties of maximum likelihood estimators and likelihood ratio tests under nonstandard conditions. *Journal of the American Statistical Association*, 82, 605–610.

Shah, B. V., Barnwell, B. G., and Bieler, G. S. (2002). SUDAAN User's Manual, Release 8.0.1. Research Triangle Institute, Research Triangle Park, NC.

Sheih, G. (2001). Sample size calculation for logistic and Poisson regression. *Biometrika*, 88, 1193–1199.

Skinner, C. J., Holt, D., and Smith, T. M. F. (1989). *Analysis of Complex Surveys*, Wiley Inc., New York.

Skrondal, A. (2003). Interaction as departure from additivity in case-control studies: A cautionary note. *American Journal of Epidemiology*, 158, 251–258.

Skrondal, A., and Rabe-Hesketh, S. (2009). Prediction in multilevel generalized linear models. *Journal of the Royal Statistical Society, Series A*, 172, 659–687.

Snijders, T., and Bosker, R. (1999). *Multilevel Analysis, An Introduction to Basic and Advanced Multilevel Modeling*, SAGE publications, London.

Spiegelhalter, D., Best, N., Carlin, B., and van der Linde, A. (2002). Bayesian measures of model complexity and fit. *Journal of the Royal Statistical Society, Series B*, 64, 583–639.

Spiegelman, D., and Hertzmark, E. (2005). Easy SAS calculation for risk or prevalence ratios and differences. *American Journal of Epidemiology*, 162, 199–200.

SPSS for Windows, Release 20.0. (2012). SPSS Inc., Chicago.

Stallard, N. (2009). Simple tests for the external validation of mortality prediction scores. *Statistics in Medicine*, 28, 377–388.

StataCorp. (2011). *Stata: Release 12*. Statistical Software Stata Corporation, College Station, TX.

Stiratelli, R., Laird, N., and Ware, J. (1984). Random-effects models for serial observations with binary response. *Biometrics*, 40, 961–971.

Stukel, T. A. (1988). Generalized logistic models. *Journal of the American Statistical Association*, **83**, 426–431.

Sturdivant, R. X. (2005). Goodness-of-fit in hierarchical logistic regression models. Unpublished doctoral dissertation, University of Massachusetts, Amherst, MA.

Sturdivant, R. X., and Hosmer, D. W. (2007). A smoothed residual based goodness-of-fit statistic for logistic hierarchical regression models. *Computational Statistics and Data Analysis*, **51**, 3898–3912.

Sturdivant, R. X., Rotella, J. J., and Russell, R. E. (2007). A smoothed residual based goodness-of-fit statistic for nest survival models. *Studies in Avian Biology*, **34**, 45–54.

Su, J. Q., and Wei, L. J. (1991). A lack-of-fit test for the mean function in a generalized linear model. *Journal of the American Statistical Association*, **86**, 420–426.

Surgeon General (1964). *Smoking and Health. Report on the Advisory Committee to the Surgeon General of the Public Heath Service*, U.S. Department of Health, Education and Welfare, Washington, DC.

Tarone, R. E. (1985). On heterogeneity tests based on efficient scores. *Biometrika*, **72**, 91–95.

TenHave, T., and Ratcliffe, S. (2004). Deviations from the population-averaged versus cluster-specific relationship for clustered binary data. *Statistical Methods in Medical Research*, **13**, 3–16.

Thomas, A. (2004). BRugs User Manual. Available from http://www.openbugs.info/w /UserContributedCode.

Thomas, D. R., and Rao, J. N. K. (1987). Small-sample comparisons of level and power for simple goodness-of-fit statistics under cluster sampling. *Journal of the American Statistical Association*, **82**, 630–636.

Tjur, T. (2009). Coefficients of determination in logistic regression models – A new proposal: The coefficient of discrimination. *American Statistician*, **63**, 366–372.

Tritchler, D. (1984). An algorithm for exact logistic regression. *Journal of the American Statistical Association*, **79**, 709–711.

Truett, J., Cornfield, J., and Kannel, W. (1967). A multivariate analysis of the risk of coronary heart disease in Framingham. *Journal of Chronic Diseases*, **20**, 511–524.

Tsiatis, A. A. (1980). A note on a goodness-of-fit test for the logistic regression model. *Biometrika*, **67**, 250–251.

van Buuren, S., Brand, P., Groothuis-Oudshoorn, C., and Rubin, D. (2006). Fully conditional specification in multivariate imputation. *Journal of Statistical Computation and Simulation*, **76**, 1049–1064.

VanderWeele, T. J. (2009). Sufficient cause interactions and statistical interactions. *Epidemiology*, **20**, 6–13.

VanderWeele, T. J., and Vansteelandt, S. (2010). Odds ratios for mediation analysis for a dichotomous outcome. *American Journal of Epidemiology*, **172**, 1339–1348.

Venzon, D. J., and Moolgavkar, S. H. (1988). A method for computing profile-likelihood based confidence intervals. *Applied Statistics*, **37**, 87–94.

Verbeke, G., and Molenberghs, G. (2009). *Linear Mixed Models for Longitudinal Data*. Springer, New York.

Vittinghof, E., and McCulloch, C. E. (2006). Relaxing the rule of ten events per variable in logistic and Cox regression. *American Journal of Epidemiology*, **165**, 710–718.

Vonesh, E., Chinchilli, V., and Pu, K. (1996). Goodness-of-fit in generalized nonlinear mixed-effects models. *Biometrics*, **52**, 572–587.

Weesie, J. (1998). Windmeijer's goodness-of-fit test for logistic regression. *Stata Technical Bulletin*, **STB-44**, 22–27.

Welsch, R. (1986). Discussion of paper by S. Chatterjee and A. S. Hadi. *Statistical Science*, **1**, 403–405.

White, H. (1982). Maximum likelihood estimation of misspecified models. *Econometrika*, **50**, 1–25.

White, H. (1989). *Estimation Inference and Specification Analysis*, Cambridge University Press, New York.

White, I., Royston, P., and Wood, A. (2011). Multiple imputation using chained equations: Issues and guidance for practice. *Statistics in Medicine*, **30**, 377–399.

Whitemore, A. S. (1981). Sample size for logistic regression with small response probability. *Journal of the American Statistical Association*, **76**, 27–32.

Williams, D. (1975). The analysis of binary responses from toxicological experiments involving reproduction and teratogenicity. *Biometrics*, **31**, 949–952.

Williamson, E., Morely, R., Lucas, A., and Carpenter, J. (2011). Propensity scores: From naïve enthusiasm to intuitive understanding. *Statistical Methods in Medical Research*, **21**, 273–293.

Windmeijer, F. A. G. (1990). The asymptotic distribution of the sum of weighted squared residuals in binary choice models. *Statistica Neerlandica*, **44**, 69–78.

Wolfe, R. (1998). Continuation-ratio models for ordinal response data. *Stata Technical Bulletin*, **STB-44**, 18–21.

Wolfinger, R., and O'Connell, M. (1993). Generalized linear mixed models: a pseudo-likelihood approach. *Journal of Statistical Computation and Simulation*, **48**, 233–243.

Wong, G., and Mason, W. (1985). The hierarchical logistic regression model for multilevel analysis. *Journal of the American Statistical Association*, **80**, 513–524.

Wood, A., White, I. and Royston, P. (2008). How should variable selection be performed with multiply imputed data. *Statistics in Medicine*, **27**, 3227–3246.

Xu, H. (1996). Extensions of the Hosmer-Lemeshow goodness-of-fit test. Unpublished Masters Thesis, School of Public Health and Health Sciences, University of Massachusetts, Amherst, MA.

Zadnik, K., Mutti, D. O., Friedman, N. E., and Adams, A. J. (1993). Initial cross-sectional results from the Orinda Longitudinal Study of Myopia. *Optometry and Vision Science*, **70**, 750–758.

Zadnik, K., Satariano, W. A., Mutti, D. O., Sholtz, R. I., and Adams, A. J. (1994). The effect of parental history of myopia on children's eye size. *Journal of the American Medical Association*, **271**, 1323–1327.

Zeger, S., and Liang, K. (1986). Longitudinal data analysis for discrete and continuous outcomes. *Biometrics*, **42**, 121–130.

Zeger, S. L., Liang, K-Y., and Albert, P. A. (1988). Models for longitudinal data: A generalized estimating equation approach. *Biometrics*, **44**, 1049–1060.

Zhang, B. (1999). A chi-squared goodness-of-fit for logistic regression models based on case-control data. *Biometrika*, **86**, 531–539.

Zhang, H., Lu, N., Feng, C., Thurston, S., Yinglin, X., Zhu, L., and Tu, X. (2011). On fitting generalized linear mixed-effects models for binary responses using different statistical packages. *Statistics in Medicine*, **30**, 2562–2572.

Zhang, J., and Yu, K. F. (1998). What's the relative risk? *Journal of the American Medical Association*, **280**, 1690–1691.

Zou, G. (2004). A modified Poisson regression approach to prospective studies with binary data. *American Journal of Epidemiology*, **154**, 702–706.

Index

Applied Logistic Regression, Third Edition.
David W. Hosmer, Jr., Stanley Lemeshow, and Rodney X. Sturdivant.
© 2013 John Wiley & Sons, Inc. Published 2013 by John Wiley & Sons, Inc.

>

WILEY SERIES IN PROBABILITY AND STATISTICS
ESTABLISHED BY WALTER A. SHEWHART AND SAMUEL S. WILKS

Editors: *David J. Balding, Noel A. C. Cressie, Garrett M. Fitzmaurice,*
Harvey Goldstein, Iain M. Johnstone, Geert Molenberghs, David W. Scott,
Adrian F. M. Smith, Ruey S. Tsay, Sanford Weisberg
Editors Emeriti: *Vic Barnett, J. Stuart Hunter, Joseph B. Kadane, Jozef L. Teugels*

The *Wiley Series in Probability and Statistics* is well established and authoritative. It covers many topics of current research interest in both pure and applied statistics and probability theory. Written by leading statisticians and institutions, the titles span both state-of-the-art developments in the field and classical methods.

Reflecting the wide range of current research in statistics, the series encompasses applied, methodological and theoretical statistics, ranging from applications and new techniques made possible by advances in computerized practice to rigorous treatment of theoretical approaches.

This series provides essential and invaluable reading for all statisticians, whether in academia, industry, government, or research.

† ABRAHAM and LEDOLTER · Statistical Methods for Forecasting
  AGRESTI · Analysis of Ordinal Categorical Data, *Second Edition*
  AGRESTI · An Introduction to Categorical Data Analysis, *Second Edition*
  AGRESTI · Categorical Data Analysis, *Third Edition*
  ALTMAN, GILL, and McDONALD · Numerical Issues in Statistical Computing for the
    Social Scientist
  AMARATUNGA and CABRERA · Exploration and Analysis of DNA Microarray and
    Protein Array Data
  ANDĚL · Mathematics of Chance
  ANDERSON · An Introduction to Multivariate Statistical Analysis, *Third Edition*
* ANDERSON · The Statistical Analysis of Time Series
  ANDERSON, AUQUIER, HAUCK, OAKES, VANDAELE, and WEISBERG ·
    Statistical Methods for Comparative Studies
  ANDERSON and LOYNES · The Teaching of Practical Statistics
  ARMITAGE and DAVID (editors) · Advances in Biometry
  ARNOLD, BALAKRISHNAN, and NAGARAJA · Records
* ARTHANARI and DODGE · Mathematical Programming in Statistics
* BAILEY · The Elements of Stochastic Processes with Applications to the Natural
    Sciences
  BAJORSKI · Statistics for Imaging, Optics, and Photonics
  BALAKRISHNAN and KOUTRAS · Runs and Scans with Applications
  BALAKRISHNAN and NG · Precedence-Type Tests and Applications
  BARNETT · Comparative Statistical Inference, *Third Edition*
  BARNETT · Environmental Statistics
  BARNETT and LEWIS · Outliers in Statistical Data, *Third Edition*
  BARTHOLOMEW, KNOTT, and MOUSTAKI · Latent Variable Models and Factor
    Analysis: A Unified Approach, *Third Edition*
  BARTOSZYNSKI and NIEWIADOMSKA-BUGAJ · Probability and Statistical
    Inference, *Second Edition*
  BASILEVSKY · Statistical Factor Analysis and Related Methods: Theory and
    Applications
  BATES and WATTS · Nonlinear Regression Analysis and Its Applications
  BECHHOFER, SANTNER, and GOLDSMAN · Design and Analysis of Experiments for
    Statistical Selection, Screening, and Multiple Comparisons

*Now available in a lower priced paperback edition in the Wiley Classics Library.
†Now available in a lower priced paperback edition in the Wiley–Interscience Paperback Series.

BEIRLANT, GOEGEBEUR, SEGERS, TEUGELS, and DE WAAL · Statistics of Extremes: Theory and Applications

BELSLEY · Conditioning Diagnostics: Collinearity and Weak Data in Regression

† BELSLEY, KUH, and WELSCH · Regression Diagnostics: Identifying Influential Data and Sources of Collinearity

BENDAT and PIERSOL · Random Data: Analysis and Measurement Procedures, *Fourth Edition*

BERNARDO and SMITH · Bayesian Theory

BERZUINI, DAWID, and BERNARDINELL · Causality: Statistical Perspectives and Applications

BHAT and MILLER · Elements of Applied Stochastic Processes, *Third Edition*

BHATTACHARYA and WAYMIRE · Stochastic Processes with Applications

BIEMER, GROVES, LYBERG, MATHIOWETZ, and SUDMAN · Measurement Errors in Surveys

BILLINGSLEY · Convergence of Probability Measures, *Second Edition*

BILLINGSLEY · Probability and Measure, *Anniversary Edition*

BIRKES and DODGE · Alternative Methods of Regression

BISGAARD and KULAHCI · Time Series Analysis and Forecasting by Example

BISWAS, DATTA, FINE, and SEGAL · Statistical Advances in the Biomedical Sciences: Clinical Trials, Epidemiology, Survival Analysis, and Bioinformatics

BLISCHKE and MURTHY (editors) · Case Studies in Reliability and Maintenance

BLISCHKE and MURTHY · Reliability: Modeling, Prediction, and Optimization

BLOOMFIELD · Fourier Analysis of Time Series: An Introduction, *Second Edition*

BOLLEN · Structural Equations with Latent Variables

BOLLEN and CURRAN · Latent Curve Models: A Structural Equation Perspective

BOROVKOV · Ergodicity and Stability of Stochastic Processes

BOSQ and BLANKE · Inference and Prediction in Large Dimensions

BOULEAU · Numerical Methods for Stochastic Processes

* BOX and TIAO · Bayesian Inference in Statistical Analysis

BOX · Improving Almost Anything, *Revised Edition*

* BOX and DRAPER · Evolutionary Operation: A Statistical Method for Process Improvement

BOX and DRAPER · Response Surfaces, Mixtures, and Ridge Analyses, *Second Edition*

BOX, HUNTER, and HUNTER · Statistics for Experimenters: Design, Innovation, and Discovery, *Second Editon*

BOX, JENKINS, and REINSEL · Time Series Analysis: Forcasting and Control, *Fourth Edition*

BOX, LUCEÑO, and PANIAGUA-QUIÑONES · Statistical Control by Monitoring and Adjustment, *Second Edition*

* BROWN and HOLLANDER · Statistics: A Biomedical Introduction

CAIROLI and DALANG · Sequential Stochastic Optimization

CASTILLO, HADI, BALAKRISHNAN, and SARABIA · Extreme Value and Related Models with Applications in Engineering and Science

CHAN · Time Series: Applications to Finance with R and S-Plus®, *Second Edition*

CHARALAMBIDES · Combinatorial Methods in Discrete Distributions

CHATTERJEE and HADI · Regression Analysis by Example, *Fifth Edition*

CHATTERJEE and HADI · Sensitivity Analysis in Linear Regression

CHERNICK · Bootstrap Methods: A Guide for Practitioners and Researchers, *Second Edition*

CHERNICK and FRIIS · Introductory Biostatistics for the Health Sciences

CHILÈS and DELFINER · Geostatistics: Modeling Spatial Uncertainty, *Second Edition*

CHOW and LIU · Design and Analysis of Clinical Trials: Concepts and Methodologies, *Second Edition*

CLARKE · Linear Models: The Theory and Application of Analysis of Variance

---

*Now available in a lower priced paperback edition in the Wiley Classics Library.

†Now available in a lower priced paperback edition in the Wiley–Interscience Paperback Series.

CLARKE and DISNEY · Probability and Random Processes: A First Course with
Applications, *Second Edition*
* COCHRAN and COX · Experimental Designs, *Second Edition*
COLLINS and LANZA · Latent Class and Latent Transition Analysis: With Applications
in the Social, Behavioral, and Health Sciences
CONGDON · Applied Bayesian Modelling
CONGDON · Bayesian Models for Categorical Data
CONGDON · Bayesian Statistical Modelling, *Second Edition*
CONOVER · Practical Nonparametric Statistics, *Third Edition*
COOK · Regression Graphics
COOK and WEISBERG · An Introduction to Regression Graphics
COOK and WEISBERG · Applied Regression Including Computing and Graphics
CORNELL · A Primer on Experiments with Mixtures
CORNELL · Experiments with Mixtures, Designs, Models, and the Analysis of Mixture
Data, *Third Edition*
COX · A Handbook of Introductory Statistical Methods
CRESSIE · Statistics for Spatial Data, *Revised Edition*
CRESSIE and WIKLE · Statistics for Spatio-Temporal Data
CSÖRGŐ and HORVÁTH · Limit Theorems in Change Point Analysis
DAGPUNAR · Simulation and Monte Carlo: With Applications in Finance and MCMC
DANIEL · Applications of Statistics to Industrial Experimentation
DANIEL · Biostatistics: A Foundation for Analysis in the Health Sciences, *Eighth Edition*
* DANIEL · Fitting Equations to Data: Computer Analysis of Multifactor Data,
Second Edition
DASU and JOHNSON · Exploratory Data Mining and Data Cleaning
DAVID and NAGARAJA · Order Statistics, *Third Edition*
* DEGROOT, FIENBERG, and KADANE · Statistics and the Law
DEL CASTILLO · Statistical Process Adjustment for Quality Control
DeMARIS · Regression with Social Data: Modeling Continuous and Limited Response
Variables
DEMIDENKO · Mixed Models: Theory and Applications
DENISON, HOLMES, MALLICK and SMITH · Bayesian Methods for Nonlinear
Classification and Regression
DETTE and STUDDEN · The Theory of Canonical Moments with Applications in
Statistics, Probability, and Analysis
DEY and MUKERJEE · Fractional Factorial Plans
DILLON and GOLDSTEIN · Multivariate Analysis: Methods and Applications
* DODGE and ROMIG · Sampling Inspection Tables, *Second Edition*
* DOOB · Stochastic Processes
DOWDY, WEARDEN, and CHILKO · Statistics for Research, *Third Edition*
DRAPER and SMITH · Applied Regression Analysis, *Third Edition*
DRYDEN and MARDIA · Statistical Shape Analysis
DUDEWICZ and MISHRA · Modern Mathematical Statistics
DUNN and CLARK · Basic Statistics: A Primer for the Biomedical Sciences,
Fourth Edition
DUPUIS and ELLIS · A Weak Convergence Approach to the Theory of Large Deviations
EDLER and KITSOS · Recent Advances in Quantitative Methods in Cancer and Human
Health Risk Assessment
* ELANDT-JOHNSON and JOHNSON · Survival Models and Data Analysis
ENDERS · Applied Econometric Time Series, *Third Edition*
† ETHIER and KURTZ · Markov Processes: Characterization and Convergence
EVANS, HASTINGS, and PEACOCK · Statistical Distributions, *Third Edition*

---

*Now available in a lower priced paperback edition in the Wiley Classics Library.
†Now available in a lower priced paperback edition in the Wiley–Interscience Paperback Series.

---

*Now available in a lower priced paperback edition in the Wiley Classics Library.

†Now available in a lower priced paperback edition in the Wiley–Interscience Paperback Series.

* HOAGLIN, MOSTELLER, and TUKEY · Understanding Robust and Exploratory
Data Analysis

HOCHBERG and TAMHANE · Multiple Comparison Procedures

HOCKING · Methods and Applications of Linear Models: Regression and the Analysis
of Variance, *Second Edition*

HOEL · Introduction to Mathematical Statistics, *Fifth Edition*

HOGG and KLUGMAN · Loss Distributions

HOLLANDER and WOLFE · Nonparametric Statistical Methods, *Second Edition*

HOSMER, LEMESHOW, and STURDIVANT · Applied Logistic Regression, *Third
Edition*

HOSMER, LEMESHOW, and MAY · Applied Survival Analysis: Regression Modeling
of Time-to-Event Data, *Second Edition*

HUBER · Data Analysis: What Can Be Learned From the Past 50 Years

HUBER · Robust Statistics

† HUBER and RONCHETTI · Robust Statistics, *Second Edition*

HUBERTY · Applied Discriminant Analysis, *Second Edition*

HUBERTY and OLEJNIK · Applied MANOVA and Discriminant Analysis,
Second Edition

HUITEMA · The Analysis of Covariance and Alternatives: Statistical Methods for
Experiments, Quasi-Experiments, and Single-Case Studies, *Second Edition*

HUNT and KENNEDY · Financial Derivatives in Theory and Practice, *Revised Edition*

HURD and MIAMEE · Periodically Correlated Random Sequences: Spectral Theory
and Practice

HUSKOVA, BERAN, and DUPAC · Collected Works of Jaroslav Hajek—
with Commentary

HUZURBAZAR · Flowgraph Models for Multistate Time-to-Event Data

JACKMAN · Bayesian Analysis for the Social Sciences

† JACKSON · A User's Guide to Principle Components

JOHN · Statistical Methods in Engineering and Quality Assurance

JOHNSON · Multivariate Statistical Simulation

JOHNSON and BALAKRISHNAN · Advances in the Theory and Practice of Statistics: A
Volume in Honor of Samuel Kotz

JOHNSON, KEMP, and KOTZ · Univariate Discrete Distributions, *Third Edition*

JOHNSON and KOTZ (editors) · Leading Personalities in Statistical Sciences: From the
Seventeenth Century to the Present

JOHNSON, KOTZ, and BALAKRISHNAN · Continuous Univariate Distributions,
Volume 1, *Second Edition*

JOHNSON, KOTZ, and BALAKRISHNAN · Continuous Univariate Distributions,
Volume 2, *Second Edition*

JOHNSON, KOTZ, and BALAKRISHNAN · Discrete Multivariate Distributions

JUDGE, GRIFFITHS, HILL, LÜTKEPOHL, and LEE · The Theory and Practice of
Econometrics, *Second Edition*

JUREK and MASON · Operator-Limit Distributions in Probability Theory

KADANE · Bayesian Methods and Ethics in a Clinical Trial Design

KADANE AND SCHUM · A Probabilistic Analysis of the Sacco and Vanzetti Evidence

KALBFLEISCH and PRENTICE · The Statistical Analysis of Failure Time Data, *Second
Edition*

KARIYA and KURATA · Generalized Least Squares

KASS and VOS · Geometrical Foundations of Asymptotic Inference

† KAUFMAN and ROUSSEEUW · Finding Groups in Data: An Introduction to Cluster
Analysis

KEDEM and FOKIANOS · Regression Models for Time Series Analysis

KENDALL, BARDEN, CARNE, and LE · Shape and Shape Theory

KHURI · Advanced Calculus with Applications in Statistics, *Second Edition*

*Now available in a lower priced paperback edition in the Wiley Classics Library.

†Now available in a lower priced paperback edition in the Wiley–Interscience Paperback Series.

KHURI, MATHEW, and SINHA · Statistical Tests for Mixed Linear Models
* KISH · Statistical Design for Research
KLEIBER and KOTZ · Statistical Size Distributions in Economics and Actuarial Sciences
KLEMELÄ · Smoothing of Multivariate Data: Density Estimation and Visualization
KLUGMAN, PANJER, and WILLMOT · Loss Models: From Data to Decisions, *Fourth Edition*
KLUGMAN, PANJER, and WILLMOT · Student Solutions Manual to Accompany Loss Models: From Data to Decisions, *Fourth Edition*
KOSKI and NOBLE · Bayesian Networks: An Introduction
KOTZ, BALAKRISHNAN, and JOHNSON · Continuous Multivariate Distributions, Volume 1, *Second Edition*
KOTZ and JOHNSON (editors) · Encyclopedia of Statistical Sciences: Volumes 1 to 9 with Index
KOTZ and JOHNSON (editors) · Encyclopedia of Statistical Sciences: Supplement Volume
KOTZ, READ, and BANKS (editors) · Encyclopedia of Statistical Sciences: Update Volume 1
KOTZ, READ, and BANKS (editors) · Encyclopedia of Statistical Sciences: Update Volume 2
KOWALSKI and TU · Modern Applied U-Statistics
KRISHNAMOORTHY and MATHEW · Statistical Tolerance Regions: Theory, Applications, and Computation
KROESE, TAIMRE, and BOTEV · Handbook of Monte Carlo Methods
KROONENBERG · Applied Multiway Data Analysis
KULINSKAYA, MORGENTHALER, and STAUDTE · Meta Analysis: A Guide to Calibrating and Combining Statistical Evidence
KULKARNI and HARMAN · An Elementary Introduction to Statistical Learning Theory
KUROWICKA and COOKE · Uncertainty Analysis with High Dimensional Dependence Modelling
KVAM and VIDAKOVIC · Nonparametric Statistics with Applications to Science and Engineering
LACHIN · Biostatistical Methods: The Assessment of Relative Risks, *Second Edition*
LAD · Operational Subjective Statistical Methods: A Mathematical, Philosophical, and Historical Introduction
LAMPERTI · Probability: A Survey of the Mathematical Theory, *Second Edition*
LAWLESS · Statistical Models and Methods for Lifetime Data, *Second Edition*
LAWSON · Statistical Methods in Spatial Epidemiology, *Second Edition*
LE · Applied Categorical Data Analysis, *Second Edition*
LE · Applied Survival Analysis
LEE · Structural Equation Modeling: A Bayesian Approach
LEE and WANG · Statistical Methods for Survival Data Analysis, *Third Edition*
LePAGE and BILLARD · Exploring the Limits of Bootstrap
LESSLER and KALSBEEK · Nonsampling Errors in Surveys
LEYLAND and GOLDSTEIN (editors) · Multilevel Modelling of Health Statistics
LIAO · Statistical Group Comparison
LIN · Introductory Stochastic Analysis for Finance and Insurance
LITTLE and RUBIN · Statistical Analysis with Missing Data, *Second Edition*
LLOYD · The Statistical Analysis of Categorical Data
LOWEN and TEICH · Fractal-Based Point Processes
MAGNUS and NEUDECKER · Matrix Differential Calculus with Applications in Statistics and Econometrics, *Revised Edition*
MALLER and ZHOU · Survival Analysis with Long Term Survivors
MARCHETTE · Random Graphs for Statistical Pattern Recognition

Software

PIANTADOSI · Clinical Trials: A Methodologic Perspective, *Second Edition*

POURAHMADI · Foundations of Time Series Analysis and Prediction Theory

POWELL · Approximate Dynamic Programming: Solving the Curses of Dimensionality, *Second Edition*

POWELL and RYZHOV · Optimal Learning

PRESS · Subjective and Objective Bayesian Statistics, *Second Edition*

PRESS and TANUR · The Subjectivity of Scientists and the Bayesian Approach

PURI, VILAPLANA, and WERTZ · New Perspectives in Theoretical and Applied Statistics

† PUTERMAN · Markov Decision Processes: Discrete Stochastic Dynamic Programming

QIU · Image Processing and Jump Regression Analysis

* RAO · Linear Statistical Inference and Its Applications, *Second Edition*

RAO · Statistical Inference for Fractional Diffusion Processes

RAUSAND and HØYLAND · System Reliability Theory: Models, Statistical Methods, and Applications, *Second Edition*

RAYNER, THAS, and BEST · Smooth Tests of Goodnes of Fit: Using R, *Second Edition*

RENCHER and SCHAALJE · Linear Models in Statistics, *Second Edition*

RENCHER and CHRISTENSEN · Methods of Multivariate Analysis, *Third Edition*

RENCHER · Multivariate Statistical Inference with Applications

RIGDON and BASU · Statistical Methods for the Reliability of Repairable Systems

* RIPLEY · Spatial Statistics

* RIPLEY · Stochastic Simulation

ROHATGI and SALEH · An Introduction to Probability and Statistics, *Second Edition*

ROLSKI, SCHMIDLI, SCHMIDT, and TEUGELS · Stochastic Processes for Insurance and Finance

ROSENBERGER and LACHIN · Randomization in Clinical Trials: Theory and Practice

ROSSI, ALLENBY, and McCULLOCH · Bayesian Statistics and Marketing

† ROUSSEEUW and LEROY · Robust Regression and Outlier Detection

ROYSTON and SAUERBREI · Multivariate Model Building: A Pragmatic Approach to Regression Analysis Based on Fractional Polynomials for Modeling Continuous Variables

* RUBIN · Multiple Imputation for Nonresponse in Surveys

RUBINSTEIN and KROESE · Simulation and the Monte Carlo Method, *Second Edition*

RUBINSTEIN and MELAMED · Modern Simulation and Modeling

RYAN · Modern Engineering Statistics

RYAN · Modern Experimental Design

RYAN · Modern Regression Methods, *Second Edition*

RYAN · Statistical Methods for Quality Improvement, *Third Edition*

SALEH · Theory of Preliminary Test and Stein-Type Estimation with Applications

SALTELLI, CHAN, and SCOTT (editors) · Sensitivity Analysis

SCHERER · Batch Effects and Noise in Microarray Experiments: Sources and Solutions

* SCHEFFE · The Analysis of Variance

SCHIMEK · Smoothing and Regression: Approaches, Computation, and Application

SCHOTT · Matrix Analysis for Statistics, *Second Edition*

SCHOUTENS · Levy Processes in Finance: Pricing Financial Derivatives

SCOTT · Multivariate Density Estimation: Theory, Practice, and Visualization

* SEARLE · Linear Models

† SEARLE · Linear Models for Unbalanced Data

† SEARLE · Matrix Algebra Useful for Statistics

† SEARLE, CASELLA, and McCULLOCH · Variance Components

SEARLE and WILLETT · Matrix Algebra for Applied Economics

SEBER · A Matrix Handbook For Statisticians

† SEBER · Multivariate Observations

* WHITTAKER · Graphical Models in Applied Multivariate Statistics

WINKER · Optimization Heuristics in Economics: Applications of Threshold Accepting

WOODWORTH · Biostatistics: A Bayesian Introduction

WOOLSON and CLARKE · Statistical Methods for the Analysis of Biomedical Data, *Second Edition*

WU and HAMADA · Experiments: Planning, Analysis, and Parameter Design Optimization, *Second Edition*

WU and ZHANG · Nonparametric Regression Methods for Longitudinal Data Analysis

YIN · Clinical Trial Design: Bayesian and Frequentist Adaptive Methods

YOUNG, VALERO-MORA, and FRIENDLY · Visual Statistics: Seeing Data with Dynamic Interactive Graphics

ZACKS · Stage-Wise Adaptive Designs

* ZELLNER · An Introduction to Bayesian Inference in Econometrics

ZELTERMAN · Discrete Distributions—Applications in the Health Sciences

ZHOU, OBUCHOWSKI, and McCLISH · Statistical Methods in Diagnostic Medicine, *Second Edition*